D1567882

Arterial Disorders

Adel Berbari • Giuseppe Mancia
Editors

Arterial Disorders

Definition, Clinical Manifestations,
Mechanisms and Therapeutic Approaches

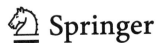 Springer

Editors
Adel Berbari
American University of Beirut
Medical Center
Beirut
Lebanon

Giuseppe Mancia
University of Milano Bicocca IRCCS
Istituto Auxologico Italiano
Milan
Italy

ISBN 978-3-319-14555-6   ISBN 978-3-319-14556-3   (eBook)
DOI 10.1007/978-3-319-14556-3

Library of Congress Control Number: 2015935349

Springer Cham Heidelberg New York Dordrecht London

Printed on acid-free paper

Springer is part of Springer Science+Business Media (www.springer.com)

Preface

Cardiovascular disorders account for the increased morbidity and mortality that accompanies a large number of diseases, including diabetes mellitus, obesity, hypertension, nephropathies and rheumatoid arthritis. Recent progress in knowledge has led to an increased understanding of the pathophysiologic mechanisms that underlie vascular alterations in these diseases, the evidence being that a wide range of factors are likely to participate to a variable degree in each of them. Aim of this book is to describe the physiology of macro- and microcirculation together with their interactions. It is also to discuss the structural and functional alterations that macro- and microcirculation develop with diseases, with attention to their hemodynamic, metabolic, humoral, hormonal, inflammatory, as well as genetic or environmental nature. Emphasis is placed on recent notions, such as the involvement of arterial stiffness in the initiation and progression of atherosclerosis, as well as in the age-related alterations of systemic and renal vasculature; the importance of mineral-bone-vascular interactions; the diagnostic and prognostic significance of new noninvasive measures of vascular structure and function in the retina and the kidney; the role of toxemia in pregnancy; and the modern perception of diabetes as a vascular disease. Some chapters are also devoted to the anatomy and the factors involved in atherosclerosis, arteriosclerosis and remodeling of precapillary resistance vessels, and to the vascular changes and interactions with respiratory processes in pulmonary hypertension. Evaluation procedures as well as the full range of available therapeutic options, including lifestyle modifications and pharmacologic approaches, are described and appraised. We hope that clinicians with a specific interest in arterial diseases, but also those operating in other areas of medicine, will find this comprehensive update useful and timely.

Beirut, Lebanon   Adel E. Berbari
Milan, Italy   Giuseppe Mancia

Contents

Part I

Introductory Aspects

Definition and Epidemiology of Arterial Disease

Reza Aghamohammadzadeh, Danielle Ormandy, and Anthony M. Heagerty

1.1 Introduction

Cardiovascular diseases (CVDs) are the number one cause of death globally and account for around a third of all deaths worldwide [1, 2]. In 2008, an estimated 17.3 million people died from these conditions which is 48 % of noncommunicable diseases; of these, 6.2 million were a consequence of stroke and 7.3 million due to coronary artery disease [3]. In the UK alone, 160,000 people died of CVD in 2001 [4]. The number of deaths from CVDs is predicted to rise to around 23 million by 2030 [5], thus highlighting the need for better understanding of these disorders and exploration of new treatment and prevention strategies both at individual and population level. Developing countries will suffer a similar fate if steps are not taken urgently.

As the name suggests, cardiovascular diseases are a consequence of pathobiological processes afflicting the heart and blood vessels. A number of disorders pertaining to the heart are also vascular in origin; these include coronary artery disease and microvascular disease within the myocardium. Arterial disorders can be split into coronary, cerebrovascular and peripheral disorders based on the vascular bed, but from a pathological perspective, the underlying processes can be grouped into five categories: atherosclerosis, arterial stiffness, endothelial dysfunction, neurohormonal

R. Aghamohammadzadeh (✉) • A.M. Heagerty
Institute of Cardiovascular Sciences, University of Manchester,
46 Grafton Street, Manchester M13 9NT, UK
e-mail: Reza.zadeh@manchester.ac.uk; Tony.heagerty@manchester.ac.uk

D. Ormandy
Institute of Cardiovascular Sciences, Central Manchester University Hospitals NHS
Foundation Trust (Manchester Royal Infirmary), Oxford Road, Manchester M13 9WL, UK
e-mail: Danielle.ormandy@doctors.org.uk

© Springer International Publishing Switzerland 2015
A. Berbari, G. Mancia (eds.), *Arterial Disorders:
Definition, Clinical Manifestations, Mechanisms and Therapeutic Approaches*,
DOI 10.1007/978-3-319-14556-3_1

interactions and vascular remodelling. These processes often coexist in a range of disorders including diabetes mellitus, hypertension, obesity and chronic kidney disease.

1.2   Pathophysiology

Cardiovascular disorders are a heterogeneous group of diseases which share common underlying pathological manifestations. Atherosclerosis is a complex phenomenon and itself a result of a combination of pathological processes including inflammation and endothelial damage. Far from a simplistic view that atherosclerosis is lipid driven and predominantly a cholesterol-related disorder, more recently a number of inflammatory cells have been implicated in the process including monocytes [6], macrophages [7], neutrophils [8] and dendritic cells [9], and further exploration of novel chemokines including CCL2 [10], CCL17 and macrophage migration inhibitory factor [10] can yet advance our understanding of the disorder. A better understanding of the role of inflammation in atherosclerosis can in theory lead to the introduction of immunomodulators alongside statins to treat those with difficult-to-control atherogenic dyslipidaemia.

Endothelial dysfunction is characterised by processes which result in attenuated endothelial vasodilatation, either by reducing the bioavailability of nitric oxide or by increasing levels of endothelium-derived vasoconstrictor and prothrombotic factors [11]. Endothelial dysfunction has been described in diabetes mellitus [12–14], hypertension [15, 16], aging [17–19], chronic kidney disease [20] and obesity [21, 22] and contributes to formation of atherosclerotic plaques and vascular stiffness.

Vascular remodelling is an adaptive process in response to long-term changes in the haemodynamic environment that ultimately may contribute to vascular and circulatory disorders. Four main processes have been implicated in remodelling: cell growth, cell death, cell migration and extracellular matrix production or degradation [23]. The specific type of remodelling depends on the disease process necessitating the change within the vasculature. Eutrophic remodelling (rearrangement of the same cellular material around a narrowed lumen resulting in increased media/lumen ratio) has been described in patients with essential hypertension [24] and hypertrophic remodelling (increase in wall thickness or media cross-sectional area and preservation of the lumen diameter) in individuals with diabetes [25–27]. Similarly, obese patients exhibit an increase in media-to-lumen ratio in keeping with hypertrophic remodelling [28], and persistent weight loss following weight-loss surgery regresses these vascular changes [29].

Over the past 10 years, microRNAs have emerged as a rapidly advancing domain offering much promise to enhance our understanding of the pathobiology of CVDs at the molecular and cellular level. MicroRNAs are small noncoding RNAs involved in post-transcriptional gene regulation by binding to mRNA sequences resulting in a reduction of protein expression or leading to mRNA degradation [30]. The potential involvement of microRNAs has been reported in atherosclerosis [31, 32], endothelial cell function [30] and arterial remodelling [33], as well as in disorders such as peripheral arterial disease [34], stroke [35], obesity [36] and aortic disease [37]. A better understanding of the role of microRNAs in cardiovascular disorders will no doubt lead to development of future therapies [38].

1.3   Investigating Arterial Disorders

Over the years, a variety of techniques have been utilised to study the micro- and macro-circulation at molecular, cellular and tissue level. These include functional assessments of vessel wall and luminal changes using wire and pressure myography, arterial stiffness studies using pulse wave velocity measurements as well as high-resolution ultrasound assessment of endothelial function using flow-mediated dilatation, evaluation of reactive hyperaemia using gauge-strain plethysmography and more recently, pulse amplitude tonometry [39, 40]. One of the most recent developments in the field of cardiovascular investigations is the emergence of retinal artery imaging as a means of assessment and monitoring of arterial disease. The retinal microcirculation offers a noninvasive and easily accessible window to the human microvasculature. Advances in imaging technology using computer-based analysis of retinal photographs allow for reproducible means for quantification of retinal vascular calibre. Changes in retinal vascular calibre are associated with age, ethnicity and genetic factors [41]. Changes such as narrowing of retinal arteriolar calibre, enhanced arteriolar wall reflex and wider venular calibre are associated with the metabolic syndrome [42, 43], waist circumference [44, 45], higher triglyceride levels [45], diabetes and hypertension [44, 46] as well as stroke [47, 48], coronary microvascular disease [49] and coronary artery disease [50]. Retinal microvascular changes can predict subsequent vascular events following ischaemic stroke [51]. These changes are also observed in the paediatric and adolescent population [52–54]. Retinal microvascular signs such as venular dilatation are associated with CKD both in the presence and absence of diabetes, thus reinforcing the link between renal and retinal microvasculature independently of diabetes [55].

1.4   Risk Factors

Identifying major risk factors for arterial disorders with the aim of developing new therapies and public health strategies to reduce cardiovascular mortality and morbidity has been at the forefront of efforts by major healthcare, academic, pharmaceutical and governmental bodies. However, despite our best efforts, cardiovascular diseases are on the rise, and controlling and treating their risk factors remain a major challenge.

Obesity has emerged as a major global healthcare burden and a symptom of our unhealthy lifestyles. In the most simplistic terms, obesity is a result of the imbalance between calories consumed versus calories expended. The worldwide prevalence of obesity has nearly doubled between 1998 and 2008. Over half a billion adults over 20 were obese in 2008 (10 % of all men and 14 % of all women) [56]. The obesity prevalence tripled from 7 % in lower-middle-income countries to 24 % in upper-middle-income countries. In low- and medium-income countries, there is a positive correlation between socioeconomic status and obesity; however, in the European Union, there seems to be an inverse relationship between education and obesity/ BMI [57–60]. These trends most likely reflect the growing awareness of the detrimental effects of obesity on health in the developed countries which should extend to the developing countries in the not-too-distant future and help reduce the mortality rate from 2.8 million deaths each year (2008) as a result of overweight and obesity [1]. In the context of the metabolic syndrome, obesity often coexists with hypertension, diabetes and high cholesterol. There is an intricate interplay between the components of the metabolic syndrome which is evident from both cellular and epidemiological data. For example, those with a raised waist circumference are twice as likely to have high blood pressure [61]. The interplay between adipose tissue and adjacent vasculature has been studied in the context of perivascular adipose tissue and adipokines with vasoactive properties. White adipocytes are the main constituents of perivascular adipose tissue (PVAT) which surrounds a large proportion of blood vessels in the human body and secretes molecules known as adipokines. Healthy PVAT exerts a vasorelaxant effect mediated via a number of potential candidates including adiponectin [62], nitric oxide [63], hydrogen sulphide [64] and methyl palmitate [65]. In obesity, the vasorelaxant effect is not observed thus, in theory, contributing to increased resting tone in peripheral small arteries. Interestingly, weight loss following bariatric (weight loss) surgery restores the PVAT vasorelaxant effect with its potential beneficial effects on resting BP [66]. These recent data are encouraging as they indicate the potential for reversal of a degree of the obesity-induced cardiovascular damage.

Smoking is thought to cause around 10 % of cardiovascular diseases worldwide [1]. Globally, there are more than one billion smokers, and despite a decrease in the use of tobacco products in high-income countries, the total number of smokers is increasing given that 80 % of the world's smokers live in low- and middle-income countries. Smoking kills 5.4 million people a year and has resulted in 100 million deaths in the twentieth century [67]. Smoking cessation is very effective at reducing mortality, and in those with coronary heart disease, it leads to a 36 % reduction in crude relative risk of mortality [68]. The recent emergence and popularity of E-cigarettes has proven controversial given that they may be a helpful aid to smoking cessation, but the hype around the new products might lead to a renewed interest in nicotine-based products and in some cases serve as an introduction to cigarette smoking. The true effect of E-cigarettes on health and on smoking trends will become apparent in the next decade.

The aging population of the world is another risk factor for cardiovascular disease and one which has no prescribed treatment. The developed countries, and to a certain extent the developing countries, have fallen victim to their own economic success. Improved quality of life, falling birth rates and longer life expectancies have resulted in increasingly old populations in the developed countries. In 2010, at least 20 % of the populations of the more industrialised countries were over the age of 65, and by 2050, one billion people will be over the age of 65 worldwide [69].

Age-related vascular changes have been well documented. These include luminal enlargement with wall thickening, arterial stiffness and endothelial dysfunction. Arterial stiffness is the reduced capability of a blood vessel to dilate and constrict in response to changes in pressure. Both a linear relationship between age and stiffness [70] as well as an accelerated stiffening between ages 50 and 60 have been described [71]. The aetiology of endothelial dysfunction in aging is multifaceted and includes a reduction in endothelial nitric oxide synthase activity leading to a reduction in endothelial vasodilation, as well as a decline in the integrity of the endothelium as a barrier and loss of the ability of endothelial cells to proliferate and migrate after tissue injury [72]. Aging is one CVD risk factor that cannot be curbed; however, new treatment strategies to fight the effects of aging might help alleviate the burden of an increasingly old population.

In 2008, around 40 % of adults had raised blood pressure [73], and it accounts for nearly 13 % of all deaths (7.5 million) worldwide [1]. Hypertension is a major risk factor for ischaemic heart disease (IHD) and haemorrhagic stroke with 54 % of stroke and 47 % of IHD attributable to hypertension. Eighty percent of this burden occurred in low-income and middle-income countries [74]. Moreover, blood pressure levels have been shown to be positively and progressively related to coronary heart disease and stroke [75]. In those older than 50, every increment of 20/10 mmHg results in a doubling of cardiovascular risk, starting as low as 115/75 mmHg [76]. This highlights the importance of effective control of blood pressure which might be addressed using a combination of antihypertensive drugs as well stressing the importance of compliance.

Dyslipidaemia is another major cardiovascular risk factor. In 2008, 39 % of adults had raised total cholesterol and an estimated 2.6 million deaths were attributed to this risk factor alone. In high-income countries, 50 % of the population had raised total cholesterol which is double that of low-income countries, with 2.6 million deaths annually [1]. The Framingham study first reported a link between high cholesterol and increased coronary heart disease in the 1960s [77], and more recently, lipoprotein (a) which is an LDL-like particle has been independently associated with CHD and stroke [78]. Various treatment strategies have aimed to reduce CVD risk in those with dyslipidaemia, but statins have been the most significant players in this field. Recent controversy around statin use has threatened to derail the success of preventing cardiovascular mortality by treating high cholesterol. The authors of a paper published in 2013 by the British Medical Journal [79] had indicated that statin therapy in low-risk individuals does not result in a reduction in all-cause mortality or serious illness whilst conveying an 18 % risk of side effects. The subsequent media reports have no doubt concerned physicians, as sensationalist headlines could potentially affect patient compliance with medication.

Cardiovascular disease is the leading cause of morbidity and mortality in people with diabetes, and diabetes is a significant contributor to cardiovascular risk. In 2001, just under a million deaths were directly caused by diabetes, and nearly 1.5 million deaths from ischaemic heart disease and 700,000 deaths from stroke were attributed to high blood glucose [80]. However, with the emergence of better treatment strategies and patient education, the tide might just be changing. In the past two decades, the difference in CVD complications in people with and without diabetes has narrowed substantially. In 1990, the rates of acute myocardial infarction and stroke were three to four times higher in those with diabetes as compared with the general population; however, by 2010, this difference had been reduced to less than double that of the general population without diabetes [81]. Moreover, since the 1990s, there has been a 3–5 % decline in the rates of acute myocardial infarction, cardiovascular mortality and all-cause mortality in patients with diabetes [82]. This might be a result of earlier detection of diabetes, as well as more effective drugs with fewer side effects and a renewed emphasis on patient education.

Arguably, urbanisation has been the most significant contributor to the growing cardiovascular mortality worldwide. As of 2010, more than half of the world's population live in cities. The advent of globalisation and urbanisation coupled with the emergence of 21 megacities around the world (>10 million) has led to the realisation that inhabitants of cities are at a greater cardiovascular risk than their rural counterparts simply by the virtue of the fact that their lifestyles have changed beyond recognition. Reduced physical activity, the use of motorised transportation, air pollution, sedentary jobs, stress of commuting to work, increased rates of smoking and readily available 'junk food' consisting of high calorie and high salt and sugar foods with low nutritional value, all contribute to increases in blood pressure, obesity and cardiovascular risk in general [69]. Air pollution in particular has been linked with increased incident stroke risk [83], and high residential traffic exposure has been linked with increased blood pressure in a recent comprehensive meta-analysis of European population-based cohorts [84].

Cardiovascular diseases are no different to other disorders in that prevention is better than cure. The World Health Organization 'best buy' interventions for treatment and prevention of CVD would cost around 11–13 billion dollars annually which is a significant saving considering that in the next 25 years, the cost of not investing in CVD prevention and treatment is predicted to be as much as $47 trillion worldwide [69]. These 'best buys' include protecting people from tobacco smoke and banning smoking in public places, warning about the dangers of tobacco use, enforcing bans on tobacco advertising and sponsorship, raising taxes on tobacco, restricting access to retailed alcohol, enforcing bans on alcohol advertising, raising taxes on alcohol, reducing salt intake and salt content of food, replacing trans fat in food with polyunsaturated fat and promoting public awareness about diet and physical activity, including through mass media. These might seem intuitive and straightforward; however, pressure from multinational companies with vested interest and difficulty in changing lifestyle habits that have been formed over many years make it a formidable challenge and one which will not be easily achieved; however, in high-income countries, focus on prevention and improved treatment following cardiovascular events has resulted in significantly reduced rates of mortality [1].

References

1. Alwan A (2011) World Health Organisation: global status report on noncommunicable diseases 2010. World Health Organization, Geneva

2. Mendis S, Lindholm LH, Anderson SG et al (2011) Total cardiovascular risk approach to improve efficiency of cardiovascular prevention in resource constrain settings. J Clin Epidemiol 64:1451–1462
3. Mendis S, Puska P, Norrving B (2011) Global atlas on cardiovascular disease prevention and control. World Health Organisation, Geneva
4. Foundation BH (2014) Cardiovascular disease. (cited 24 Jun 2014); Available from: http://www.bhf.org.uk/heart-health/conditions/cardiovascular-disease.aspx
5. Mathers C, Loncar D (2006) Projections of global mortality and burden of disease from 2002 to 2030. PLoS Med 3(11):e442
6. Woollard KJ, Geissmann F (2010) Monocytes in atherosclerosis: subsets and functions. Nat Rev Cardiol 7(2):77–86
7. Moore KJ, Sheedy FJ, Fisher EA (2013) Macrophages in atherosclerosis: a dynamic balance. Nat Rev Immunol 13(10):709–721
8. Zernecke A, Bot I, Djalali-Talab Y et al (2008) Protective role of CXC receptor 4/CXC ligand 12 unveils the importance of neutrophils in atherosclerosis. Circ Res 102(2):209–217
9. Weber C, Noels H (2011) Atherosclerosis: current pathogenesis and therapeutic options. Nat Med 17(11):1410–1422
10. Zernecke A, Weber C (2012) Improving the treatment of atherosclerosis by linking anti-inflammatory and lipid modulating strategies. Heart 98(21):1600–1606
11. Hadi HA, Carr CS, Al Suwaidi J (2005) Endothelial dysfunction: cardiovascular risk factors, therapy, and outcome. Vasc Health Risk Manag 1(3):183–198
12. Clarkson P, Celermajer DS, Donald AE et al (1996) Impaired vascular reactivity in insulin-dependent diabetes mellitus is related to disease duration and low density lipoprotein cholesterol levels. J Am Coll Cardiol 28(3):573–579
13. Skrha J, Vackva I, Kvasnicka J et al (1990) Plasma free N-terminal fibronectin 30-kDa domain as a marker of endothelial dysfunction in type 1 diabetes mellitus. Eur J Clin Invest 20(2):171–176
14. Hadi HA, Suwaidi JA (2007) Endothelial dysfunction in diabetes mellitus. Vasc Health Risk Manag 3(6):853–876
15. Hamasaki S, Al Suwaidi J, Higano ST et al (2000) Attenuated coronary flow reserve and vascular remodeling in patients with hypertension and left ventricular hypertrophy. J Am Coll Cardiol 35(6):1654–1660
16. Yoshida M, Imalzumi T, Ando S et al (1991) Impaired forearm vasodilatation by acetylcholine in patients with hypertension. Heart Vessels 6(4):218–223
17. Taddei S, Virdis A, Ghiadoni L et al (2001) Age-related reduction of NO availability and oxidative stress in humans. Hypertension 38(2):274–279
18. Versari D, Daghini E, Virdis A et al (2009) The ageing endothelium, cardiovascular risk and disease in man. Exp Physiol 94(3):317–321
19. Virdis A, Ghiadoni L, Giannarelli C, Taddei S et al (2010) Endothelial dysfunction and vascular disease in later life. Maturitas 67(1):20–24
20. Stehouwer CD, Smulders YM (2006) Microalbuminuria and risk for cardiovascular disease: analysis of potential mechanisms. J Am Soc Nephrol 17(8):2106–2111
21. Prieto D, Contreras C, Sanchez A (2014) Endothelial dysfunction, obesity and insulin resistance. Curr Vasc Pharmacol 12(3):412–426
22. Toda N, Okamura T (2013) Obesity impairs vasodilatation and blood flow increase mediated by endothelial nitric oxide: an overview. J Clin Pharmacol 53(12):1228–1239
23. Gibbons GH, Dzau VJ (1994) The emerging concept of vascular remodeling. N Engl J Med 330(20):1431–1438
24. Mulvany MJ (2012) Small artery remodelling in hypertension. Basic Clin Pharmacol Toxicol 110(1):49–55
25. Endemann DH, Pu Q, DeCiuceis C et al (2004) Persistent remodeling of resistance arteries in type 2 diabetic patients on antihypertensive treatment. Hypertension 43(2):399–404
26. Schofield I, Malik R, Izzard A et al (2002) Vascular structural and functional changes in type 2 diabetes mellitus: evidence for the roles of abnormal myogenic responsiveness and dyslipidemia. Circulation 106(24):3037–3043

27. Rosei EA, Rizzoni D (2010) Small artery remodelling in diabetes. J Cell Mol Med 14(5):1030–1036
28. Rizzoni D, De Ciuceis C, Porteri E et al (2012) Structural alterations in small resistance arteries in obesity. Basic Clin Pharmacol Toxicol 110(1):56–62
29. De Ciuceis C, Porteri E, Rizzoni D et al (2011) Effects of weight loss on structural and functional alterations of subcutaneous small arteries in obese patients. Hypertension 58(1):29–36
30. Sun X, Belkin N, Feinberg MW (2013) Endothelial microRNAs and atherosclerosis. Curr Atheroscler Rep 15(12):372
31. Madrigal-Matute J, Rotllan N, Arand JF, Fernandez-Hernando C (2013) MicroRNAs and atherosclerosis. Curr Atheroscler Rep 15(5):322
32. Rayner KJ, Moore KJ (2012) The plaque "micro" environment: microRNAs control the risk and the development of atherosclerosis. Curr Atheroscler Rep 14(5):413–421
33. Zampetaki A, Dudek K, Mayr M (2013) Oxidative stress in atherosclerosis: the role of microRNAs in arterial remodeling. Free Radic Biol Med 64:69–77
34. Imanishi T, Akasaka T (2013) MicroRNAs in peripheral artery disease. Curr Top Med Chem 13(13):1589–1595
35. Koutsis G, Siasos G, Spengos K (2013) The emerging role of microRNA in stroke. Curr Top Med Chem 13(13):1573–1588
36. Hulsmans M, Holvoet P (2013) MicroRNAs as early biomarkers in obesity and related metabolic and cardiovascular diseases. Curr Pharm Des 19(32):5704–5717
37. Vavuranakis M, Kariori M, Vrachatis D et al (2013) MicroRNAs in aortic disease. Curr Top Med Chem 13(13):1559–1572
38. Quiat D, Olson EN (2013) MicroRNAs in cardiovascular disease: from pathogenesis to prevention and treatment. J Clin Invest 123(1):11–18
39. Celermajer DS (2008) Reliable endothelial function testing: at our fingertips? Circulation 117(19):2428–2430
40. Tousoulis D, Antoniades C, Stefanadis C (2005) Evaluating endothelial function in humans: a guide to invasive and non-invasive techniques. Heart 91(4):553–558
41. Sun C, Wang JJ, Mackey DA, Wong TY (2009) Retinal vascular caliber: systemic, environmental, and genetic associations. Surv Ophthalmol 54(1):74–95
42. Nguyen TT, Wong TY (2006) Retinal vascular manifestations of metabolic disorders. Trends Endocrinol Metab 17(7):262–268
43. Wong TY, Duncan BB, Golden SH et al (2004) Associations between the metabolic syndrome and retinal microvascular signs: the atherosclerosis risk in communities study. Invest Ophthalmol Vis Sci 45(9):2949–2954
44. Zhao Y, Yang K, Wang F et al (2012) Associations between metabolic syndrome and syndrome components and retinal microvascular signs in a rural Chinese population: the Handan Eye study. Graefes Arch Clin Exp Ophthalmol 250(12):1755–1763
45. Kawasaki R, Tielsh JM, Wang JJ et al (2008) The metabolic syndrome and retinal microvascular signs in a Japanese population: the Funagata study. Br J Ophthalmol 92(2):161–166
46. Ding J, Wai KL, McGeechan K et al (2014) Retinal vascular caliber and the development of hypertension: a meta-analysis of individual participant data. J Hypertens 32(2):207–215
47. Kawasaki R, Xie J, Cheung N et al (2012) Retinal microvascular signs and risk of stroke: the Multi-Ethnic Study of Atherosclerosis (MESA). Stroke 43(12):3245–3251
48. Cheung CY, Tay WT, Ikram MK et al (2013) Retinal microvascular changes and risk of stroke: the Singapore Malay Eye study. Stroke 44(9):2402–2408
49. Wang L, Wong TY, Sharrett AR et al (2008) Relationship between retinal arteriolar narrowing and myocardial perfusion: multi-ethnic study of atherosclerosis. Hypertension 51(1):119–126
50. Al-Fiadh AH, Farouque O, Kawasaki R et al (2014) Retinal microvascular structure and function in patients with risk factors of atherosclerosis and coronary artery disease. Atherosclerosis 233(2):478–484
51. De Silva DA, Manzano JJ, Liu EY et al (2011) Retinal microvascular changes and subsequent vascular events after ischemic stroke. Neurology 77(9):896–903

52. Taylor B, Rochtchina E, Wang JJ et al (2007) Body mass index and its effects on retinal vessel diameter in 6-year-old children. Int J Obes (Lond) 31(10):1527–1533
53. Cheung N, Saw SM, Islam FM et al (2007) BMI and retinal vascular caliber in children. Obesity (Silver Spring) 15(1):209–215
54. Murgan I, Beyer S, Kotliar KE et al (2013) Arterial and retinal vascular changes in hypertensive and prehypertensive adolescents. Am J Hypertens 26(3):400–408
55. Liew G, Mitchell P, Wong TY, Wang JJ (2012) Retinal microvascular signs are associated with chronic kidney disease in persons with and without diabetes. Kidney Blood Press Res 35(6):589–594
56. Finucane MM, Stevens GA, Cowan MJ et al (2011) National, regional, and global trends in body-mass index since 1980: systematic analysis of health examination surveys and epidemiological studies with 960 country-years and 9.1 million participants. Lancet 377(9765): 557–567
57. Gutierrez-Fisac JL, Regidor E, Banegas JR, Rodriguez A (2002) The size of obesity differences associated with educational level in Spain, 1987 and 1995/97. J Epidemiol Community Health 56(6):457–460
58. Martinez JA, Kearney JM, Kafatos A et al (1999) Variables independently associated with self-reported obesity in the European Union. Public Health Nutr 2(1A):125–133
59. Sundquist J, Johansson SE (1998) The influence of socioeconomic status, ethnicity and lifestyle on body mass index in a longitudinal study. Int J Epidemiol 27(1):57–63
60. van Lenthe FJ, Schrijvers CTM, Droomers M et al (2004) Investigating explanations of socioeconomic inequalities in health: the Dutch GLOBE study. Eur J Public Health 14(1):63–70
61. The NHS Information Centre LS (2011) Statistics on obesity, physical activity and diet: England, 2011. http://www.hsic.gov.uk. Published 24 Feb 2011
62. Greenstein AS, Khavandi K, Withers SB et al (2009) Local inflammation and hypoxia abolish the protective anticontractile properties of perivascular fat in obese patients. Circulation 119(12):1661–1670
63. Gil-Ortega M, Stucchi P, Guzman-Ruiz R et al (2010) Adaptative nitric oxide overproduction in perivascular adipose tissue during early diet-induced obesity. Endocrinology 151(7): 3299–3306
64. Gao YJ, Lu C, Su L-Y et al (2007) Modulation of vascular function by perivascular adipose tissue: the role of endothelium and hydrogen peroxide. Br J Pharmacol 151(3):323–331
65. Lee YC, Chang HH, Chiang CL et al (2011) Role of perivascular adipose tissue-derived methyl palmitate in vascular tone regulation and pathogenesis of hypertension. Circulation 124(10):1160–1171
66. Aghamohammadzadeh R, Greenstein AS, Yadav R et al (2013) Effects of bariatric surgery on human small artery function: evidence for reduction in perivascular adipocyte inflammation, and the restoration of normal anticontractile activity despite persistent obesity. J Am Coll Cardiol 62(2):128–135
67. Jha P, Chaloupka FJ (1999) Curbing the epidemic: governments and the economics of tobacco control. The World Bank. Tob Control 8(2):196–201
68. Critchley JA, Capewell S (2003) Mortality risk reduction associated with smoking cessation in patients with coronary heart disease: a systematic review. JAMA 290(1):86–97
69. Laslett LJ, Alagona P Jr, Clark BA 3rd et al (2012) The worldwide environment of cardiovascular disease: prevalence, diagnosis, therapy, and policy issues: a report from the American College of Cardiology. J Am Coll Cardiol 60(25 Suppl):S1–S49
70. Avolio AP, Chen SG, Wang RP et al (1983) Effects of aging on changing arterial compliance and left ventricular load in a northern Chinese urban community. Circulation 68(1):50–58
71. McEniery CM, Yasmin, Hall IR et al (2005) Normal vascular aging: differential effects on wave reflection and aortic pulse wave velocity: the Anglo-Cardiff Collaborative Trial (ACCT). J Am Coll Cardiol 46(9):1753–1760
72. North BJ, Sinclair DA (2012) The intersection between aging and cardiovascular disease. Circ Res 110(8):1097–1108

73. WHO (2011) Blood pressure. Available from: http://www.who.int/gho/ncd/risk_factors/blood_pressure_prevalence/en/index.html. (cited 17 Jul 2011)
74. Lawes CM, Vander Hoorn S, Rodgers A et al (2008) Global burden of blood-pressure-related disease, 2001. Lancet 371(9623):1513–1518
75. Whitworth JA, WHO, ISH Writing Group (2003) 2003 World Health Organization (WHO)/International Society of Hypertension (ISH) statement on management of hypertension. J Hypertens 21(11):1983–1992
76. Chobanian AV, Bakris GL, Black HR et al (2003) Seventh report of the joint national committee on prevention, detection, evaluation, and treatment of high blood pressure. Hypertension 42(6):1206–1252
77. Kannel WB, Castelli WP, Gordon T, McNamara PM (1971) Serum cholesterol, lipoproteins, and the risk of coronary heart disease. The Framingham study. Ann Intern Med 74(1):1–12
78. Emerging Risk Factors Collaboration, Erqou S, Kaptoge S et al (2009) Lipoprotein(a) concentration and the risk of coronary heart disease, stroke, and nonvascular mortality. JAMA 302(4):412–423
79. Abramson JD, Rosenberg HG, Jewell N, Wright JM (2013) Should people at low risk of cardiovascular disease take a statin? BMJ 347:f6123
80. Danaei G, Lawes CM, Vander Hoorn S et al (2006) Global and regional mortality from ischaemic heart disease and stroke attributable to higher-than-optimum blood glucose concentration: comparative risk assessment. Lancet 368(9548):1651–1659
81. Gregg EW, Li Y, Wang J et al (2014) Changes in diabetes-related complications in the United States, 1990–2010. N Engl J Med 370(16):1514–1523
82. Booth GL, Kapral MK, Fung K, Tu JV (2006) Recent trends in cardiovascular complications among men and women with and without diabetes. Diabetes Care 29(1):32–37
83. Stafoggia M, Cesaroni G, Peters A et al (2014) Long-term exposure to ambient air pollution and incidence of cerebrovascular events: results from 11 European cohorts within the ESCAPE project. Environ Health Perspect. doi:10.1289/ehp.1307301
84. Fuks KB, Weinmayr G, Foraster M et al (2014) Arterial blood pressure and long-term exposure to traffic-related air pollution: an analysis in the European Study of Cohorts for Air Pollution Effects (ESCAPE). Environ Health Perspect. doi:10.1289/ehp.1307725

Overview of the Normal Structure and Function of the Macrocirculation and Microcirculation

2

Wilmer W. Nichols, Kevin S. Heffernan, and Julio A. Chirinos

Abbreviations

(ED – Tr)	Systolic duration of reflected wave
AIx	Augmentation index (AP/PP)
AP	Reflected pressure wave amplitude
CFR	Coronary blood flow reserve
DPTI/SPTI	Supply/demand or subendocardial viability ratio
DPTI	Diastolic pressure time index
ED	Ejection duration
Ew	Wasted LV pressure energy (or effort)
GTF	Generalized transfer function
LV	Left ventricle
LVH	Left ventricular hypertrophy
MAP	Mean arterial pressure
$\bar{Q}$	Mean blood flow
P1	Forward pressure wave amplitude
P_i	Inflection point

W.W. Nichols (✉)
Department of Medicine/Cardiology, University of Florida,
1600 SW Archer Road, Gainesville, FL 32610, USA
e-mail: nichoww@medicine.ufl.edu

K.S. Heffernan
Department of Exercise Science, Syracuse University, Syracuse, NY 13224, USA
e-mail: ksheffer@syr.edu

J.A. Chirinos
Department Medicine/Cardiology, University of Pennsylvania,
University and Woodland Avenues, Philadelphia, PA 19104, USA
e-mail: Julio.Chirinos@uphs.upenn.edu

© Springer International Publishing Switzerland 2015
A. Berbari, G. Mancia (eds.), *Arterial Disorders:
Definition, Clinical Manifestations, Mechanisms and Therapeutic Approaches*,
DOI 10.1007/978-3-319-14556-3_2

PP	Pulse pressure
PWV	Pulse wave velocity
RM	Reflected wave magnitude (AP/P1)
SMC	Smooth muscle cells
SPTI	Systolic pressure time index
Tr	Round trip travel time of the pressure wave to and from the lower body reflection site
Z_1	First (or fundamental) aortic input impedance modulus
Z_c	Characteristic impedance

"However eloquent may be the words of a writer, he cannot in a page convey as clear an idea of the rhythm of the heart as a simple pulse-tracing; and if writers had given us more pulse-tracings, their works would have been greatly enhanced in value". James Mackenzie, 1902

2.1   Introduction

It is impossible to discuss the "normal" structure and function of the arterial system without considering the changes that occur with advancing age. Normal arterial structure and function is very different for a young person compared to an older person. Furthermore, it is of paramount importance to understand normal arterial function at all ages in order to recognize abnormal function in cardiovascular disease. In this chapter, we consider normality as meaning "without disease" and focus our discussion on the structure and function of the arterial system over a wide age range beginning in adult youth and continuing to old age.

There are numerous misconceptions in the conventional approach to quantifying arterial function and ventricular/vascular coupling. Believing these misconceptions as true may lead to ineffective treatment. The main misconception arises from the reliance on the sphygmomanometer for measurement of systolic and diastolic blood pressures in the brachial artery. This approach implies that the arterial system behaves as a model that does not take into consideration nonuniform elastic arteries or arterial wave reflections. Also, it does not allow for pressure wave transmission and amplification along the arterial tree, but considers that the pressure measured in the arm is the same in all arteries, including the aorta, and under all conditions. Of course, we now know that this is not true; the pressure is not the same in all arteries. As the pressure wave travels from the heart along the arteries of the macrocirculation, both systolic and pulse pressures increase markedly due to wave reflections. Thus, both systolic and pulse pressures are greater in the arm and leg than in the ascending aorta; in young adults this difference in pressure (pressure gradient) can be 20–30 mmHg. These facts must be considered before completely understanding the working relationship between the heart and the arterial system. Our approach in this chapter is to consider the heart as a pump and the viscoelastic arterial system, including wave reflections, as its load with both static and dynamic components.

The function of the left ventricle (LV) is to pump blood (the cardiac output) through the macrocirculation of the systemic arterial tree to the microcirculation. If the ventricle is ideally matched to its afterload, ventricular/vascular coupling and cardiac efficiency are optimal and myocardial oxygen consumption is minimal [1–4]. The amount of energy and thus the oxygen used by the LV to produce the cardiac output is dependent not only on the contractile properties of the myocardium but also on the physical properties and wave reflections of the arterial system. Thus, the arterial system constitutes the external vascular "afterload" placed on the ventricle during fiber shortening and ejection. Since the ventricle ejects a pulsatile blood flow into a distensible arterial buffering system, the load has both static (nonpulsatile) and dynamic (pulsatile) components. The static (or resistive) component is dependent primarily upon blood viscosity and arteriolar caliber (microcirculation), while the dynamic (or compliant) component is dependent on the elastic properties of the large arteries (macrocirculation) and pulse wave reflections. In this chapter, LV arterial load is characterized in the frequency domain by the aortic input impedance, since it is a function of systemic vascular resistance, central aortic stiffness, and wave reflections and since it selectively describes the arterial system [2, 3, 5]. However, since input impedance requires measurement of both pulsatile pressure and pulsatile flow in the ascending aorta and use of Fourier analysis, a simpler time-domain approach is also presented [3]. Each load component is defined in terms of the impedance spectra and pressure wave morphology and is related to the geometric and structural variables that are likely to change with advancing age. Also, the effects of increasing individual load components on LV function, coronary blood flow reserve, and pulse pressure amplification are discussed.

2.2 Macrocirculation and Microcirculation (Structure)

The macro- and microcirculations of the systemic arterial tree are composed of different types of blood vessels, each with a distinct link between structure and function. The macrocirculation (large elastic and muscular arteries) transports oxygen, metabolites, and nutrient-rich blood from the LV to the microcirculation (prearterioles, arterioles, and capillaries) where it is distributed to the organs and tissues of the body to meet their metabolic requirements at rest and during periods of stress. The deoxygenated blood and waste products return to the right ventricle via the venous system. The arterial and venous systems are linked through a complex network of capillaries [5].

The walls of arteries (large, medium, and small) are composed of living cells and their products including stiff collagen and compliant elastic fibers which directly imparts elasticity and strength to the vessel wall [6]; collagen fibers are 500–1,000 times stiffer than elastic fibers. Larger arteries have small blood vessels within their walls known as the vasa vasorum to provide them with oxygen-rich blood and nutrients [7]. Since the pressure within systemic arteries is relatively high, the vasa vasorum must function in the outer layers of the vessel wall. The structure of the vasa vasorum varies with the size, function, and location of the arteries. Cells need to be within a few cell-widths of a capillary to stay alive. In the largest arteries, the vasa vasorum penetrates the outer layer and middle layer almost to the inner layer. In smaller arteries it penetrates only the outer layer. Endogenous and exogenous vasoactive agents are delivered to the smooth muscle cells (SMC) in the arterial wall through the vasa vasorum. In the microcirculation, the vessels' own circulation nourishes the walls directly and they have no vasa vasorum at all [7]. The confinement of the vasa vasorum to the outer layers of arteries, along with the higher intraluminal pressure, may be the reason that arterial diseases are more common than venous diseases, since its location makes it more difficult to nourish the cells of the arteries and remove waste products. There are also minute nerves within the walls of arteries that alter contraction and relaxation of the SMC. These minute nerves are known as the nervi vasorum. All arteries have the same basic structure despite variations in the proportions of their structural components [8, 9]. They are composed of three layers, or tunicae, which are from the inside out: the intima, the media, and the adventitia (or tunica externa). The tunica intima is composed of epithelial and connective tissue layers. Lining the tunica intima is the specialized simple squamous cells called the endothelium, which is continuous throughout the entire vascular system, including the lining of the chambers of the heart. Damage to this endothelial lining and exposure of blood to the collagenous fibers beneath is one of the primary triggers of clot formation. Up until the late 1970s, the vascular endothelium was considered as a passive lining of flat cells that separated the load-bearing elements of the vascular media from the flowing blood. Over the subsequent 40 plus years, it has become apparent that the endothelium produces a host of chemical substances, notably nitric oxide, endothelin-1, prostacyclin, and angiotensinogen, which are designed to maintain homeostasis through effects on elements of blood in the lumen, on the intimal surface which is exposed to blood, within the tunica intima itself, and on vascular SMC in the tunica media [3, 10, 11]. Also, a multitude of studies have now shown that the endothelium is physiologically critical to such activities as helping to regulate capillary exchange and altering arterial blood flow and pressure [12–15]. Endothelial cells synthesize, store, and release vasoactive substances in response to increased shear stress produced by increases in blood flow velocity [16, 17]. Also, these substances are delivered through the vasa vasorum and can constrict and relax the SMC within the walls of the arteries and arterioles to increase or decrease both pulsatile and mean blood pressure [3]. Next to the endothelium is the basement membrane, or basal lamina, that effectively binds the endothelium to the connective tissue. The basement membrane provides strength while maintaining flexibility, and it is permeable, allowing materials to pass through it. The thin outer layer of the tunica intima contains a small amount of areola connective tissue that consists primarily of elastic fibers to provide the vessel with additional flexibility; it also contains some collagenous fibers to provide additional strength [9].

In larger arteries, there is also a thick, distinct layer of elastic fibers known as the internal elastic lamina at the boundary with the tunica media. Like the other components of the tunica intima, the internal elastic membrane provides structure while allowing the vessel to stretch. It is permeated with small openings that allow exchange of materials between the various layers. Microscopically, the lumen and the entire tunica intima of an artery will normally appear wavy because of the partial constriction of the SMC in the tunica media, the next layer of the arterial wall. The tunica media is the substantial middle layer of the arterial wall. It is generally the thickest layer in arteries. The tunica media consists of layers of SMC supported by connective tissue that is primarily made up of elastic fibers, most of which are arranged in circular sheets. Toward the outer portion of the tunica media, there are also layers of longitudinal SMC [18, 19]. Contraction and relaxation of the circular SMC increase and decrease the stiffness of the artery, respectively. Specifically in large conduit arteries, vasoconstriction increases stiffness and pulse wave propagation as the SMC in the walls of the tunica media contract, making the lumen smaller and increasing pulse blood pressure [3]. Vasoconstriction in arterioles reduces their caliber and causes an increase in vascular resistance and mean arterial blood pressure. Similarly, vasodilation decreases stiffness and reduces pulse wave propagation as the SMC relax, allowing the lumen to widen and pulse blood pressure to decrease. Vasodilation in arterioles increases their caliber and causes a decrease in vascular resistance and mean arterial blood pressure. Both vasoconstriction and vasodilation are regulated in part by the nervi vasorum that runs within the adventitia of the arterial wall. Most arteries and arterioles in the body are innervated by sympathetic adrenergic nerves, which release norepinephrine as a neurotransmitter. Some blood vessels are innervated by parasympathetic cholinergic or sympathetic cholinergic nerves both of which release acetylcholine as their primary neurotransmitter. Neurotransmitter binding to the adrenergic and cholinergic receptors activates signal transduction pathways that cause the observed changes in vascular function. Nervous control over arteries tends to be more generalized than the specific targeting of individual arteries. Hormones and local chemicals such as those released from the endothelium also affect SMC in the arterial wall; some are vasodilators [20], while others are vasoconstrictors [21]. Together, these neural and chemical mechanisms increase or decrease blood flow and arterial pressure in response to changing body conditions, from exercise to hydration and other forms of stress. The layers of SMC in the tunica media are supported by a framework of collagenous fibers that also binds the tunica media to the tunica intima and externa. Along with the collagenous fibers are large numbers of elastic fibers that appear as wavy lines. Separating the tunica media from the outer tunica externa in larger arteries is the external elastic membrane. This structure is not usually seen in smaller arteries. The tunica externa is a substantial sheath of connective tissue composed primarily of collagenous fibers. Some bands of elastic fibers are found here as well. The outer layers of the tunica externa are not distinct but rather blend with the surrounding connective tissue outside the artery, helping to hold the vessel in relative position [9].

2.3 Macrocirculation

2.3.1 Elastic Arteries

Arteries of the macrocirculation have relatively thick walls that can withstand the high pressure of blood ejected from the LV. However, those closer to the heart have the thickest walls, containing a high percentage of elastic fibers and a lower percentage of collagen fibers and SMC in all three of their layers, especially the tunica media. This type of artery is known as an elastic artery. Arteries larger than approximately 5.0 mm in diameter are typically elastic. These include the aorta (thoracic and abdominal), brachiocephalic, carotids, proximal subclavians, and proximal iliacs. Their abundant elastic fibers allow them to expand, as blood pumped from the LV passes through them, and then to recoil after the surge has passed. The collagen fibers in the adventitia prevent elastic arteries from stretching beyond their physiological limits during systole. The SMC are arranged in a spiral around the long axis of the vessels. These lamellae, and the large size of the media, are the most striking histological feature of elastic arteries. In addition to elastin, the SMC of the media secrete reticular and fine collagen fibers and proteoglycans (all not identifiable). The distribution of elastin and collagen differs strikingly between the central and peripheral arteries. In the proximal aorta, elastin is the dominant component, while in the abdominal aorta the content reverses, and in peripheral arteries collagen dominates [22–25]. The transition occurs rapidly over a few centimeters of the lower thoracic aorta just above the diaphragm and over a similar distance in the branches leaving the aortic arch. With advancing age elastic arteries become stiffer and, therefore, expansion and recoil are limited. When this occurs, the impedance to blood flow increases and pulsatile blood pressure rises, which in turn requires the LV to work harder in an attempt to overcome the boost in pressure to maintain the volume of blood expelled by each heartbeat [3, 26]. Artery walls become thicker in response to this chronic increase in pressure and the larger elastic arteries dilate and elongate [27]. The elastic recoil of the vascular wall helps to maintain the pressure gradient that drives the blood through the arterial system. At low levels of arterial blood pressure, wall stress is supported by compliant elastin fibers, while at higher levels of pressure, wall stress is supported by stiff collagen fibers. This transition from elastic to collagen fibers occurs at a mean blood pressure of about 120 mmHg [3]. An elastic artery is also known as a conducting artery, because the large diameter of the lumen enables it to accept a large volume of blood from the LV and distribute it to smaller muscular artery branches and finally to the microcirculation.

2.3.2 Muscular Arteries

Further from the LV, the percentage of elastic fibers in an artery's tunica intima decreases and the amount of collagen fibers and SMC in its tunica media increases [22, 23, 28]. The artery at this point is described as a muscular artery. The diameter of muscular arteries typically ranges from 0.1 to 5.0 mm. These include distal subclavians, axillaries, brachials, ulnars, and radials of the arms and femorals, popliteals, posterior tibials, and dorsalis pedises of the thighs and legs. The length of muscular arteries in the lower body of humans is about twice that of the elastic aorta. Their thick tunica media with numerous SMC allows muscular arteries to play a major role in vasoconstriction and vasodilation [29]. Also, their decreased quantity of elastic fibers and increased quantity of collagen fibers limit their ability to expand and alter wave propagation [22, 30]. Notice that although the distinctions between elastic and muscular arteries are important, there is no "line of demarcation" where an elastic artery suddenly becomes muscular. Rather, there is a gradual transition as the arterial tree repeatedly branches. In turn, muscular arteries branch to distribute blood to the vast network of the microcirculation. For this reason, a muscular artery is also known as a distributing artery.

2.4   Microcirculation

2.4.1   Arterioles

An arteriole is a very small artery that leads to a capillary. Arterioles have the same three layers as the larger arteries, but the thickness of each is greatly diminished. The critical endothelial lining of the tunica intima is intact. The tunica media is restricted to one or two SMC layers in thickness. The tunica externa remains but is very thin. With a lumen 10–150 μm in diameter, arterioles are critical in slowing down—or resisting—blood flow and, thus, causing a substantial increase in resistance and a marked fall in mean blood pressure. Because of this, the arterioles are referred to as resistance vessels; also, vascular pulsations are highly damped in the pre-arterioles and arterioles. The muscle fibers in arterioles are normally slightly contracted, causing arterioles to maintain a consistent SMC tone. In reality, all arteries exhibit some degree of vascular tone due to the partial contraction of SMC. The importance of the arterioles is that they will be the primary site of both resistance and regulation of mean arterial blood pressure and blood flow. The precise diameter of the lumen of an arteriole at any given moment is determined by neural and chemical controls, and vasoconstriction and vasodilation in the arterioles are the primary mechanisms for blood pressure control and distribution of blood flow to the capillary bed [9, 31].

2.4.1.1 Capillaries

A capillary is a microscopic channel that supplies blood to the tissues themselves, a process called perfusion. Exchange of gases (oxygen and carbon dioxide) and other substances occurs in the capillaries between the blood and the surrounding cells and their interstitial fluid. The diameter of a capillary lumen ranges from 5.0 to 10 μm; the smallest are just barely wide enough for an erythrocyte to squeeze through. Flow through capillaries and arterioles are described as the microcirculation. The wall of a capillary consists of the endothelial layer surrounded by a basement membrane with occasional smooth muscle fibers. There is some variation in wall structure: In a large capillary, several endothelial cells bordering each other may line the lumen; in a small capillary, there may be only a single cell layer that wraps around to contact itself. For capillaries to function, their walls must be leaky, allowing substances to pass through [9, 31].

2.5   Macrocirculation (Function)

When the LV contracts, it generates both internal and external "energy"; the external energy (or power) wave is the product of both forward-traveling pressure and flow waves in the ascending aorta which causes a pulsatile change in vessel diameter as they travel [5]. These pressure and flow waves are propagated along the arterial tree at a finite velocity of about 400 cm/s in youth to about 1,500 cm/s in old age [3]. Their morphology (or shape) depends upon the physical properties of both the macrocirculation and microcirculation and also upon their location within the arterial tree [3]. As noted above, the arterial tree can be separated into three anatomical regions, and since the LV is a pulsatile pump, each region has a distinct and separate function: (1) The large elastic arteries of the macrocirculation, especially the aorta, serve as a buffering reservoir or Windkessel that stores blood during systole and expels it to the peripheral circulation during diastole so that the capillaries of the microcirculation receive a steady or continuous flow of blood during the entire cardiac cycle [32]. (2) The large elastic arteries plus the muscular arteries in the lower body, by altering SMC tone, modify the speed of travel of pressure and flow waves along their length and determine, to a great extent, when the reflected wave arrives back at the heart; the arrival time also depends upon reflection site distance. (3) The pre-arterioles and arterioles of the microcirculation, by changing their caliber, alter peripheral resistance and, therefore, aid in the maintenance of mean arterial blood pressure. Increased stiffness of the central elastic arteries occurs over time and acute alterations in wall properties are passive, while changes in the muscular arteries and arterioles (contraction and relaxation) most often occur acutely and alterations in wall properties are active [33]. Increased arterial stiffness causes an increase in pulse wave velocity (PWV) which causes early return of reflected pressure and flow waves from peripheral reflecting sites to the heart [2–5, 34, 35]; PWV is segment related and increases with distance from the heart. This mechanism augments central aortic systolic (and pulse) pressure, which increases arterial wall stress, elevates pulsatile afterload, and increases LV mass and may potentiate the development of atherosclerosis [36–41]. Such studies have suggested that logical treatment for lowering blood pressure should focus not only on arteriolar caliber and peripheral resistance of the microcirculation but also on arterial stiffness, pulse wave propagation, and wave reflections of the macrocirculation [42–44]. Indeed, previous meta-analyses reports have shown that aortic stiffness and wave reflections are independent predictors of adverse cardiovascular events and outcomes [45–47]. A logical approach to understanding and treatment of the changes in cardiovascular, cerebrovascular, and renovascular function is to consider the interaction between the heart as a pump and the arterial system as its load.

2.5.1   Ventricular/Vascular Coupling and Ventricular Afterload

The mechanical "afterload" imposed by the systemic circulation (macro- and micro-circulations) to the pumping LV is composed of a static (or steady) and a dynamic (or pulsatile) component (Fig. 2.1) and is an important determinant of normal

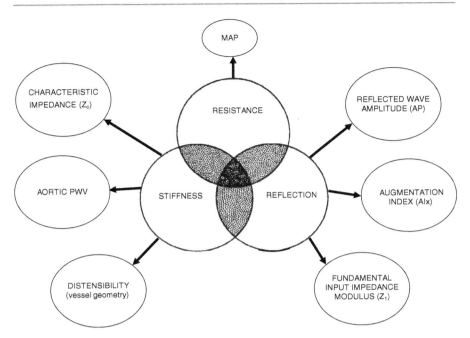

Fig. 2.1 Illustration showing the three components of LV "afterload" and their measurements. The non-pulsatile or static component is total peripheral resistance or mean arterial pressure and the dynamic or pulsatile components are wall stiffness and wave reflections. Measurements of arterial stiffness include characteristic impedance (Z_c), pulse wave velocity (PWV), and distensibility; measurements of wave reflection include reflected wave amplitude (AP), augmentation index (AIx = AP/PP), reflection magnitude (RM = AP/P1), and amplitude of the first (or fundamental) harmonic input impedance moduli (Z_1). Changes in any (or all) of these load components can alter ventricular performance

cardiovascular function and a key pathophysiological factor in various cardiac and vascular disease states. Pulsatile LV afterload is largely determined by the elastic properties of the macrocirculation (characteristic impedance and forward pressure wave amplitude) and wave reflection characteristics (reflected wave amplitude and first harmonic of input impedance modulus) of the arterial tree; the steady component of afterload is determined by the microcirculation (peripheral resistance and mean arterial pressure) [3, 48–50]. Although brachial arterial pressure (systolic, diastolic, and pulse) is taken as a useful surrogate of arterial function and LV afterload in clinical practice, it should be recognized that LV afterload cannot be fully described in terms of brachial cuff (systolic and diastolic) pressure alone, but should be assessed from central aortic pulsatile pressure or aortic input impedance derived from central aortic pressure and flow waves [2–5].

The forward-traveling pressure and flow waves generated by the LV are transmitted by the macrocirculation and are partially reflected at sites of impedance change or mismatch, such as points of branching and/or tortuosity, change in lumen diameter (taper), and physical properties along the macrocirculation system [2, 3, 35, 51, 52].

Multiple small reflections are transmitted back toward the LV and merge into a larger "net" reflected wave, composed of the contributions of all the smaller backward scattered reflected waves. This reflected wave is most often a single discrete wave, originating from an "effective" reflection site, but is actually the resultant of multiple scattered reflections, originating from distributed reflection sites in the lower body [3, 53]. In addition to hemodynamic phenomena related to wave travel and reflections, the large elastic arteries exert a buffering function, which depends on its stiffness and allows them to accommodate additional blood volume during systole without excessive increases in pressure and in turn to release that excess volume throughout diastole without excessive drops in blood pressure [2, 54].

2.5.2 Quantification of LV Afterload

Fourier analyses of ascending aortic pulsatile pressure–flow relations (i.e., aortic input impedance spectra) allow the quantification of various components of LV pulsatile load and "steady" or "resistive" load in the frequency domain (Figs. 2.2 and 2.3) [2, 3, 55–57]. The steady component of afterload depends largely on mean arterial pressure and the peripheral resistance, which in turn depends on arteriolar caliber (microcirculation), the total number of arterioles that are present "in parallel," and blood viscosity [3, 57, 58]. Therefore, the steady afterload component can be affected by arteriolar tone, arteriolar remodeling, microvascular rarefaction, endothelial function, and changes in blood viscosity. Pulsatile LV afterload is, in contrast, predominantly influenced by the properties of larger macrocirculation arteries (both elastic and muscular) and wave reflections. Although pulsatile LV afterload is fairly complex and cannot be expressed as a single numeric measure, key indices of pulsatile LV afterload can be quantified and summarized using relatively simple principles and mechanical models of the systemic circulation, using time-resolved ascending aortic pressure and flow waves [57, 58]. The large majority of the early studies on LV pulsatile load were performed in dogs and rats with cuff-type flow probes implanted on the ascending aorta and pressure measured with fluid-filled catheter–manometer systems [59] or high-fidelity pressure catheter transducers [60]. Later invasive studies in humans were performed using high-fidelity pressure–velocity catheters [61–65]. Noninvasive assessment of central aortic pressure can now be achieved using high-fidelity applanation arterial tonometry at the carotid artery or by using a generalized transfer (GTF) function to synthesize an aortic pressure waveform from the radial (or brachial) pressure waveform [3, 66, 67]. Pulsatile aortic blood flow can also be measured noninvasively in humans, using pulsed wave Doppler ultrasound [68–70] or phase-contrast magnetic resonance imaging [71]. The most convenient method to assess aortic inflow is pulsed wave Doppler interrogation of the LV outflow tract, given that systolic LV volume outflow equals proximal aortic volume inflow [70]. As stated above, LV afterload can be assessed in the frequency domain from the aortic input impedance spectra (calculated from the harmonic components of central aortic pressure and flow waves) or estimated in the time domain from the central aortic pressure wave (Figs. 2.2 and 2.3) [3, 4, 48–50, 72–74]. Input impedance is the

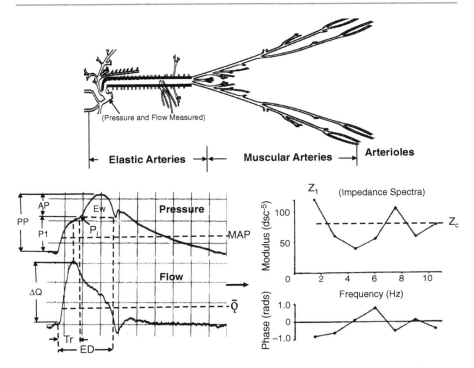

Fig. 2.2 Illustration showing the arterial tree of an older individual with a stiff aorta. Invasive measurements of blood pressure and flow velocity obtained in the ascending aorta (*bottom left*) and input impedance spectra (*bottom right*) obtained from these measurements are shown. AP is the reflected wave amplitude, $P1$ is the forward wave amplitude, PP is the pulse pressure, P_i is the inflection point, Ew is the wasted LV energy, ΔQ is the peak flow, Tr is the travel time of the pressure wave, ED is the ejection duration, MAP is the mean arterial pressure, $\bar{Q}$ is the mean flow, $MAP/\bar{Q}$ is the peripheral resistance and the impedance at zero frequency (not shown), Z_1 is the amplitude of the fundamental harmonic of impedance moduli, and Z_c is the characteristic impedance

"summed" mechanical load imposed by all vessels downstream of a particular point (and which can be fully assessed by measuring pulsatile flow and pressure at that particular point) [3, 49, 55, 59, 73, 75–77]. Therefore, "aortic input impedance" represents the summed mechanical load impeding LV ejection and represents the "gold standard" for representation of LV afterload [3]. It should be noted that aortic input impedance is not exclusively determined by aortic properties alone, but depends on the physical characteristics of both the macro- and microcirculations and wave reflections [2, 3]. Key parameters of pulsatile LV afterload include the characteristic impedance (Z_c) of the ascending aorta and the amplitude and timing of wave reflections (Figs. 2.2 and 2.3) [3, 34, 53, 78, 79]. The characteristic impedance of an artery is a "local" property and can be intuitively calculated as the average of higher harmonics of the aortic input impedance moduli spectrum [61]. Aortic Z_c can also be computed in the time domain as the slope of the early systolic pressure–flow relation or as the ratio ($P1/\Delta Q$) [3] where P1 is the amplitude of the forward-traveling

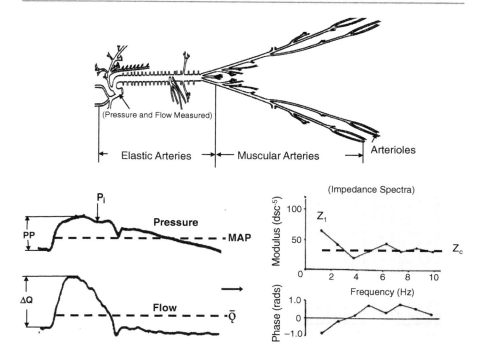

Fig. 2.3 Illustration showing the arterial tree of a young adult with a compliant aorta. Invasive measurements of blood pressure and flow velocity obtained in the ascending aorta (*bottom left*) and input impedance spectra (*bottom right*) obtained from these measurements are shown. *AP* is the reflected wave amplitude, *P1* is the forward wave amplitude, *PP* is the pulse pressure, *Pi* is the inflection point, *Ew* is the wasted LV energy, ΔQ is the peak flow, *Tr* is the travel time of pressure wave, *ED* is the ejection duration, *MAP* is the mean arterial pressure, $\bar{Q}$ is the mean flow, $MAP/\bar{Q}$ is the peripheral resistance and the impedance at zero frequency (not shown), Z_1 is the amplitude of the fundamental harmonic of impedance moduli, and Z_c is the characteristic impedance

pressure wave and ΔQ is the peak aortic blood flow velocity. An estimate of wave reflection amplitude can be obtained from the aortic input impedance spectrum as the first (or fundamental) harmonic of the impedance moduli (Z_1) [3, 61]. It is important to note that the large majority of LV energy (>80 %) is contained within the first and second harmonics; therefore, logical therapy to reduce LV energy (internal and external) should focus on these lower harmonics [5] which are influenced by reflected wave amplitude (AP) in the time domain. Wave reflections are usually assessed via wave separation analysis, based on the superposition principle that reflected waves, by virtue of adding to forward pressure and subtracting from forward flow, distort the linear relationship between the increase in pressure and the increase in flow that is seen in early systole (as a result of the forward wave generated by ventricular contraction) when the pulsatile pressure–flow relation is assumed to be governed purely by ascending aortic Z_c (see below).

2.5.3 Effect of Arterial Stiffness and Wave Reflections on LV Afterload

The stiffness of various arterial segments of the macrocirculation have complex effects on LV afterload, through their effects on the early aortic systolic pressure rise, the total compliance of the arterial tree, and the velocity at which the pulse waves travel forward in the arteries and reflected waves travel backward toward the heart [2, 3, 50, 72]. In early systole, the forward-traveling energy (flow) pulse from LV contraction produces a forward-traveling pressure wave in the aortic root just distal to the valve. If proximal aortic Z_c is high due to a stiff wall, a small aortic diameter, or both, the early part of the pressure wave (P1) (Figs. 2.2 and 2.3) increase is relatively large for any given early systolic flow wave [3, 49, 52, 54]. The time of arrival of the reflected wave at the proximal aorta from the lower body depends on the location of major reflection sites and on PWV along the macrocirculation. Both the forward- and backward-traveling waves are propagated along the macrocirculation at a similar velocity [2, 3, 80, 81]; some investigators have suggested that these velocities may be different and the location of the reflection site may be elusive [82]. Aortic PWV is directly related to the stiffness of the aortic wall (square root of elastic modulus) and inversely proportional to the square root of aortic diameter [3, 52, 83, 84]. Stiffer arteries of the macrocirculation conduct forward- and backward-traveling waves at a greater velocity than compliant arteries and therefore promote an earlier arrival of the reflected wave for any given distance to reflection sites [53, 79, 85–88]. Distance to the major reflection site is strongly dependent on body height (or length) and both elastic and muscular artery stiffness of the macrocirculation. When the elastic arteries become very stiff, for example, with old age, PWV can increase to levels that cause an apparent distal shift of the major reflection site [89]. This usually occurs when elastic artery stiffness matches or exceeds muscular artery stiffness. However, this distal shift of the reflection site does not cause a reduction in wave reflection amplitude or augmentation index [3]. In the presence of normal LV systolic function, typical ill effects of increased amplitude and propagation of the reflected wave on the aortic (and LV) pressure waveform include a mid-to-late systolic shoulder which causes an increase in systolic and pulse aortic pressure and the area under the pressure curve during systole; this area represents the systolic pressure time index (SPTI) [3, 79]. The total arterial compliance of the systemic macrocirculation depends on the summed compliance of the various arterial segments. The compliance of individual segments is linearly proportional to vessel volume (or radius³) and, for any given "relative" vessel geometry (wall volume/lumen volume ratio), linearly and inversely proportional to wall stiffness (Young's elastic modulus). The interaction between the stiffness and geometry (including taper) of the macrocirculation also impacts location of the major reflection site and amplitude and duration of the reflected wave. Reflected waves that arrive during LV ejection increase the mid-to-late LV systolic workload, SPTI, wasted LV energy (or effort, Ew), and myocardial oxygen demand [1, 3, 4, 40, 41, 60, 90]. It has been proposed that the chronic increase in elastic artery stiffness with age increases wave reflection amplitude and pulse pressure and promotes an excessive penetration of pulsatility further into the microcirculation of target organs with high flow rates such as the heart, the brain, and the kidneys [56, 91–94]. This process reduces the number of SMC [95] and causes endothelial dysfunction [94] which leads to attenuation of the reserve capacity of the vascular bed. Indeed, aortic stiffness and wave reflection amplitude are both inversely related to coronary blood flow reserve (CFR) [96] (see below). An increase in arterial pulsatility resulting from arterial stiffness and wave reflection amplitude has little effect on the systemic arterial circulation to most bodily tissues because their flow is determined by the mean pressure gradient and because cells are protected by the vasoconstricted small arteries and arterioles upstream [56]. Brain and kidney cells receive no such protection because arterial vessels remain somewhat dilated. The large increase in arterial pulsatility is applied to all the distributing arteries in these organs while mean flow is maintained [97]. Brain and kidney arteries of all sizes, including pre-arterioles, are thus subjected to higher pulsatile circumferential stress and higher longitudinal shear stress. Their ability to withstand increased stresses depends on their resilience, and this is markedly decreased in a number of diseases, particularly diabetes mellitus [3, 98]. Increased stiffness of large elastic arteries thus promotes a "setup" for small arterial disease and the types of changes elucidated by Byrom [97, 99] over 50 years ago. Byrom's work was initially conducted in rats but was applied to the small-vessel disease seen in human hypertension. He showed that damage to small arteries could be induced by increased pulsatile stress and could lead to tearing of their endothelium and SMC with disruption of the vessel wall. He thus explained development of small arterial dilations and aneurysms and the features of lipohyalinosis and of fibrinoid necrosis as seen in the brains and kidneys of hypertensive disease. Byrom further showed that these changes were largely reversible when disrupting forces were reduced [99].

It should be noted that although the timing of arrival of reflected waves from the lower body to the heart is influenced by arterial (both elastic and muscular) stiffness, the relationship between arterial stiffness and reflected wave transit time is relatively poor, presumably given the wide variability in the distance to wave reflection sites. Furthermore, there is not a direct correlation between aortic stiffness and wave reflection amplitude or augmentation index (AIx) over the entire life span [3]. Changes in elastic artery and muscular artery PWV do not always parallel each other. For example, during the aging process elastic artery PWV (and AIx) increases markedly, while muscular artery PWV changes very little. Also, during vasoconstrictor administration (without a large increase in mean arterial pressure) elastic artery PWV changes very little, while muscular artery PWV increases markedly and causes a large increase in AIx [3]. PWV is a measure of arterial stiffness while AIx is an index of the net effect of wave reflection on late systolic and pulse pressure.

Various indices of pulsatile LV afterload are useful because they are meant to be purely reflective of arterial properties and wave reflection. However, arterial load should always be interpreted by considering interactions between arteries as a load and the LV as a pump [3, 100] and also between myocardial elements and instantaneous LV geometry and the time-varying load imposed by both macro- and microcirculations. Wall stress represents the time-varying mechanical load experienced by the contractile elements in the myocardium (myocardial afterload).

Throughout systole, myocardial fiber activation results in the development of tension (stress) and shortening of myocardial segments, which results in progressive ejection of blood from the LV cavity and wall thickening. During early ejection, active development of fiber cross-bridges occurs in the electrically activated myocardium and peak myocardial wall stress occurs [101]. Myocardial fiber shortening and ejection of blood determine a progressive change in LV geometry which causes a drop in myocardial stress (despite rising pressure) during mid-to-late systole [3]. This shift in the pressure–stress relation is related to the ejection process itself and appears to be favorable for the myocardium to handle the additional load imposed by wave reflections and increased LV wasted energy, but may be insufficient and/or compromised in the setting of wave reflections of early onset of large amplitude [102] and in the presence of lower LV ejection fractions or abnormal LV ejection patterns [101, 103]. This may be important, because the myocardium appears to be particularly vulnerable to late systolic loading.

As expected from physiologic principles, various arterial properties affect time-varying myocardial wall stress differently. Whereas systemic vascular resistance is an important determinant of wall stress throughout systole, Z_c selectively affects early systole and peak systolic wall stress, wave reflections, and total arterial compliance correlate with myocardial stress in mid and late systole and significantly influence the area under the stress curve generated for any given flow output [104].

An increase in the pulsatile component of afterload causes an undesirable mismatch between the ventricle and arterial system, which increases myocardial oxygen demand and decreases cardiac efficiency [1, 105, 106]. These changes in ventricular/vascular coupling promote the development of LV hypertrophy (LVH) and often lead to both systolic and diastolic myocardial dysfunction [103, 107–111]. Indeed, Jankowski et al. [108] reported that the pulsatile but not the steady component of LV load predicted cardiovascular events in coronary patients. Several lines of evidence support the importance of the LV loading sequence (and not just "absolute" load) in LV remodeling and failure [40, 60, 90]. Late systolic loading (and increase in wasted LV energy) has been shown to induce much more pronounced LVH and fibrosis in an animal model compared to early systolic loading, at identical peak LV pressure levels [60]. Increased late systolic load has also been shown to exert more profound adverse effects on ventricular relaxation than early systolic load, for any given level of peak LV pressure [60]. Consistent with available animal data, changes in wave reflection magnitude (RM = AP/P1) have been reported to correlate with regression of LVH in response to antihypertensive therapy [40], and reflection magnitude has been shown to be strongly associated with incident heart failure and mortality in the general population [45, 82].

2.5.4 Pressure Differences Within the Arterial Tree and Pulse Pressure Amplification

As the pressure wave travels from the heart along the arteries of the macrocirculation, both systolic and pulse pressures (PP) increase markedly, while mean pressure decreases only slightly (−2 mmHg) due to wave reflection and viscous damping [3, 112]

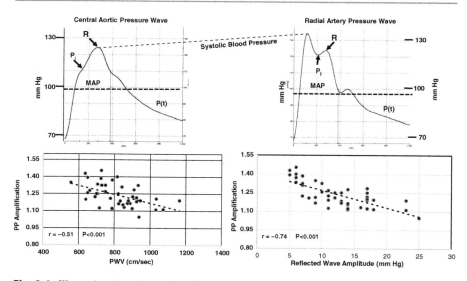

Fig. 2.4 Illustration showing noninvasive measurements of radial artery pressure (*upper right*) and synthesized central aortic pressure (*upper left*). *Pi* is the inflection point, *R* is the peak of the reflected wave, and *MAP* is the mean arterial pressure. *Lower panels* show that PP amplification (radial PP/aortic PP) is significantly inversely related to both aortic PWV (*lower left*) and reflected wave amplitude (AP) (*lower right*)

(Fig. 2.4). Thus, both systolic and pulse pressures are greater in the arm and leg than in the ascending aorta [3, 87]. This mechanism (PP amplification) ensures that pulsatile load is lower in the elastic ascending aorta versus peripheral muscular arteries and, therefore, minimizes excessive LV pressure energy and subsequent pulsatile afterload [41]. PP amplification (i.e., peripheral PP/central PP) is determined by a combination of factors including LV contractility and ejection duration, heart rate, arterial stiffness (elastic moduli), arterial caliber (and taper), arterial path length, timing and magnitude of wave reflections, and tone of the microcirculation (vascular resistance) [3, 86, 112–115]. From about 30 years of age onward, central aortic PP is the sum of a forward-traveling wave (P1) and a reflected wave (AP) (Fig. 2.2); therefore, PP amplification is influenced by both central aortic stiffness and wave reflection. These factors are interassociated, making it difficult to determine specific primary modulators. Overall, it would appear that wave reflection amplitude explains the largest proportion of the variance in PP amplification with PWV (arterial stiffness) and heart rate making additional notable contributions [112, 115, 116]. Indeed, the degree of amplification is age- and elastic artery stiffness-dependent and decreases as aortic stiffness and wave reflection amplitude increase (Fig. 2.4) [116, 117]. This difference between central and peripheral pressure progression may explain why central aortic pressure tends to be a better predictor of cardiovascular events and outcome than peripheral brachial pressure [118–121]. Since peripheral muscular arteries stiffen little with age [122–125], elastic properties of these vessels alter amplification along the vessels minimally. Thus, transmission (propagation) characteristics in the upper limbs remain relatively constant [126]. However, PP amplification in the proximal elastic aorta is markedly influenced by acute changes in SMC tone of muscular arteries. Increased SMC tone (contraction) increases wave reflection amplitude and reduces PP amplification, while decreased tone (relaxation) has the opposite effect. Reduced PP amplification occurs with aging [3, 86, 117, 127], obesity, and arterial disease (hypertension, diabetes, hypercholesterolemia, coronary artery disease, renal disease) and is associated with traditional cardiovascular risk factors [128, 129] and overall vascular burden [130]. Moreover, PP amplification is associated with overt target organ damage and regression of target organ damage with therapy (i.e., LVH regression with antihypertensive therapy and exercise conditioning) [131], and it independently predicts future cardiovascular mortality [132, 133]. Thus, PP amplification has been proposed as a potential mechanical biomarker of cardiovascular risk and global arterial function. Racial differences in PP amplification have been reported with African American men having lower amplification than their white peers [134] related to increased arterial stiffness and wave reflections [81]. Sex differences in PP amplification also exist, with women (particularly postmenopausal women) having lower values than men [135]. Reasons for this difference have been ascribed to a host of factors including shorter stature in women (reduced height resulting in attenuated arterial path length and movement of reflection sites more proximal), increased PWV affecting timing of the return of the reflected pressure wave, increased aortic taper, and arterial impedance mismatch affecting wave reflection amplitude [3, 136]. Sex differences in PP amplification have been linked to LV diastolic dysfunction in women [111]. In men and women over age 55 years, the mortality impact of PP amplification is threefold higher in women compared to men [137]. Since wave reflections do not alter PP in younger adults, amplification declines as diastolic blood pressure rises, offering insight into well-noted observations that peripheral PP is unrelated to cardiovascular risk in this age cohort [126]. Conversely, loss of PP amplification with aging results in peripheral pressures more closely approximating central pressures, hence increasing the ability of peripheral PP to accurately predict CV risk in older adults [126]. In older adults, PP amplification is predictive of heart failure, ischemic heart disease, atrial fibrillation, and mortality [132, 137]. In young healthy adults, it is also possible for PP amplification to result in spurious systolic hypertension [138]. Seen in taller men with compliant elastic arteries, wave reflections are markedly attenuated and PP amplification profound [139, 140]. The clinical implications of this elevated PP amplification in this population remain to be determined [138]. As noted above, heart rate also makes a notable contribution to PP amplification and this is most likely via effects on wave reflection [141, 142]. With slower heart rate and prolonged systolic ejection duration, there is greater temporal overlap between forward and reflected pressure waves causing an increase in reflected wave amplitude and AIx [3]. It is estimated that for every 10 bpm reduction in HR, there is an increase in AIx of 4 % [142]. This in turn results in a reduction in PP amplification. Medications that reduce heart rate such as β-blockers are associated with reduced PP amplification because these drugs cause an increase in wave reflection amplitude [143, 144]. Interestingly, lifestyle modification that results in bradycardia such as habitual aerobic exercise could possibly result in reduced PP amplification owing to HR-mediated increase in PP from increased wave reflection coupled with reduced arterial stiffness [134, 145]. As stated above, PP amplification is usually calculated as the ratio of the amplitude of the PP between a proximal and distal site. Alternative methods include calculation of absolute PP differences from peripheral to central sites (peripheral PP – central PP) and expressed as the absolute difference from peripheral to central sites relative to the central site [(peripheral PP – central PP)/central PP]. An issue that remains to be resolved pertains to methodology for obtaining central and peripheral PP appraisal. Although the gold standard for PP measurement remains invasive recordings, this is not practical for routine clinical use. Current studies noting clinical utility of PP amplification have calculated central PP noninvasively either via (1) synthesized aortic pressure waves derived from radial pressure waves and a GTF; (2) carotid pressure waves as a surrogate for aortic pressure calibrated against brachial mean and diastolic pressure [112]. While both methods are valid and have merit, neither is without flaw. When using the GTF approach, radial pressure waves are usually calibrated against brachial systolic and diastolic blood pressure, an approach that assumes that pulse pressure in the brachial and radial arteries are identical to each other (i.e., no brachial-to-radial amplification). When using synthesized aortic pressure waves from the GTF approach and brachial pressures obtained from an oscillometric cuff as done in the Anglo-Cardiff Collaborative Trial (ACCT), amplification varies from 1.7 in the young (<20 years of age) to 1.2 in the elderly (>80 years of age) [123]. These results are similar to those reported by Bia et al. [127] over the same age range in the CUiiDARTE Project and those collected by Nichols et al. [3]. When carotid and/or radial pressure waves obtained from applanation tonometry are calibrated against brachial diastolic and tonometric mean pressures (the latter being obtained from a brachial artery tonometric waveform), as was done in the Asklepios Study, PP amplification values tend to be lower [116]. Although not without limitation, measurement of PP amplification from noninvasive central and peripheral pulse recordings has proven superior to brachial cuff measures alone when assessing cardiovascular disease (CVD) burden, identifying individuals at risk for CVD events, and monitoring response to therapy [130, 132].

2.5.4.1 Components of the Central Aortic Pressure Wave

Figures 2.2 and 2.3 show invasively measured high-fidelity ascending aortic pressure and flow velocity waves in a normal young adult and a middle-aged human. The measured aortic pressure (P) and flow (Q) waves are determined by the interaction (or algebraic sum) of an LV-ejected forward-traveling "incident" wave and a later arriving backward-traveling reflected wave from the lower body [2, 3, 80, 146]. The characteristics of the forward-traveling wave depend, primarily, upon the elastic properties (Z_c) of the ascending aorta and are not influenced by wave reflections [3, 67, 147]. Two visible demarcations usually occur on the initial upstroke of the central aortic pressure wave in middle-aged (Fig. 2.2) and older individuals with stiff aortas and elevated Z_c: the first shoulder (P1) and the inflection point (P_i). These demarcation points occur at an earlier age in patients with hypertension. The first (or early) shoulder is generated by LV ejection and occurs at peak blood flow velocity, while the inflection point occurs later and denotes the initial upstroke of the reflected pressure wave; this wave represents the second (or mid-to-late) systolic shoulder [3, 148, 149]. The first shoulder is an estimate of incident (or forward-traveling) wave with amplitude P1, while the second shoulder is generated by the reflected pressure wave from the lower body with amplitude AP and duration (ED – Tr); ED is ejection duration and Tr is the round trip travel time of the pressure wave to and from the lower body reflection site [3]; AP increases in parallel with the first aortic input impedance moduli (Z_1). When the first shoulder and P_i occur simultaneously (or merge), as often occurs in older individuals and patients with severe hypertension, no demarcation is visible. Therefore, if pressure and flow velocity are measured simultaneously, the initial upstroke of the reflected wave, P1, and P_i can be determined and AP, AIx, and RM calculated. If flow velocity is not measured and P_i is not visible, a method that uses the second derivative of the pulse to identify P_i is used. In this method, P_i occurs at the second peak of the second derivative; the fourth derivative has also been used [3]. In younger individuals with compliant aortas and reduced Z_c, the second systolic shoulder occurs much later (after peak systolic pressure) than the first and is usually of lower amplitude (Fig. 2.3) [3, 62]; Z_1 is also reduced in this cohort. In a system with no reflections, the flow and pressure waves are similar in shape (see Fig. 2.3). The characteristics of the reflected wave depend upon a more complex set of determinants than the forward wave, namely, the physical properties (stiffness, taper and branching) of all the arteries in the macrocirculation, especially those in the aorta and lower body, PWV, Tr, and distance to the major "effective" reflection site [2, 3, 62, 74, 148–152]. Augmentation index (AIx = AP/PP), an estimate of wave reflection strength and its contribution to central PP, is related to arterial properties via changes in PWV from the heart to the termination of the microcirculation in the lower body. The magnitude of wave reflection can also be expressed by the reflection magnitude (RM = AP/P1) [52]. Increased arterial stiffness increases PWV (and Z_c) and causes early return (Tr decreases) of the reflected wave from the lower body reflecting sites to the heart during systole when the ventricle is still ejecting blood [2, 3, 53, 72, 101, 153]. As Tr decreases, both AP and systolic duration (ED – Tr) increase. This mechanism augments ascending aortic systolic pressure and PP [108, 154–157], an effect that increases arterial wall stress, potentiates the development of coronary artery atherosclerosis, elevates LV afterload, and increases LV mass and oxygen demand while decreasing stroke volume [1, 87, 131, 148]. Since the reflected wave and associated boost in pressure (LV and aortic) does not contribute positively to ejection of blood, the effect of the extra workload is wasted (pressure) energy (or effort) (Ew) (Fig. 2.2) [103, 148, 158–160] the ventricle must generate to overcome AP. Thus, the ventricle shifts from a flow source to a pressure source which uses extra oxygen to generate less flow, and therefore, efficiency decreases [3]. Accordingly, optimal treatment for high central systolic pressure and PP (pulsatile component of LV load) should focus not only on increasing arteriolar caliber and reducing peripheral resistance of the microcirculation but also on reducing arterial stiffness, Z_c, PWV, systolic wave reflection (and Z_1), and Ew [161, 162]. Correct calculation of variables from the pressure wave (i.e., AIx, forward and reflected wave amplitude and travel time, distance to reflection sites, RM, and Ew) depends on the accurate determination of the inflection point, P_i, on the aortic pressure wave (see above) [3, 70]. Also, care must be taken not to use AIx as a measure of arterial stiffness because of its dependence on wave reflections, heart rate, ejection duration, and body height [3]. Since invasive recordings of ascending aortic pressure waves and pulse wave analysis can only be made in a selected number of patients in the cardiac catheterization laboratory, techniques have been developed recently that enable the noninvasive determination of the above variables [66, 115] in large cohorts with similar results [144, 156, 163–166]. For example, large population studies such as the Baltimore Longitudinal Study of Aging [167, 168], Framingham [169], Anglo-Cardiff (ACCT) [123, 129], and many other aging studies [117, 125] and reviews [85, 162] observed that age is an important determinant of arterial properties and wave reflection characteristics that influence dramatic changes in the macrocirculation. In youth, the reflected wave from the lower body travels at a reduced PWV and arrives at the heart in diastole (Fig. 2.3) which aids coronary artery and myocardial perfusion, but with increasing age (Fig. 2.2), the elastic arteries stiffen, increase Z_c (and PWV), and cause the reflected wave to arrive at the heart during systole (second shoulder) with greater amplitude, systolic duration, and Z_1. This modification in wave reflection characteristics contributes to a decrease in stroke output (negative reflected flow wave contributing to flow deceleration) and a corresponding decline in cardiac output [168]. Aortic systolic pressure and PP increase, whereas diastolic pressure increases to middle age and then decreases in later life [3, 125]. Because of increased central elastic artery stiffness and PWV measured as carotid–femoral PWV, the reflected wave from the lower body migrates into systole and increases aortic AP, AIx, and RM; in the radial and brachial artery, since stiffness changes very little with age [123, 125], the forward to reflected wave (from the hand region) ratio remains essentially unchanged. Tr decreases with age, whereas (ED – Tr) increases causing Ew and myocardial oxygen demand to increase markedly. Arterial stiffness and wave reflection characteristics are amplified in older individuals and in patients with systemic hypertension [125, 170], thereby causing a reduction in PP amplification (Fig. 2.4). In a system with no reflections or one in which the reflected wave arrives after peak systolic pressure and with low amplitude, an increase in aortic stiffness alone only causes an increase in aortic PP (for a given stroke volume), with little change in wave contour (see Fig. 2.3). Major changes in aortic pressure wave contour are due to alterations in amplitude and timing of wave reflections from the macrocirculation, including both elastic and muscular arteries (including arterioles). LV afterload, central aortic and brachial artery systolic, and PP, SPTI, RM, and AIx are increased by elastic artery stiffening and increased wave reflection amplitude, all of which are alterations associated with aging and resulting in LVH [60, 131] and arterial wall damage [127]—major cardiovascular, cerebrovascular, and renovascular risk factors [56, 154, 155]. Major cardiovascular risk factors resulting from increased aortic stiffness and wave reflection (LV afterload) include coronary artery atherosclerosis, decreased coronary blood flow and coronary flow

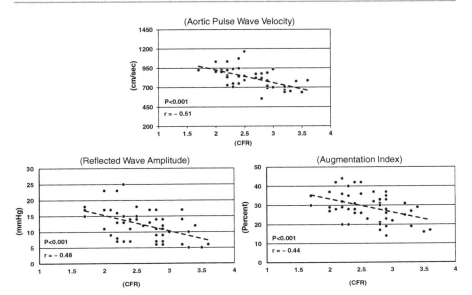

Fig. 2.5 Graphs showing the effects of aortic PWV (*upper*), reflected wave amplitude (AP) (*lower left*), and augmentation index (AIx) (*lower right*) on coronary flow reserve (*CFR*). All three of these variables are significantly inversely related to CFR

reserve (CFR) (Fig. 2.5), LVH, heart failure, and mortality. An explanation for the progression from normal LV systolic function to severe failure is available on the basis of the argument proposed by Westerhof and O'Rourke [107] and Nichols et al. [3]. This explanation has been effectively used to characterize mechanical pumps, with the LV seen to act as a flow source (powerful ejection) in youth when the ventricle is optimally matched to a compliant arterial system and power generation is minimal and wasted energy is zero. Under these circumstances the reflected wave arrives in diastole and aids in coronary artery perfusion and CFR. The age-related increase in elastic artery stiffness (and PWV) causes the reflected wave to arrive earlier to the heart and boost pressure in mid-to-late systole and places an extra pulsatile workload on the LV causing it to generate more force, which is wasted energy [103]. These changes in arterial properties and wave reflection characteristics cause the LV to change from a flow source to a combined flow and pressure source (ejection limited by pressure achieved) as hypertension develops. As the elastic arteries become stiffer, LV pressure increases and causes an increase in systolic pressure time index (SPTI) and myocardial oxygen demand. Sustained elevation and prolongation of mid-to-late systolic augmentation results in LVH [3], which is associated with progressive degenerative changes in the myocytes such that these weaken and develop less force with each contraction. The weakened, hypertrophied fibers lengthen and the LV dilates, with augmented systolic pressure and stroke output initially being somewhat maintained at greater muscle length and LV volume through the Frank–Starling mechanism [3].

2.5.4.2 III Effects of Increased Aortic Stiffness and Wave Reflections on the Coronary Microcirculation

The concept of coronary blood flow reserve (CFR) was introduced to reflect the maximal oxygen delivery capacity during increasing myocardial oxygen demand. Since myocytes extract large amounts (70–80 %) of oxygen from the blood at rest, the best way of meeting increasing oxygen demand is by increasing coronary blood flow [171, 172]. An increase in coronary blood flow can be accomplished by decreasing coronary microvascular resistance, as occurs with elevated myocardial oxygen demand, or increasing oxygen supply by increasing coronary artery perfusion pressure. At rest, there is significant autoregulation in the coronary microvascular bed which ensures sufficient blood supply to the myocytes under a wide range of oxygen demand and perfusion pressure. Thus, resting coronary blood flow is mainly under control of tissue metabolic demand [173]. To test the maximum flow reserve capacity, the autoregulation must be uncoupled, which will create a linear relationship between perfusion pressure and coronary flow [174–177]. Thus, CFR in humans is usually measured during either exercise challenge or pharmacological stimuli such as dobutamine or adenosine [178]; in animals CFR is measured as reactive hyperemia following 10 or 20 s of total coronary artery occlusion and release [179]. Hemodynamically significant lesions in the epicardial coronary arteries (macrocirculation) are known to cause reduced CFR [178–180]. Furthermore, numerous recent studies have shown that some individuals (especially women) with normal epicardial coronary arteries have reduced CFR [181–187]. CFR is defined as the ratio of blood flow at maximal (or near maximal) vasodilation and basal (or resting) blood flow [175]. Vasodilation results from relaxation of SMC of the microcirculation and is associated with endothelial function. Therefore, in the absence of obstructive epicardial coronary artery disease, a reduction in CFR is frequently used as an index of "microvascular dysfunction" [185–188]; however, this association has been questioned by some. CFR is strongly dependent upon changes in the plateau level of basal perfusion and coronary flow. For example, in LVH resulting from chronically elevated afterload, total basal coronary blood flow is increased, but maximal flow does not change; therefore, CFR is reduced [175, 177, 189, 190]. Conditions that increase myocardial oxygen demand increase basal coronary blood flow and deplete a portion of the total reserve capacity of the microcirculation and, therefore, reduce CFR [172].

To fully appreciate the importance of coronary microvascular physiology (and pathophysiology), it must be realized that coronary blood flow changes dramatically during the cardiac cycle. Since the rhythmic contraction of the LV compresses and squeezes the coronary vessels and throttles blood flow during systole, the majority of flow (about 80 %) occurs during relaxation (or diastole) [191]. As central aortic stiffness and wave reflection amplitude increase, central systolic blood pressure rises, PP widens, and LV wall stress and myocardial oxygen demand increase, while aortic diastolic pressure decreases [123, 192, 193]. These alterations in pulsatile load cause LVH independent of change in the steady load component [60, 194]. Such abnormalities in ventricular/vascular coupling unbalance the favorable myocardial oxygen supply/demand ratio and promote myocardial ischemia and contractile dysfunction [3]. Information regarding the ill effects of aortic stiffening and wave reflections on the coronary circulation has come primarily from experimental animal models where the aorta was artificially stiffened or replaced with a rigid tube [26, 195–197]. In these studies when the heart ejected into a stiff or noncompliant aorta, systolic pressure and PP, wasted LV energy, and myocardial oxygen demand increased and diastolic pressure decreased, but coronary blood flow also increased in response to the marked increase in oxygen demand [26]. However, increased aortic stiffness and wave reflection caused a decrease in CFR [189, 196], and during increased myocardial contractility, subendocardial blood flow was impaired and the subendocardial electrocardiogram showed signs of ischemia [195]. These undesirable alterations in ventricle/vascular coupling were enhanced in the presence of a high-grade coronary artery stenosis [195] and during reductions in aortic diastolic blood pressure. During total coronary artery occlusion and myocardial ischemia, increased aortic stiffness caused marked enhancement in cardiac dysfunction [196]. In more recent experimental rat studies, Hachamovitch et al. [198] and Gosse and Clementy [190] found that age and hypertension, conditions associated with increased aortic stiffness and wave reflection, produced LVH and adversely affected the coronary circulation and CFR. These changes in coronary hemodynamics in response to increased aortic stiffness increase the potential for ischemic episodes, especially in the subendocardial region [198]. From these experimental animal studies, it appears that both acute and chronic preparations with artificially stiffened aortas or other interventions that increase myocardial oxygen demand have increased resting coronary blood flow and reduced CFR.

Several studies in humans have confirmed and expanded the findings in experimental animal models. The age-related increase in aortic stiffness and wave reflection, in healthy volunteers with presumably normal coronary arteries, causes an increase in LV afterload and resting coronary blood flow, but a decrease in CFR [199]. The majority of older patients have increased aortic stiffness and wave reflection which causes increased systolic blood pressure and decreased diastolic pressure resulting in isolated systolic hypertension so that aggressive treatment to lower blood pressure, especially those with macro- and/or microvascular anomalies, is more difficult [200]. Under these conditions the myocardium is primarily and linearly dependent upon coronary perfusion pressure for myocardial blood supply because autoregulation is exhausted; however, the jeopardized region may receive some blood flow through collaterals [201]. In other studies, significant correlations between CFR and increased aortic stiffness and wave reflection amplitude were demonstrated in different patient populations, some with [202] and others without [181–184] CAD. The decrease in coronary blood flow and CFR in CAD results predominantly from narrowing of epicardial coronary arteries, while reduction in CFR in patients with normal or nonobstructive CAD is more difficult to explain. Therefore, one must consider other factors than coronary artery narrowing such as myocardial oxygen demand [191, 202], diastole pressure time index (DPTI) [203], coronary pressure gradient, and coronary artery endothelial function [204]. Arterial stiffness and wave reflection affect all four of these variables and can readily explain angina pectoris even in the absence of macrovascular epicardial coronary artery atherosclerosis [205,

206]. Increased stiffness of central elastic arteries with aging and/or vasoconstriction of peripheral muscular arteries increases central aortic pressure (systolic and pulse) to a much greater extent than brachial cuff pressure because of wave reflection [3, 74]; central and brachial diastolic pressures decrease in parallel. These hemodynamic changes cause an increase in myocardial oxygen demand during systole while decreasing coronary artery perfusion in diastole. Such chronic changes in LV afterload are associated with an undesirable imbalance in the myocardial oxygen supply/demand ratio which is exacerbated in LVH and can lead to ischemia and angina even in the absence of coronary atherosclerosis [207]. Similarly, a marked increase in heart rate in the face of increased aortic stiffness can reduce coronary perfusion and precipitate myocardial stunning [208]. Aortic stiffness and wave reflection can have a profound influence on coronary blood flow and CFR through an elevation in systolic pressure, a slowing in LV relaxation, and a reduction in diastolic pressure [209]. These effects can be estimated as the "subendocardial viability ratio" (DPTI/SPTI) which has been shown to be directly related to CFR [191, 210]. Clinical information on the effects of arterial stiffness and wave reflection on epicardial coronary artery blood flow waveforms and CFR has come from both invasive (Doppler catheter or guidewire) and noninvasive (transesophageal and transthoracic Doppler echocardiography) measurements [96, 182–184]. Regardless of the method used to measure coronary blood flow velocity and aortic stiffness, the results are similar—aortic stiffness and wave reflection amplitude are both inversely related to CFR in the presence or absence of CAD (Fig. 2.5). Results from the Dallas Heart Study [207] showed that angina among women in the general population is common and is not necessarily associated with subclinical atherosclerosis. However, angina in the absence of subclinical atherosclerosis is not related to traditional atherosclerotic risk factors but is associated with clinical, inflammatory, and vascular factors that reflect endothelial dysfunction and increased aortic stiffness and wave reflection, suggesting a distinct vascular etiology and alternative potential therapeutic targets. Furthermore, coronary microvascular dysfunction, if it exists, in some cases, however, may be independent of the endothelium [211]. Thus, Reis et al. [212] of the Women's Ischemic Syndrome Evaluation (WISE) study group reported that of 159 women without significant obstructive CAD undergoing invasive studies, 74 (47 %) had what they defined as subnormal coronary flow responses to intracoronary adenosine (CFR < 2.5). Age and the number of years postmenopausal correlated inversely with reduced CFR, but not lipid and hormone levels, blood pressure, or left ventricular ejection fraction. A more recent report from the WISE study group found that, compared with a reference group, WISE participants with normal epicardial coronaries had higher aortic systolic and pulse BP and ejection duration. These differences were associated with an increase in reflected wave amplitude and systolic duration. These modifications in wave reflection characteristics were associated with an increase in SPTI and wasted LV energy and a decrease in PP amplification, subendocardial viability ratio, and diastolic pressure time fraction [213]. Subsequent data from this WISE study group showed that aortic PWV was elevated and CFR was reduced. Furthermore, there was a significant inverse relationship between CFR and indices of aortic stiffness and wave reflections (Fig. 2.5), variables that increase myocardial oxygen demand and basal coronary blood flow. Therefore, it is difficult to say with certainty that microvascular dysfunction was present. Support for this conclusion was published recently by Pauly et al. [181]. These authors showed, in a substudy of WISE, that treatment with an ACE inhibitor, an agent that reduces arterial stiffness and wave reflections, improved CFR. In light of these findings, we tend to agree with O'Rourke's suggestion that "decreased coronary flow reserve" should be used instead of "microvascular dysfunction" [191], since none of the above studies actually measured microvascular function.

References

1. Namasivayam M, Adji A, O'Rourke MF (2011) Influence of aortic pressure wave components determined noninvasively on myocardial oxygen demand in men and women. Hypertension 57:193–200
2. Westerhof N, Stergiopulos N, Noble MIM (2010) Snapshots of hemodynamics, 2nd edn. Springer, New York
3. Nichols WW, O'Rourke MF, Vlachopoulos C (2011) McDonald's blood flow in arteries: theoretic, experimental and clinical principles, 6th edn. Edward Arnold, London
4. Salvi P (2012) Pulse waves how vascular hemodynamics affects blood pressure. Springer, Lexington
5. Milnor WR (1990) Cardiovascular physiology. Oxford University Press, New York
6. Tsamis A, Krawiec JT, Vorp DA (2013) Elastin and collagen fibre microstructure of the human aorta in ageing and disease: a review. J R Soc Interface 10:20121004
7. Mulligan-Kehoe MJ, Simons M (2014) Vasa vasorum in normal and diseased arteries. Circulation 129:2557–2566
8. Wolinsky H, Glagov S (1969) Comparison of abdominal and thoracic aortic medial structure in mammals. Deviation of man from the usual pattern. Circ Res 25:677–686
9. OpenStax College (2013) Structure and function of blood vessels. OpenStax-CNX. http://cnx.org/content/m46597/1.4
10. Vane JR, Anggård EE, Botting RM (1990) Regulatory functions of the vascular endothelium. N Engl J Med 323:27–36
11. Celermajer DS (1997) Endothelial dysfunction: does it matter? Is it reversible? J Am Coll Cardiol 30:325–333
12. Deanfield J, Donald A, Ferri C, Working Group on Endothelin and Endothelial Factors of the European Society of Hypertension et al (2005) Endothelial function and dysfunction. Part I: methodological issues for assessment in the different vascular beds: a statement by the Working Group on Endothelin and Endothelial Factors of the European Society of Hypertension. J Hypertens 23:7–17
13. Deanfield JE, Halcox JP, Rabelink TJ (2007) Endothelial function and dysfunction: testing and clinical relevance. Circulation 115:1285–1295
14. Vanhoutte PM, Shimokawa H, Tang EH, Feletou M (2009) Endothelial dysfunction and vascular disease. Acta Physiol (Oxf) 196:193–222
15. Tomiyama H, Yamashina A (2010) Non-invasive vascular function tests: their pathophysiological background and clinical application. Circ J 74:24–33
16. Burnstock G (1999) Release of vasoactive substances from endothelial cells by shear stress and purinergic mechanosensory transduction. J Anat 194:335–342
17. Pyke KE, Tschakovsky ME (2005) The relationship between shear stress and flow-mediated dilatation: implications for the assessment of endothelial function. J Physiol 568:357–369
18. Gasser TC, Ogden RW, Holzapfel GA (2006) Hyperelastic modelling of arterial layers with distributed collagen fibre orientations. J R Soc Interface 3:15–35

19. Timmins LH, Wu Q, Yeh AT et al (2010) Structural inhomogeneity and fiber orientation in the inner arterial media. Am J Physiol Heart Circ Physiol 298:H1537–H1545
20. Vanhoutte PM, Mombouli JV (1996) Vascular endothelium: vasoactive mediators. Prog Cardiovasc Dis 39:229–238
21. Hoffmann E, Assennato P, Donatelli M et al (1998) Plasma endothelin-1 levels in patients with angina pectoris and normal coronary angiograms. Am Heart J 135:684–688
22. Harkness ML, Harkness RD, McDonald DA (1957) The collagen and elastin content of the arterial wall in the dog. Proc R Soc Lond B Biol Sci 146:541–551
23. Fischer GM, Llaurado JG (1966) Collagen and elastin content in canine arteries selected from functionally different vascular beds. Circ Res 19:394–399
24. Armentano RL, Levenson J, Barra JG et al (1991) Assessment of elastin and collagen contribution to aortic elasticity in conscious dogs. Am J Physiol 260:H1870–H1877
25. Wagenseil JE, Mecham RP (2012) Elastin in large artery stiffness and hypertension. J Cardiovasc Transl Res 5:264–273
26. Saeki A, Recchia F, Kass DA (1995) Systolic flow augmentation in hearts ejecting into a model of stiff aging vasculature. Influence on myocardial perfusion-demand balance. Circ Res 76:132–141
27. O'Rourke MF, Nichols WW (2005) Aortic diameter, aortic stiffness, and wave reflection increase with age and isolated systolic hypertension. Hypertension 45:652–658
28. Wagenseil JE, Mecham RP (2009) Vascular extracellular matrix and arterial mechanics. Physiol Rev 89:957–989
29. Vanhoutte PM, Rubanyi GM, Miller VM, Houston DS (1986) Modulation of vascular smooth muscle contraction by the endothelium. Annu Rev Physiol 48:307–320
30. Schlatmann TJ, Becker AE (1977) Histologic changes in the normal aging aorta: implications for dissecting aortic aneurysm. Am J Cardiol 39:13–20
31. Guyton AC, Hall JE (2000) Textbook of medical physiology, 10th edn. Saunders, Philadelphia
32. Boudoulas H, Stefanadis C (2009) The aorta: structure, function, dysfunction and diseases. Informa Healthcare, New York
33. Boutouyrie P, Bussy C, Hayoz D et al (2000) Local pulse pressure and regression of arterial wall hypertrophy during long-term antihypertensive treatment. Circulation 101:2601–2606
34. O'Rourke MF, Hashimoto J (2007) Mechanical factors in arterial aging: a clinical perspective. J Am Coll Cardiol 50:1–13
35. O'Rourke MF, Yaginuma T (1984) Wave reflections and the arterial pulse. Arch Intern Med 144:366–371
36. Stary HC, Blankenhorn DH, Chandler AB et al (1992) A definition of the intima of human arteries and of its atherosclerosis-prone regions. A report from the Committee on Vascular Lesions of the Council on Arteriosclerosis, American Heart Association. Circulation 85:391–405
37. Bouthier JD, De Luca N, Safar ME, Simon AC (1985) Cardiac hypertrophy and arterial distensibility in essential hypertension. Am Heart J 109:1345–1352
38. Isnard RN, Pannier BM, Laurent S et al (1989) Pulsatile diameter and elastic modulus of the aortic arch in essential hypertension: a noninvasive study. J Am Coll Cardiol 13:399–405
39. Marchais SJ, Guerin AP, Pannier BM et al (1993) Wave reflections and cardiac hypertrophy in chronic uremia. Influence of body size. Hypertension 22:876–883
40. Hashimoto J, Westerhof BE, Westerhof N et al (2008) Different role of wave reflection magnitude and timing on left ventricular mass reduction during antihypertensive treatment. J Hypertens 26:1017–1024
41. Hashimoto J, Nichols WW, O'Rourke MF, Imai Y (2008) Association between wasted pressure effort and left ventricular hypertrophy in hypertension: influence of arterial wave reflection. Am J Hypertens 21:329–333
42. O'Rourke M (1990) Arterial stiffness, systolic blood pressure, and logical treatment of arterial hypertension. Hypertension 15:339–347

43. Nichols WW (1994) Determinants of systolic hypertension in older persons. In: Hosoda S, Yaginuma T, Sugawara M, Taylor MG, Caro CG (eds) Recent progress in cardiovascular mechanics. Harwood Academic Publishers, Australia, pp 315–332
44. London GM, Pannier B, Vicaut E et al (1996) Antihypertensive effects and arterial haemodynamic alterations during angiotensin converting enzyme inhibition. J Hypertens 14: 1139–1146
45. Zamani P, Jacobs DR Jr, Segers P et al (2014) Reflection magnitude as a predictor of mortality: the multi-ethnic study of atherosclerosis. Hypertension 64:958–964. doi:10.1161/HYPERTENSIONAHA.114.03855
46. Ben-Shlomo Y, Spears M, Boustred C et al (2014) Aortic pulse wave velocity improves cardiovascular event prediction: an individual participant meta-analysis of prospective observational data from 17,635 subjects. J Am Coll Cardiol 63:636–646
47. Vlachopoulos C, Aznaouridis K, O'Rourke MF et al (2010) Prediction of cardiovascular events and all-cause mortality with central haemodynamics: a systematic review and meta-analysis. Eur Heart J 31:1865–1871
48. Chirinos JA (2013) Ventricular-arterial coupling: invasive and non-invasive assessment. Artery Res 7:2–14
49. Mitchell GF (2009) Clinical achievements of impedance analysis. Med Biol Eng Comput 47:153–163
50. Chirinos JA, Segers P (2010) Noninvasive evaluation of left ventricular afterload: part 1: pressure and flow measurements and basic principles of wave conduction and reflection. Hypertension 56:555–562
51. Segers P, Stergiopulos N, Westerhof N (2000) Quantification of the contribution of cardiac and arterial remodeling to hypertension. Hypertension 36:760–765
52. Westerhof N, Westerhof BE (2013) CrossTalk proposal: forward and backward pressure waves in the arterial system do represent reality. J Physiol 591:1167–1169
53. O'Rourke MF (1999) Mechanical principles. Arterial stiffness and wave reflection. Pathol Biol (Paris) 47:623–633
54. Westerhof N, Lankhaar JW, Westerhof BE (2009) The arterial windkessel. Med Biol Eng Comput 47:131–141
55. Segers P, Verdonck P (2002) Principles of vascular physiology. In: Lanzer P, Topol E (eds) Pan vascular medicine: integrated clinical management. Springer, Berlin, pp 116–137
56. O'Rourke MF, Safar ME (2005) Relationship between aortic stiffening and microvascular disease in brain and kidney: cause and logic of therapy. Hypertension 46:200–204
57. Ooi H, Chung W, Biolo A (2008) Arterial stiffness and vascular load in heart failure. Congest Heart Fail 14:31–36
58. Westerhof N, Elzinga G, van den Bos GC (1973) Influence of central and peripheral changes on the hydraulic input impedance of the systemic arterial tree. Med Biol Eng 11:710–723
59. O'Rourke MF, Taylor MG (1967) Input impedance of the systemic circulation. Circ Res 20:365–380
60. Kobayashi S, Yano M, Kohno M et al (1996) Influence of aortic impedance on the development of pressure-overload left ventricular hypertrophy in rats. Circulation 94:3362–3368
61. Nichols WW, Conti CR, Walker WE, Milnor WR (1977) Input impedance of the systemic circulation in man. Circ Res 40:451–458
62. Murgo JP, Westerhof N, Giolma JP, Altobelli SA (1980) Aortic input impedance in normal man: relationship to pressure wave forms. Circulation 62:105–116
63. Murgo JP, Westerhof N, Giolma JP, Altobelli SA (1981) Effects of exercise on aortic input impedance and pressure wave forms in normal humans. Circ Res 48:334–343
64. Merillon JP, Motte G, Masquet C et al (1982) Relationship between physical properties of the arterial system and left ventricular performance in the course of aging and arterial hypertension. Eur Heart J 3(Suppl A):95–102
65. Laskey WK, Kussmaul WG (1987) Arterial wave reflection in heart failure. Circulation 75:711–722

66. Pauca AL, O'Rourke MF, Kon ND (2001) Prospective evaluation of a method for estimating ascending aortic pressure from the radial artery pressure waveform. Hypertension 38: 932–937
67. Stergiopulos N, Westerhof BE, Westerhof N (1998) Physical basis of pressure transfer from periphery to aorta: a model-based study. Am J Physiol 274:H1386–H1392
68. Mitchell GF, Lacourciere Y, Ouellet JP et al (2003) Determinants of elevated pulse pressure in middle-aged and older subjects with uncomplicated systolic hypertension: the role of proximal aortic diameter and the aortic pressure-flow relationship. Circulation 108:1592–1598
69. Li W, Ahn AC (2012) Pulsatile hemodynamics of hypertension: systematic review of aortic input impedance. J Hypertens 30:1493–1499
70. Segers P, Rietzschel ER, De Buyzere ML et al (2007) Assessment of pressure wave reflection: getting the timing right! Physiol Meas 28:1045–1056
71. Gatehouse PD, Keegan J, Crowe LA et al (2005) Applications of phase-contrast flow and velocity imaging in cardiovascular MRI. Eur Radiol 15:2172–2184
72. Chirinos JA, Segers P (2010) Noninvasive evaluation of left ventricular afterload: part 2: arterial pressure-flow and pressure-volume relations in humans. Hypertension 56:563–570
73. Segers P, Rietzschel ER, De Buyzere ML et al (2008) Three- and four-element windkessel models: assessment of their fitting performance in a large cohort of healthy middle-aged individuals. Proc Inst Mech Eng H 222:417–428
74. O'Rourke MF (2009) Time domain analysis of the arterial pulse in clinical medicine. Med Biol Eng Comput 47:119–129
75. Kim SY, Hinkamp TJ, Jacobs WR et al (1995) Effect of an inelastic aortic synthetic vascular graft on exercise hemodynamics. Ann Thorac Surg 59:981–989
76. Yin FC, Weisfeldt ML, Milnor WR (1981) Role of aortic input impedance in the decreased cardiovascular response to exercise with aging in dogs. J Clin Invest 68:28–38
77. Yaginuma T, Avolio A, O'Rourke M et al (1986) Effect of glyceryl trinitrate on peripheral arteries alters left ventricular hydraulic load in man. Cardiovasc Res 20:153–160
78. O'Rourke M (1989) Systolic blood pressure: arterial compliance and early wave reflection, and their modification by antihypertensive therapy. J Hum Hypertens 3(Suppl 1):47–52
79. O'Rourke MF (1999) Wave travel and reflection in the arterial system. J Hypertens Suppl 17:S45–S47
80. Westerhof N, Sipkema P, van den Bos GC, Elzinga G (1972) Forward and backward waves in the arterial system. Cardiovasc Res 6:648–656
81. Chirinos JA, Kips JG, Jacobs DR Jr et al (2012) Arterial wave reflections and incident cardiovascular events and heart failure: MESA (Multiethnic Study of Atherosclerosis). J Am Coll Cardiol 60:2170–2177
82. Westerhof BE, van den Wijngaard JP, Murgo JP, Westerhof N (2008) Location of a reflection site is elusive: consequences for the calculation of aortic pulse wave velocity. Hypertension 52:478–483
83. Chirinos JA (2012) Arterial stiffness: basic concepts and measurement techniques. J Cardiovasc Transl Res 5:243–255
84. Laurent S, Cockcroft J, Van Bortel L et al (2006) Expert consensus document on arterial stiffness: methodological issues and clinical applications. Eur Heart J 27:2588–2605
85. O'Rourke MF (2007) Arterial aging: pathophysiological principles. Vasc Med 12:329–341
86. O'Rourke MF, Blazek JV, Morreels CL Jr, Krovetz LJ (1968) Pressure wave transmission along the human aorta. Changes with age and in arterial degenerative disease. Circ Res 23: 567–579
87. Nichols WW, Denardo SJ, Wilkinson IB et al (2008) Effects of arterial stiffness, pulse wave velocity, and wave reflections on the central aortic pressure waveform. J Clin Hypertens (Greenwich) 10:295–303
88. Filipovský J, Tichá M, Cífková R et al (2005) Large artery stiffness and pulse wave reflection: results of a population-based study. Blood Press 14:45–52
89. Sugawara J, Hayashi K, Tanaka H (2010) Distal shift of arterial pressure wave reflection sites with aging. Hypertension 56:920–925

90. Hashimoto J, Watabe D, Hatanaka R et al (2006) Enhanced radial late systolic pressure augmentation in hypertensive patients with left ventricular hypertrophy. Am J Hypertens 19: 27–32
91. Mitchell GF (2008) Effects of central arterial aging on the structure and function of the peripheral vasculature: implications for end-organ damage. J Appl Physiol 105:1652–1660
92. Hashimoto J (2014) Central hemodynamics and target organ damage in hypertension. Tohoku J Exp Med 233:1–8
93. Muiesan ML, Salvetti M, Rizzoni D et al (2013) Pulsatile hemodynamics and microcirculation: evidence for a close relationship in hypertensive patients. Hypertension 61:130–136
94. Tousoulis D, Simopoulou C, Papageorgiou N et al (2014) Endothelial dysfunction in conduit arteries and in microcirculation. Novel therapeutic approaches. Pharmacol Ther 144:253–267
95. Tümer N, Toklu HZ, Muller-Delp JM et al (2014) The effects of aging on the functional and structural properties of the rat basilar artery. Physiol Rep 2:e12031
96. Saito M, Okayama H, Nishimura K et al (2008) Possible link between large artery stiffness and coronary flow velocity reserve. Heart 94:e20
97. Byrom FB (1954) The pathogenesis of hypertensive encephalopathy and its relation to the malignant phase of hypertension; experimental evidence from the hypertensive rat. Lancet 267:201–211
98. Schram MT, Kostense PJ, Van Dijk RA et al (2002) Diabetes, pulse pressure and cardiovascular mortality: the Hoorn Study. J Hypertens 20:1743–1751
99. Byrom F (1969) The hypertensive vascular crisis: an experimental study. Heinemann, London
100. Kawaguchi M, Hay I, Fetics B, Kass DA (2003) Combined ventricular systolic and arterial stiffening in patients with heart failure and preserved ejection fraction: implications for systolic and diastolic reserve limitations. Circulation 107:714–720
101. Chirinos JA, Segers P, Gupta AK et al (2009) Time-varying myocardial stress and systolic pressure-stress relationship: role in myocardial-arterial coupling in hypertension. Circulation 119:2798–2807
102. Nichols WW, Petersen JW, Denardo SJ, Christou DD (2013) Arterial stiffness, wave reflection amplitude and left ventricular afterload are increased in overweight individuals. Artery Res 7:222–229
103. Denardo SJ, Nandyala R, Freeman GL et al (2010) Pulse wave analysis of the aortic pressure waveform in severe left ventricular systolic dysfunction. Circ Heart Fail 3:149–156
104. Chirinos JA, Segers P, Gillebert TC, on behalf of the Asklepios Investigators et al (2012) Arterial properties as determinants of time-varying myocardial stress in humans. Hypertension 60:64–70
105. Kelly RP, Tunin R, Kass DA (1992) Effect of reduced aortic compliance on cardiac efficiency and contractile function of in situ canine left ventricle. Circ Res 71:490–502
106. Guelen I, Mattace-Raso FU, van Popele NM et al (2008) Aortic stiffness and the balance between cardiac oxygen supply and demand: the Rotterdam Study. J Hypertens 26:1237–1243
107. Westerhof N, O'Rourke MF (1995) Haemodynamic basis for the development of left ventricular failure in systolic hypertension and for its logical therapy. J Hypertens 13:943–952
108. Jankowski P, Kawecka-Jaszcz K, Czarnecka D, Aortic Blood Pressure and Survival Study Group et al (2008) Pulsatile but not steady component of blood pressure predicts cardiovascular events in coronary patients. Hypertension 51:848–855
109. Weber T, Auer J, Lamm G et al (2007) Arterial stiffness, central blood pressures, and wave reflections in cardiomyopathy-implications for risk stratification. J Card Fail 13:353–359
110. Weber T, O'Rourke MF, Ammer M et al (2008) Arterial stiffness and arterial wave reflections are associated with systolic and diastolic function in patients with normal ejection fraction. Am J Hypertens 21:1194–1202
111. Russo C, Jin Z, Palmieri V et al (2012) Arterial stiffness and wave reflection: sex differences and relationship with left ventricular diastolic function. Hypertension 60:362–368
112. Avolio AP, Van Bortel LM, Boutouyrie P et al (2009) Role of pulse pressure amplification in arterial hypertension: experts' opinion and review of the data. Hypertension 54:375–383

113. O'Rourke MF (1970) Influence of ventricular ejection on the relationship between central aortic and brachial pressure pulse in man. Cardiovasc Res 4:291–300
114. Sugawara J, Hayashi K, Yokoi T, Tanaka H (2008) Age-associated elongation of the ascending aorta in adults. JACC Cardiovasc Imaging 1:739–748
115. Miyashita H (2012) Clinical assessment of central blood pressure. Curr Hypertens Rev 8:80–90
116. Segers P, Mahieu D, Rietzschel E et al (2009) Amplification of the pressure pulse in the upper limb in healthy, middle-aged men and women. Hypertension 54:414–420
117. Wojciechowska W, Stolarz-Skrzypek K, Tikhonoff V, European Project On Genes In Hypertension (Epogh) Investigators et al (2012) Age dependency of central and peripheral systolic blood pressures: cross-sectional and longitudinal observations in European populations. Blood Press 21:58–68
118. Roman MJ, Devereux RB, Kizer JR et al (2007) Central pressure more strongly relates to vascular disease and outcome than does brachial pressure: the Strong Heart Study. Hypertension 50:197–203
119. Roman MJ, Devereux RB, Kizer JR et al (2009) High central pulse pressure is independently associated with adverse cardiovascular outcome the strong heart study. J Am Coll Cardiol 54:1730–1734
120. Pini R, Cavallini MC, Palmieri V et al (2008) Central but not brachial blood pressure predicts cardiovascular events in an unselected geriatric population: the ICARe Dicomano Study. J Am Coll Cardiol 51:2432–2439
121. Wang KL, Cheng HM, Sung SH et al (2010) Wave reflection and arterial stiffness in the prediction of 15-year all-cause and cardiovascular mortalities: a community-based study. Hypertension 55:799–805
122. Bortolotto LA, Hanon O, Franconi G et al (1999) The aging process modifies the distensibility of elastic but not muscular arteries. Hypertension 34:889–892
123. McEniery CM, Yasmin, Hall IR, ACCT Investigators et al (2005) Normal vascular aging: differential effects on wave reflection and aortic pulse wave velocity: the Anglo-Cardiff Collaborative Trial (ACCT). J Am Coll Cardiol 46:1753–1760
124. McEniery CM, Wilkinson IB, Avolio AP (2007) Age, hypertension and arterial function. Clin Exp Pharmacol Physiol 34:665–671
125. Choi CU, Kim EJ, Kim SH et al (2010) Differing effects of aging on central and peripheral blood pressures and pulse wave velocity: a direct intra- arterial study. J Hypertens 28:1252–1260
126. Wilkinson IB, Franklin SS, Hall IR et al (2001) Pressure amplification explains why pulse pressure is unrelated to risk in young subjects. Hypertension 38:1461–1466
127. Bia D, Zócalo Y, Farro I et al (2011) Integrated evaluation of age-related changes in structural and functional vascular parameters used to assess arterial aging, subclinical atherosclerosis, and cardiovascular risk in Uruguayan adults: CUiiDARTE Project. Int J Hypertens 2011:587303
128. Wykretowicz A, Rutkowska A, Krauze T et al (2012) Pulse pressure amplification in relation to body fatness. Br J Clin Pharmacol 73:546–552
129. McEniery CM, Yasmin, McDonnell B, Anglo-Cardiff Collaborative Trial Investigators et al (2008) Central pressure: variability and impact of cardiovascular risk factors: the Anglo-Cardiff Collaborative Trial II. Hypertension 51:1476–1482
130. Nijdam ME, Platinga Y, Hulsen HT et al (2008) Pulse pressure amplification and risk of cardiovascular disease. Am J Hypertens 21:388–392
131. Hashimoto J, Imai Y, O'Rourke MF (2007) Indices of pulse wave analysis are better predictors of left ventricular mass reduction than cuff pressure. Am J Hypertens 20:378–384
132. Benetos A, Gautier S, Labat C et al (2012) Mortality and cardiovascular events are best predicted by low central/peripheral pulse pressure amplification but not by high blood pressure levels in elderly nursing home subjects: the PARTAGE (Predictive Values of Blood Pressure and Arterial Stiffness in Institutionalized Very Aged Population) Study. J Am Coll Cardiol 60:1503–1511

133. Benetos A, Thomas F, Joly L et al (2010) Pulse pressure amplification a mechanical bio-marker of cardiovascular risk. J Am Coll Cardiol 55:1032–1037
134. Heffernan KS, Fahs CA, Iwamoto GA et al (2009) Resistance exercise training reduces central blood pressure and improves microvascular function in African American and white men. Atherosclerosis 207:220–226
135. Regnault V, Thomas F, Safar ME et al (2012) Sex difference in cardiovascular risk: role of pulse pressure amplification. J Am Coll Cardiol 59:1771–1777
136. Cecelja M, Jiang B, McNeill K et al (2009) Increased wave reflection rather than central arterial stiffness is the main determinant of raised pulse pressure in women and relates to mismatch in arterial dimensions: a twin study. J Am Coll Cardiol 54:695–703
137. Salvi P, Safar ME, Labat C et al (2010) Heart disease and changes in pulse wave velocity and pulse pressure amplification in the elderly over 80 years: the PARTAGE Study. J Hypertens 28:2127–2133
138. Hulsen HT, Nijdam ME, Bos WJ et al (2006) Spurious systolic hypertension in young adults; prevalence of high brachial systolic blood pressure and low central pressure and its determinants. J Hypertens 24:1027–1032
139. Mahmud A, Feely J (2003) Spurious systolic hypertension of youth: fit young men with elastic arteries. Am J Hypertens 16:229–232
140. O'Rourke MF, Vlachopoulos C, Graham RM (2000) Spurious systolic hypertension in youth. Vasc Med 5:141–145
141. Laurent P, Albaladejo P, Blacher J et al (2003) Heart rate and pulse pressure amplification in hypertensive subjects. Am J Hypertens 16:363–370
142. Wilkinson IB, Mohammad NH, Tyrrell S et al (2002) Heart rate dependency of pulse pressure amplification and arterial stiffness. Am J Hypertens 15:24–30
143. Mackenzie IS, McEniery CM, Dhakam Z et al (2009) Comparison of the effects of antihypertensive agents on central blood pressure and arterial stiffness in isolated systolic hypertension. Hypertension 54:409–413
144. Manisty CH, Hughes AD (2013) Meta-analysis of the comparative effects of different classes of antihypertensive agents on brachial and central systolic blood pressure, and augmentation index. Br J Clin Pharmacol 75:79–92
145. Laurent P, Marenco P, Castagna O et al (2011) Differences in central systolic blood pressure and aortic stiffness between aerobically trained and sedentary individuals. J Am Soc Hypertens 5:85–93
146. Adji A, Hirata K, Hoegler S, O'Rourke MF (2007) Noninvasive pulse waveform analysis in clinical trials: similarity of two methods for calculating aortic systolic pressure. Am J Hypertens 20:917–922
147. Westerhof BE, Guelen I, Westerhof N et al (2006) Quantification of wave reflection in the human aorta from pressure alone: a proof of principle. Hypertension 48:595–601
148. Nichols WW, Edwards DG (2001) Arterial elastance and wave reflection augmentation of systolic blood pressure: deleterious effects and implications for therapy. J Cardiovasc Pharmacol Ther 6:5–21
149. O'Rourke MF, Pauca AL (2004) Augmentation of the aortic and central arterial pressure waveform. Blood Press Monit 9:179–185
150. Segers P, Rietzschel ER, De Buyzere ML et al (2007) Noninvasive (input) impedance, pulse wave velocity, and wave reflection in healthy middle-aged men and women. Hypertension 49:1248–1255
151. Segers P, Verdonck P (2000) Role of tapering in aortic wave reflection: hydraulic and mathematical model study. J Biomech 33:299–306
152. Segers P, De Backer J, Devos D et al (2006) Aortic reflection coefficients and their association with global indexes of wave reflection in healthy controls and patients with Marfan's syndrome. Am J Physiol Heart Circ Physiol 290:H2385–H2392
153. Hirata K, Kawakami M, O'Rourke MF (2006) Pulse wave analysis and pulse wave velocity: a review of blood pressure interpretation 100 years after Korotkov. Circ J 70:1231–1239
154. Chirinos JA, Zambrano JP, Chakko S et al (2005) Relation between ascending aortic pressures and outcomes in patients with angiographically demonstrated coronary artery disease. Am J Cardiol 96:645–648

155. Chirinos JA, Zambrano JP, Chakko S et al (2005) Aortic pressure augmentation predicts adverse cardiovascular events in patients with established coronary artery disease. Hypertension 45:980–985
156. Frimodt-Møller M, Kamper AL, Strandgaard S et al (2012) Beneficial effects on arterial stiffness and pulse-wave reflection of combined enalapril and candesartan in chronic kidney disease–a randomized trial. PLoS One 7:e41757
157. Weber T, Auer J, O'Rourke MF et al (2004) Arterial stiffness, wave reflections, and the risk of coronary artery disease. Circulation 109:184–189
158. Nichols WW (2005) Clinical measurement of arterial stiffness obtained from noninvasive pressure waveforms. Am J Hypertens 18:3S–10S
159. Martin JS, Casey DP, Gurovich AN et al (2011) Association of age with timing and amplitude of reflected pressure waves during exercise in men. Am J Hypertens 24:415–420
160. Casey DP, Beck DT, Nichols WW et al (2011) Effects of enhanced external counterpulsation on arterial stiffness and myocardial oxygen demand in patients with chronic angina pectoris. Am J Cardiol 107:1466–1472
161. Ghiadoni L, Bruno RM, Stea F et al (2009) Central blood pressure, arterial stiffness, and wave reflection: new targets of treatment in essential hypertension. Curr Hypertens Rep 11:190–196
162. O'Rourke MF, Adji A, Namasivayam M, Mok J (2011) Arterial aging: a review of the pathophysiology and potential for pharmacological intervention. Drugs Aging 28:779–795
163. Agabiti-Rosei E, Mancia G, O'Rourke MF et al (2007) Central blood pressure measurements and antihypertensive therapy: a consensus document. Hypertension 50:154–160
164. Namasivayam M, McDonnell BJ, McEniery CM, O'Rourke MF, Anglo-Cardiff Collaborative Trial Study Investigators (2009) Does wave reflection dominate age-related change in aortic blood pressure across the human life span? Hypertension 53:979–985
165. Nelson MR, Stepanek J, Cevette M et al (2010) Noninvasive measurement of central vascular pressures with arterial tonometry: clinical revival of the pulse pressure waveform? Mayo Clin Proc 85:460–472
166. Nunan D, Wassertheurer S, Lasserson D et al (2012) Assessment of central haemodynamics from a brachial cuff in a community setting. BMC Cardiovasc Disord 12:48. doi:10.1186/1471-2261-12-48
167. Lakatta EG, Levy D (2003) Arterial and cardiac aging: major shareholders in cardiovascular disease enterprises: Part II: the aging heart in health: links to heart disease. Circulation 107:346–354
168. Mitchell GF, Parise H, Benjamin EJ et al (2004) Changes in arterial stiffness and wave reflection with advancing age in healthy men and women: the Framingham Heart Study. Hypertension 43:1239–1245
169. Lakatta EG, Levy D (2003) Arterial and cardiac aging: major shareholders in cardiovascular disease enterprises: Part I: aging arteries: a "set up" for vascular disease. Circulation 107:139–146
170. Safar ME (2008) Pulse pressure, arterial stiffness and wave reflections (augmentation index) as cardiovascular risk factors in hypertension. Ther Adv Cardiovasc Dis 2:13–24
171. Gould KL, Kirkeeide RL, Buchi M (1990) Coronary flow reserve as a physiologic measure of stenosis severity. J Am Coll Cardiol 15:459–474
172. Gan LM, Wikström J, Fritsche-Danielson R (2013) Coronary flow reserve from mouse to man–from mechanistic understanding to future interventions. J Cardiovasc Transl Res 6:715–728
173. Westerhof N, Boer C, Lamberts RR, Sipkema P (2006) Cross-talk between cardiac muscle and coronary vasculature. Physiol Rev 86:1263–1308
174. Hoffman JI (1987) A critical view of coronary reserve. Circulation 75(Suppl 1):I6–I11
175. Hoffman JI (1984) Maximal coronary flow and the concept of coronary vascular reserve. Circulation 70:153–159
176. Klocke FJ (1987) Measurements of coronary flow reserve: defining pathophysiology versus making decisions about patient care. Circulation 76:1183–1189

177. Knaapen P, Camici PG, Marques KM et al (2009) Coronary microvascular resistance: methods for its quantification in humans. Basic Res Cardiol 104:485–498
178. Gould KL, Lipscomb K, Hamilton GW (1974) Physiologic basis for assessing critical coronary stenosis. Instantaneous flow response and regional distribution during coronary hyperemia as measures of coronary flow reserve. Am J Cardiol 33:87–94
179. Feldman RL, Nichols WW, Pepine CJ, Conti CR (1979) Influence of aortic insufficiency on the hemodynamic significance of a coronary artery narrowing. Circulation 60:259–268
180. Feldman RL, Nichols WW, Pepine CJ, Conti CR (1978) Hemodynamic significance of the length of a coronary arterial narrowing. Am J Cardiol 41:865–871
181. Pauly DF, Johnson BD, Anderson RD et al (2011) In women with symptoms of cardiac ischemia, non-obstructive coronary arteries, and microvascular dysfunction, angiotensin-converting enzyme inhibition is associated with improved microvascular function: a double-blind randomized study from the National Heart, Lung and Blood Institute Women's Ischemia Syndrome Evaluation (WISE). Am Heart J 162:678–684
182. Leung MC, Meredith IT, Cameron JD (2006) Aortic stiffness affects the coronary blood flow response to percutaneous coronary intervention. Am J Physiol Heart Circ Physiol 290: H624–H630
183. Ikonomidis I, Lekakis J, Papadopoulos C et al (2008) Incremental value of pulse wave velocity in the determination of coronary microcirculatory dysfunction in never-treated patients with essential hypertension. Am J Hypertens 21:806–813
184. Nemes A, Forster T, Csanády M (2007) Reduction of coronary flow reserve in patients with increased aortic stiffness. Can J Physiol Pharmacol 85:818–822
185. Dimitrow PP, Galderisi M, Rigo F (2005) The non-invasive documentation of coronary microcirculation impairment: role of transthoracic echocardiography. Cardiovasc Ultrasound 3:18
186. Camici PG, Crea F (2007) Coronary microvascular dysfunction. N Engl J Med 356: 830–840
187. Crea F, Camici PG, Bairey Merz CN (2014) Coronary microvascular dysfunction: an update. Eur Heart J 35:1101–1111
188. Beyer AM, Gutterman DD (2012) Regulation of the human coronary microcirculation. J Mol Cell Cardiol 52:814–821
189. O'Gorman DJ, Thomas P, Turner MA, Sheridan DJ (1992) Investigation of impaired coronary vasodilator reserve in the guinea pig heart with pressure induced hypertrophy. Eur Heart J 13:697–703
190. Gosse P, Clementy J (1995) Coronary reserve in experimental myocardial hypertrophy. Eur Heart J 16(Suppl I):22–25
191. O'Rourke MF (2008) How stiffening of the aorta and elastic arteries leads to compromised coronary flow. Heart 94:690–691
192. Franklin SS, Gustin W 4th, Wong ND et al (1997) Hemodynamic patterns of age-related changes in blood pressure. The Framingham Heart Study. Circulation 96:308–315
193. Franklin SS, Chow VH, Mori AD, Wong ND (2011) The significance of low DBP in US adults with isolated systolic hypertension. J Hypertens 29:1101–1118
194. Morita S, Asou T, Kuboyama I et al (2002) Inelastic vascular prosthesis for proximal aorta increases pulsatile arterial load and causes left ventricular hypertrophy in dogs. J Thorac Cardiovasc Surg 124:768–774
195. Watanabe H, Ohtsuka S, Kakihana M, Sugishita Y (1993) Coronary circulation in dogs with an experimental decrease in aortic compliance. J Am Coll Cardiol 21:1497–1506
196. Ohtsuka S, Kakihana M, Watanabe H, Sugishita Y (1994) Chronically decreased aortic distensibility causes deterioration of coronary perfusion during increased left ventricular contraction. J Am Coll Cardiol 24:1406–1414
197. Kass DA, Saeki A, Tunin RS, Recchia FA (1996) Adverse influence of systemic vascular stiffening on cardiac dysfunction and adaptation to acute coronary occlusion. Circulation 93:1533–1541
198. Hachamovitch R, Wicker P, Capasso JM, Anversa P (1989) Alterations of coronary blood flow and reserve with aging in Fischer 344 rats. Am J Physiol 256:H66–H73

199. Czernin J, Müller P, Chan S et al (1993) Influence of age and hemodynamics on myocardial blood flow and flow reserve. Circulation 88:62–69
200. Beckett NS, Peters R, Fletcher AE, HYVET Study Group et al (2008) Treatment of hypertension in patients 80 years of age or older. N Engl J Med 358:1887–1898
201. Cruickshank JM (1988) Coronary flow reserve and the J curve relation between diastolic blood pressure and myocardial infarction. BMJ 297:1227–1230
202. Fukuda D, Yoshiyama M, Shimada K et al (2006) Relation between aortic stiffness and coronary flow reserve in patients with coronary artery disease. Heart 92:759–762
203. Sarnoff SJ, Braunwald E, Welch GR Jr et al (1958) Hemodynamic determinants of oxygen consumption of the heart with special reference to the tension-time index. Am J Physiol 192:148–156
204. Ferro G, Duilio C, Spinelli L et al (1995) Relation between diastolic perfusion time and coronary artery stenosis during stress-induced myocardial ischemia. Circulation 92:342–347
205. Al Suwaidi J, Higano ST, Holmes DR Jr et al (2001) Obesity is independently associated with coronary endothelial dysfunction in patients with normal or mildly diseased coronary arteries. J Am Coll Cardiol 37:1523–1528
206. Johnson BD, Shaw LJ, Pepine CJ et al (2006) Persistent chest pain predicts cardiovascular events in women without obstructive coronary artery disease: results from the NIH-NHLBI-sponsored Women's Ischaemia Syndrome Evaluation (WISE) study. Eur Heart J 27:1408–1415
207. Banks K, Puttagunta D, Murphy S et al (2011) Clinical characteristics, vascular function, and inflammation in women with angina in the absence of coronary atherosclerosis: the Dallas Heart Study. JACC Cardiovasc Imaging 4:65–73
208. Ishibashi K, Osamura T, Yamahara Y (2009) Myocardial stunning with partial aneurysmal formation generated during the recovering process of tachycardia-induced cardiomyopathy. J Cardiol 54:121–127
209. Wu MS, Chang CY, Chang RW, Chang KC (2012) Early return of augmented wave reflection impairs left ventricular relaxation in aged Fisher 344 rats. Exp Gerontol 47:680–686
210. Tsiachris D, Tsioufis C, Syrseloudis D et al (2012) Subendocardial viability ratio as an index of impaired coronary flow reserve in hypertensives without significant coronary artery stenoses. J Hum Hypertens 26:64–70
211. Cannon RO 3rd (2009) Microvascular angina and the continuing dilemma of chest pain with normal coronary angiograms. J Am Coll Cardiol 54:877–885
212. Reis SE, Holubkov R, Conrad Smith AJ, WISE Investigators et al (2001) Coronary microvascular dysfunction is highly prevalent in women with chest pain in the absence of coronary artery disease: results from the NHLBI WISE study. Am Heart J 141:735–741
213. Nichols WW, Denardo SJ, Johnson BD et al (2013) Increased wave reflection and ejection duration in women with chest pain and nonobstructive coronary artery disease: ancillary study from the Women's Ischemia Syndrome Evaluation. J Hypertens 31:1447–1454

Part II

Classification and Clinical Manifestations of Arterial Disease

Atherosclerosis

3

Michael Hristov and Christian Weber

Atherosclerosis as an enduring inflammatory disease of the arterial wall is characterised by an imbalanced lipid metabolism and a maladaptive immune response resulting in sub-endothelial lipoprotein retention and endothelial activation with migration of immune and smooth muscle cells to the inflamed intima. This leads to formation of atheromas with chronic vascular stenosis and tissue ischemia which is often complicated by acute atherothrombotic events such as myocardial infarction or stroke. Even today, atherosclerosis and its consequences remain the leading causes of mortality and morbidity in the industrialised nations.

3.1 Traditional Risk Factors and Pathogenesis of Plaque Formation

Atherosclerotic lesions develop preferentially in vascular segments with slowed or disturbed blood flow, e.g. arterial bifurcations and branching sites. This arterial environment in combination with traditional risk factors such as hypertension, smoking and diabetes or other pathogens (immune complexes, toxins, viruses, etc.) may favour non-denuding endothelial dysfunction or even denuding injury with exposure of matrix proteoglycans and platelet activation. Accordingly, this so-called "response-to-injury" hypothesis has provided a fundamental framework in the pathogenesis of atherosclerosis to address numerous questions about cellular interactions and the nature of inflammatory mediators they produce [1].

M. Hristov • C. Weber (✉)
Department of Vascular Medicine, Institute for Cardiovascular Prevention,
Ludwig-Maximilians-University (LMU), Pettenkoferstr. 9, Munich 80336, Germany
e-mail: michael.hristov@med.uni-muenchen.de; christian.weber@med.uni-muenchen.de

© Springer International Publishing Switzerland 2015
A. Berbari, G. Mancia (eds.), *Arterial Disorders:*
Definition, Clinical Manifestations, Mechanisms and Therapeutic Approaches,
DOI 10.1007/978-3-319-14556-3_3

Early atherosclerotic lesions (known as *fatty streaks*) do not affect the vascular lumen and consist predominantly of focal lipid deposition, T lymphocytes and monocytes that transform to macrophages and lipid-loaded foam cells [1–4]. Indeed, almost each leukocyte sub-population ranging from lymphocytes, monocytes and neutrophils to dendritic or mast cells can be found at varying numbers inside the lesion during different stages [4]. Epidemiological data have further acknowledged leukocytosis as independent risk factor and predictor of cardiovascular events [5].

The continuous cell infiltration, proliferation and necrosis with accumulation of cell debris and cholesterol crystals result in lesion growth, and the *fatty streaks* transform gradually into stenotic plaques. These fibrous plaques contain an acellular necrotic core that is covered by a fibrous cap of dense connective tissue consisting of collagen, intimal smooth muscle cells (SMCs) and macrophages [1–3]. The "shoulder" regions of the plaques are often infiltrated by T lymphocytes and mast cells, which release proteolytic enzymes and proinflammatory mediators that may facilitate plaque destabilisation [3, 6]. Moreover, because of increasing plaque volume, the overlaying endothelial monolayer may be stretched quite thin and becomes more permeable or can even rupture.

Advanced stable fibroatheromas are covered by a dense, tension-resistant fibrous cap and contain few inflammatory cells [6, 7]. These plaques typically associate with chronic tissue ischemia that can be partially compensated by the growth of collateral vessels. In contrast, vulnerable plaques have a thin fibrous cap with more inflammatory cells than SMCs next to relative large and "soft" necrotic core. These plaques are more prone to erosion or rupture with subsequent occlusive atherothrombotic complications.

Dyslipidaemia with elevated circulating low-density lipoprotein (LDL) levels is another cardinal risk factor for the development and progression of atherosclerotic plaques. Due to increased endothelial permeability at predilection sites, LDL is easily embedded in the sub-endothelial space [2]. A variety of biochemical modifications occur there and enhance its pro-atherogenic action [2, 8]. Most important is the oxidation of LDL by reactive oxygen species or enzymes such as myeloperoxidase or lipoxygenases released from surrounding inflammatory cells [3]. Products of oxidised LDL (oxLDL) are chemotactic for monocytes but cytotoxic to endothelial cells. OxLDL is taken up at enhanced rates by macrophages, thus contributing to foam cell formation. Moreover, oxLDL can inhibit macrophage egress from the lesion but induce expression of adhesion molecules or deposition of chemokines on activated endothelial cells which further accelerates the recruitment of leukocytes. This accelerated leukocyte recruitment in conjunction with insufficient egress drives a continuous, oxLDL-mediated cell overload and lesion growth.

To complement the above traditional risk factors, a search for genetic variants linked with coronary artery disease (CAD) has flourished. Several genome-wide association studies (GWASs) have created an enormous wealth of data on susceptibility loci. The characterisation of these CAD-associated loci (9p21.3, 10q11.21, etc.) should provide new insight in the molecular mechanisms driving atherosclerosis and its outcomes and should open new fields for cardiovascular research [9].

3.2 Inflammatory Mediators in Atherogenic Cell Recruitment

Atherogenic recruitment of leukocytes involves rolling, firm adhesion, migration and trans-endothelial diapedesis [10]. This sequential cascade is controlled by chemokines, which are chemotactic cytokines divided into four groups according to their conserved cysteines and corresponding G protein-coupled receptors: C, CC, CXC and CX_3C [11, 12]. Considering the diversity of various leukocytes recruited during the atherogenic process, the abundance in the chemokine system has been perceived to confer robustness and specificity [13]. At a site of inflammation, particular leukocyte subsets may be recruited by a signature combination of chemokines engaging in heterophilic interactions, facilitated by a local repertoire of proteoglycans with differential binding affinities for these chemokines [4, 12, 13]. Soluble chemokines mediate direct leukocyte recruitment while surface-immobilised chemokines on activated endothelial cells trigger leukocyte arrest and activation of integrins. Numerous studies using antagonists or gene-deficient mice for important chemokines and/or their respective receptors have generated valuable insights into receptor-ligand axes with specific and combined contributions to atherogenesis [12]. Some of these crucial axes are CCR2-CCL2 (also known as monocyte chemotactic protein-1) and CCR5-CCL5 (also known as RANTES). Other chemokines and receptors appear rather involved in cell homeostasis and associate with reduced atheroprogression and plaque stabilisation, e.g. CXCL12 (also known as stromal cell-derived factor-1) and CXCR4/CXCR7, CX_3CL1 (also known as fractalkine) and CX_3CR1 or the dendritic cell chemokine CCL17 [12–14]. Finally, the combined action of chemokines such as the CCL5-CXCL4 (also known as platelet factor-4) heteromer can result in synergistic effects during atherogenic leukocyte recruitment [15].

Advanced human atherosclerotic lesions show an up-regulation of macrophage migration inhibitory factor (MIF) in macrophages and endothelial cells, which express MIF also in response to oxLDL [16]. Multiple mouse studies have confirmed the atheroprogressive function of MIF, which is probably linked to its versatile proinflammatory properties at crucial checkpoints in atherogenesis [3]. Macrophages can secret further proinflammatory mediators with implication in atherogenesis such as interleukin-1-beta (IL-1β) and tumour necrosis factor-alpha (TNF-α) [2, 6]. They are another robust source of platelet-derived growth factor (PDGF), which is one of the more important candidates coordinating the proliferative response of intimal SMCs [17].

Type I interferons (IFNs) have been implicated in atherogenesis as other important myeloid effector cytokines. Hence, treatment of atherosclerosis-prone mice with IFN-β increases lesion size, macrophage content and CCL5 plasma levels, whereas myeloid deficiency of the receptor for type I IFNs (IFNAR1) was associated with stable plaques [18]. Signalling through IFN-β-IFNAR1 interaction triggers CCL5 production by macrophages, thus increasing the CCR5-mediated monocyte recruitment [18]. This explains a correlation between up-regulated type I IFN signalling and CCL5 expression in advanced human lesions [3, 18].

Co-stimulatory and co-inhibitory signalling molecules fine-tune immune reactions by regulating inflammatory phenotypes and responses of T lymphocytes and antigen-presenting cells. For the prominent co-stimulatory pair CD40-CD40L, both receptor and ligand are expressed by lesional cell types and highly up-regulated in advanced human plaques [3, 19]. Mouse studies have revealed a plaque-destabilising function for CD40-CD40L signalling, attributable to the induction of multiple inflammatory factors [19]. Notably, repeated injection of CD40L-deficient platelets specifically implicated platelet CD40L in atherogenesis by mediating proinflammatory leukocyte-platelet interactions and regulatory T-cell homeostasis without compromising systemic immune responses or inducing haemorrhage [20].

3.3   The Role of Scavenger and Toll-Like Receptors (TLRs)

Although the major uptake of modified LDL in macrophages is mediated by scavenger receptor A (SR-A) and CD36, the genetic deletion of these receptors has yielded varying effects on experimental atherosclerosis [3, 21]. Combined deficiency of SR-A and CD36 in *Apoe−/−* mice has implicated both receptors in athero-progression by inducing proinflammatory gene expression and macrophage apoptosis rather than foam cell formation [22]. TLR4 and TLR6 cooperate with CD36 in this inflammatory response to atherogenic lipids: oxLDL sequestered by CD36 induces intracellular CD36-TLR4-TLR6 heteromerisation, thus activating the transcription factor NF-κB and the secretion of chemokines [23]. Accordingly, a sustained oxidative burst and apoptosis elicited by oxLDL with continuous stress of the endoplasmic reticulum through combined signalling of CD36 with TLR2-TLR6 may similarly occur in lesional macrophages with intracellular accumulation of free cholesterol [24, 25].

3.4   Activated Platelets

Chronic inflammation associates with elevated platelet counts and platelet activation. Similar to leukocytosis, the thrombocytosis has been considered as risk factor for atherosclerosis. Platelets are activated by shear flow, oxLDL or hyperglycaemia. Upon activation they release membrane microparticles next to a broad arsenal of soluble components with relevance not only to coagulation and wound healing but also to immune response [26, 27]. The intravenous injection of activated platelets leads to a rapid progression of atherosclerotic lesions in mouse models that can be explained by a transfer of inflammatory chemokines such as CXCL4 and CCL5 [28]. As mentioned above, both chemokines may form a heteromer with synergistic effect on monocyte recruitment [15]. Disrupting this interaction by a designed synthetic peptide in vivo resulted in decreased atherosclerotic lesion formation, and the genetic deficiency of CCL5 and CXCL4 has been found to reduce plaque formation in mice [15]. Furthermore, the P-selectin-mediated adhesion of platelets to monocytes under coronary flow conditions results in circulating complexes with increased adhesion to endothelial cells and immigration into the arterial wall [29]. These monocyte-platelet aggregates are increased in patients with CAD end especially after myocardial infarction [30].

3.5   Concluding Remarks and Perspectives for Prevention and Therapy

The currently available non-invasive therapy against atherosclerosis and especially CAD is usually restricted to controlling body weight, blood pressure, glycaemia, LDL cholesterol and triglyceride levels as well as platelet aggregation to prevent advanced thrombotic complications. Patients but also healthy individuals are further encouraged to follow general lifestyle recommendations including physical activity, smoking cessation and balanced diet. So far, the positive dietary effects of cold-water oily fish, red wine and olive oil consumption on CAD have been well documented [31, 32].

However, these established strategies do not fully address the inflammatory and immune mechanisms driving atheroprogression. Thus, emerging and future concepts in the treatment of atherosclerosis are urgently required. In this regard, several lessons from experimental animal models could help to develop novel, more powerful therapeutics such as inhibitors of chemokine heteromerisation, receptor antagonists, artificial lipoprotein complexes or even vaccination [13, 33–35]. Such a pioneering drug development requires stringent evaluation of effectiveness which has to rely on surrogate markers. Although a variety of cellular, soluble, imaging or functional biomarkers are available, their predictability remains partially limited. Hence, new biomarkers should be developed to complement existing ones and multiple biomarker panels should be combined in an integrated approach with higher predictive potential. Associated GWASs and transcriptional, proteomic or metabolic profiling may facilitate this search.

Moreover, there is an urgent need for improved imaging techniques, as current modalities (intravascular ultrasound, carotid intima-media thickness, quantitative coronary angiography and computed tomography) are often invasive and provide only quantitative but incomplete morphological data of atherosclerotic lesions. As cellular and molecular composition better reflects plaque pathology compared to size, highly advanced imaging techniques, such as high-resolution magnetic resonance and positron-emission tomography, will be required. The development of new molecular imaging with specific biological functions could add another dimension to plaque imaging, including monitoring the activation of endothelial cells and macrophages. If successful, this will be of tremendous value for drug development and testing efficacy, allowing detailed mechanistic insights into therapeutic effects at early stages, as well as imaging-based clinical outcome studies.

References

1. Ross R (1999) Atherosclerosis-an inflammatory disease. N Engl J Med 340:115–126
2. Hansson GK (2005) Inflammation, atherosclerosis, and coronary artery disease. N Engl J Med 352:1685–1695
3. Weber C, Noels H (2011) Atherosclerosis: current pathogenesis and therapeutic options. Nat Med 17:1410–1422
4. Weber C, Zernecke A, Libby P (2008) The multifaceted contributions of leukocyte subsets to atherosclerosis: lessons from mouse models. Nat Rev Immunol 8:802–815
5. Madjid M, Awan I, Willerson JT et al (2004) Leukocyte count and coronary heart disease: implications for risk assessment. J Am Coll Cardiol 44:1945–1956
6. Hansson GK, Libby P (2006) The immune response in atherosclerosis: a double-edged sword. Nat Rev Immunol 6:508–519
7. Libby P, Aikawa M (2002) Stabilization of atherosclerotic plaques: new mechanisms and clinical targets. Nat Med 8:1257–1262
8. Witztum JL, Berliner JA (1998) Oxidized phospholipids and isoprostanes in atherosclerosis. Curr Opin Lipidol 9:441–448
9. Schunkert H, König IR, Kathiresan S et al (2011) Large-scale association analysis identifies 13 new susceptibility loci for coronary artery disease. Nat Genet 43:333–338
10. Weber C, Fraemohs L, Dejana E (2007) The role of junctional adhesion molecules in vascular inflammation. Nat Rev Immunol 7:467–477
11. Luster AD (1998) Chemokines–chemotactic cytokines that mediate inflammation. N Engl J Med 338:436–445
12. Zernecke A, Weber C (2014) Chemokines in atherosclerosis: proceedings resumed. Arterioscler Thromb Vasc Biol 34:742–750
13. Koenen RR, Weber C (2010) Therapeutic targeting of chemokine interactions in atherosclerosis. Nat Rev Drug Discov 9:141–153
14. Weber C, Meiler S, Döring Y et al (2011) CCL17-expressing dendritic cells drive atherosclerosis by restraining regulatory T cell homeostasis in mice. J Clin Invest 121:2898–2910
15. Koenen RR, von Hundelshausen P, Nesmelova IV et al (2009) Disrupting functional interactions between platelet chemokines inhibits atherosclerosis in hyperlipidemic mice. Nat Med 15:97–103
16. Bernhagen J, Krohn R, Lue H et al (2007) MIF is a noncognate ligand of CXC chemokine receptors in inflammatory and atherogenic cell recruitment. Nat Med 13:587–596
17. Doran AC, Meller N, McNamara CA (2008) Role of smooth muscle cells in the initiation and early progression of atherosclerosis. Arterioscler Thromb Vasc Biol 28:812–819
18. Goossens P, Gijbels MJ, Zernecke A et al (2010) Myeloid type I interferon signaling promotes atherosclerosis by stimulating macrophage recruitment to lesions. Cell Metab 12:142–153
19. Lievens D, Eijgelaar WJ, Biessen EA et al (2009) The multi-functionality of CD40L and its receptor CD40 in atherosclerosis. Thromb Haemost 102:206–214
20. Lievens D, Zernecke A, Seijkens T et al (2010) Platelet CD40L mediates thrombotic and inflammatory processes in atherosclerosis. Blood 116:4317–4327
21. Greaves DR, Gordon S (2009) The macrophage scavenger receptor at 30 years of age: current knowledge and future challenges. J Lipid Res 50:S282–S286
22. Manning-Tobin JJ, Moore KJ, Seimon TA et al (2009) Loss of SR-A and CD36 activity reduces atherosclerotic lesion complexity without abrogating foam cell formation in hyperlipidemic mice. Arterioscler Thromb Vasc Biol 29:19–26
23. Stewart CR, Stuart LM, Wilkinson K et al (2010) CD36 ligands promote sterile inflammation through assembly of a Toll-like receptor 4 and 6 heterodimer. Nat Immunol 11:155–161
24. Seimon TA, Nadolski MJ, Liao X et al (2010) Atherogenic lipids and lipoproteins trigger CD36-TLR2-dependent apoptosis in macrophages undergoing endoplasmic reticulum stress. Cell Metab 12:467–482

25. Tabas I (2010) Macrophage death and defective inflammation resolution in atherosclerosis. Nat Rev Immunol 10:36–46
26. Weber C (2005) Platelets and chemokines in atherosclerosis: partners in crime. Circ Res 96:612–616
27. von Hundelshausen P, Weber C (2007) Platelets as immune cells: bridging inflammation and cardiovascular disease. Circ Res 100:27–40
28. Huo Y, Schober A, Forlow SB et al (2003) Circulating activated platelets exacerbate atherosclerosis in mice deficient in apolipoprotein E. Nat Med 9:61–67
29. Freedman JE, Loscalzo J (2002) Platelet-monocyte aggregates: bridging thrombosis and inflammation. Circulation 105:2130–2132
30. Tapp LD, Shantsila E, Wrigley BJ et al (2012) The CD14++CD16+ monocyte subset and monocyte-platelet interactions in patients with ST-elevation myocardial infarction. J Thromb Haemost 10:1231–1241
31. Saravanan P, Davidson NC, Schmidt EB et al (2010) Cardiovascular effects of marine omega-3 fatty acids. Lancet 376:540–550
32. Hernáez Á, Fernández-Castillejo S, Farràs M et al (2014) Olive oil polyphenols enhance high-density lipoprotein function in humans: a randomized controlled trial. Arterioscler Thromb Vasc Biol 34:2115–2119
33. Zhao Q (2010) Dual targeting of CCR2 and CCR5: therapeutic potential for immunologic and cardiovascular diseases. J Leukoc Biol 88:41–55
34. Nissen SE, Tsunoda T, Tuzcu EM et al (2003) Effect of recombinant ApoA-I Milano on coronary atherosclerosis in patients with acute coronary syndromes: a randomized controlled trial. JAMA 290:2292–2300
35. Nilsson J, Hansson GK, Shah PK (2005) Immunomodulation of atherosclerosis: implications for vaccine development. Arterioscler Thromb Vasc Biol 25:18–28

Arteriosclerosis/Large Artery Disease

4

Michael F. O'Rourke

To a student of medical history, it is fascinating to reflect on how careful our predecessors were in classification of diseases and how lazy and careless we have become. In recent times, all forms of arterial disease are generally considered to cause ill effects through narrowing and restriction of blood flow. All such disease is considered to be a form of atherosclerosis. The effects of arterial stiffening are usually set aside and overlooked or forgotten. Coronary artery disease is synonymous with coronary atherosclerosis. The AHA Journal Arteriosclerosis was renamed Arteriosclerosis, Thrombosis, and Vascular Biology (ATVB). The journal Atherosclerosis has retained its name but both it and ATVB now carry the same type of content.

The late nineteenth-century physicians were more careful in their terminology. William Osler's textbook *Principles and Practice of Medicine* [1] (first published in 1892) had great influence. After Councilman, Osler described three types of arteriosclerosis, on the basis of pathology. The first – nodular arteriosclerosis – corresponds to what we call atherosclerosis today. The second – diffuse arteriosclerosis – was predominantly a medial disease in young to middle-aged adults and probably corresponds to the arterial consequences of chronic severe hypertension, a condition which was untreatable in 1900 but rarely encountered today, whereas senile arteriosclerosis was the condition seen in elderly persons where the aorta and large arteries were dilated with thickened stiff walls and with disorganisation of the orderly arrangement of elastin in the arterial media. "Elderly" in Osler's day probably meant over 60 (an age that became particularly significant in the controversy following publication of his essay on "the Fixed Period" [2]). In modern times, a far greater proportion of the population lives to well over 60 years, so that one would expect senile arteriosclerosis to be far more common than in 1890–1920. Yet "senile

M.F. O'Rourke
Department of Cardiology, Victor Chang Cardiac Research Institute, St Vincent's
Hospital, University of New South Wales, Victoria Street, Sydney, NSW 2010, Australia
e-mail: m.orourke@unsw.edu.au

© Springer International Publishing Switzerland 2015
A. Berbari, G. Mancia (eds.), *Arterial Disorders:*
Definition, Clinical Manifestations, Mechanisms and Therapeutic Approaches,
DOI 10.1007/978-3-319-14556-3_4

arteriosclerosis" or "arteriosclerosis" is not listed in textbook indices or in subject titles for American Heart Association, American College of Cardiology or European Society of Cardiology meetings. The lonely lot of researchers offering abstracts for such meetings has to make do with "hypertension", which was referred to as high blood pressure in Osler's day and diagnosed from the radial artery pulse, as felt at the wrist or recorded by a sphygmogram.

Similar problems with terminology hinder communication between researchers and clinicians who are interested in Alzheimer's disease and how this condition is defined [3]. To many physicians and psychiatrists today, Alzheimer's disease is dementia which is not caused by vascular disease, i.e. "if it has a vascular cause, it is not Alzheimer's disease" [3]. It is instructive to read Alzheimer's first description of a case [4] in which severe dementia in an older man was not associated with any cerebral pathology at autopsy but was associated with arteriosclerosis. The views of Osler and Councilman were followed at the time (1907), and it is probable that Alzheimer's reference was to senile arteriosclerosis with stiffening and dilation of the thoracic aorta and with no particular abnormality of the intracranial or carotid arteries. Alzheimer's emphasis in describing this condition was absence of obvious abnormalities at autopsy to explain it [4].

I find myself to be part of the problem. Despite railing against imprecise wording in medicine [5], I find in the Index of our 6th edition of *McDonald's Blood Flow in Arteries* [6] the word "arteriosclerosis" to state succinctly "see atherosclerosis". In Osler's time, senile or physiological arteriosclerosis and high blood pressure were diagnosed on the basis of pulse wave contour – from high and prolonged pressure in late systole, "the tidal wave is prolonged and too much sustained" [7], and "the pulse (of high tension) is slow in its ascent, enduring, subsides slowly, and in the interval between the beats, the vessel remains full and firm" [8]. Osler emphasised that the (radial) "pulse of high tension" is similar to the pulse in arteriosclerosis but that a test could be used to distinguish between the two (which are often combined) "(if) when the radial (artery) is compressed with the index finger, the artery can be felt beyond the point of compressions, its walls are sclerosed" [8].

The difference between senile arteriosclerosis and atherosclerosis could not be more stark (Table 4.1). Atherosclerosis is initially and predominantly an intimal disease which may or may not secondarily involve the media. It occurs predominantly in small- to medium-sized arteries and preferentially at sites where there are high and changing patterns of pulsatile shear throughout the cardiac cycle – at flow dividers below a branch in coronary arteries and at or about the carotid sinus in the neck [6]. It occurs predominantly in Western rather than Eastern societies, more commonly in males than females, and has well-known and accepted "risk factors" [9]. In all but one site (the infrarenal aorta, where abdominal aortic aneurysms arise), it causes clinical effects through narrowing of arteries, limiting or preventing arterial flow to the organ or tissue beyond. Finally, arteriosclerosis is diffuse, affecting the thoracic aorta almost exclusively and uniformly, whereas atherosclerosis creates individual discrete lesions, with normal segments between "nodules".

Table 4.1 Key differences between arteriosclerosis and atherosclerosis

Arteriosclerosis	Atherosclerosis
Stiffens aorta	Little effect
Dilates aorta	Occludes
Media	Intima
Diffuse	Focal
Age and blood pressure	Cholesterol and smoking
Cushion function	*Conduit function*

The key functions of the arterial system are first as a conduit, to distribute blood to tissues and organs of the body according to need and at an appropriately high pressure, and, second, to cushion the pulsations generated by the heart, so that blood can flow through the organs and tissues of the body in a near-steady, non-pulsatile stream Arteriosclerosis predominantly affects cushioning function; atherosclerosis predominantly affects conduit function. Arteriosclerosis is caused by the pulsations of the artery, with elastin fibre fatigue, then fracture, with greatest damage in the vessel (the proximal aorta) which pulsates most. Ill effects are on the heart upstream, whose load is increased but whose coronary flow in diastole is limited. Distal effects are on small arteries in vasodilated organs – notably brain and kidney – from tearing of smooth muscle cells and haemorrhage and from dislodgement of endothelial cells and thromboses (pulse wave encephalopathy, pulse wave nephropathy). Atherosclerosis predominantly affects conduit function by limiting or obstructing flow to critical organs and tissues

Arteriosclerosis as it affects the aorta is illustrated in a schematic form prepared with Seymour Glagov (Fig. 4.1).

In an editorial questioning the "comfort zone" of physicians [10], the Emeritus invasive cardiologist Spencer King referred to the future developments he expects to see from the use of engineering principles in this field. While concentrating on hydraulic factors and shear stresses which are involved in development of and damage to atherosclerotic plaques and which precipitate coronary acute events, he alluded to the predictability of other diseases, on the basis of engineering principles. One of them is arteriosclerosis, which Osler described as follows:

As an *involution process* arterio-sclerosis is an accompaniment of old age, and is the expression of the natural wear and tear to which the tubes are subjected. Longevity is a vascular question, which has been well expressed in the axiom that "a man is only as old as his arteries." To a majority of men, death comes primarily or secondarily through this portal. The onset of what may be called physiological arterio-sclerosis depends, in the first place, upon the quality of arterial tissue (vital rubber) which the individual has inherited, and secondly upon the amount of wear and tear to which he has subjected it. [1]

The engineering principles that apply to development of arteriosclerosis from "wear and tear" (now quantifiable in terms of S/N (strain/cycle number) curves) are easier to understand than those that apply to rupture of an atherosclerotic plaque.

Fig. 4.1 Conceptual view of a young normal proximal aorta (*left*) and an elderly arteriosclerotic aorta (*right*) showing (*above*) dilation and wall thickening. *Below* is shown the orderly pattern of thick elastin fibres in the normal aorta with some muscular cells and collagenous fibres as wavy elements that do not bear any load at normal arterial pressure. In the thickened stretched arteriosclerotic wall at right, elastin fibres are fractured and fragmented. Collagenous fibres are stretched, and there is accumulation of amorphous material in the wall. The intima is thickened by hyperplasia of endothelial cells (Cartoon prepared by M O'Rourke and S Glagov. From Ref. [9])

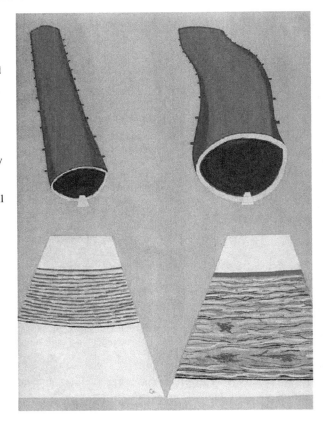

4.1 Cause of Arteriosclerosis

In seeking a cause for arteriosclerosis and an explanation for its development, one has to explain:

- Why it predominantly affects the proximal thoracic aorta and not the peripheral muscular arteries
- Why it affects the media of the aorta and not the intima or adventitia
- Why it decreases distensibility of the aorta or (as put another way) why it increases aortic stiffness
- Why it is associated with dilation of the aorta as well as increased stiffness
- Why its major cause is aging

These issues are explicable and predictable on the basis of engineering principles of material fatigue, alluded to by Osler [1, 8] and King [10], as applied to inanimate objects, such as ships, bridges, aeroplane wing spars and even dance floors [6]. Each material object which is subjected to stretch or bending has a characteristic strain

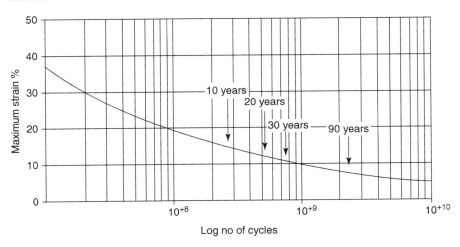

Fig. 4.2 Strain/cycle number (S/N) curve for natural rubber showing the relationship between distention and cycle number at which fracture of the rubber element is expected. The ascending aorta medial elastin fibres (if similar to natural rubber) which pulsate around 15 % with each beat would be expected to show evidence of fracture between 500 and 800 million cycles, corresponding to 20–30 years of life, whereas the distal muscular arteries which pulsate by <5 % with each beat would not be expected to show fracture in a lifetime of 100 years (From Ref. [6])

(S)/cycle number (N) or S/N curve. Natural rubber has properties similar to those of arterial elastin (indeed Osler referred to "vital rubber" as well as the effects of "wear and tear") [1]. An S/N curve is shown in Fig. 4.2. The graph plots the properties of natural rubber in terms of the number of cycles of expansion to which it needs to be subjected in relation to the extent of strain, before fracture would be expected. The heart's cycle is repeated some 30 million times per year and so some 1 billion times in 30 years. With the proximal thoracic aorta in youth stretching by some 15 % with each beat of the heart, one would expect that fracture of elastin fibres would begin to occur at age 30 years and progress steadily thereafter. One would also expect that peripheral muscular arteries (which dilate by <3 % at each cycle), or larger arteries such as the femoral, carotid or brachial which dilate by 3–5 % per cycle [11], would show little change in physical properties in a lifetime of 90 years.

Such an explanation fits with the disorganisation of the elastin network in the aortic media with age (Fig. 4.1), and as seen in histology and pathology texts. This is regarded as a normal aging process "physiological arteriosclerosis", unless extreme and unless associated with areas of medionecrosis, which is the substrate for aortic weakening and aortic dissection in the elderly [1, 6].

The explanation accounts for confining this process to the media since the intima and adventitia contain no elastin fibres (and do not oppose applied stress). It accounts for distension of the aorta since fracture of structural elements causes stretch. It accounts for increased stiffness of the aorta, since cycles of stretch are transferred to and borne by the collagenous fibres in the wall which have much higher modulus of elasticity (stiffness) than elastin. Physical damage to the proximal aorta is stressed here, whereas others such as Lakatta and colleagues tend to concentrate on cellular and molecular changes with aging [12]. I favour the physical (engineering) hypothesis since it explains the issues listed above. I see the physical damage to be primary and the chemical/cellular changes to be secondary and part of the attempt to repair the damaged aorta.

4.2   Effects of Aortic Change in Arteriosclerosis

Fracture of elastin elements in the aortic wall cause increase in elastic modulus. This appears to increase four- to tenfold over an average lifetime and so be greater than any other measurable effect of aging [6]. Stiffening of the aorta from change in elastic modulus increases aortic pulse wave velocity by an amount that depends on the square root of aortic modulus according to the classic Moens-Korteweg equation [6]:

$$\text{Pulse wave velocity } (\text{PWV}) = \sqrt{\frac{Eh}{2r\rho}}$$

where E is Young's modulus of the wall, h is the wall thickness, r is the vessel radius and ρ is the blood density.

Hence, a ninefold increase in aortic modulus would increase aortic PWV threefold, and this explains the increase in aortic PWV with age from ~5 M/s to around 15 M/s at 90 years of age (Fig. 4.3).

Increase in aortic PWV explains another characteristic change in the pulse waveform in older persons, with wave reflection returning early and augmenting the pressure wave in late systole. This is seen in Fig. 4.4 and is the cause of the change in

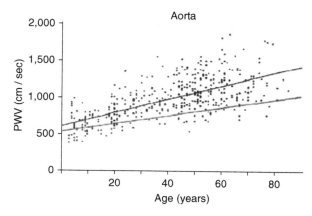

Fig. 4.3 Change in "aortic" carotid-femoral PWV with age in urban Beijing (individual data points and *upper regression line*), where hypertension is prevalent and salt intake high [13], and in rural Guangdong province where hypertension is less prevalent and salt intake is low (*regression line at bottom*). In Beijing, PWV increased approximately threefold between zero and 80 years. In rural Guangdong, PWV increased around twofold over the same period [13, 14] (From Ref. [9])

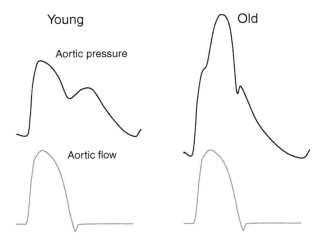

Fig. 4.4 Schematic drawing of ascending aortic pressure waves (*top*) in a young (*left*) and old (*right*) subject for the same ejection (flow) wave from the heart (*bottom, red*). Increase in pressure from foot to initial peak or shoulder at ~100 msec later is higher in the old subject and attributable to high aortic characteristic impedance (Zc), while augmentation in late systole is due to early return of the reflected wave from peripheral sites, caused by increase in aortic PWV. In the younger subject, the initial pressure peak at ~100 msec forms the systolic peak, and the reflected wave returns at the end of systole and boosts coronary blood flow. In both young and old subjects, there is just one single spurt of blood from the LV into the aorta, but two distinct pressure pulses are created. The second pressure pulse must be due to wave reflection

radial artery pulse wave described by Mahomed, Broadbent, Osler and other physicians 100 years ago [6]: "The tidal wave is prolonged and too much sustained" [7]; "The pulse is slow in its ascent, enduring, subsides slowly" [8].

4.3   Clinical Effects of Arteriosclerosis

Ill effects of arteriosclerosis are apparent in the shape of the arterial pulse waveform in the time domain (Fig. 4.4), as shown by Mahomed, Mackenzie and others over 100 years ago and by ourselves [15] and by Murgo [16], Gourgon [17] and others in the frequency domain 30–40 years ago. With respect to the heart, Taylor (40–50 years ago) pointed out that in the mammalian kingdom, impedance of the systemic circulation is "tuned" to heart rate and energy of pressure and flow waves in the ascending aorta [18, 19]. This is evident in the matching of heart rate and major harmonic components of the aortic flow wave to very low values of impedance modulus at normal heart rate in rabbits but not in humans beyond youth (Fig. 4.5) [6, 21, 22]. In middle-aged humans, this relationship is distorted as a consequence of increased aortic stiffening over the (average) 44 years of life in Murgo's patients [16, 21, 22], such that impedance modulus is markedly increased over the frequency band that normally contains the greatest energy of the ascending aortic flow wave.

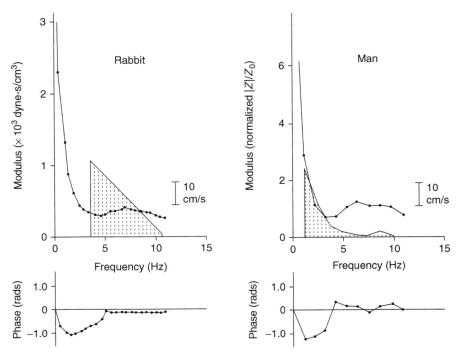

Fig. 4.5 Modulus (*upper*) and phase (*lower*) of ascending aortic impedance in a rabbit (*left*) (Data from Ref. [20]) and in a middle-aged human (*right*) with human data from Murgo et al. [16]. The *dotted area* shows the amplitude of flow harmonics between first and second for the rabbit (at 4–11 Hz) and between first and eighth harmonic for the human (1–10 Hz). "Tuning" of LV to arterial tree is ideal for the rabbit but is not apparent by middle age in humans. Efficient vascular/ventricular interaction in the rabbit is apparent as correspondence between minimal value of impedance with highest energy of the aortic flow wave. Inefficient vascular/ventricular interaction in the middle-aged human is apparent as impedance minimum disassociated from highest energy of the aortic flow wave. Inefficient timing of the arterial system to the LV in the human is attributable to high aortic stiffness, resulting in high Zc and aortic PWV. Despite the rabbit's body length being about one quarter that of a human, aortic stiffening in the human causes return of wave reflection to be similar in rabbit and man, with minimal value of impedance and phase crossover at 4–5 Hz in both

Despite the far greater size and length of the human body, impedance modulus in the ascending aorta is almost identical to that of the rabbit (Fig. 4.5). Such changes in ascending aortic impedance with aging and hypertension were confirmed in humans by Nichols [23], Gourgon [17], Merillon [24] and others and modelled by O'Rourke and Avolio [22].

The aortic change with aging, i.e. arteriosclerosis, leads to marked increase in aortic and left ventricular (LV) systolic pressure with that corresponding to peak systolic flow ejection increasing two- to threefold (from increase in Zc) and with this increase further augmented by the reflected pressure wave from the peripheral sites by up to another 40 %. Pulse pressures of near 100 mmHg are only occasionally seen for the ascending aorta of old subjects since dilation of the ascending aorta with age reduces flow velocity for the same stroke volume. The fall in peak flow velocity in the aorta, seen in normal older subjects, is due partly to aortic dilation and partly from reduced capacity for the LV to expel blood against such high pressure [25–27].

Arteriosclerosis thus increases work of the heart and the pressure required by the LV to expel spurts of flow into the ascending aorta. From this results LV hypertrophy [6], the "cardiomyopathy of overload" [28], with resultant LV failure (most often with near-normal LV ejection fraction). Also resulting is predisposition to angina pectoris even in the absence of epicardial coronary narrowing, caused by a combination of increased LV requirement for blood and decreased capacity for coronary supply caused by prolonged ejection period of the hypertrophied ventricle and with correspondingly reduced time for perfusion, together with delayed relaxation and the lowered pressure gradient across the coronary vascular bed. There is no need to postulate "microvascular dysfunction" to explain angina pectoris in elderly arteriosclerotic patients with normal coronary angiograms [6].

4.4   The Cerebral and Renal Circulation in Arteriosclerosis

Alzheimer was the first to describe the presence of arteriosclerosis in patients with dementia and to whom his name was given, as previously pointed out. A mechanistic explanation for this condition and for its development and associated cerebral microscopic pathology is that arteriosclerosis prevents effective cushioning of the arterial pulse, so that pressure pulsations of very high amplitude (up to 100 mmHg) enter into and pass through the large dilated arteries of the brain and into the small delicate arteries, arterioles, capillaries and venules of the brain, causing excessive stretching and rupture of the media with resulting microbleeds widely throughout the brain [3, 29] – a condition referred as "pulse wave encephalopathy" by neuroradiologists [30, 31]. Absorption of blood from the brain leaves pigment that is changed into the amyloid plaques and tangles that are characteristic of dementia of the Alzheimer type [3].

Similar damage is seen in the kidney with age, and this can be attributed to the same mechanism [32].

The "arteriosclerotic continuum" or "aging continuum" [33] (Fig. 4.6) has been proposed by O'Rourke, Safar and Dzau as a complement to the "atherosclerotic continuum" [34] to explain progression from atherosclerotic risk factors to end-stage heart disease together with dementia and renal failure in older humans. Later stages of the "aging continuum" dovetail into the last part of the "atherosclerotic continuum", leading on to the same termination.

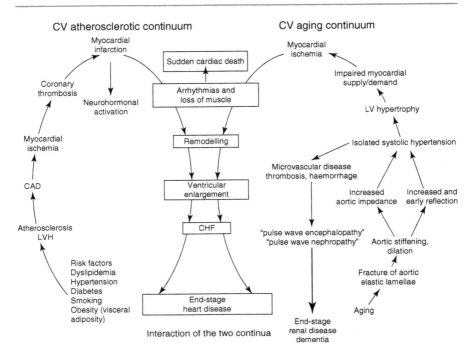

Fig. 4.6 The cardiovascular continuum described by Dzau et al. [34] (*left*) is an atherosclerotic process developing from risk factors, coronary atherosclerosis, coronary obstruction, myocardial damage and scarring, cardiac failure and end-stage heart disease. This can be extended by considering the cardiovascular aging continuum (*right*), which begins with aging and aortic stiffening [33], leading on to LV hypertrophy, myocardial ischemia and the same myocardial damage and resulting in cardiac failure (often with preserved LV contraction) and end-stage heart disease. This aging continuum also includes microvascular disease in brain and kidney, with the comorbidities of dementia and end-stage renal disease which are often seen in end-stage cardiac disease in the elderly [33]

References

1. Osler W (1906) The principles and practice of medicine, 6th edn. Appleton, New York, p 848
2. Osler W (1906) Aequanimitas: with other addresses to medical students, nurses and practitioners of medicine, 2nd edn. HK Lewis, London, pp 391–411
3. Stone J, Johnstone D, Mitrofanis J, O'Rourke M (2015) The mechanical cause of age-related dementia: the brain is destroyed by the pulse. J Alzheimer's Disease. 44:355–373
4. Alzheimer A (1907) Über eine eigenartige Erkrankung der Hirnrinde. Allg Z Psychiatr 64:146–148
5. O'Rourke MF (2014) Robust reflections and radical thoughts: perspectives of a medical journal editor. Int Med J 44:325–330
6. Nichols WW, O'Rourke MF, Vlachopoulos C (2011) McDonald's blood flow in arteries, 6th edn. Hodder Arnold, London
7. Mahomed FA (1872) The physiology and clinical use of the sphygmograph. Med Time Gaz 1:62–64

8. Osler W (1898) The principles and practices of medicine, 3rd edn. Appleton, New York
9. O'Rourke MF, Hashimoto J (2007) Mechanical factors in arterial aging: a clinical perspective. J Am Coll Cardiol 50:1–13
10. King SB (2014) Getting outside of our comfort zone. JACC Cardiovasc Int 7:825–826
11. Boutouyrie P, Laurent S, Benetos A et al (1992) Opposing effects of ageing on distal and proximal large arteries in hypertensives. J Hypertens Suppl 10(6):S87–S91
12. Lakatta EG (2003) Arterial and cardiac aging: major shareholders in cardiovascular enter-prises. Part III: cellular and molecular clues to heart and arterial aging. Circulation 107:490–497
13. Avolio AP, Chen S-G, Wang R-P et al (1983) Effects of aging on changing arterial compliance and left ventricular load in a northern Chinese urban community. Circulation 68:50–58
14. Avolio AP, Deng F-Q, Li W-Q et al (1985) Effects of aging on arterial distensibility in popula-tions with high and low prevalence of hypertension: comparison between urban and rural com-munities in China. Circulation 71:202–210
15. O'Rourke MF (1970) Arterial haemodynamics in hypertension. Circ Res 26/27(Suppl 2): 123–133
16. Murgo JP, Westerhof N, Giolma JP, Altobelli SA (1980) Aortic input impedance in normal man: relationship to pressure wave forms. Circulation 62:105–116
17. Merillon JP, Fontenier GJ, Lerallut JF et al (1982) Aortic input impedance in normal man and arterial hypertension: its modification during changes in aortic pressure. Cardiovasc Res 16:646–656
18. Taylor MG (1964) Wave travel in arteries and the design of the cardiovascular system. In: Attinger EO (ed) Pulsatile blood flow. McGraw-Hill, New York, pp 343–367
19. Taylor MG (1967) The elastic properties of arteries in relation to the physiological functioning of the arterial system. Gastroenterology 52:358–363
20. Avolio AP, O'Rourke MF, Mang K et al (1976) A comparative study of pulsatile arterial hemodynamics in rabbits and guinea pigs. Am J Physiol 230:868–875
21. Taylor MG (1966) The input impedance of an assembly of randomly branching elastic tubes. Biophys J 6:29–51
22. O'Rourke MF, Avolio AP (1980) Pulsatile flow and pressure in human systemic arteries: studies in man and in a multi-branched model of the human systemic arterial tree. Circ Res 46:363–372
23. Nichols WW, O'Rourke MF, Avolio AP et al (1985) Effects of age on ventricular/vascular coupling. Am J Cardiol 55:1179–1184
24. Merillon JP, Motte G, Masquet C et al (1982) Relationship between physical properties of the arterial system and left ventricular performance in the course of aging and arterial hyperten-sion. Eur Heart J 3(Suppl A):95–102
25. Miyashita H, Ikeda U, Tsuruya Y et al (1994) Noninvasive evaluation of the influence of aortic wave reflection on left ventricular ejection during auxotonic contraction. Heart Vessels 9:30–39
26. Westerhof N, O'Rourke MF (1995) The hemodynamic basis for the development of left ventricular failure in systolic hypertension. J Hypertens 13:943–952
27. Adji A, Kachenoura N, Bollache E et al (2014) Effect of aging on ascending aortic flow measured by non-invasive MRI. Hypertension 63:e143
28. Katz AM (1990) Cardiomyopathy of overload. A major determinant of prognosis in congestive heart failure. N Engl J Med 322:100–110
29. O'Rourke MF, Safar ME (2005) Relationship between aortic stiffening and microvascular disease in brain and kidney: cause and logic of therapy. Hypertension 46:200–204
30. Bateman GA (2004) Pulse wave encephalopathy: a spectrum hypothesis incorporating Alzheimer's disease, vascular dementia and normal pressure hydrocephalus. Med Hypo 62: 182–187
31. Henry Feugeas MC, DeMarco G, Peretti II et al (2005) Age-related cerebral white matter changes and pulse-wave encephalopathy: observations with three-dimensional MRI. Magn Reson Imaging 23:929–937

32. Hashimoto J, Ito S (2011) Central pulse pressure and aortic stiffness determine renal hemody-namics: pathophysiological implication for microalbuminuria in hypertension. Hypertension 58:839–846
33. O'Rourke MF, Safar ME, Dzau V (2010) The cardiovascular continuum extended: aging effects on the aorta and microvasculature. Vasc Med 15:461–468
34. Dzau VJ, Antman EM, Black HR et al (2006) The cardiovascular disease continuum validated: clinical evidence of improved patient outcomes: part I: pathophysiology and clinical trial evidence (risk factors through stable coronary artery disease). Circulation 114:2850–2870

Vascular Changes in the Microcirculation: Arterial Remodeling and Capillary Rarefaction

5

Carmine Savoia and Ernesto L. Schiffrin

5.1 Introduction

Blood pressure load and numerous hormonal and locally acting agents mediate vascular damage associated with elevated blood pressure, leading to the complications of hypertension that include stroke, myocardial infarction as a consequence of accelerated atherosclerosis [1], heart failure, and chronic kidney disease, the latter resulting from nephroangiosclerosis. Increased peripheral resistance as a result of changes in small arteries and arterioles has been classically presented as the mechanism for blood pressure elevation in essential hypertension. However, this occurs primarily in younger individuals. In older people, especially after age 50–60, aging and cardiovascular risk factors contribute to stiffen the wall of large arteries such as the aorta and other elastic vessels, which leads to elevated systolic blood pressure.

C. Savoia, MD
Cardiology Unit and Clinical and Molecular Medicine Department,
Faculty of Medicine and Psychology, Sant'Andrea Hospital, Sapienza
University of Rome, Via di Grottarossa, 1035, Rome 00189, Italy
e-mail: carmine.savoia@uniroma1.it

E.L. Schiffrin, C.M., MD, PhD, FRSC, FRCPC, FACP (✉)
Lady Davis Institute for Medical Research and Department of Medicine,
Sir Mortimer B. Davis-Jewish General Hospital, McGill University,
B-127, 3755 Côte-Ste-Catherine Rd., Montreal, QC H3T 1E2, Canada
e-mail: ernesto.schiffrin@mcgill.ca

© Springer International Publishing Switzerland 2015
A. Berbari, G. Mancia (eds.), *Arterial Disorders:*
Definition, Clinical Manifestations, Mechanisms and Therapeutic Approaches,
DOI 10.1007/978-3-319-14556-3_5

5.2   Mechanisms of Remodeling of the Vasculature

Chronically elevated blood pressure initiates a number of complex signal transduction cascades that lead to remodeling of the vasculature [2]. A critical regulator of vascular tone is the endothelium [3], which becomes dysfunctional in people with high blood pressure. As a result, vasodilation is diminished, and in addition, there develops a pro-inflammatory and prothrombotic state. Endothelial dysfunction is a key early determinant of progression of atherosclerosis and is independently associated with increased cardiovascular risk [4]. Low-grade inflammation localized in the vascular wall and perivascular fat also contributes to the mechanisms of hypertension [5] and participates in the initiation and progression of atherosclerosis [6, 7] (see Chap. 3).

Activation of the renin-angiotensin-aldosterone system (RAAS) plays a significant role in the pathophysiology of hypertension [2, 8]. Angiotensin (Ang) II, one of the final products and major mediators of the RAAS, induces vascular remodeling and injury by several mechanisms including vasoconstriction, cell growth, oxidative stress, and inflammation. Ang II induces hyperplasia and hypertrophy of vascular smooth muscle cells (VSMCs) of resistance arteries of patients with essential hypertension and small arteries from hypertensive rats. Ang II and aldosterone, as well as endothelin-1 (ET-1) produced by the endothelium, enhance reactive oxygen species (ROS) generation by stimulating reduced nicotinamide adenine dinucleotide phosphate (NADPH) oxidase and expression of its subunits by pathways that involve c-Src, protein kinase C, phospholipase A_2, and phospholipase D. NADPH oxidase is indeed the major source of ROS in the vascular wall and is expressed in endothelial cells, VSMCs, fibroblasts, and monocytes/macrophages [9–11], although uncoupled nitric oxide (NO) synthase, xanthine oxidase, myeloperoxidase, cytochrome P450 enzymes, and mitochondria are also involved in generating vascular oxidative stress. Increased ROS generation induced by Ang II, aldosterone, and ET-1 contributes to vascular remodeling through VSMC proliferation and hypertrophy and collagen deposition and by modulating cytokine release and pro-inflammatory transcription factors such as NF-κB, as well as by reducing the bioavailability of NO.

Aldosterone increases as well as tissue angiotensin-converting enzyme activity is enhanced [12] and upregulates angiotensin receptors [13], thus potentiating effects of other components of the RAAS. Indeed, aldosterone and other mineralocorticoids affect blood vessels in the heart and kidneys by inducing oxidative stress and impairing endothelial function [13], which can be blunted by mineralocorticoid antagonism. Some of aldosterone's actions may be mediated by stimulation of endothelial production of ET-1 [14].

Ang II, aldosterone, and ET-1 trigger endothelial dysfunction and vascular inflammation by inducing oxidative stress, which upregulates inflammatory mediators in the endothelium and stimulates immune cells such as T effector lymphocytes [15]. Ang II and aldosterone as well as ET-1 stimulate fibrosis via TGF beta. Vasoconstriction induced by Ang II thus becomes embedded in the enhanced collagen deposited in the vascular wall [1, 2, 16]. Collagen I and III mRNA and collagen protein synthesis by fibroblasts are increased in vessels from essential hypertensive patients [17], contributing to thickening of the media in hypertrophic remodeling and reorganization of components of the vascular wall in eutrophic remodeling [18–21]. Reduction in the activity of matrix metalloproteinases (MMPs) may also participate in the stiffening of the vascular wall as collagen and other extracellular matrix components are not degraded and consequently collagen type IV and V and fibronectin accumulate in resistance arteries [22]. MMP-1 and MMP-3 activity is reduced in SHR before hypertension is established [23]. In hypertensive patients with increased vascular type I collagen, serum concentrations of MMP-1 are reduced [24]. Ang II stimulates hyperplasia and hypertrophy of VSMCs [25, 26]. Other processes participating in remodeling of blood vessels include apoptosis, cell elongation, reorganization, and inflammation [25–29]. Also, inflammation in perivascular fat with enhanced generation of tumor necrosis factor (TNF)-alpha and reduced adiponectin, which has anticontractile and thus antihypertensive properties [30, 31], is critically involved in small artery remodeling [32].

Myogenic tone, the intrinsic ability of vessels to constrict in response to increases in intraluminal pressure, participates early on in the alterations occurring in the arterial wall [33]. Among the mechanisms involved in the control of myogenic tone are changes in intracellular calcium, protein kinases, diacylglycerol, modulation of transient receptor potential-like channels, and ion transport [34]. Structural narrowing of the lumen may amplify vasoconstriction. Constriction may be a consequence of increased concentration of specific agents at the level of receptors, greater receptor density, or postreceptor signaling alterations associated with enhanced Ang II signaling leading to increased ROS generation and enhanced constriction and vessel growth [25, 28, 34, 35].

Endothelial dysfunction is involved in the initiation of vascular inflammation and development of atherosclerosis [36]. The number of circulating endothelial progenitor cells (EPCs), a bone marrow–derived population of cells capable of developing into competent mature endothelial cells, is an important determinant of endothelial function [37]. Decreased EPC numbers are associated with arterial stiffness and decreased endothelial function [38]. Endothelial dysfunction is not only accompanied by reduced vasodilation and increased endothelium-dependent contraction but also by cell proliferation, platelet activation, vascular permeability, and a pro-inflammatory and prothrombotic vascular phenotype. Detachment of endothelial cells (anoikis), increases in circulating microparticles derived from the endothelium, and reduced endothelial progenitor cells contribute also to dysfunction and remodeling of the microcirculation in hypertension [39].

Endothelial dysfunction promotes vascular inflammation through generation of ROS and by the production of vasoconstrictor agents, adhesion molecules, and growth factors [40, 41]. Inflammation is central in cardiovascular disease and could be involved in triggering myocardial and cerebrovascular ischemia [36, 42]. Blood pressure itself [43] or activation of the RAAS [26, 32] may induce an inflammatory process characterized by increased expression of adhesion molecules VCAM-1 (vascular cell adhesion molecule 1) and ICAM-1 (intercellular adhesion molecule 1) on endothelial cells, leukocyte extravasation, increased oxidative stress, cytokine production, and activation of immune cells and pro-inflammatory signaling pathways. Greater expression of adhesion molecules on the endothelial cell membrane and accumulation of monocyte/macrophages, dendritic cells, natural killer (NK) cells, and B and T lymphocytes are some of the mechanisms that participate in the inflammatory response in the vascular wall [44]. Patients with cardiovascular disease present indeed increased expression and plasma concentration of inflammatory markers and mediators [41, 45, 46]. High levels of inflammatory mediators, particularly IL-6, ICAM-1, and C-reactive protein (CRP), may be independent risk factors for the development of hypertension [47, 48] and have been associated with increased risk of diabetes [49] and cardiovascular disease. CRP levels correlate with insulin resistance, systolic blood pressure, pulse pressure, and hypertension [49, 50] and with markers of endothelial dysfunction (plasma levels of von Willebrand factor, tissue plasminogen activator, and cellular fibronectin) [51].

A role of innate immunity in mechanisms that contribute to the low-grade inflammatory response in hypertension has also been described. In an osteopetrotic mouse model that is deficient in vascular macrophages because of a mutation in the mCSF gene (*csf1*), neither Ang II nor DOCA-salt induced hypertension or vascular remodeling [5]. Dendritic cells, which are antigen presenting cells originating in the bone marrow but present in other tissues, including the vasculature, are critically involved in activation of adaptive immune responses. As such, their presence in the vasculature in hypertension and atherosclerosis suggests that they are associated with disease onset and progression through priming of T cells in cardiovascular disease in response to danger-associated molecular patterns (DAMPs) [52]. Recent evidence also suggests that different subsets of T lymphocytes may be involved in the mechanisms leading to the inflammatory response described in cardiac and metabolic diseases when an imbalance exists between the pro-inflammatory T helper lymphocytes (Th) 1, Th2, and Th17 and the anti-inflammatory T regulatory (Treg) subsets [44]. Mice deficient in T and B lymphocytes presented blunted hypertensive response to Ang II and DOCA-salt as well as reduced vascular remodeling in response to Ang II [53]. Effector T cell but not B lymphocyte adoptive transfer corrected the lack of response to Ang II. The central and pressor effects of Ang II are also critical for T-cell activation and development of vascular inflammation [54]. One of the mechanisms whereby T lymphocytes participate in hypertension and peripheral inflammation is in response to increased oxidative stress [55]. We recently showed that adaptive immunity could be enhanced as a result of a genetic predisposition with loci on chromosome 2 (which carries many pro-inflammatory genes) in a consomic strain of rats (SSBN2), which contains the genetic background of hypertensive Dahl-salt-sensitive rats and chromosome 2 from Brown-Norway normotensive rats [56]. The presence of the normotensive chromosome 2 was associated with upregulation of Treg markers, which were depressed in the Dahl-salt-sensitive rats. Enhanced Treg (CD8+ and CD4+ lymphocytes which were CD25+) and increased expression of Foxp3 (transcription factor that is a marker of Treg) as well as IL-10 and TGF-beta production (typically produced by Treg) were found in consomic rats, and the opposite in Dahl rats. Thus Treg decrease and T effector upregulation are associated to increased blood pressure and vascular inflammation. The potential protective role of Treg in cardiovascular disease is supported by the more recent evidence that adoptive transfer of Treg cells ameliorated cardiac damage and improved electric remodeling in Ang II-infused mice, independently of blood pressure-lowering effects [57], suggesting a role of T regulatory lymphocytes in the pathogenesis of blood pressure-induced cardiovascular remodeling. We have also recently shown that Treg adoptive transfer lowered blood pressure and protected from vascular remodeling in mice infused with either angiotensin II [58] or aldosterone [59].

Interestingly, inflammation may activate the RAAS, which in turn may further contribute to vascular remodeling and hypertension. Activators of nuclear receptors, such as the peroxisome proliferator-activated receptors (PPARs), downregulate the vascular inflammatory response in experimental animals [60] and decrease serum markers of inflammation in humans [61]. Thus, PPARs may be endogenous modulators of the inflammatory process involved in vascular structural changes occurring in hypertension. On the other hand, Ang II downregulates PPARs through activation of nuclear factor (NF)-κB [62]. Also, gene inactivation of PPAR gamma was shown to be associated with enhanced responses to Ang II including greater hypertrophic and inflammatory response as well as enhanced endothelial dysfunction [63].

Arterial aging is a predominant risk factor for the onset of cardiovascular diseases such as hypertension; on the other hand, hypertension is an important factor in accelerated aging of the vasculature, resulting in premature cardiovascular disease. The hypertensive vascular phenotype and the age-associated changes in blood vessels are similar. They include structural changes consisting in increased arterial wall thickness, reduced compliance, increased stiffness, and decreased lumen diameter and an associated pro-inflammatory phenotype [64, 65]. These structural changes are associated with impaired endothelial function, caused by oxidative stress and decreased production of vasodilators (NO and prostacyclins). The activation of the RAS and increased oxidative stress, decreased telomerase activity and telomere shortening, DNA damage, and genomic instability are all important promoters of cellular senescence [64].

5.3   Remodeling of Small Resistance Arteries and Arterioles in Hypertension

As mentioned above, increased peripheral vascular resistance appears to be a mechanism for diastolic or systo-diastolic hypertension found mostly in younger individuals with essential hypertension [65] which results mostly from resistance to flow in small arteries (with a lumen diameter of 100–300 μm) and arterioles (smaller than 100 μm) [1, 18]. Since according to Poiseuille's law resistance is inversely related to the fourth power of the radius of the blood vessel, small decreases in the lumen diameter will increase resistance to a significant degree. Remodeling of resistance arteries (reduced vascular lumen with increased media thickness not correlated with stiffness changes) may be functional, mechanical, and structural [1]. Increases in the media-to-lumen ratio (M/L) are typical and the most reproducible parameter to compare changes in small arteries in subjects followed in repeat studies and when comparing different subjects [1, 18]. Our work has suggested that

Fig. 5.1 Remodeling of small arteries and arterioles in hypertension is inward (smaller lumen) and could be eutrophic, with no increase in the media cross-sectional area despite a thickened media (in essential hypertension), or it could be hypertrophic, in which case the media cross-sectional area is increased (generally associated with severe or secondary forms of hypertension). In both, media-to-lumen ratio (M/L) is greater than in normotension. Media cross-sectional area is calculated as $\pi r_o^2 - \pi r_i^2$

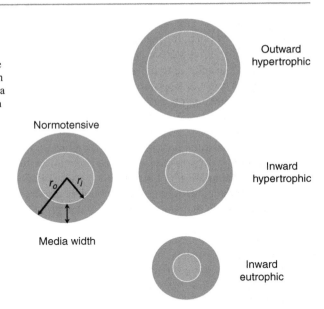

increased M/L of small arteries may be the most prevalent and possibly the earliest alteration that occurs in the cardiovascular system of hypertensive patients aged less than 60 years of age [16] and may be much more frequent than and in fact precede endothelial dysfunction in humans. Enhanced M/L of small arteries has been demonstrated to be associated with increased cardiovascular events, especially in high-risk patients [66].

In stage 1 hypertension in individuals younger than 60 years, eutrophic remodeling of small arteries and arterioles is usually found (Fig. 5.1). In this type of remodeling, the outer diameter and the lumen are reduced, but the media cross section does not increase; thus there is no vascular hypertrophy [1, 18]. Smooth muscle cells are rearranged around a smaller lumen leading to increased media width and M/L. Whether vascular smooth muscle cells are increased in volume, length, or number remains a subject of controversy. Media growth toward the lumen combined with enhanced apoptosis in the periphery of the vessel may also contribute to these changes [32]. The smaller lumen decreases circumferential tension, according to Laplace's law, and the increased media width reduces media stress, which protects the vessel's wall from the effects of elevated blood pressure. When blood pressure elevation is severe or of long duration, increased wall stress results in hypertrophic remodeling of small arteries and arterioles as smooth muscle cell growth becomes greater than apoptosis and media cross-sectional area is enhanced [1, 67, 68]. Eutrophic and hypertrophic remodeling may be found in the same experimental animals in different arteries. Interestingly, hypertrophic remodeling of resistance arteries is found, particularly in humans, in renovascular hypertension [68], diabetes [69, 70], and acromegaly [71]. In experimental animals, hypertrophic

Fig. 5.2 Folkow's model shows that at each level of vascular constriction (e.g., at the level of the *dashed vertical line*), resistance to blood flow is increased more in eutrophic remodeling than in hypertrophic remodeling; and in the latter, resistance to flow is greater than in vessels from normotensive subjects

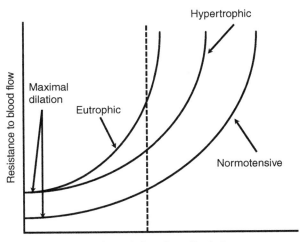

% Constriction of small arteries

remodeling can be demonstrated in those hypertensive models that are associated with excess endothelin, such as one-kidney one-clip renovascular hypertension, DOCA-salt hypertension, aldosterone-salt hypertension, and Dahl-salt-sensitive hypertension. Folkow's model (Fig. 5.2) demonstrates that at all levels of vascular constriction, arteries with eutrophic remodeling generate more resistance to blood flow than arteries with hypertrophic remodeling, which in turn, generate more resistance than those from normotensive animals.

5.4   Rarefaction of Arterioles and Capillaries

Rarefaction is another type of remodeling that is found in hypertension. It occurs at the level of small arterioles with a lumen diameter smaller than 40 μm and capillaries [1]. With rarefaction, the density of arterioles and capillaries in tissues is diminished and consequently vascular resistance is increased [72, 73] and tissue perfusion is impaired [74]. Arteriolar rarefaction is functional initially as a result of vasoconstriction, and later anatomical and permanent, followed by rarefaction of capillaries with decreased tissue perfusion. Decreases in tissue perfusion have been associated with vascular complications and cardiovascular events [75].

Conclusion

Vascular remodeling and endothelial dysfunction in small resistance arteries are features regularly reported in hypertension. Functional, structural, and mechanical alterations of resistance arteries are probably the earliest alterations in the vasculature found in hypertensive subjects younger than 60 years of age. They take the form of eutrophic inward remodeling accompanied by endothelial dysfunction associated eventually to enhanced stiffness. These changes have been shown to have prognostic significance with respect to outcomes. They could contribute through wave reflection to increases in stiffness of large arteries and thus to systolic hypertension and the increased pulse pressure found in older subjects with hypertension. Alternatively, increased large artery stiffness could increase pulsatility, which when conducted into the microcirculation, may cause injury and remodeling of small arteries and arterioles. Activation of the RAAS plays a key role in vascular remodeling and endothelial dysfunction through redox-sensitive pathways that promote growth and inflammation in the blood vessel wall.

Disclosure This study was supported by CIHR grants 13570, 37917, 82790, and 102606, a Canada Research Chair on Hypertension and Vascular Research from the CRC/CIHR Program of the Government of Canada, and a Canada Fund for Innovation grant, all to ELS.

References

1. Schiffrin EL (2004) Remodeling of resistance arteries in essential hypertension and effects of antihypertensive treatment. Am J Hypertens 17:1192–1200
2. Schiffrin EL, Touyz RM (2004) From bedside to bench to bedside: role of renin angiotensin aldosterone system in remodeling of resistance arteries in hypertension. Am J Physiol Heart Circ Physiol 287:H435–H446
3. Endemann DH, Schiffrin EL (2004) Endothelial dysfunction. J Am Soc Nephrol 15: 1983–1992
4. Lerman A, Zeiher AM (2005) Endothelial function: cardiac events. Circulation 111:363–368
5. De Ciuceis C, Amiri F, Brassard P et al (2005) Reduced vascular remodeling, endothelial dysfunction, and oxidative stress in resistance arteries of angiotensin II-infused macrophage colony-stimulating factor-deficient mice: evidence for a role in inflammation in angiotensin-induced vascular injury. Arterioscler Thromb Vasc Biol 25:2106–2113
6. Savoia C, Schiffrin EL (2007) Reduction of C-reactive protein and the use of the antihypertensives. Vasc Health Risk Manag 3(6):975–983
7. Savoia C, Schiffrin EL (2006) Inflammation in hypertension. Curr Opin Nephrol Hypertens 2:152–158
8. Kranzhofer R, Schmidt J, Pfeiffer CA et al (1999) Angiotensin induces inflammatory activation of human vascular smooth muscle cells. Arterioscler Thromb Vasc Biol 19:1623–1629
9. Fukui T, Ishizaka N, Rajagopalan S et al (1997) p22phox mRNA expression and NAD(P)H oxidase activity are increased in aortas from hypertensive rats. Circ Res 80:45–51
10. Griendling KK, Sorescu D, Lassegue B, Ushio-Fukai M (2000) Modulation of protein kinase activity and gene expression by reactive oxygen species and their role in vascular physiology and pathophysiology. Arterioscler Thromb Vasc Biol 20:2175–2183
11. Touyz RM, Chen X, Tabet F et al (2002) Expression of a functionally active gp91phox-containing neutrophil-type NAD(P)H oxidase in smooth muscle cells from human resistance arteries: regulation by angiotensin II. Circ Res 90:1205–1213
12. Harada E, Yoshimura M, Yasue H et al (2001) Aldosterone induces angiotensin-converting enzyme gene expression in cultured neonatal rat cardiocytes. Circulation 104:137–139
13. Schiffrin EL, Gutkowska J, Genest J (1984) Effect of angiotensin II on deoxycorticosterone infusion on vascular angiotensin II receptors in rats. Am J Physiol Heart Circ Physiol 246: H608–H614
14. Pu Q, Fritsch Neves M, Virdis A, Touyz RM, Schiffrin EL (2003) Endothelin antagonism on aldosterone-induced oxidative stress and vascular remodeling. Hypertension 42:49–55
15. Idris-Khodja N, Mian MOR, Paradis P, Schiffrin EL (2014) Dual roles of adaptive immunity in hypertension. Eur Heart J 35:1238–1244

16. Park JB, Schiffrin EL (2001) Small artery remodeling is the most prevalent (earliest?) form of target organ damage in mild essential hypertension. J Hypertens 19:921–930
17. Delva P, Lechi A, Pastori C et al (2002) Collagen I and III mRNA gene expression and cell growth potential of skin fibroblasts in patients with essential hypertension. J Hypertens 20:1393–1399
18. Schiffrin EL (1992) Reactivity of small blood vessels in hypertension: relation with structural changes. Hypertension 19(Suppl 2):II-1–II-9
19. Schiffrin EL, Deng LY (1999) Structure and function of resistance arteries of hypertensive patients treated with a β-blocker or a calcium channel antagonist. J Hypertens 14:1247–1255
20. Intengan HD, Thibault G, Li JS, Schiffrin EL (1999) Resistance artery mechanics, structure and extracellular components in spontaneously hypertensive rats effects of angiotensin receptor antagonism and converting enzyme inhibition. Circulation 100:2267–2275
21. Intengan HD, Deng LY, Li JS, Schiffrin EL (1999) Mechanics and composition of human subcutaneous resistance arteries in essential hypertension. Hypertension 33:569–574
22. Marchesi C, Dentali F, Nicolini F et al (2012) Plasma levels of matrix metalloproteinases and their inhibitors in hypertension: a systematic review and meta-analysis. J Hypertens 30:3–16
23. Intengan HD, Schiffrin EL (2000) Structure and mechanical properties of resistance arteries in hypertension role of adhesion molecules and extracellular matrix determinants. Hypertension 36:312–318
24. Laviades C, Varo N, Fernandez J et al (1998) Abnormalities of the extracellular degradation of collagen type I in essential hypertension. Circulation 98:535–540
25. Touyz RM, Schiffrin EL (2000) Signal transduction mechanisms mediating the physiological and pathophysiological actions of angiotensin II in vascular smooth muscle cells. Pharmacol Rev 52:639–672
26. Schiffrin EL, Touyz RM (2003) Multiple actions of angiotensin II in hypertension: benefits of AT1 receptor blockade. J Am Coll Cardiol 42(5):911–913
27. Nurnberger J, Keflioglu-Scheiber A, Opazo Saez AM et al (2002) Augmentation index is associated with cardiovascular risk. J Hypertens 20:2407–2414
28. Touyz RM, Deng LY, He G et al (1999) Angiotensin II stimulates DNA and protein synthesis in vascular smooth muscle cells from human arteries: role of extracellular signal-regulated kinases. J Hypertens 17:907–916
29. Diep QN, Li JS, Schiffrin EL (1999) In vivo study of AT1 and AT2 angiotensin receptors in apoptosis in rat blood vessels. Hypertension 34:617–624
30. Marchesi C, Ebrahimian T, Angulo O et al (2009) Endothelial NO synthase uncoupling and perivascular adipose oxidative stress and inflammation contribute to vascular dysfunction in a rodent model of metabolic syndrome. Hypertension 54:1384–1392
31. Greenstein AS, Khavandi K, Withers SB et al (2009) Local inflammation and hypoxia abolish the protective anticontractile properties of perivascular fat in obese patients. Circulation 119:1661–1670
32. Savoia C, Schiffrin EL (2007) Vascular inflammation in hypertension and diabetes: molecular mechanisms and therapeutic intervention. Clin Sci 112:375–384
33. Izzard AS, Bund SJ, Heagerty AM (1996) Myogenic tone in mesenteric arteries from spontaneously hypertensive rats. Am J Physiol (Heart Circ Physiol) 270:H1–H6
34. Touyz RM, Yao G, Schiffrin EL (2003) c-Src induces phosphorylation and translocation of p47phox role in superoxide generation by Ang II in human vascular smooth muscle cells. Arterioscler Thromb Vasc Biol 23:981–987
35. Intengan HD, Schiffrin EL (2001) Vascular remodeling in hypertension – roles of apoptosis, inflammation, and fibrosis. Hypertension 38:581–587
36. Libby P, Tabas I, Fredman G, Fisher EA (2014) Inflammation and its resolution as determinants of acute coronary syndromes. Circ Res 114:1867–1879
37. Urbich C, Dimmeler S (2004) Endothelial progenitor cells: characterization and role in vascular biology. Circ Res 95(4):343–353
38. Hill JM, Zalos G, Halcox JP et al (2003) Circulating endothelial progenitor cells, vascular function, and cardiovascular risk. N Engl J Med 348(7):593–600

39. Burger D, Schock S, Thompson CS et al (2013) Microparticles: biomarkers and beyond. Clin Sci 124:423–441
40. Ross R (1999) Atherosclerosis – an inflammatory disease. N Engl J Med 340:115–126
41. Ridker PM (2014) Inflammation, C-reactive protein, and cardiovascular disease: moving past the marker versus mediator debate. Circ Res 114:594–595
42. Luna JM, Moon YP, Liu KM et al (2014) High-sensitivity C-reactive protein and interleukin-6–dominant inflammation and ischemic stroke risk: the Northern Manhattan Study. Stroke 45:979–987
43. Wung BS, Cheng JJ, Chao YJ et al (1996) Cyclical strain increases monocyte chemotactic protein-1 secretion in human endothelial cells. Am J Physiol 270:H1462–H1468
44. Schiffrin EL (2010) T lymphocytes: a role in hypertension? Curr Opin Nephrol Hypertens 19:181–186
45. Sesso HD, Buring JE, Rifai N et al (2003) C-reactive protein and the risk of developing hypertension. J Am Med Assoc 290:2945–2951
46. Preston RA, Ledford M, Materson BJ et al (2002) Effects of severe, uncontrolled hypertension on endothelial activation: soluble vascular cell adhesion molecule-1, soluble intercellular adhesion molecule-1 and von Willebrand factor. J Hypertens 20:871–877
47. Blake GJ, Rifai N, Buring JE, Ridker PM (2003) Blood pressure, C-reactive protein, and risk of future cardiovascular events. Circulation 108:2993–2999
48. Thorand B, Lowel H, Schneider A et al (2003) C-reactive protein as a predictor for incident diabetes mellitus among middle-aged men: results from the MONICA Augsburg cohort study, 1984–1998. Arch Intern Med 163:93–99
49. Barzilay JI, Peterson D, Cushman M et al (2004) The relationship of cardiovascular risk factors to microalbuminuria in older adults with or without diabetes mellitus or hypertension: the cardiovascular health study. Am J Kidney Dis 44:25–34
50. Chae CU, Lee RT, Rifai N, Ridker PM (2001) Blood pressure and inflammation in apparently healthy men. Hypertension 38:399–403
51. Engstrom G, Janzon L, Berglund G et al (2002) Blood pressure increase and incidence of hypertension in relation to inflammation-sensitive plasma protein. Arterioscler Thromb Vasc Biol 22:2054–2058
52. Christ A, Temmerman L, Legein B et al (2013) Dendritic cells in cardiovascular diseases: epiphenomenon, contributor, or therapeutic opportunity. Circulation 128:2603–2613
53. Guzik TJ, Hoch NE, Brown KA et al (2007) Role of T cell in the genesis of angiotensin II induced hypertension and vascular dysfunction. J Exp Med 204:2449–2460
54. Marvar PJ, Thabet SR, Guzik TJ et al (2010) Central and peripheral mechanisms of T-lymphocyte activation and vascular inflammation produced by angiotensin II-induced hypertension. Circ Res 107:263–270
55. Lob HE, Marvar PJ, Guzik TJ et al (2010) Induction of hypertension and peripheral inflammation by reduction of extracellular superoxide dismutase in the central nervous system. Hypertension 55:277–283
56. Viel EC, Lemarié CA, Benkirane K et al (2011) Immune regulation and vascular inflammation in genetic hypertension. Am J Physiol Heart Circ Physiol 298(3):H938–H944
57. Kvakan HKM, Quadri F, Park J-K et al (2009) Regulatory T cells ameliorate angiotensin II-induced cardiac damage. Circulation 119:2904–2912
58. Barhoumi T, Kasal DAB, Li MW et al (2011) T regulatory lymphocytes prevent angiotensin II-induced hypertension and vascular injury. Hypertension 57:469–476
59. Kasal DAB, Barhoumi T, Li MW et al (2012) T regulatory lymphocytes prevent aldosterone-induced vascular injury. Hypertension 59:324–330
60. Diep QN, Amiri F, Touyz RM et al (2002) PPARa activator effects on Ang II-induced vascular oxidative stress and inflammation. Hypertension 40:866–871
61. Haffner SM, Greenberg AS, Weston WM et al (2002) Effect of rosiglitazone treatment on nontraditional markers of cardiovascular disease in patients with type 2 diabetes mellitus. Circulation 106:679–684
62. Tham DM, Martin-McNulty B, Wang YX et al (2002) Angiotensin II is associated with activation of NF-kappaB mediated genes and down regulation of PPARs. Physiol Genomics 11:21–30

63. Marchesi C, Rehman A, Rautureau Y et al (2013) Protective role of vascular smooth muscle cell PPARγ in angiotensin II-induced vascular disease. Cardiovasc Res 97:562–570

64. Wang M, Zhang J, Jiang LQ, Spinetti G, Pintus G, Monticone R, Kolodgie FD, Virmani R, Lakatta EG (2007) Proinflammatory profile within the grossly normal aged human aortic wall. Hypertension 50:219–227

65. Schiffrin EL (2007) The vascular phenotypes in hypertension: relation to the natural history of hypertension. J Am Soc Hypertens 1:56–67

66. Rizzoni D, Porteri E, Boari G et al (2003) Prognostic significance of small artery structure in hypertension. Circulation 108:2230–2235

67. Sharifi AM, Schiffrin EL (1998) Apoptosis in vasculature of spontaneously hypertensive rats effect of an angiotensin converting enzyme inhibitor and a calcium channel antagonists. Am J Hypertens 11:1108–1116

68. Rizzoni D, Porteri E, Guelfi D et al (2000) Cellular hypertrophy in subcutaneous small arteries of patients with renovascular hypertension. Hypertension 25:931–935

69. Rizzoni D, Porteri E, Guelfi D et al (2001) Structural alteration in subcutaneous small arteries of normotensive and hypertensive patients with non insulin-dependent diabetes mellitus. Circulation 103:1238–1244

70. Endemann DH, Pu Q, De Ciuceis C et al (2004) Persistent remodeling of resistance arteries in type 2 diabetic patients on antihypertensive treatment. Hypertension 43:399–404

71. Rizzoni D, Porteri E, Giustina A et al (2004) Acromegalic patients show the presence of hypertrophic remodeling of subcutaneous small resistance arteries. Hypertension 43:561–565

72. Prewitt RL, Chen II, Dowell R (1982) Development of microvascular rarefaction in the spontaneously hypertensive rat. Am J Physiol (Heart Circ Physiol) 243:H243–H251

73. Greene AS, Tonellato PJ, Lui J et al (1989) Microvascular rarefaction and tissue vascular resistance in hypertension. Am J Physiol (Heart Circ Physiol) 256:H126–H131

74. Greene AS, Tonellato PJ, Zhang Z et al (1992) Effect of microvascular rarefaction on tissue oxygen delivery in hypertension. Am J Physiol (Heart Circ Physiol) 262:H1486–H1493

75. Levy B, Schiffrin EL, Mourad JJ et al (2008) Impaired tissue perfusion: a pathology common to hypertension, obesity and diabetes. Circulation 118:968–976

Part III

Pathogenetic Mechanisms in Arterial Disease

Perinatal Programming of Cardiovascular Disease

6

Maria Franco

6.1 Fetal Programming: Early Origins of Adult Disease

Impairment of intrauterine environment during critical periods may result in perturbations in growth and development of the fetus. Barker et al. have originally proposed the hypothesis that several chronic adult diseases can be programmed in early life [1]. These authors examined the mortality records of 5,654 men who were born during 1911–1930 in Hertfordshire (UK) [1]. In this report was found that the men with the lowest weights at birth subsequently had the highest death rates from ischemic heart disease [1]. In addition, a retrospective study of babies born during the Dutch famine of 1945 has demonstrated a significant association between cardiovascular disease (CVD) and early nutritional impairment during gestation [2]. In this programming concept, stimulus or injury during the critical period of development can result in the permanent changes in physiology and the metabolism and produces persistent effects throughout life. Afterward, Hales and Barker suggested the "Thrifty Phenotype Hypothesis" or "Economic Phenotype" to explain the biological basis of the fetal origin hypothesis. In this context, impairment of fetal environment can result in a physiological adaptive response that promotes early survival at the detrimental of later health [3, 4]. In fact, poor nutritional conditions during pregnancy can alter the development of a fetus to prepare him or her to survive in an environment with low nutritional resources. The main basis of this hypothesis is that the deleterious effects are more pronounced when there is a significant difference between the early nutritional deficiency and later nutritional intake. Reduced growth, represented mainly by low birth weight, is the major result of a suboptimal

M. Franco, PhD
Division of Nephrology, School of Medicine, Federal University
of São Paulo, São Paulo, Brazil
e-mail: maria.franco@unifesp.br

© Springer International Publishing Switzerland 2015
A. Berbari, G. Mancia (eds.), *Arterial Disorders:*
Definition, Clinical Manifestations, Mechanisms and Therapeutic Approaches,
DOI 10.1007/978-3-319-14556-3_6

intrauterine environment and is associated with chronic conditions in adulthood, such as type 2 diabetes, hypertension, and CVD [5].

The fetal growth is complex and delicate. There are three stages associated with the development of the fetus. During the first stage (cellular hyperplasia), cells multiply in the fetus's organs, and this occurs from the beginning of development through the early part of the fourth month. In the second stage (hyperplasia and hypertrophy), cells continue to multiply and the organs grow. During the third stage (hypertrophy) (after 32 weeks), growth occurs quickly and the baby gains weight. If this delicate process of development is disturbed or interrupted, the baby can suffer from restricted growth.

Low-birth-weight babies are defined as infant whose weight at birth is ≤2,500 g, which could be due to the intrauterine growth restriction (IUGR) or prematurity. Infants who are delivered before 37 weeks (gestational age: inadequate) are termed preterm. On the other hand, infants with history of low birth weight and adequate gestational age (37–42 weeks) are termed with IUGR or small for gestational age (SGA). IUGR resulting in SGA infants can be due to many known and unknown factors either acting alone or in combination. The fetal growth is determined not only by the substrate availability but also by the integrity of physiologic processes necessary to ensure the transfer of nutrients and oxygen to the developing fetus.

6.2   Fetal Programming of Hypertension

6.2.1   Renal Mechanisms

There is evidence that people whose birth weight was low have a congenital deficit in the nephron number and are more susceptible to the development of renal disease [6, 7]. Several ultrasound studies that examined the fetal kidney have supported these findings [8, 9]. In Australian aborigines, a population in which renal failure is several times higher than in the Australian Caucasian population, an ultrasound study showed that in 174 children aged between 5 and 18 years, birth weight was related to the kidney volume; individuals of lower weight at birth appeared to have thinner kidneys of normal length, suggesting decreased nephron number [9]. In the human, nephrogenesis is complete around 32–34 week of gestation, and therefore, a nephron deficit presented at birth would persist through life. A kidney with a reduced nephron number becomes more susceptible to renal injury and functional decline. Interestingly, other studies have shown a direct relation between birth weight and the number of nephrons with 250,000 more glomeruli per kidney per kilogram increased in birth weight [10, 11]. In addition, early catch-up kidney growth was observed in small for gestational age infants, suggesting either an accelerated renal maturation process or early compensatory kidney hypertrophy in this group of infants [12]. In fact, nephrogenesis requires a perfect balance of many factors that can be disturbed by intrauterine growth restriction, leading to an impairment of the nephron number. The compensatory hyperfiltration in the remaining nephrons results in glomerular and systemic hypertension, which hastens injury to functioning glomeruli and perpetuates the vicious cycle of ongoing nephron loss [7]. These observations indicated that during its period of development, the kidney can be influenced quite dramatically by alterations in the intrauterine environment that lead to impairment of nephrogenesis.

Increasing evidence is available also concerning the effect of fetal growth restriction on impairment of renal function in children and adults [13–16]. The assessment of renal function is important to detect the extension, as well as the progression, of nephropathy. Moderate renal metabolic disturbance was found in SGA children between 4 and 12 years of age [15]. Giapros et al. [16] found early catch-up kidney growth in SGA children, suggesting an accelerated renal maturation process or early compensatory kidney hypertrophy in these infants. Recent evidence highlighting the importance of low birth weight on renal function was described in SGA children with high levels of cystatin C [17]. In this context, the lower birth weight appears to be associated with early impairment of renal function in 8–13-year-old children, and this is consistent with the high incidence of lower number of nephrons in cases of fetal growth restriction and with high prevalence of metabolic and cardiovascular disease in later life [17]. Plasma cystatin C was proposed as a novel surrogate marker of GFR. Cystatin C is a low-molecular-weight protein that functions as an extracellular inhibitor of cysteine protease. It has been suggested that elevated cystatin C levels may be a more sensitive indicator of renal dysfunction than conventional creatinine-based measures [18, 19]. In fact, the serum cystatin C concentration already increases with mildly reduced GFR of 70–90 ml/min, i.e., in the "creatinine-blind" range [20]. Moreover, several studies concluded that cystatin C performed better than serum creatinine and even better than equations estimating GFR based on creatinine [17–20].

Several evidences derived from animal studies indicate that changes in fetal environment may affect renal development [21–24]. In fact, Merlet-Benichou et al. described a reduction in nephron number in offspring of rats submitted to substantial protein restriction in utero [21]. Other study showed that 50 % of protein restriction intake during pregnancy produces offspring with a reduced number of glomeruli, glomerular hypertrophy, and hypertension in adulthood [22]. In addition, Langley-Evans et al. demonstrated in rats that the prenatal exposure to a maternal low-protein diet in mid–late gestation induces an impairment of nephrogenesis and hypertension in adult life [23]. Nwagwu et al. [24] have shown that low-protein diet in utero induced increased blood urea, urinary output, and urinary albumin excretion in resulting offspring. It has been also shown that the induction of IUGR by uteroplacental insufficiency produces a significant reduction in glomeruli number in the full-term fetal kidneys [25]. It has been suggested that some aspects of nephrogenesis, which begins around day 12 of gestation and is not complete until 8 days after birth, are basically a maladaptive process leading to the subsequent development of hypertension.

Additional evidence comes from some studies developed by Lucas et al. [26–28]. These authors demonstrated that when pregnant rats were subjected to 50 % of food restriction during the first or second half or throughout pregnancy, the renal function of the offspring was impaired 3 months after birth. Morphometric evaluation showed that the number of glomeruli was significantly decreased both in newborn and adult offspring, irrespective of the period in which restriction was imposed. Glomerular diameter showed a significant increase in every studied group, which characterized a compensatory hypertrophy in the remaining nephrons. These findings led us to raise the hypothesis that fetal undernutrition could be the determinant of the early appearance of glomerulosclerosis in adult life. In fact, in a subsequent study when renal function studies were performed in 18-month-old intrauterine undernourished rats, a significant decrease in GFR and renal plasma flow levels was observed when compared to normal controls at the same age. The GFR values were very similar in 3-month-old intrauterine undernourished rats and in control animals, which means that the age-related decline in GFR was manifested earlier in young adults because of a significant decrease in the number of glomeruli. Increased blood pressure levels were observed from 8 weeks on while proteinuria began to increase later, in 9-month-old animals. Histological evaluation of kidney sections showed a markedly increase in glomerulosclerosis and tubulointerstitial lesions in 18-month-old intrauterine undernourished rats. Immunohistochemical studies revealed that an accelerated process of glomerulosclerosis took place in those rats, with high expression levels of fibronectin, desmin, and L-actin in both glomeruli and Bowman's capsule as well as in interstitial areas. These findings led us to conclude that the age-induced renal changes could be accelerated in this model of fetal undernutrition, with renal structural changes occurring early in life.

It is well established that the intrarenal renin–angiotensin system (RAS) plays an important role in the normal morphological development of the kidney [29]. In fact, all components of the RAS are expressed from early in gestation in the rat and human in meso- and metanephrons [25]. Thus, changes in this system programmed in utero may be responsible for the renal alterations observed in animals submitted to intrauterine undernutrition. Some studies have demonstrated that renal renin and tissue angiotensin II mRNA levels were significantly reduced in newborn submitted to low-protein diet in utero, suggesting that maternal malnutrition promoted suppression of the newborn intrarenal RAS and this could affect nephrogenesis, resulting in a lower total number of nephrons [25, 30]. In addition, other study also found that blockade of the AT_1 receptor during the first 12 days of postnatal life (i.e., period of nephrogenesis) promotes in a decreased number of glomeruli and reduced renal function [31]. In addition, angiotensin II can stimulate the expression of Pax-2 (homeobox 2 gene), which might be important in kidney development and repair. This process occurs through AT2 receptor and modifying nephrogenesis and kidney development [32]. Other studies suggest a negative interaction between fetal exposure to glucocorticoids and intrarenal RAS [32].

In kidneys from the offspring of rats given a low-protein diet during pregnancy, an increased expression of several genes has been detected, including those encoding sodium transporters. Manning and Vehaskari [33] suggested that inappropriate sodium retention and expansion of extracellular volume could be involved in hypertension observed in rats submitted to intrauterine undernutrition. In a subsequent study, Manning et al. [34] demonstrated that some tubular sodium-related transporters as bumetanide-sensitive Na–K–2Cl cotransporter (BSC1) and thiazide-sensitive

Na–Cl cotransporter (TSC) were increased at different ages, suggesting that transcriptional upregulation of Na+ transport could originate hypertension in this model. It thus appears that, when nephrogenesis is compromised, the nephrons have an increased capacity to retain salt and water. This is likely to contribute to the development of hypertension.

6.2.2 Extrarenal Mechanisms

The vascular dysfunction may result from fetal programming of the vascular wall by adverse intrauterine environment. The underlying mechanism linking fetal life factors to vascular function remains unclear. It has been postulated that fetal programming alters NO formation leading to endothelium dysfunction by impairment of vasodilatory capacity and consequently to the development of hypertension and other CVDs. Clinical studies have demonstrated considerably association between low birth weight and endothelial dysfunction. Leeson et al. [35] and Franco et al. [36], using a noninvasive method to evaluate endothelium-dependent dilatation in the brachial artery, reported a positive association of low birth weight with impaired endothelial function in young children. These studies were performed in the absence of clinical complications and cardiovascular risk factors. On the other hand, Goodfellow et al. [37] and Leeson et al. [38] reported the same correlation between impaired endothelium-dependent relaxation and low birth weight in young adult, suggesting that the impact of prenatal growth on vascular disease does not operate through modification of acquired risk factors. Experimental data confirm the clinical findings. In fact, impaired responses to different endothelium-dependent agonists have been consistently demonstrated in different vascular beds isolated from rats submitted to fetal undernutrition. Holemans et al. [39] and Ozaki et al. [40] demonstrated that maternal undernutrition during pregnancy caused abnormal endothelium-dependent response in both mesenteric arteries and skeletal circulation from resulting male offspring. In another study, Franco et al. have shown that fetal undernutrition induced impaired endothelium-dependent vasodilation in vivo in the mesenteric circulation [41] and in aortic rings [42] of the adult male offspring. The same authors also demonstrated that severe restriction of all dietary constituents during pregnancy aggravates the already existing endothelial dysfunction in aortic rings isolated from spontaneously hypertensive rat offspring [43]. Lamireau et al. [44] found that maternal protein deprivation is associated with diminished NO-dependent relaxation of cerebral microvasculature. In addition, the impairment of the endothelial function is also described in female offspring submitted to both low-protein diet and global nutrient restriction in utero [39, 42, 45].

Reduced activity and gene expression of endothelial nitric oxide synthase (eNOS) have been described in aortic rings isolated from rats submitted to intrauterine undernutrition [42]. Alves et al. [46] demonstrated that the urinary excretion of NOx (NO_2+NO_3) was lower in these rats. Furthermore, reduction in NO synthesis by alterations in NOS activity via tetrahydrobiopterin cofactor was also observed in mesenteric vascular bed isolated from intrauterine undernourished rats [47]. Taken together, these data suggest that fetal programming can promote impairment of the endothelial function, in part, by decrease in NO synthesis. Confirming these experimental findings, clinical investigations also reported reduction in both NO concentration and NOS activity. In pregnancies complicated by fetal growth restriction, a reduction in the NOS activity and fetoplacental NO synthesis was observed [48–50]. In addition, children with low birth weight have a lower urinary NO concentration, suggesting that alterations to NO pathways could contribute to adult disease [51]. The same authors also described that NO levels are significantly correlated with both systolic blood pressure levels and vascular function in these children [51].

The NO bioavailability may be modified by reactive oxygen species (ROS), such as superoxide anion. An increase in superoxide concentration putatively leads to the scavenging of NO and to the cellular damage associated with endothelial dysfunction [52]. Vascular reactivity studies performed in mesenteric arteriolar bed found that topic application of SOD and MnTMPyP (a cell-permeable metalloporphyrin SOD mimetic) corrected the decreased endothelium-dependent relaxation induced by intrauterine undernutrition [53]. These authors also demonstrated that intrauterine undernutrition markedly attenuated the superoxide dismutase (SOD) activity and increased superoxide anion concentrations [53]. Confirming these findings, the treatment of intrauterine undernourished rats with both vitamins C and E promoted reduction in the blood pressure levels, and the antihypertensive effects of these antioxidant vitamins were accompanied by improved endothelium-dependent vasodilation and decreased superoxide anion concentration [54]. In addition, we have found that NADPH oxidase inhibition attenuated superoxide anion generation and ameliorated vascular function in rats submitted to intrauterine undernutrition. Although it is not clear which mechanisms are responsible for the increase in NADPH oxidase activity, a decrease in superoxide anion generation after losartan treatment associated with an increased production of angiotensin II was observed, suggesting a role of angiotensin II-mediated superoxide production via activation of NADPH oxidase [41]. Clinical studies also described oxidative imbalances associated with fetal programming. In fact, Gupta et al. [55] demonstrated that the activity of the SOD, catalase, and glutathione was lower, indicating deficient antioxidant defense mechanism in cord blood of the newborn with low birth weight. Furthermore, there is evidence of oxidative stress in low-birth-weight children as evidenced by increased lipid peroxidation [56]. The same authors also found increased erythrocyte SOD activity in these children, suggesting an important compensatory mechanism that protects these children against the excessive production of superoxide radicals [56]. Although a mechanism was not identified for the increased oxidative status found a decade after the insult caused by adverse fetal life, these observations contribute to a better understanding of the link between birth weight and later development of hypertension, and they have implications for health risks in children.

References

1. Barker DJ, Winter PD, Osmond C et al (1989) Weight in infancy and death from ischaemic heart disease. Lancet 2:577–580
2. Roseboom TJ, van der Meulen JH, Ravelli AC et al (2001) Effects of prenatal exposure to the Dutch famine on adult disease in later life: an overview. Twin Res 4:293–298
3. Gluckman PD, Hanson MA (2004) The developmental origins of the metabolic syndrome. Trends Endocrinol Metab 15:183–187
4. McMillen IC, Robinson JS (2005) Developmental origins of the metabolic syndrome: prediction. Plast Program Physiol Rev 85:571–633
5. Jarvelin M-R (2000) Fetal and infant markers of adult heart disease. Heart 84:219–226
6. Brenner BM, Garcia DL, Anderson S (1998) Glomeruli and blood pressure: less of one, more the other? Am J Hypertens 1:335–347
7. Schreuder M, Delemarre-van de Waal H, Van Wijk A (2006) Consequences of intrauterine growth restriction for the kidney. Kidney Blood Press Res 29:108–125
8. Konje JC, Bell SC, Morton JJ, deChazal R, Taylor D (1996) Human fetal kidney morphometry during gestation and the relationship between weight, kidney morphometry and plasma active renin concentration at birth. Clin Sci 91:169–175
9. Spencer J, Wang Z, Hoy W (2001) Low birth weight and reduced renal volume in Aboriginal children. Am J Kidney Dis 375:915–920
10. Feig DI, Nakagawa T, Karumanchi SA (2004) Hypothesis: uric acid, nephron number, and the pathogenesis of essential hypertension. Kidney Int 66:281–287
11. Hoy WE, Hughson MD, Bertram JF et al (2005) Nephron number, hypertension, renal disease, and renal failure. J Am Soc Nephrol 16:2557–2564
12. Giapros V, Drougia A, Hotoura E et al (2006) Kidney growth in small-for-gestational-age infants: evidence of early accelerated renal growth. Nephrol Dial Transplant 21:3422–3427
13. Hoy WE, Rees M, Kile M et al (1999) A new dimension to the Barker hypothesis: low birth weight and susceptibility to renal disease. Kidney Int 56:1072–1077
14. Nelson RG, Morgenstern H, Bennett PH (1998) Birth weight and renal disease in Pima Indians with type 2 diabetes mellitus. Am J Epidemiol 148:650–656
15. Monge M, García-Nieto VM, Domenech E et al (1998) Study of renal metabolic disturbances related to renal lithiasis at school age in very-low-birth-weight children. Nephron 79:269–273
16. Giapros V, Papadimitriou P, Challa A, Andronikou S (2007) The effect of intrauterine growth retardation on renal function in the first two months of life. Nephrol Dial Transplant 22:96–103
17. Franco MC, Nishida SK, Sesso R (2008) GFR estimated from cystatin C versus creatinine in children born small for gestational age. Am J Kidney Dis 51:925–932
18. Hoek FJ, Kemperman FA, Krediet RT (2003) A comparison between cystatin C, plasma creatinine and the Cockcroft and Gault formula for the estimation of glomerular filtration rate. Nephrol Dial Transplant 18:2024–2031
19. Coll E, Botey A, Alvarez L (2000) Serum cystatin C as a new marker for non invasive estimation of glomerular filtration rate and as a marker for early renal impairment. Am J Kidney Dis 36:29–34
20. Filler G, Bokenkamp A, Hofmann W et al (2005) Cystatin C as a marker of GFR-history, indications, and future research. Clin Biochem 38:1–8
21. Merlet-Benichou C, Gilbert T, Muffat MJ et al (1994) Intrauterine growth retardation leads to a permanent nephron deficit in the rat. Pediatr Nephrol 8:175–180
22. Woods LL (2000) Fetal origins of adult hypertension: a renal mechanism? Curr Opin Nephrol Hypertens 9:419–425
23. Langley-Evans SC, Welham SJM, Jackson AA (1999) Fetal exposure to a maternal low protein diet impairs nephrogenesis and promotes hypertension in the rat. Life Sci 64:965–974

24. Nwagwu MO, Cook A, Langley-Evans SC (2000) Evidence of progressive deterioration of renal function in rats exposed to a maternal low-protein diet in utero. Br J Nutr 83:79–85

25. McMillen IC, Robinson JS (2005) Developmental origins of the metabolic syndrome: prediction, plasticity, and programming. Physiol Rev 85:571–633

26. Lucas SRR, Gil ZF, Silva VLC, Miraglia SM (1991) Functional and morphometric evaluation of intrauterine undernutrition on kidney development of the progeny. Braz J Med Biol Res 24:967–970

27. Lucas SRR, Silva VLC, Miraglia SM, Gil FZ (1997) Functional and morphometric evaluation of offspring kidney after intrauterine undernutrition. Pediatr Nephrol 11:719–723

28. Lucas SRR, Miraglia SM, Gil FZ, Coimbra TM (2001) Intrauterine food restriction as a determinant of nephrosclerosis. Am J Kidney Dis 37:467–476

29. Guron G, Friberg P (2000) An intact renin–angiotensin system is a prerequisite for normal renal development. J Hypertens 18:123–137

30. Franco MCP, Nigro D, Fortes ZB et al (2003) Intrauterine undernutrition–renal and vascular origin of hypertension. Cardiovasc Res 60:228–234

31. Woods LL, Ingelfinger JR, Nyengaard JR, Rasch R (2001) Maternal protein restriction suppresses the newborn renin–angiotensin system and programs adult hypertension in rats. Pediatr Res 49:460–467

32. Zandi-Nejad K, Luyckx VA, Brenner BM (2006) Adult hypertension and kidney disease: the role of fetal programming. Hypertension 47:502–508

33. Manning J, Vehaskari VM (2001) Low birth weight associated adult hypertension in the rat. Pediatr Nephrol 16:417–422

34. Manning J, Beutler K, Knepper MA, Vehaskari VM (2002) Upregulation of renal BSC1 and TSC in prenatally programmed hypertension. Am J Physiol 283:F202–F206

35. Leeson CPM, Whincup PH, Cook DG et al (1997) Flow-mediated dilatation in 9–11 year old children: the influence of intrauterine and childhood factors. Circulation 96:2233–2238

36. Franco MC, Christofalo DM, Sawaya AL et al (2006) Effects of low birth weight in 8- to 13-year-old children: implications in endothelial function and uric acid levels. Hypertension 48(1):45–50

37. Goodfellow J, Bellamy MF, Gorman ST et al (1998) Endothelial function is impaired in fit young adults of low birth weight. Cardiovasc Res 40:600–606

38. Leeson CPM, Kattenhorn M, Morley R et al (2001) Impact of low birth weight and cardiovascular risk factors on endothelial function in early adult life. Circulation 103:1264–1268

39. Holemans K, Gerber R, Meurrens K et al (1999) Maternal food restriction in the second half of pregnancy affects vascular function but not blood pressure of rat female offspring. Br J Nutr 81:73–79

40. Ozaki T, Nishina P, Hanson MA, Poston L (2001) Dietary restriction in pregnant rats causes gender-related hypertension and vascular dysfunction in offspring. J Physiol 530(1):141–158

41. Franco MC, Akamine EH, Di Marco GS et al (2003) NADPH oxidase and enhanced superoxide generation in intrauterine undernourished rats: involvement of the renin-angiotensin system. Cardiovasc Res 59:767–775

42. Franco MCP, Dantas APV, Arruda RMP et al (2002) Intrauterine undernutrition: expression and activity of the endothelial nitric oxide synthase in male and female adult offspring. Cardiovasc Res 56:145–153

43. Franco MCP, Arruda RMMP, Fortes ZB et al (2002) Severe nutritional restriction in pregnant rats aggravates hypertension, altered vascular reactivity and renal development in spontaneously hypertensive rats offspring. J Cardiovasc Pharmacol 29(3):369–377

44. Lamireau D, Nuyt AM, Hou X et al (2002) Altered vascular function in fetal programming of hypertension. Stroke 33(12):2992–2998

45. Franco MC, Akamine EH, Rebouças N et al (2007) Long-term effects of intrauterine malnutrition on vascular function in female offspring: implications of oxidative stress. Life Sci 80(8):709–715

46. Alves GM, Barão MA, Nascimento Gomes G et al (2002) L-Arginine effects on blood pressure and renal function of intrauterine restricted rats. Pediatr Nephrol 17(10):856–862

47. Franco MC, Fortes ZB, Akamine EH et al (2004) Tetrahydrobiopterin improves endothelial dysfunction and vascular oxidative stress in microvessels of intrauterine undernourished rats. J Physiol 558:239–248
48. Rutherford RA, McCarthy A, Sullivan MH et al (1995) Nitric oxide synthase in human placenta and umbilical cord from normal, intrauterine growth-retarded and pre-eclamptic pregnancies. Br J Pharmacol 116:3099–3109
49. Hata T, Hashimoto M, Manabe A et al (1998) Maternal and fetal nitric oxide synthesis is decreased in pregnancies with small for gestational age infants. Hum Reprod 13:1070–1073
50. Schiessl B, Strasburger C, Bidlingmaier M et al (2006) Plasma and urine concentrations of nitrite/nitrate and cyclic Guanosinemonophosphate in intrauterine growth restricted and pre-eclamptic pregnancies. Arch Gynecol Obstet 274:150–154
51. Franco MC, Higa EM, D'Almeida V et al (2007) Homocysteine and nitric oxide are related to blood pressure and vascular function in small-for-gestational-age children. Hypertension 50(2):396–402
52. Harrison DG (1997) Cellular and molecular mechanism of endothelial cell dysfunction. J Clin Invest 100:2153–2157
53. Franco MCP, Dantas APV, Akamine HE et al (2002) Enhanced oxidative stress as a potential mechanism underlying the programming of hypertension *in utero*. J Cardiovasc Pharmacol 40:501–509
54. Franco Mdo C, Akamine EH, Aparecida de Oliveira M et al (2003) Vitamins C and E improve endothelial dysfunction in intrauterine-undernourished rats by decreasing vascular superoxide anion concentration. J Cardiovasc Pharmacol 42(2):211–217
55. Gupta P, Narang M, Banerjee BD, Basu S (2004) Oxidative stress in term small for gestational age neonates born to undernourished mothers: a case control study. BMC Pediatr 20:4–14
56. Franco MC, Kawamoto EM, Gorjão R et al (2007) Biomarkers of oxidative stress and antioxidant status in children born small for gestational age: evidence of lipid peroxidation. Pediatr Res 62:204–208

Hemodynamic and Mechanical Factors Acting on Arteries

7

Pierre Boutouyrie, Hélène Beaussier, and Stéphane Laurent

7.1 Mechanical Forces Acting on Arteries

Arteries are permanently exposed to mechanical stress [1]. Mechanical stress can be divided according to its nature, either tensile stress or shear stress. Tensile stress corresponds to changes in dimension according to changes in forces applied on the vessel. Shear stress is of a different nature; it corresponds to the friction of viscous fluid (here the blood) on the inner surface of the vessel (here the endothelium). It is to be noted that direct measurement of stress is difficult in vivo and that stress is most of the time deduced from stretch (elongation) and force (derived from pressure). Stress can also be derived from mechanical modelling.

7.1.1 Tensile Stress

Tensile stress is represented by a tensor comprising stress along the three axes in a cylindrical symmetry [2]: elongation stress (z axis), circumferential stress (circumference) and compressive stress (radius). Because arteries are markedly anisotropic (i.e. different mechanical properties along the axes of the vessel wall), the behaviour of the artery is complex and best described by energy function [3–6].

P. Boutouyrie (✉) • S. Laurent
Department of Pharmacology, Université Paris Descartes, HEGP,
Assistance Publique Hôpitaux de Paris, Institut national de la santé et de la recherche médicale (INSERM) U970, 20 rue Leblanc, Paris 75015, France
e-mail: pierre.boutouyrie@egp.aphp.fr

H. Beaussier
Department of Clinical Research, Hôpital Saint Joseph, Paris, France

© Springer International Publishing Switzerland 2015
A. Berbari, G. Mancia (eds.), *Arterial Disorders:*
Definition, Clinical Manifestations, Mechanisms and Therapeutic Approaches,
DOI 10.1007/978-3-319-14556-3_7

7.1.2 Longitudinal Stress

Arteries are stretched longitudinally. When arteries are dissected and removed from the body, their length decreases by an average of 20 % [2]. Arteries are maintained in place by tethering from side branches, adherence of the adventitia to surrounding tissues, so it is questionable whether the arterial wall bears all the stress involved by the elongation [6]. Although measurement of longitudinal stretch is possible experimentally [2], or noninvasively by speckle tracking [7], its role in physiology is still debated. There is at least one arterial segment which is very influenced by longitudinal stretch, the ascending aorta, because of the heart pulling on the aorta during systole. The influence of longitudinal stretch on the global behaviour of the aorta is still a matter of active research.

7.1.3 Circumferential Wall Stress

Here again, arteries exhibit residual stress at zero pressure. The artery remains cylindrical at zero pressure, and when cut longitudinally, the arterial segment ring opens with an opening angle. This angle depends from residual stress and conditions of the behaviour of the artery [8]. Then stress is proportional to the blood pressure, proportional to diameter and inversely proportional to the thickness of the vessel. This is the classical Laplace law (Fig. 7.1), generalized by the Lamé equations. The elastic modulus in the circumferential direction is in the range of 10^6 Pa. The typical strain is in the range of 10 % during cardiac cycle for elastic arteries. It decreases when getting farther from the heart [9, 10].

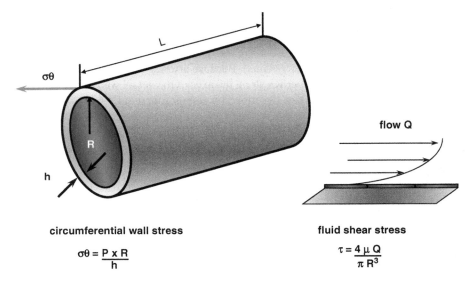

circumferential wall stress

$$\sigma\theta = \frac{P \times R}{h}$$

fluid shear stress

$$\tau = \frac{4\,\mu\,Q}{\pi\,R^3}$$

Fig. 7.1 Forces exerting on arteries

7.1.4   Radial Stress

Although arteries are mainly composed of water and thus hardly compressible, the arterial wall is submitted to compressive stress during life. The compressive modulus is very high, similar to that of water, in the range of 10^9 Pa, thus radial strain is negligible [11].

7.1.5   Shear Stress

Shear stress is linked to the friction of blood on the endothelium. Blood velocity is relatively low (lower than 2 m/s), and blood has a complex viscosity behaviour, being non-Newtonian, i.e., viscosity decreases with increasing shear rates. Altogether, shear stress has a low amplitude, in the range of 10^1 Pa, albeit of great physiological importance because determining the secretion of active substances by the endothelium. An extensive recent review has been published on the topic [12].

7.2   Integrated Wall Mechanics

The main function of large arteries is to conduct blood from the heart to the organs that necessitate a certain amount of blood for performing their task. This function makes it necessary to have a potential energy allowing directing the blood flow toward the organ which needs it at a certain time. This potential energy is represented by blood pressure (equivalent to the elevated water tank). Moreover, the circulation is alternative, the heart pumping the blood during one third of the time (systole) and resting two thirds of the time (diastole). Nevertheless, blood is flowing constantly throughout the body, with a pulsatile pattern on the arterial site and more continuous on the venous side. The second most important function of the arteries is to store energy during the heart contraction through elastic deformation and to restore this energy during diastole. The thermodynamic advantage of such system is huge, because elasticity buffers the oscillations of pressure generated by the heart, and pressure has a high energetic cost. Second, energy storage and restitution are almost at zero energetic cost because arteries have pseudo pure elastic behaviour (energy dissipation through wall viscosity is small in vivo on healthy arteries [13]). Last, the volume of blood stored under elastic deformation during systole acts as an instant reservoir, allowing very fast adaptation of flow to increased demand in some territories. For instance, if the whole blood flow was generated by the heart, any acute increase in blood demand by exercise, for instance, would have to be compensated immediately by the pump (the heart), at the cost of increased ventricular work. The electric equivalent is a well-designed sound amplifier, with lamps or transistor giving limited current, loading capacitors with very fast current restitution, buffering transient needs of current generated by the music or the bad impedance curves of loudspeakers.

The high integration of regulation of blood flow is also observed at the level of the arterial wall. The arterial wall is rich in vascular smooth muscle cells. These cells are sensitive to stress. They are able to contract in response to increase in stress (myogenic response) [14]. This is of very high importance on medium to small arteries, because any increase in pressure tending to dilate the artery will be counteracted by a vasoconstriction, limiting the effect of pressure. As said before, this phenomenon is particularly marked at the level of medium to small arteries and plays a major role in the autoregulation of local blood flows in organs such as the kidney, the brain and the digestive tract.

Arteries are also sensitive to shear stress. Through the seminal work of Furchgott [15] and followers, the endothelium has been shown to be indispensable to the modulation of the effect of several substances (acetylcholine, bradykinin, etc.) since their vasoconstrictive effect is reversed to vasodilatation in the presence of intact endothelium [12]. This seminal observation has been shown to be related to the secretion of NO by the endothelium. Since then, many endothelium-derived substances, either vasodilatory (NO, prostacyclin, EDHF) or vasoconstrictive (endothelin), have been put in evidence. One of the major physiological stimuli for endothelial activation is blood flow. Increase in blood flow through peripheral vasodilatation increases shear stress at the level of the upstream arterial bed, leading to the paracrine secretion of vasoactive substances, mainly NO [12]. The resultant is a potent vasodilatation, appearing with a delay of several seconds and lasting several minutes after cessation of the peripheral vasodilatation. When combined with myogenic tone, peripheral blood flows are highly autoregulated, and the role of large arteries is to provide a steady load while at the same time buffering pressure oscillations and allowing a permanent reservoir pressure for providing adequate flow to organs.

Small arteries and arterioles are predominantly muscular. Because of their small diameter, even small vasoconstrictions will induce large increase in vascular resistance because of its dependence on the third power of diameter. Thus small arteries and arterioles are the major site of peripheral resistance. These arteries have also very prominent myogenic response and endothelium-modulated response.

7.2.1   Trophic Response to Mechanical Stress

Mechanical stress is the major trophic factor for large arteries. Mechanical stress induces synthesis of extracellular matrix, smooth muscle cell growth, proliferation and migration until a new equilibrium is found. The regulated parameter appears to be the circumferential wall stress. The potency of pulsatile stress is much larger than steady stress [16]. In humans, the associations of large arteries remodelling with local pulse pressure have been found to be stronger than with mean blood pressure [17].

7.3   Small-Large Arteries Crosstalk

It is convenient to interpret the circulation by opposing large arteries (conduit, compliance) to small arteries (resistance). This view is of course a caricature. As developed before, the function of large arteries is to conduct blood, buffer pulsatile

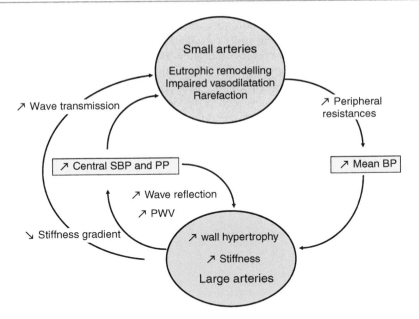

Fig. 7.2 Large and small arteries interplay

pressure and provide a reservoir pressure to maintain blood flow. Another function of large arteries is to provide sufficient pressure wave reflection to filter them out and maintain them low at the site of medium-sized arteries [18]. Indeed, because of their elasticity, the pressure wave propagates at a finite speed and partially reflects on bifurcations and geometric patterns. The role of the stiffness gradient from the central compartment (the more elastic) to the periphery (the stiffer) helps to confine reflected waves within the large arteries and to protect small arteries from excessive pulsatility. This is a double-edged sword, because more proximal reflection can alter LV function; however, less distal reflection will decrease pulsatility in the microvasculature and protect small arteries from remodelling and weakening [18]. On the other hand, remodelling of small arteries and subsequent vasoconstriction will increase blood pressure and wave reflections and therefore contribute to stiffen the proximal compartment (Fig. 7.2). Medium-sized arteries sit in between, and the lack of stiffening with ageing and blood pressure of medium-sized arteries has been seen as a compensatory mechanism to compensate for the increased proximal stiffness.

For these reasons, a real crosstalk between large and small arteries occurs during physiological ageing and cardiovascular diseases [19] (Fig. 7.2).

Alteration of endothelial function and myogenic response must be integrated in the scene, because they occur in parallel with alterations of the wall properties. The general view is that similar functionality can be achieved with a higher energy cost, the LV being the only source of energy; it will hypertrophy and alter its diastolic and then systolic function to achieve similar peripheral blood flow. The second view is that for similar peripheral perfusion, stiff vessels lacking autoregulation will lead to increased perfusion pressure in order to maintain sufficient blood flow to organs. Indeed, increased arterial stiffness has been shown to precede hypertension in the Framingham heart study [20]. The final view is that when the organism is subjected to stress because of concomitant illness (dehydration, heat shock, etc.), the autoregulation of blood flow to organs such as the kidney, the brain and the heart will be overrun, and such a situation which should be easily overcome by otherwise healthy subjects will lead to organ failure in patients with increased stiffness and dysfunctional autoregulation of arterial calibre.

Conclusion

The arterial system is constantly subject to hemodynamic stresses. These stresses play a paramount role in physiology and pathology. Large and small arteries are narrowly interconnected in terms of physiology. Ageing and cardiovascular risk factors alter the interplay between small and large arteries, leading to disease.

Glossary

Compliance Change in volume for a change in pressure. Expresses the elasticity of a chamber.

Distensibility Compliance normalized to initial volume.

Elastic modulus Either incremental elastic modulus (if reference dimension unknown) or Young's elastic modulus (if reference dimension known). Ratio of stress to stretch: expresses the stiffness of the wall material.

Pressure Force per unit of surface.

Stress Force per unit of surface (same unit as pressure).

Stretch Elongation, defined from a reference dimension, synonymous to strain.

References

1. Nichols WW, O'Rourke MF (2011) McDonald's blood flow in arteries: theoretical, experimental and clinical principles. Hodder Arnold, London, pp 195–225
2. Han HC, Fung YC (1995) Longitudinal strain of canine and porcine aortas. J Biomech 28: 637–641
3. Wilson JS, Baek S, Humphrey JD (2012) Importance of initial aortic properties on the evolving regional anisotropy, stiffness and wall thickness of human abdominal aortic aneurysms. J R Soc Interface 9:2047–2058
4. Masson I, Beaussier H, Boutouyrie P et al (2011) Carotid artery mechanical properties and stresses quantified using in vivo data from normotensive and hypertensive humans. Biomech Model Mechanobiol 10:867–882
5. Humphrey JD, Yin FC (1987) A new constitutive formulation for characterizing the mechanical behavior of soft tissues. Biophys J 52:563–570
6. Humphrey JD, Eberth JF, Dye WW, Gleason RL (2009) Fundamental role of axial stress in compensatory adaptations by arteries. J Biomech 42:1–8

7. Jackson ZS, Gotlieb AI, Langille BL (2002) Wall tissue remodeling regulates longitudinal tension in arteries. Circ Res 90:918–925
8. Fung YC (1991) What are the residual stresses doing in our blood vessels? Ann Biomed Eng 19:237–249
9. Boutouyrie P, Laurent S, Benetos A et al (1992) Opposing effects of ageing on distal and proximal large arteries in hypertensives. J Hypertens Suppl 10:S87–S91
10. Benetos A, Laurent S, Hoeks AP et al (1993) Arterial alterations with aging and high blood pressure. A noninvasive study of carotid and femoral arteries. Arterioscler Thromb 13:90–97
11. Nichols WW, O'Rourke MF (2005) McDonald's blood flow in arteries: theoretical, experimental and clinical principles. Hodder Arnold, London
12. Chiu JJ, Chien S (2011) Effects of disturbed flow on vascular endothelium: pathophysiological basis and clinical perspectives. Physiol Rev 91:327–387
13. Boutouyrie P, Bezie Y, Lacolley P et al (1997) In vivo/in vitro comparison of rat abdominal aorta wall viscosity. Influence of endothelial function. Arterioscler Thromb Vasc Biol 17:1346–1355
14. Davis MJ, Hill MA (1999) Signaling mechanisms underlying the vascular myogenic response. Physiol Rev 79:387–423
15. Furchgott RF, Zawadzki JV (1980) The obligatory role of endothelial cells in the relaxation of arterial smooth muscle by acetylcholine. Nature 288:373–376
16. Lehoux S, Castier Y, Tedgui A (2006) Molecular mechanisms of the vascular responses to haemodynamic forces. J Intern Med 259:381–392
17. Boutouyrie P, Bussy C, Lacolley P et al (1999) Association between local pulse pressure, mean blood pressure, and large-artery remodeling. Circulation 100:1387–1393
18. Briet M, Boutouyrie P, Laurent S, London GM (2012) Arterial stiffness and pulse pressure in CKD and ESRD. Kidney Int 82:388–400
19. Laurent S, Boutouyrie P (2015) Structural factor of hypertension: large and small artery alterations. Circ Res. doi: 10.1161/CIRCRESAHA.116.303596
20. Kaess BM, Rong J, Larson MG et al (2012) Aortic stiffness, blood pressure progression, and incident hypertension. JAMA 308:875–881

Role of Metabolic Factors: Lipids, Glucose/Insulin Intolerance

8

Guanghong Jia, Annayya R. Aroor, and James R. Sowers

8.1 Introduction

The main cause of arterial disease (AD) is hardening of the arteries or atherosclerosis due to a thickening of the artery lining from fatty deposits or plaques. There are several different symptoms, depending on the location of the AD. It most commonly affects the arteries in the heart, brain, and legs [1]. Diabetes is associated with a two- to fourfold increase in the risk of developing coronary artery disease (CAD). Diabetic patients presenting with unstable angina are more likely to develop myocardial infarction. The mortality caused by myocardial infarction in diabetic patients is more than in nondiabetic individuals [2]. Similarly, diabetes increases the risk of stroke and stroke-related mortality [3]. Meanwhile, diabetes is a major risk factor for the development of peripheral arterial disease, which is typically caused by progressive narrowing of the arteries in the lower extremities [4]. Thus, AD is the major cause of mortality and significant morbidity in diabetes and cardiorenal metabolic syndrome (CRS).

G. Jia • A.R. Aroor
Division of Endocrinology, Diabetes, and Metabolism, Diabetes Cardiovascular Center,
Department of Medicine, University of Missouri School of Medicine, Columbia, MO, USA

Harry S. Truman Memorial Veterans Hospital, Columbia, MO, USA

J.R. Sowers, MD (✉)
Division of Endocrinology, Diabetes, and Metabolism, Diabetes Cardiovascular Center,
Department of Medicine, University of Missouri School of Medicine, Columbia, MO, USA

Department of Medical Pharmacology and Physiology, University of Missouri,
D109 Diabetes Center HSC, One Hospital Drive, Columbia, MO 65212, USA

Harry S. Truman Memorial Veterans Hospital, Columbia, MO, USA
e-mail: sowersj@health.missouri.edu

© Springer International Publishing Switzerland 2015
A. Berbari, G. Mancia (eds.), *Arterial Disorders:*
Definition, Clinical Manifestations, Mechanisms and Therapeutic Approaches,
DOI 10.1007/978-3-319-14556-3_8

Epidemiologic evidence supports the hypothesis that diabetes adds to the impact of individual risk factors, such as hypertension and hyperlipidemia, for the prediction of excess AD [3]. It was suggested that integrative effects of elevated glucose, insulin, and triglycerides may have a considerable impact on AD and play an important role in the early pathophysiology of AD in patients with type 2 diabetes [5]. In individuals with the CRS and those with clinical diabetes, AD has been observed in all age groups, including children. Indeed, obese children prematurely manifest signs of AD [6]. In individuals 40 years and older, multiple logistic and linear regression analyses from a total of 2,188 individuals demonstrated that AD was independently associated with insulin resistance (IR) in middle-aged adults [7]. In elderly people without diabetes mellitus, the Rotterdam study found that impaired fasting glucose was associated with increased AD [8]. Therefore, glycemic control, low-density cholesterol-lowering therapy, blood pressure lowering, and comprehensive approaches targeting multiple metabolic risk factors to reduce cardiovascular risk may therefore account for the clinical beneficial effects in obese and diabetic patients with AD. In the present review, we will discuss the roles of metabolic factors in the pathogenesis of AD and provide a better understanding of potential therapeutic strategies.

8.2   Risk Factors for AD in CRS

Several metabolic risk factors such as hyperglycemia, IR, dyslipidemia, obesity, fructose, and uric acid may initiate and accelerate artery impairment (Fig. 8.1).

8.2.1   Hyperglycemia and IR

Hyperglycemia, a hallmark of diabetes, has been implicated in the development of vascular cell dysfunction including vascular smooth muscle cells (VSMCs) and endothelial cells (ECs) via mechanisms of protein kinase C (PKC) activation, activation of the hexosamine, and advanced glycation end products (AGEs). These pathways are believed to mediate vascular dysfunction through the unifying mechanism of reactive oxygen species (ROS) overproduction, most notably increases in O_2^- [9]. Studies have also shown that elevated glucose concentration may activate the tissue renin–angiotensin–aldosterone system (RAAS), and this plays an important role in the pathogenesis of vascular complications of diabetes [10, 11]. In vivo exposure of healthy human subjects to an acute glucose load leads to attenuated endothelium-dependent vascular relaxation [12]. This impaired endothelial relaxation is associated with increased oxidative stress, adhesion molecule expression, vascular permeability, and plasma levels of plasminogen activator inhibitor-1 [12]. In vitro, both high glucose and angiotensin II (Ang II) induced a progressive increase in Ang II receptor type 1 receptor 1 (AT-1R) expression on the cultured human ECs. Furthermore, high glucose enhanced Ang II-mediated peroxisome proliferation-activated receptor-γ inactivation and expression of pro-inflammatory adhesion molecules via signaling through the AT-1R [13]. With chronic exposure to elevated

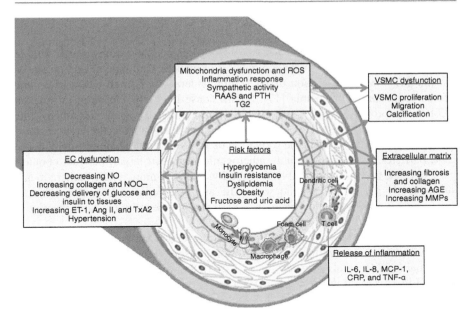

Fig. 8.1 Proposed the interaction of metabolic risk factors, adaptive metabolic response, and AD in CRS. Risk factors for AD such as hyperglycemia, insulin resistance, dyslipidemia, fructose, and uric acid induce the adaptive metabolic responses including mitochondria dysfunction, ROS, inflammation response, sympathetic activity, RAAS, PTH, and TG2, resulting in the pathophysiological abnormalities in ECs, VSMCs, and extracellular matrix on CRS. *Abbreviations*: *AD* arterial disease, *RAAS* renin–angiotensin–aldosterone system, *PTH* Parathyroid hormone, *AGE* advanced glycation end products, *TG2* tissue transglutaminase, *ROS* reactive oxygen species, *IL* interleukin, *TNF* tumor necrosis factor, *NO* nitric oxide, $ONOO^-$ peroxynitrite, *ET-1* endothelin-1, *Ang II* angiotensin II, *TxA2* thromboxane A2, *MCP-1* monocyte chemotactic protein-1, *CRP* C-reactive protein, *MMP* matrix metalloproteinase

plasma glucose, the resulting glucotoxicity may activate mitogen-activated protein kinase (MAPK) thus increasing secretion of inflammatory cytokines and inhibiting phosphatidylinositol 3-kinase (PI3K)/protein kinase B (Akt) signaling leading to reduced nitric oxide (NO) production and endothelial dysfunction [13].

IR, a metabolic risk factor in patients with normal glucose tolerance and even after adjustment for known risk factor such as low-density lipoprotein (LDL), triglycerides (TG), high-density lipoprotein cholesterol (HDL), and systolic blood pressure, is frequently present in obesity, hypertension, dyslipidemia, and AD [14]. In nonobese subjects without diabetes, IR predicted the development of cardiovascular disease (CVD) independently of other known risk factors. In another group of subjects without diabetes or impaired glucose tolerance, patients with IR had a 2.5-fold increase in CVD risk. These data indicate that IR itself promotes atherogenesis [15]. Our study has found that abnormal insulin metabolic signaling is an important contributor to AD. In this regard, IR is typically accompanied by reduced PI3K-NO pathway and heightened MAPK-endothelin-1 (ET-1) pathway [16].

8.2.2 Dyslipidemia and Obesity

Lipid abnormalities play an important part in raising the cardiovascular risk in patients with diabetes. The main components of diabetic dyslipidemia are increased plasma TG, low concentration of HDL, preponderance of small dense LDL, and excessive postprandial lipemia [17]. Small, dense LDL, the elevation in remnant TG-rich lipoprotein particles, and the low HDL are the most powerful atherogenic components. The coexistence of these factors strongly aggravates the lipid accumulation in the arterial wall and the formation of atherosclerotic plaques. Small, dense LDL particles are held to be more atherogenic than their larger, buoyant counterparts because they are more liable to oxidation and may more readily adhere to and subsequently invade the arterial wall. The atherogenicity of LDL may also be enhanced by nonenzymatic glycation [18]. Thus, the benefits of statin therapy in type 2 diabetics can no longer be questioned.

Obesity has a strong association with atherogenic dyslipidemia. In a large series of 26,000 overweight children, concentrations of one or more of the lipids were abnormal in 32 %, total cholesterol in 14.1 %, LDL-C in 15.8 %, HDL-C in 11.1 %, and TG in 14.3 % of those in whom data were available [19]. Indeed, overweight and obesity are associated with development of CRS which is a constellation of risk factors, such as IR, dyslipidemia, and high blood pressure [16]. The development of AD in obese patients can be attributed to a number of factors including proinflammatory cytokines, inappropriate activation of RAAS, vasoconstriction from increased sympathetic nervous system (SNS) activation, and dysregulation in adipokine production and secretion [20]. These data suggest that obesity and dyslipidemia are involved in AD in CRS.

8.2.3 Fructose and Uric Acid

The increasing fructose consumption has led to a rise in obesity from 13 to 34 % since 1960 and the subsequent rise in diagnosed type 2 diabetes from 5 to 8 % since 1988 [21]. In children, the intake of artificially sweetened beverages was found to be positively associated with adiposity [22]. A prospective cohort analyses of non-diabetic women in the Nurses' Health Study II concluded that higher consumption of sugar-sweetened beverages is associated with greater magnitude of weight gain and an increased risk for the development of type 2 diabetes [22]. In the Framingham Heart Study, the relationship between soft drink consumption and cardiovascular risk factors was evaluated in 6,039 participants; consumption of more than one can of soft drink per day was significantly associated with the prevalence of CRS [23]. Thus, fructose has been implicated in promoting obesity and CRS by altering appetite, inducing leptin resistance, and resulting in increased food intake. Recently, The Third National Health and Nutrition Examination Survey (NHANES III) report has indicated that consumption of sugar-sweetened beverages is significantly associated with plasma uric acid concentrations [23]. Thus, a novel hypothesis has been proposing to link fructose intake, hyperuricemia, and AD in CRS.

8.3   EC Dysfunction Initiates AD

Forming a vast interface between blood and surrounding tissues, the endothelium forms a monolayer comprising the innermost lining of blood vessels. The arterial endothelium provides a continuous barrier between the elements of blood and the arterial wall and is a critical component to vascular homeostasis, actively responding to biochemical and physical stimuli through the release of a diverse set of vasoactive substances [24]. Endothelial damage and thickening of the intima-media layers induced by risk factors we discussed above are early events in the AD process. For example, LDL particles invade the endothelium and become oxidized, creating risk for a subsequent inflammatory response and ultimately CVD. Monocytes enter the artery wall from the bloodstream with platelets adhering to the area of insult, differentiate into macrophages, and eventually form foam cells. Foam cells die and further propagate the inflammatory process [25] (Fig. 8.1).

NO, a most significant endothelium-derived mediator, plays multiple roles in preventing AD. NO diffuses into neighboring VSMCs, activating guanylyl cyclase and producing cyclic guanosine monophosphate (cGMP) and activating kinases responsible for vascular relaxation [16]. NO also inhibits platelet aggregation, smooth muscle cell proliferation, and nuclear transcription of leukocyte-adhesion molecules including vascular cell adhesion molecule (VCAM) and intercellular adhesion molecule (ICAM) [9]. Indeed, vascular homeostasis is tightly controlled by EC secreting the vasodilatory substances, such as NO, endothelium-derived hyperpolarizing factor (EDHF), prostacyclin (PGI$_2$), and vasoconstrictory substances, such as ET-1, Ang II, and thromboxane A2 (TxA2) [26]. These EC-secreting vasoactivity substances have been proposed to mediate the AD in CRS, including continued activation of the SNS; increased production and activity of vasoconstrictors, such as ET-1, Ang II, and TxA2; and impaired endothelium-dependent relaxation [27]. Thus, endothelial dysfunction has been suggested as a common underlying mechanism in AD with IR, hyperinsulinemia, and CRS.

8.4   Dysregulation of VSMCs and Vascular Extracellular Matrix Promotes AD

Following the EC dysfunction, the metabolic abnormalities that characterize diabetes, hyperglycemia, free fatty acids, and IR provoke the impairment of the function and structures in blood vessels include VSMC and extracellular vascular matrix (Fig. 8.1).

8.4.1   VSMC Dysfunction

The impact of CRS on vascular function is not only limited to the ECs but also to VSMCs, which are the predominant cell type found in the arterial wall and are essential for the structural and functional integrity of the vessel. Diabetes increases PKC activity, NF-kappaB (NF-κB) production, and generation of oxygen-derived free radicals in VSMCs and heightens migration of VSMCs into atherosclerotic lesions, where they replicate and produce extracellular matrix—important steps in mature lesion formation [28]. Dysregulation of VSMC function is exacerbated by impairments in SNS function. Studies from the Zucker obese insulin-resistant rat have shown that VSMCs from these rats manifested greater concentrations of ROS and impaired activation of the NO/cGMP/protein kinase G (PKG) pathway when compared to VSMC from the lean, insulin-sensitive Zucker rats [29]. Our recent data also showed excessive serine phosphorylation of insulin receptor substrate (IRS-1) as a key mechanism underlying cellular IR in VSMCs. Furthermore, after treatment with aldosterone or Ang II, VSMCs show increased activation of p70 S6 kinase 1 signaling pathway, increased proteasome degradation of IRS-1, and attenuated insulin-induced Akt phosphorylation and glucose uptake [30]. These observations provide a biochemical basis to the IR in VSMCs in the development of AD.

8.4.2   VSMC Calcification

Studies conducted in the United States have revealed that calcium deposits in arterial walls are reported in nearly 30 % of Americans over 45 years of age [31]. Vascular calcification risk factors are similar to those of atherosclerosis including hypertriglyceridemia, increased LDL, decreased HDL, obesity, and hypertension. It has also been shown that diabetes and renal failure contribute significantly to higher risk of accumulation of calcium depositions in the vessel wall [32]. Calcification of vessels reduces their elasticity, affecting hemodynamic parameters of the cardiovascular system. Vascular calcification is an active and complex process that involves numerous mechanisms responsible for calcium deposits in arterial walls. They lead to an increase in arterial stiffness and in pulse wave velocity, which in turn increases CVD morbidity and mortality. We have known that VSMCs can differentiate from a quiescent, contractile phenotype to a proliferative, synthetic phenotype following arterial injury and in atherosclerotic diseases [33]. Indeed, VSMCs are capable of osteoblast transdifferentiation in calcifying arteries [34]. Epidemiological data have shown that higher insulin levels in diabetes can independently predicate arterial calcification [35]. The mechanisms of insulin involved in arterial calcification in these clinical settings are still controversial. Furthermore, it has been demonstrated that insulin enhances the calcification of VSMCs in vitro [36]. In this regard, insulin promotes alkaline phosphatase activity, osteocalcin expression, and the formation of mineralized nodules in VSMCs by increased receptor expression of NF-κB ligand (RANKL) through extracellular signal-regulated protein kinases 1 and 2 (Erk ½) activation [37]. However, others suggest that insulin attenuated VSMC calcification induced by high phosphate conditions [38]. These contradictory results may be explained by different cell types or different experimental conditions.

8.4.3   Elastin, Collagen, and Advanced Glycation End Products

Elastin is the most abundant protein in the walls of the arteries, which are subjected to pulsatile pressure generated by cardiac contraction. Matrix metalloproteinases (MMPs) have an important role in the degradation of elastin [39]. Recently, it was reported that in the arterial vasculature from chronic kidney disease patients, the presence of diabetes markedly upregulated MMP-2 and -9, and this adaption is strongly associated with elastic fiber degradation and AD. The increase in MMPs in diabetic vessels was also accompanied by pronounced generation of angiostatin, and the reduction of microvascular density was associated with impaired vasorelaxation [40]. In addition, the degradation of elastin also induces the overexpression of transforming growth factor beta (TGF-β). TGF-β1 not only plays an important role in osteoblast differentiation but also accelerates the calcification of VSMCs [39]. Meanwhile, hyperglycemia may cause changes in the type or structure of elastin and/or collagen in the arterial wall through nonenzymatic glycosylation of proteins that generate AGE. AGE may form irreversible cross-links between long-lived proteins such as collagen, leading to accumulation of stiffer molecules that are less susceptible to hydrolytic turnover [41]. These data confirm that the interaction among MMPs, elastin, collagen, and AGE plays a key role in the development of AD with CRS.

8.5   Misregulation of Adaptive Metabolic Responses Aggravate to the Progression of AD

Misregulation of an adaptive metabolic response contributes to the risk factors related CRS and dysfunction of ECs, VSMCs, and extracellular vascular matrix in AD (Fig. 8.1).

8.5.1   Mitochondria Dysfunction and ROS

Mitochondria are essential for intermediary metabolism as well as energy production and normally provide more than 90 % of the cellular energy [42]. It has been established that mitochondrial respiratory chain function is responsible for energy metabolism and adenosine triphosphate (ATP) production through the tricarboxylic acid (TCA) cycle, coupling of oxidative phosphorylation (OXPHOS), and electron transfer [43]. Mitochondria dysfunction is recognized as playing a central role in the development of various abnormalities, including disturbed glucose homeostasis, IR, abdominal fat accumulation, dyslipidemia, hypertension, and associated cardiac and renal pathology. ROS production occurs mainly at complex I and complex III in mitochondria [44]. Under conditions of glucose and fatty acid overnutrition, nutrient overflow into cells prompts electrons transferring to oxygen without ATP production and further favors a state of increased ROS, which potentially leads to oxidative damage within mitochondria [45]. Therefore, ROS generated from mitochondria damages proteins, DNA, and lipid in membrane components, which result in mitochondrial dysfunction. Although this review is concerned with mitochondrial ROS, it should be recognized that the considerable amount of ROS is derived from outside of mitochondria, such as oxygen radicals from peroxisomal β-oxidation of fatty acids, nicotinamide adenine dinucleotide phosphate (NADPH) oxidase, xanthine oxidase, arachidonic acid metabolism, microsomal P-450 enzymes, and prooxidant heme molecule [46].

8.5.2 Adaptive Immunity and Inflammation Response

Atherosclerosis is a chronic inflammatory disease of the arterial wall characterized by an innate and adaptive immune system, which is composed of diverse cellular components including granulocytes, mast cells, monocytes, macrophages, dendritic cells (DCs), and natural killer cells [47]. Upon activation, partly in response to immunological stimuli from the local microenvironment as well as systemic circulation, macrophages polarize into classical (M1) or alternative (M2) phenotypes [48]. M1 macrophages are found in advanced lesions where they accumulate a large amount of lipids, which promotes their differentiation into foam cells. Meanwhile, M1 macrophages secrete tumor necrosis factor alpha (TNF-α), interleukin (IL)-6, and metalloproteinases, which exacerbate and destabilize lesion development. However, M2 macrophages predominate in the early stages of atherosclerosis and are characterized by IL-10 secretion and smaller amounts of accumulated lipids; these events are atheroprotective and can reduce plaque development [49].

DC precursors or monocytes are recruited to lesions where they differentiate into DCs. The DC population is heterogeneous and can be divided into four major categories: conventional DCs (cDCs), plasmacytoid DCs (pDCs), monocyte-derived DCs, and Langerhans cells [50]. DC accumulation in regions prone to AD suggests that their recruitment accounts for an initial inflammatory or immune activation. The exact localization and origin of vascular DCs, however, is still under debate [51]. In general, immature and semimature DCs uptake lipids and other intimal antigens, thus preventing them from eliciting pro-inflammatory signaling in other artery wall cells. Toll-like receptor (TLR) ligation by ligands such as oxLDL induces DC maturation. Under hyperlipidemic conditions, lipid uptake and efferocytosis likely lead to DC-foam cell formation, and mature DCs and foam cells emigrate from the vessel wall in a C-C chemokine receptor type 7 (CCR7)-dependent manner, clearing inflammatory cells, lipids, and apoptotic cell debris from the intimal space and preventing necrosis and persistent inflammation. Mature CD11b+ DCs likely expand regulatory T cells (Tregs) and CD4+ effector T cells within the artery wall [52]. CD4$^+$CD25$^+$Foxp3$^+$ Tregs can protect the pro-inflammatory activation of vascular cells. The mechanisms by which Tregs protect against inflammation are thought to be mediated, at least in part, by directing cell-to-cell interactions as well as through the secretion of soluble anti-inflammatory cytokines, including IL-10 TGF-β [53]. Thus, further studies are required to understand the role of adaptive immunity and inflammation response in AD with CRS.

8.5.3 Sympathetic Activity

The role of increased SNS activity in IR with CRS is increasingly recognized. Individuals with central obesity show increased sympathetic nervous activity. Increased sympathetic outflow has been reported in obese nonhypertensive individuals with the determination of circulating catecholamines, urinary norepinephrine (NE), and muscle sympathetic nerve activity (MSNA) [54]. Multiple neurohumoral mechanisms can activate the SNS in patients with CRS including direct activation of the SNS in response to the activation of higher cerebral nuclei and renal afferent nerve activation mediated by perirenal fat accumulation and kidney compression [55]. Sympathetic activation can also be triggered by reflex mechanisms such as arterial baroreceptor impairment, psychological stress, oxidative stress, obstructive sleep apnea, inflammation, and metabolic factors and dysregulated production and secretion of adipokines from visceral fat with a particular important role of leptin [20]. Although enhanced activation of SNS is an important component in IR, it is often related to activation of RAAS since the RAAS system causes sustained sympathetic overactivity by modulating central neurons in the subfornical organ of the forebrain [49]. The link between sympathetic nervous activity and AD offers new clues to identify AD and may allow for development of novel-targeted therapeutic interventions.

8.5.4 Renin–Angiotensin–Aldosterone System and Parathyroid Hormone

There is evidence that RAAS activation plays an important role in the pathogenesis of AD. In the course of RAAS-induced vascular injury, Ang II binds to its type 1 receptor to induce oxidative stress, mainly mediated by NADPH oxidase. Our study has also found that Ang II increased serine phosphorylation of IRS-1 and inhibited the insulin-stimulated phosphorylation of endothelial NO synthase through activation of S6 kinase (S6K) signaling pathway [30]. Recent data also suggests that increased mineralocorticoid receptor (MR) is associated with IR. Studies have demonstrated a relationship between MR activation and decreased insulin sensitivity in animal models and humans. For example, patients with primary hyperaldosteronism were found to have IR suggesting the contribution of MR signaling to IR [56]. Spironolactone, a blocker of the MR, has been shown to decrease local inflammation and vascular stiffness in rodent models of hypertension and IR [57, 58]. These observations suggest that inhibition of MR might be a beneficial therapeutic approach for preventing AD in diet-induced obesity and IR [58]. Thus, enhanced RAAS activation may represent a link between obesity, hypertension, dyslipidemia, and IR, features present in the AD with CRS [59]. Moreover, cross-talk between Ang II and aldosterone signaling underscores the importance of Ang II–aldosterone interactions in the development of IR, vascular dysfunction, and AD.

Parathyroid hormone (PTH) is secreted from parathyroid glands and increases the concentration of calcium in the blood. Recent research suggests that PTH is implicated in regulating RAAS which is proposed to regulate PTH hormones [60]. Ang II seems to be an acute modulator of PTH, potentially through direct stimulation of PTH release via the AT-1R. In contrast, aldosterone may be involved in the modulation of PTH in the chronic setting via indirect and direct mechanisms [61]. PTH may increase sensitization towards Ang II and directly stimulate aldosterone synthesis by binding to the PTH-related protein receptor, voltage-gated calcium channels, and the adrenocorticotropic hormone receptor [62]. Therefore, the interaction of PTH and RAAS plays a key role in the pathogenesis of AD.

8.5.5 Tissue Transglutaminase

Tissue transglutaminase (TG2) is a multifunctional protein that plays an important role in vascular function, including remodeling of resistance vessels, increased aortic stiffness with age, and arterial calcification [63]. TG2 is a link between IR and AD because of its regulation by NO availability. A study has found that bioavailability of NO impaired by inflammation cytokines and RAAS is associated with decreased TG2 S-nitrosylation [63, 64]. Thus, increased secretion of TG2 to the cell surface and extracellular matrix and enhanced cross-linking activity in isolated endothelial, smooth muscle, and fibroblast cells resulted in AD in CRS [65]. In addition, increased vascular TG2 activity was also associated with AD in high fat-fed mice that preceded hypertension [66], thereby suggesting TG2 activation and AD as an early vent in the long-term effects of obesity on the vasculature.

Conclusion

AD increases the risk of developing coronary, cerebrovascular, and peripheral arterial disease and is a major cause of disability and death in patients with diabetes mellitus and CRS. The pathophysiology of AD in diabetes and CRS involves abnormalities in ECs, VSMCs, elastin, collagen, and AGE products, which increase the risk of the adverse cardiovascular events. Elucidation of mechanisms leading to the pathophysiological alterations in vasculature will enable us to specifically target therapeutic interventions since currently available cardiovascular medications fall short at reducing AD. Future therapeutic strategies should emphasize the need to achieve control of hyperglycemia, dyslipidemia, blood pressure, obesity, and cigarette smoking, in addition to exercise therapy. A better understanding of the mechanisms leading to vascular dysfunction may unmask new strategies to reduce disability and death in these patients.

Acknowledgments   The authors would like to thank Brenda Hunter for her editorial assistance. This research was supported by NIH (R01 HL73101, R01 HL107910) and the Veterans Affairs Merit System (0018) for JRS. The authors have no conflict of interest associated with this manuscript.

Disclosure   The authors have no conflict of interest associated with this manuscript.

References

1. Krentz AJ (2003) Lipoprotein abnormalities and their consequences for patients with type 2 diabetes. Diabetes Obes Metab 5:S19–S27
2. Lüscher TF, Creager MA, Beckman JA, Cosentino F (2003) Diabetes and vascular disease: pathophysiology, clinical consequences, and medical therapy: part II. Circulation 108:1655–1661
3. Sowers JR (2013) Diabetes mellitus and vascular disease. Hypertension 61:943–947
4. Jia G, Sowers JR (2014) New thoughts in an old player: role of nitrite in the treatment of ischemic revascularization. Diabetes 63:39–41
5. Salomaa V, Riley W, Kark JD et al (1995) Non-insulin-dependent diabetes mellitus and fasting glucose and insulin concentrations are associated with arterial stiffness indexes. The ARIC Study. Atherosclerosis Risk in Communities Study. Circulation 91:1432–1443
6. Tounian P, Aggoun Y, Dubern B et al (2001) Presence of increased stiffness of the common carotid artery and endothelial dysfunction in severely obese children: a prospective study. Lancet 358:1400–1404
7. Ho CT, Lin CC, Hsu HS et al (2011) Arterial stiffness is strongly associated with insulin resistance in Chinese–a population-based study (Taichung Community Health Study, TCHS). J Atheroscler Thromb 18:122–130
8. van Popele NM, Elizabeth Hak A, Mattace-Raso FU et al (2006) Impaired fasting glucose is associated with increased arterial stiffness in elderly people without diabetes mellitus: the Rotterdam Study. J Am Geriatr Soc 54:397–404
9. Roberts AC, Porter KE (2013) Cellular and molecular mechanisms of endothelial dysfunction in diabetes. Diab Vasc Dis Res 10:472–482
10. Daemen MJ, Lombardi DM, Bosman FT, Schwartz SM (1991) Angiotensin II induces smooth muscle cell proliferation in the normal and injured rat arterial wall. Circ Res 68:450–456
11. Sodhi CP, Kanwar YS, Sahai A (2003) Hypoxia and high glucose upregulate AT1 receptor expression and potentiate ANG II-induced proliferation in VSM cells. Am J Physiol Heart Circ Physiol 284:H846–H852
12. Reusch JE, Wang CC (2011) Cardiovascular disease in diabetes: where does glucose fit in? J Clin Endocrinol Metab 96:2367–2376
13. Min Q, Bai YT, Jia G et al (2010) High glucose enhances angiotensin-II-mediated peroxisome proliferation-activated receptor-gamma inactivation in human coronary artery endothelial cells. Exp Mol Pathol 88:133–137
14. Shanik MH, Xu Y, Skrha J et al (2008) Insulin resistance and hyperinsulinemia: is hyperinsulinemia the cart or the horse? Diabetes Care 31:S262–S268
15. Du X, Edelstein D, Obici S et al (2006) Insulin resistance reduces arterial prostacyclin synthase and eNOS activities by increasing endothelial fatty acid oxidation. J Clin Invest 116:1071–1080
16. Bender SB, McGraw AP, Jaffe IZ, Sowers JR (2013) Mineralocorticoid receptor-mediated vascular insulin resistance: an early contributor to diabetes-related vascular disease? Diabetes 62:313–319
17. Carmena R, Betteridge DJ (2004) Statins and diabetes. Semin Vasc Med 4:321–332
18. Arca M, Pigna G, Favoccia C (2012) Mechanisms of diabetic dyslipidemia: relevance for atherogenesis. Curr Vasc Pharmacol 10:684–686
19. Raj M (2012) Obesity and cardiovascular risk in children and adolescents. Indian J Endocrinol Metab 16:13–19
20. Canale MP, Manca di Villahermosa S, Martino G et al (2013) Obesity-related metabolic syndrome: mechanisms of sympathetic overactivity. Int J Endocrinol 2013:865965
21. Masterjohn C, Park Y, Lee J et al (2013) Dietary fructose feeding increases adipose methylglyoxal accumulation in rats in association with low expression and activity of glyoxalase-2. Nutrients 5:3311–3328
22. Khitan Z, Kim DH (2013) Fructose: a key factor in the development of metabolic syndrome and hypertension. J Nutr 2013:682673

23. Tappy L, Lê KA (2010) Metabolic effects of fructose and the worldwide increase in obesity. Physiol Rev 90:23–46
24. Muniyappa R, Sowers JR (2012) Endothelial insulin and IGF-1 receptors: when yes means NO. Diabetes 61:2225–2227
25. Zhang Y, Sowers JR, Ren J (2012) Pathophysiological insights into cardiovascular health in metabolic syndrome. Exp Diabetes Res 2012:320534
26. Mudau M, Genis A, Lochner A, Strijdom H (2012) Endothelial dysfunction: the early predictor of atherosclerosis. Cardiovasc J Afr 23:222–231
27. Tran LT, Yuen VG, McNeill JH (2009) The fructose-fed rat: a review on the mechanisms of fructose-induced insulin resistance and hypertension. Mol Cell Biochem 332:145–159
28. Creager MA, Lüscher TF, Cosentino F, Beckman JA (2003) Diabetes and vascular disease: pathophysiology, clinical consequences, and medical therapy: part I. Circulation 108: 1527–1532
29. Doronzo G, Russo I, Mattiello L et al (2004) Insulin activates vascular endothelial growth factor in vascular smooth muscle cells: influence of nitric oxide and of insulin resistance. Eur J Clin Invest 34:664–673
30. Kim JA, Jang HJ, Martinez-Lemus LA, Sowers JR (2012) Activation of mTOR/p70S6 kinase by ANG II inhibits insulin-stimulated endothelial nitric oxide synthase and vasodilation. Am J Physiol Endocrinol Metab 302:E201–E208
31. Karwowski W, Naumnik B, Szczepański M, Myśliwiec M (2012) The mechanism of vascular calcification – a systematic review. Med Sci Monit 18:RA1–RA11
32. Townsend RR, Wimmer NJ, Chirinos JA et al (2010) Aortic PWV in chronic kidney disease: a CRIC ancillary study. Am J Hypertens 23:282–289
33. Speer MY, Yang HY, Brabb T et al (2009) Smooth muscle cells give rise to osteochondrogenic precursors and chondrocytes in calcifying arteries. Circ Res 104:733–741
34. Johnson RC, Leopold JA, Loscalzo J (2006) Vascular calcification: pathobiological mechanisms and clinical implications. Circ Res 99:1044–1059
35. Blaha MJ, DeFilippis AP, Rivera JJ et al (2011) The relationship between insulin resistance and incidence and progression of coronary artery calcification: the Multi-Ethnic Study of Atherosclerosis (MESA). Diabetes Care 34:749–751
36. Olesen P, Nguyen K, Wogensen L et al (2007) Calcification of human vascular smooth muscle cells: associations with osteoprotegerin expression and acceleration by high-dose insulin. Am J Physiol Heart Circ Physiol 292:H1058–H1064
37. Yuan LQ, Zhu JH, Wang HW et al (2011) RANKL is a downstream mediator for insulin-induced osteoblastic differentiation of vascular smooth muscle cells. PLoS One 6:e29037
38. Wang CC, Sorribas V, Sharma G et al (2007) Insulin attenuates vascular smooth muscle calcification but increases vascular smooth muscle cell phosphate transport. Atherosclerosis 195:e65–e75
39. Mizobuchi M, Towler D, Slatopolsky E (2009) Vascular calcification: the killer of patients with chronic kidney disease. J Am Soc Nephrol 20:1453–1464
40. Chung AW, Yang HH, Sigrist MK (2009) Matrix metalloproteinase-2 and -9 exacerbate arterial stiffening and angiogenesis in diabetes and chronic kidney disease. Cardiovasc Res 84: 494–504
41. Ganne S, Winer N (2008) Vascular compliance in the cardiometabolic syndrome. J Cardiometab Syndr 3:35–39
42. Gao L, Laude K, Cai H (2008) Mitochondrial pathophysiology, reactive oxygen species, and cardiovascular diseases. Vet Clin North Am Small Anim Pract 38:137–155
43. Nisoli E, Clementi E, Carruba MO, Moncada S (2007) Defective mitochondrial biogenesis: a hallmark of the high cardiovascular risk in the metabolic syndrome? Circ Res 100:795–806
44. Whaley-Connell A, Sowers JR (2011) Indices of obesity and cardiometabolic risk. Hypertension 58:991–993
45. Liu J, Shen W, Zhao B et al (2009) Targeting mitochondrial biogenesis for preventing and treating insulin resistance in diabetes and obesity: hope from natural mitochondrial nutrients. Adv Drug Deliv Rev 61:1343–1352

46. Sivitz WI, Yorek MA (2010) Mitochondrial dysfunction in diabetes: from molecular mechanisms to functional significance and therapeutic opportunities. Antioxid Redox Signal 12: 537–577
47. Chávez-Sánchez L, Espinosa-Luna JE, Chávez-Rueda K et al (2014) Innate immune system cells in atherosclerosis. Arch Med Res 45:1–14
48. Aroor A, McKarns S, Nistala R et al (2013) DPP-4 inhibitors as therapeutic modulators of immune cell function and associated cardiovascular and renal insulin resistance in obesity and diabetes. Cardiorenal Med 3:48–56
49. Aroor AR, McKarns S, Demarco VG et al (2013) Maladaptive immune and inflammatory pathways lead to cardiovascular insulin resistance. Metabolism 62:1543–1552
50. Legein B, Temmerman L, Biessen EA, Lutgens E (2013) Inflammation and immune system interactions in atherosclerosis. Cell Mol Life Sci 70:3847–3869
51. Döring Y, Zernecke A (2012) Plasmacytoid dendritic cells in atherosclerosis. Front Physiol 3:230
52. Alberts-Grill N, Denning TL, Rezvan A, Jo H (2013) The role of the vascular dendritic cell network in atherosclerosis. Am J Physiol Cell Physiol 305:C1–C21
53. He S, Li M, Ma X, Lin J, Li D (2010) CD4+CD25+Foxp3+ regulatory T cells protect the proinflammatory activation of human umbilical vein endothelial cells. Arterioscler Thromb Vasc Biol 30:2621–2630
54. Huang CJ, Webb HE, Zourdos MC, Acevedo EO (2013) Cardiovascular reactivity, stress, and physical activity. Front Physiol 7:4–314
55. Xiong XQ, Chen WW, Zhu GQ (2014) Adipose afferent reflex: sympathetic activation and obesity hypertension. Acta Physiol (Oxf) 210:468–478
56. Underwood PC, Adler GK (2013) The Renin angiotensin aldosterone system and insulin resistance in humans. Curr Hypertens Rep 15:59–70
57. Wada T, Kenmochi H, Miyashita Y et al (2010) Spironolactone improves glucose and lipid metabolism by ameliorating hepatic steatosis and inflammation and suppressing enhanced gluconeogenesis induced by high-fat and high-fructose diet. Endocrinology 151:2040–2049
58. Benetos A, Lacolley P, Safar ME (1997) Prevention of aortic fibrosis by spironolactone in spontaneously hypertensive rats. Arterioscler Thromb Vasc Biol 17:1152–1156
59. Garg R, Adler GK (2012) Role of mineralocorticoid receptor in insulin resistance. Curr Opin Endocrinol Diabetes Obes 19:168–175
60. Tomaschitz A, Ritz E, Pieske B, Rus-Machan J et al (2014) Aldosterone and parathyroid hormone interactions as mediators of metabolic and cardiovascular disease. Metabolism 63:20–31
61. Brown JM, Williams JS, Luther JM et al (2014) Human interventions to characterize novel relationships between the renin-angiotensin-aldosterone system and parathyroid hormone. Hypertension 63:273–280
62. Tomaschitz A, Ritz E, Pieske B et al (2012) Aldosterone and parathyroid hormone: a precarious couple for cardiovascular disease. Cardiovasc Res 94:10–19
63. Jung SM, Jandu S, Steppan J et al (2013) Increased tissue transglutaminase activity contributes to central vascular stiffness in eNOS knockout mice. Am J Physiol Heart Circ Physiol 305:H803–H810
64. Thomas WG (2005) Double trouble for type 1 angiotensin receptors in atherosclerosis. N Engl J Med 352:506–508
65. Santhanam L, Tuday EC, Webb AK et al (2010) Decreased S-nitrosylation of tissue transglutaminase contributes to age-related increases in vascular stiffness. Circ Res 107:117–125
66. Weisbrod RM, Shiang T, Al Sayah L et al (2013) Arterial stiffening precedes systolic hypertension in diet-induced obesity. Hypertension 62:1105–1110

Biomarkers of Vascular Inflammation and Cardiovascular Disease

9

Paul Welsh, David Preiss, Sofia Tsiropoulou, Francisco J. Rios, Adam Harvey, Maria G. Dulak-Lis, Augusto C. Montezano, and Rhian M. Touyz

9.1   Introduction

Altered vascular function is a common feature in many cardiovascular diseases such as hypertension, atherosclerosis and ischaemic heart disease and is characterised by endothelial dysfunction, arterial remodelling and vascular inflammation [1, 2]. Molecular and cellular changes associated with these processes include increased expression of cellular adhesion molecules, mitochondrial dysfunction, macrophage activation and immune dysregulation, processes that are redox sensitive and linked to oxidative stress (increased bioavailability of reactive oxygen species (ROS)) [3–7]. Inflammation is both a cause and consequence of oxidative stress because ROS stimulate inflammatory signalling pathways and induce activation of proinflammatory transcription factors such as NFκB, while at the same time, inflammatory processes stimulate ROS production and oxidative stress [8, 9] (Fig. 9.1). Because these phenomena occur early in the pathophysiology of vascular injury and become exaggerated as cardiovascular disease progresses, there is growing interest in identifying novel biomarkers of vascular inflammation and oxidative stress that could better predict the risk of cardiovascular disease, track the development of vascular injury, stratify patients to disease-targeted therapies and provide insights into mechanisms underlying pathological processes [10, 11].

P. Welsh, PhD • D. Preiss, MBBCh, PhD • S. Tsiropoulou, PhD • F.J. Rios, PhD
A. Harvey, PhD • M.G. Dulak-Lis, MSc • A.C. Montezano, PhD
R.M. Touyz, MBBCh, MD, PhD (✉)
Institute of Cardiovascular and Medical Sciences, British Heart Foundation
(BHF) Glasgow Cardiovascular Research Centre, University of Glasgow,
126 University Place, Glasgow G12 8TA, UK
e-mail: Paul.welsh@glasgow.ac.uk; David.preiss@glasgow.ac.uk;
SofiaTsiropoulou@glasgow.ac.uk; Francisco.rios@glasgow.ac.uk;
Adam.harvey@glasgow.ac.uk; Maria.dulak@glasgow.ac.uk;
Augusto.montezano@glasgow.ac.uk; Rhian.Touyz@glasgow.ac.uk

© Springer International Publishing Switzerland 2015
A. Berbari, G. Mancia (eds.), *Arterial Disorders:*
Definition, Clinical Manifestations, Mechanisms and Therapeutic Approaches,
DOI 10.1007/978-3-319-14556-3_9

115

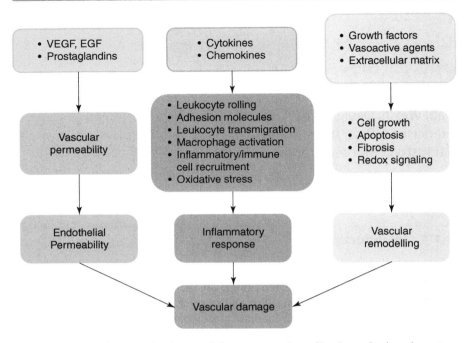

Fig. 9.1 Diagram demonstrating how proinflammatory and pro-fibrotic mechanisms impact on vascular inflammation and remodelling in vascular injury. Oxidative stress plays an important role in vascular injury. Biomarkers of these processes may provide insights into molecular mechanisms underlying vascular damage and may act as markers to predict the risk of cardiovascular disease

Many circulating biomarkers of vascular injury have been identified, including acute-phase proteins (C-reactive protein (CRP), pentraxin, amyloid A, homocysteine), inflammatory mediators (cytokines, chemokines), cellular markers of endothelial damage (microparticles, endothelial progenitor cells, microRNAs) and markers of oxidative stress (lipid peroxidation, ROS, antioxidants) [10–13]. Although the field is growing, there are still no ideal markers to predict and track vascular damage. With improved and more sensitive methodologies to measure circulating and urine biomarkers together with non-invasive vascular imaging, the domain will continue to develop, and hopefully clinically useful algorithms based on biomarkers could assist in better prediction of risk, stratification of disease and targeting of treatment. This chapter describes vascular inflammation and oxidative stress in the context of cardiovascular disease and focuses on some biomarkers that may act as clinically useful surrogates of underlying vascular injury.

9.2   Definition of a Biomarker

The term "biomarker" is a contraction of "biological marker". An NIH working group defined biomarkers as "A characteristic that is objectively measured and evaluated as an indicator of normal biological processes, pathogenic processes, or pharmacologic responses to a therapeutic intervention" [14]. Biomarkers may be useful in the early detection of vascular injury and in predicting the risk of cardiovascular disease. Biomarkers may also reflect vascular injury and hence provide insights into mechanisms underlying progression of disease. Finally, they may act as indices to better stratify patients, which should lead to more directed and mechanism-targeted treatments. Examples of biomarkers that have been included into clinical practice and may add value to classical cardiovascular risk factors include high-sensitivity CRP for cardiovascular risk prediction, glycated haemoglobin (HbA$_1$C) for the diagnosis of diabetes, N-terminal pro-B-type natriuretic peptide (NT-proBNP) for heart failure diagnosis, troponin I and troponin T for acute myocardial infarction diagnosis and microalbuminuria for kidney disease [15–19].

9.3   Vascular Inflammation

Low-grade inflammation in the vascular wall is increasingly recognised as an important contributor to the pathophysiology of cardiovascular disease [20], to the initiation and progression of atherosclerosis and to the development of hypertension [20, 21]. Inflammation participates in vascular remodelling and promotes accelerated vascular damage in aging through processes that involve increased expression of adhesion molecules (vascular cell adhesion molecule-1 (VCAM-1), intercellular adhesion molecule-1 (ICAM-1)) on the endothelial cell membrane, accumulation of monocytes/macrophages in the vascular wall and stimulation of ROS-generating enzymes, including Noxs [22–24] (Fig. 9.2). Innate immunity has been implicated to contribute to the low-grade inflammatory response in atherosclerosis and hypertension where different subsets of T lymphocytes may be involved in processes leading to inflammation [25–27]. For example, an imbalance exists between the proinflammatory Th1, Th2 and Th17 and the anti-inflammatory T regulatory (Treg) subsets of T lymphocytes [28].

9.4   Reactive Oxygen Species, Oxidative Stress
and Vascular Inflammation

ROS are formed during the reduction of oxygen and include unstable free radicals (species with an unpaired electron) such as superoxide ($O_2^{\cdot-}$) and non-free radicals, such as hydrogen peroxide (H_2O_2) [29]. ROS are generated continuously as normal

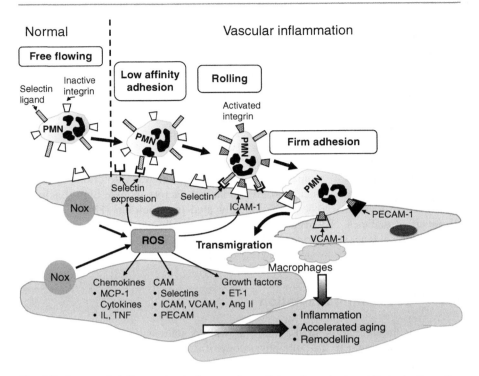

Fig. 9.2 Low-grade inflammation in the vascular wall is an important contributor to the pathophysiology of cardiovascular disease. Inflammation participates in vascular remodelling and promotes accelerated vascular damage in aging through processes that involve increased expression of adhesion molecules (vascular cell adhesion molecule-1 (*VCAM-1*), intercellular adhesion molecule-1 (*ICAM-1*), selectin, PECAM) on the endothelial cell membrane, increased rolling and adhesion of polymorphonucleocytes (*PMN*), transmigration of PMN and accumulation of monocytes/macrophages in the vascular wall. These processes are stimulated by increased generation of reactive oxygen species (*ROS*) from Noxs in endothelial and vascular smooth muscle cells (*VSMC*)

by-products of cellular metabolism and as direct products through activation of nicotinamide adenine dinucleotide phosphate (NADPH) oxidase, also called Nox [30, 31]. ROS are produced in the endothelium, throughout the vascular wall and adventitia and in perivascular fat. In the vascular system together with nitric oxide (NO), a potent endothelial-derived vasodilator, ROS play a physiological role in regulating endothelial function and vascular contraction/dilation and are important in maintaining vascular integrity [32–34]. Under pathological conditions, increased ROS levels cause cell damage and promote vascular inflammation, hypertrophy, fibrosis and increased contraction, important factors contributing to endothelial dysfunction and vascular remodelling in cardiovascular diseases [35, 36]. Molecular processes underlying ROS-induced cardiovascular injury involve activation of redox-sensitive signalling pathways [37–39]. Superoxide anion and H_2O_2 stimulate mitogen-activated protein kinases (MAPK), tyrosine kinases, Rho kinase and transcription factors (NFκB, AP-1 and HIF-1) and inactivate protein tyrosine phosphatases (PTP) [40, 41]. ROS also increase intracellular free Ca^{2+} concentration ($[Ca^{2+}]_i$) and upregulate proto-oncogene and proinflammatory gene expression and activity [42]. These phenomena occur through oxidative modification of proteins [43]. Changes in the intracellular redox state through glutathione and thioredoxin systems may also influence intracellular signalling [44].

9.4.1 Production and Metabolism of ROS in the Cardiovascular System

Enzymatic sources of ROS important in cardiovascular disease are xanthine oxidoreductase, uncoupled NO synthase (NOS), mitochondrial respiratory enzymes and NADPH oxidase [45–47], found in many cell types in the heart, kidney, vessels and central nervous system. Of the many ROS-generating enzymes, it is only NADPH oxidase that has as its primary function the formation of ROS, hence termed a "professional" ROS producer [30, 31]. NADPH oxidase was originally considered to be expressed only in phagocytic cells involved in host defence and innate immunity. It is now evident that there is a family of NADPH oxidases/Noxs that are functionally active in non-phagocytic cells, including vascular cells. The mammalian Nox family comprises seven members: Nox1, Nox2, Nox3, Nox4, Nox5, Duox1 and Duox2 [48, 49]. All are transmembrane proteins that have conserved structural properties and that transport electrons across biological membranes to reduce O_2 to $O_2^{\cdot-}$. Each isoform is encoded by separate genes. Whereas Nox1, Nox2, Nox4 and Nox5 have been identified in cardiovascular tissue [50], Nox3, found in the inner ear, and Duox1 and Duox2, found primarily in the thyroid gland, do not seem to be important in the cardiovascular system.

9.5 Biomarkers of Endothelial Dysfunction

9.5.1 Nitric Oxide (NO) and ROS

Biomarkers of impaired endothelial function reflect altered NO bioavailability, increased oxidative stress, coagulation and endothelial inflammation. NO, produced by endothelial cells, is a major determinant of endothelium-dependent vasodilation and is an inhibitor of coagulation, inflammation and oxidative stress [51–53] and consequently has been considered as an important marker reflecting endothelial status. Since NO has a short half-life, plasma levels of oxidative degradation products of NO, including nitrite (NO_2^-), nitrate (NO_3^-) and nitrosothiols, have been used as surrogate indices of NO generation [54]. In addition to assessing levels of NO and its metabolites, measurement of asymmetric dimethylarginine (ADMA), a potent endogenous inhibitor of nitric oxide synthase (NOS)-derived NO production, could also reflect NO bioavailability [55]. Plasma ADMA levels have been shown to correlate with endothelial NOS activity and to be associated with endothelial dysfunction [56, 57].

Endothelial injury is associated with increased production of $O_2^{\cdot-}$, which readily reacts with NO to form peroxynitrite ($ONOO^-$), an injurious free radical that further contributes to endothelial dysfunction [58]. Similarly, lipid peroxyl radicals react with NO and may also be a source of NO inactivation [59]. Plasma measures of endothelial oxidative stress include indices of lipid peroxidation (F_2-isoprostanes and thiobarbituric acid-reactive substances) and nitrotyrosine levels, reflecting peroxynitrite generation [60, 61]. Lipid peroxidation is increased in diseases associated with endothelial dysfunction, and there is a strong negative correlation between oxidative stress and endothelial function [62–64].

9.5.2   Endothelial Proinflammatory Markers

Because endothelial impairment is often accompanied by inflammation, proinflammatory markers have been used to reflect dysfunction. Cellular adhesion molecules play an important role in endothelial inflammation by attracting and anchoring inflammatory cells. Soluble forms of cell adhesion molecules including VCAM-1, ICAM-1 and E-selectin are found in the circulation and may reflect vascular inflammatory status and endothelial dysfunction [65]. C-reactive protein, a protein found in plasma, which rises in response to inflammation, is an independent predictor of abnormal endothelial function and cardiovascular mortality and morbidity [66, 67]. Additional circulating markers of inflammation include soluble CD40L [68] and circulating cytokines such as interleukin-6 and tumour necrosis factor-α (TNFα) [69].

9.5.3   Markers of Coagulation

Endothelial dysfunction is associated with a pro-coagulatory state and accordingly indices of coagulation may be considered as biomarkers of endothelial status. Plasminogen activator inhibitor-1 (PAI-1) is an inhibitor of fibrinolysis that is produced primarily by the endothelium [70]. P-selectin is a platelet activation marker and plasma fibrinogen levels are thought to be reflective of a pro-coagulant state. PAI-1, P-selectin and fibrinogen are increased in cardiovascular disease and correlate with endothelial dysfunction [71]. Von Willebrand factor (vWF), a glycoprotein which is secreted by endothelial cells and plays a role in coagulation, has also been proposed as a biomarker of endothelial function [72].

9.5.4   Microparticles

In addition to circulating biochemical or protein-based markers, growing evidence indicates that endothelial cell-derived fractions, including microparticles, may be reflective of endothelial dysfunction and injury. Microparticles are anuclear fragments of cellular membrane shed from stressed or damaged cells [73]. They are typically 0.1–1.0 μm in diameter and contain surface proteins and cytoplasmic material of the parent cells. Microparticles are distinguishable from other subcellular vesicles, such as exosomes and apoptotic bodies, on the basis of size, mechanism of formation and content [74].

Microparticles are identified in plasma samples by flow cytometry on the basis of size, the externalisation of phosphatidylserine and the presence of specific surface antigens. Labelling of surface antigens allows for identification of the parent cell from which the microparticles were derived. In plasma samples, microparticles of endothelial (identified by the surface presence of CD144, CD62E or CD31), platelet (CD41a, CD42b, CD62P), leukocyte (CD45, CD4, CD8, CD14) and erythrocyte (CD235a) origin are present [75–77]. Given that microparticles are released under conditions of cell stress/damage, it is not surprising that plasma levels of microparticles are increased in cardiovascular disease. Strong evidence exists to suggest that microparticles of endothelial, platelet and leukocyte origin may be reflective of endothelial dysfunction and may in fact contribute to endothelial dysfunction [78–80]. Endothelial microparticles are thought to be directly indicative of endothelial cell stress/damage and may also reflect endothelial inflammation, increased coagulation and vascular tone [81]. Platelet microparticles may indirectly reveal endothelial dysfunction by revealing increased coagulation and inflammation [82], while leukocyte microparticles may reflect inflammation, coagulation and vascular tone [83]. Microparticles of endothelial, platelet and leukocyte origin have been shown to be increased in multiple disease states associated with endothelial dysfunction including hypertension, diabetes and end-stage renal disease (reviewed in [84]). Considering the complexity of endothelial function, measuring multiple biomarkers to reflect different processes may provide a comprehensive assessment of endothelial status.

9.6   Biomarkers of Vascular Inflammation

9.6.1   Acute-Phase Response Proteins

Acute-phase proteins are a class of proteins, which are increased in response to inflammation. The phenomenon is called the acute-phase reaction [85]. Acute-phase proteins are produced by the liver in response to injury and under the control of a cascade of cytokines including IL-1β, IL-6 and TNFα. The association of elevated serum levels of acute-phase proteins with the progression of atherosclerosis, coronary artery disease, unstable angina and myocardial infarction has been documented in epidemiological studies [86, 87]. Acute-phase protein markers including CRP, pentraxin 3 (PTX3), amyloid A, homocysteine and fibrinogen are increased in cardiovascular disease and reflect generalised inflammation.

9.6.1.1 C-Reactive Protein
CRP has been the plasma biomarker of choice for a clinical index of generalised inflammation partly due to its wide dynamic range. Increased plasma CRP has been demonstrated in many cardiovascular diseases associated with endothelial dysfunction and vascular injury. Tissue necrosis is a potent inducer of CRP, and in

post-myocardial infarction, there is a significant CRP response [88]. The Emerging Risk Factors Collaboration evaluated the predictive risk of adding CRP, fibrinogen and lipid-related markers (apolipoprotein A, apolipoprotein B, apolipoprotein A-1, lipoprotein(a) or lipoprotein-associated phospholipase A2) to traditional risk factors in a meta-analysis including over 240,000 participants with no history of cardiovascular disease [89]. Adding either of these biomarkers resulted in only a modest reclassification improvement for individuals at intermediate risk versus models that included age, sex, smoking, blood pressure, diabetes and total cholesterol concentrations. CRP failed to predict incident cardiovascular disease in patients with diabetes [90]. Although initial experimental evidence suggested that CRP might itself be pro-atherogenic and cause vascular disease, later studies refuted this.

9.6.1.2 Other Acute-Phase Proteins

Besides CRP, there are other acute-phase proteins that are increased in cardiovascular disease. Pentraxin 3 appears to be more specific for vascular inflammation than CRP [91]. In patients with stable coronary artery disease, increased PTX3 levels were associated with increased risk for all-cause mortality, cardiovascular events and heart failure [92]. Elevated serum levels of homocysteine and cardiac troponins are biomarkers of myocardial injury and are elevated in patients with cardiac failure [93, 94]. Raised plasma homocysteine is associated with greater risk for more severe cardiovascular disease. Increased concentrations of plasma amyloid A and fibrinogen are linked to a large number of cardiovascular risk factors and have been associated with increased risk for coronary artery disease, thrombosis and myocardial infarction [95].

9.6.2 Cytokines

9.6.2.1 Tumour Necrosis Factor-α (TNFα)

Tumour necrosis factor-α and interleukins are proinflammatory cytokines that are upstream of the acute-phase response and are thus generally thought to be more credible causal agents in atherosclerosis and CVD. Cytokines are soluble glycoproteins produced by many cell types including cells of the vascular and immune systems [96]. They are produced in response to tissue injury or ischaemia and are responsible for controlling the innate and adaptive immune response. An increase in production of proinflammatory cytokines, such as IL-1β, IL-6 and TNFα, and a decreased production of anti-inflammatory cytokines, such as IL-10, have been observed in many diseases associated with endothelial dysfunction and vascular injury, including hypertension, heart disease, stroke and diabetes [97, 98]. As such these cytokines have been implicated as therapeutic targets and biomarkers for disease progression and prognosis.

The biology of the TNFα axis is complex and its physiological roles are still being elucidated. The TNFα precursor is membrane bound and cleaved by TNFα-converting enzyme (TACE), releasing the soluble form that binds to TNFR1 and TNFR2, expressed in most cell types [99]. TNFα signalling via

TNFR1/TNFR2 elicits signalling for cell death, survival or inflammation by recruiting specific adaptor proteins. Recruitment of adaptor proteins such as caspase-8 leads to apoptosis, while recruitment of TNF receptor-associated factor 2 (TRAF2) and receptor-interacting protein (RIP) stimulates signalling through NFκB resulting in activation of transcription factors and genes that promote inflammation [100].

9.6.2.2 Interleukin-1β (IL-1β)
Interleukin-1β is constitutively expressed in low levels and is regulated by transcription, translation, cleavage and cellular release [101]. It is synthesised as a large precursor protein and is biologically inactive until it is secreted following cleavage by caspase-1. Active IL-1β binds to IL-1R1, to induce proinflammatory signalling by stimulating Ca^{2+} channel activation, increasing expression of adhesion molecules on endothelial cells and causing impaired endothelial permeability [102].

9.6.2.3 Interleukin-6 (IL-6)
Interleukin-6 is an inflammatory cytokine that binds to class 1 cytokine receptors, inducing activation of Janus kinase (JAK), which induces activation of signal transducer and activator of transcription (STAT) family of transcription factors and RAS-RAF-MAPK pathways, leading to proinflammatory responses [103].

Increased plasma levels of IL-6 and TNFα have been demonstrated in patients with diabetes, hypertension, ischaemic heart disease and cardiac failure [104–106]. In a large prospective population-based study, a combined elevation of IL-1β and IL-6 was independently associated with an increased risk of type 2 diabetes, suggesting a role for low-grade inflammation in diabetes (EPIC) [107]. However data from the large ADVANCE clinical trial challenge the inflammatory paradigm of microvascular disease in diabetes, showing that circulating cytokines are actually not strongly associated with microvascular risk after adjusting for confounding risk factors [108].

If indeed IL-6 and TNFα are implicated in the pathogenesis of vascular inflammation and associated cardiovascular disease, then treatment targeting these cytokines should reduce cardiovascular risk. Findings from studies where anti-IL-6 and anti-TNFα biologics have been used in patients with inflammatory disease such as rheumatoid arthritis suggested reduced risk of cardiovascular disease in these patients who are at −50 % increased risk of cardiovascular disease compared to the general population [109, 110]. Data from biologics treatment registers of rheumatoid arthritis patients show that those who respond to TNF biologics have reduced rates of myocardial infarction (3.5 per 1,000 person-years) compared to nonresponders (9.4 per 1,000 person-years) [111]. Similar data have been reported in the US CORRONA database [112]. It should be highlighted that these findings are based on pharmacoepidemiology and are therefore subject to potential confounding factors. Meta-analysis of small trials failed to show a significant reduction in cardiovascular risk associated with anti-TNFα biologics [113].

9.7   Biomarkers of Oxidative Stress

Because of the key role of oxidative stress in vascular injury and cardiovascular pathology, ROS levels and redox state have been considered as promising biomarkers indicative of the disease process. However, free radicals have a very short half-life and are unstable. Hence accurately measuring $O_2^{\cdot-}$ and H_2O_2 in the circulation is complex. As such, methods have been developed to measure stable markers of ROS that reflect oxidative status. Biomarkers of oxidative stress that are currently assessed are measures of oxidation products of lipids, DNA and protein [114] (Table 9.1).

Table 9.1 Biomarkers of oxidative stress	
	Lipid peroxidation
	Malondialdehyde
	F2-isoprostanes
	4-Hydroxynonenal (4-HNE)
	OxLDL
	Pro-oxidant enzymes
	Xanthine oxidase
	Mitochondrial oxidases
	NADPH oxidases
	Antioxidant enzymes
	Superoxide dismutase
	Catalase
	Glutathione peroxidase
	GSH/GSSG ratio (thiol index)
	Nonenzymatic antioxidants
	Total antioxidant capacity
	Vitamin C
	Vitamin A
	Urate
	Bilirubin
	Thiols
	Flavonoids
	Carotenoids
	Protein/DNA oxidation
	Carbonyls
	8-Oxo-7,8-dihydroguanine
	Reactive oxygen/nitrogen species
	H_2O_2
	NO
	ONOO$^-$
	Cell-based biomarkers
	Microparticles
	Endothelial progenitor cells
	MicroRNAs

9.7.1 Lipid Peroxidation

Lipids are highly sensitive to oxidation because of their molecular structure, which is characterised by numerous reactive double bonds. Polyunsaturated fatty acids, including phospholipids, glycolipids and cholesterol, are vulnerable targets of oxidation. For instance, evidence suggests that oxidised LDL (oxLDL) is engulfed, via TLR-4, by activated macrophages, which then become cytokine-producing lipid-laden foam cells, an integral part of the atherogenic plaque. Increased ROS bioavailability triggers the process of lipid peroxidation. The most commonly studied markers of lipid peroxidation are malondialdehyde (MDA) and isoprostanes.

9.7.1.1 Malondialdehyde

Malondialdehyde is the by-product of the arachidonate cycle and a main aldehyde product of lipid peroxidation in vivo. It is formed by peroxidation of polyunsaturated fatty acids and can interact with proteins [115]. MDA can be detected by thiobarbituric acid (TBA) using a colorimetric method based on the reaction between MDA and TBA that gives a pink colour [116]. The products that are measured are termed TBA-reactive species (TBARS). The TBARS assay is amongst the most widely employed to evaluate lipid peroxidation. This assay has been extensively used as an indicator of oxidative stress in experimental and human cardiovascular disease. Plasma TBARS levels are increased in patients with coronary artery disease, hypertension, atherosclerosis, diabetes, heart failure, stroke and aging [117–120]. Cigarette smokers also have elevated levels of TBARS suggesting that pro-atherogenic and vascular injury effects of smoking are related to oxidative damage induced by lipid peroxidation [121, 122]. Some studies showed that plasma TBARS could predict cardiovascular events. For example, raised TBARS concentrations predicted carotid atherosclerotic plaque progression over a 3-year period as validated by carotid wall thickness using ultrasound [123].

9.7.1.2 Isoprostanes

F2-isoprostanes are prostaglandin-like compounds produced by nonenzymatic peroxidation of arachidonic acid, a polyunsaturated fatty acid in phospholipids of cell membranes [124]. Formation of isoprostanes is independent of the cyclooxygenase enzyme that catalyses the production of prostaglandins. F2-isoprostanes are stable end products of lipid peroxidation and can be measured in all human tissues and biological fluids, including urine, plasma and cerebrospinal fluid [125]. A metabolite of F2-isoprostanes, 8-iso-prostaglandin F2α (8-iso-PGF2α), has vasoconstrictor, cell-growth properties and platelet aggregation and as such is biologically active independently of its biomarker status. F2-isoprostanes can be assessed by gas chromatography-mass spectrometry, liquid chromatography-mass spectrometry, enzyme-linked immunosorbent assay (ELISA) and radioimmunoassay in plasma and urine [126]. Levels of F2-isoprostanes in plasma and urine correlate with ROS levels and oxidative stress in experimental and human studies [127].

Increased circulating and urine levels of F2-isoprostanes have been demonstrated in various cardiovascular diseases associated with vascular injury, including hypertension, atherosclerosis, ischaemia-reperfusion injury and cardiac failure [128–130]. In addition, in healthy individuals with risk factors, such as obesity, hyperlipidaemia and hyperhomocysteinaemia, plasma concentrations of F2-isoprostanes are elevated, suggesting that indices of lipid peroxidation may be clinically relevant biomarkers of cardiovascular risk. In support of this, a recent prospective study including 1,002 anticoagulated patients with atrial fibrillation studied over 25 months demonstrated that 8-iso-PGF2α and sNOX2-dp (a marker of Nox2 levels) correlated with cardiovascular events [131]. Using various modelling paradigms, it was shown that 8-iso-PGF2α predicted cardiovascular events and death. As such it was suggested that F2-IsoP may complement conventional risk factors in prediction of cardiovascular events.

9.7.1.3 4-Hydroxynonenal

4-Hydroxynonenal (4-HNE), an α,β-unsaturated hydroxyalkenal produced by lipid peroxidation in cells, is generated during physiological and pathophysiological conditions based on the production of ROS [132]. 4-HNE is considered as one of the most specific and sensitive measures of lipid auto-oxidation. Various methods have been developed to measure 4-HNE including HPLC and GC-MS, anti-HNE adduct antibodies and ELISA.

Higher circulating 4-HNE levels have been shown to correlate with more severe diastolic dysfunction in spontaneously hypertensive rats [133]. 4-HNE has also been associated with stroke, ischaemia-reperfusion injury and cardiac hypertrophy. Increasing experimental evidence indicates that 4-HNE may have a dual role in that it may be a marker of systemic oxidative stress and also contribute directly to the pathogenesis of cardiovascular disease [134, 135]. Despite experimental evidence linking 4-HNE and cardiovascular disease, there is a paucity of information in humans. A few studies in dialysed patients demonstrated that MDA and 4-HNE thiols correlated with severity of cardiovascular disease [136, 137].

9.7.2   Nonenzymatic Total Antioxidant Capacity

Total antioxidant capacity is a measure of the combined antioxidant effect of the nonenzymatic defences in biological fluids and does not take into account the enzymatic antioxidant systems such as superoxide dismutase, catalase, peroxidase, etc. The assay measures low molecular weight antioxidants, both water soluble and lipid soluble, and includes urate, bilirubin, vitamin C, thiols, flavonoids, carotenoids and vitamin E [138]. Experimental and clinical studies have shown, for the most part, low levels of total antioxidant capacity in various cardiovascular diseases [139–141]. Total antioxidant capacity assays have also been used extensively in human studies evaluating effects of dietary antioxidants.

A recent comprehensive study reviewed prospective cohort studies and clinical trials relating to associations between plasma/dietary antioxidants (total antioxidant capacity) and cardiovascular events [142, 143]. In long-term, large-scale, population-based cohort studies, higher levels of total antioxidant capacity were associated with a lower risk of cardiovascular disease supporting a protective effect of dietary antioxidant vitamins, carotenoids and polyphenols. However results from large randomised controlled trials failed to support long-term use of single antioxidant supplements for cardiovascular prevention due to their lack of benefit or even adverse effects on major cardiovascular events or cancer. Although antioxidant supplement use was reported to have no benefit on cardiovascular events by several large randomised controlled trials, cohort studies still supported the protective effects of dietary antioxidants in preventing cardiovascular disease. In particular antioxidant vitamins and polyphenols exhibit high antioxidant capacity in vitro and cardioprotective effects in vivo. Although total antioxidant capacity assays may shed light on dietary antioxidant effects in specific patient cohorts, there are still technical concerns regarding specificity and sensitivity of these assays, and as such, total antioxidant capacity of foods or populations should not yet be used for making decisions affecting population health [144].

9.7.3   Oxidative Modification of DNA and Proteins

DNA and proteins are highly susceptible to modifications by changes in the redox state. Protein oxidation is the process whereby amino acid residues of a protein act as electron donors and suffer an oxidative attack by an oxidising agent. This process usually leads to changes in the biological function of the protein. Oxidation of proteins can be induced by various mechanisms/stimuli including ROS, metal cations, γ-irradiation, UV light and ozone, leakage of the electron transport chain in mitochondria, oxidoreductase enzymes, products of lipid peroxidation as well as activated phagocytes [145, 146].

Protein oxidative modifications can be divided into reversible, by biological antioxidant systems, and irreversible [147]. Irreversible modification normally leads to loss of protein functionality, aggregation and consequent degradation, while reversible modification has regulatory functions. The most common type of irreversible modification is the formation of carbonyl groups. Amino acids prone to carbonylation include proline, arginine, threonine, lysine, histidine and cysteine. Assessment of the extent of such a general type of oxidation serves as a marker of increased oxidative stress [148]. On the other hand, the sulfur (S)-containing amino acids, Cys and Met, are the only amino acids which can undergo modifications that can be reversed by cellular enzymes and have, therefore, a potential regulatory role in redox signalling [147]. The most common types of oxidative modifications include nitrosylation, S-glutathionylation, sulfenylation and carbonylation [149]. Another biomarker of oxidative stress is the extent of oxidation of bases in DNA. 8-Oxo-7,8-dihydroguanine or the corresponding nucleoside is most often measured, either chromatographically or enzymatically [150], as an index of DNA oxidation.

Oxidatively modified proteins regulate the activities of several redox-sensitive proteins involved in cardiovascular homeostasis, including endothelial function, myocyte contraction, vasodilation, oxidative phosphorylation, protein synthesis and glycolytic metabolism [151, 152]. At the same time, they may serve as biomarkers of oxidative stress.

Strategies to examine protein oxidation can be classified into direct and indirect assays. Direct approaches detect oxidation by exploiting the properties of oxidised forms of proteins or structural changes induced by oxidation and use specific antibodies [153, 154] or chemoselective probes [155]. The development of cell-permeable probes provides the advantage of labelling within the system, thus preventing any artefactual labelling due to oxidation upon cell lysis [155]. Indirect approaches utilising labelled substrates are the most commonly used, as they exploit conserved biochemical properties of the reversible oxidative modifications, as well as the catalytic activity of certain proteins.

While there is growing interest in studying oxidative modifications of proteins in cardiovascular tissue in experimental models, such approaches are not yet used in the clinical setting [156, 157]. However recent studies have shown that in patients with post-acute myocardial infarction, circulating levels of fibrinogen carbonylation, a marker of modified protein structure and altered fibrinogen function, are increased compared to controls [158].

Conclusions

Epidemiological studies have identified numerous factors, such as hypertension, dyslipidaemia, smoking, obesity, sedentary lifestyle and diabetes, as risks for cardiovascular disease [159]. Controlling such risk factors to prevent cardiovascular disease is a priority in global health. Identification of new biomarkers of vascular injury and inflammation, such as those highlighted in this chapter, offers information on underlying pathology and together with classical risk factors may provide better prediction of cardiovascular disease. With the many new biomarkers that continue to be identified, it is challenging to know which should be used in the clinic. To address this, a joint task force of the American Heart Association and the American College of Cardiology recently issued guidelines on biomarkers as predictors of cardiovascular disease [160, 161]. In addition to classical risk factors including family history, haemoglobin A_1C and microalbuminuria, the task force suggested CRP, lipoprotein-associated phospholipase A2, coronary calcium, carotid intima-media thickness and ankle/brachial index as clinical markers of risk. Thus although there is tremendous enthusiasm and interest in identifying novel biomarkers to predict cardiovascular disease, the utility still remains unclear, and to date, only a few have been accepted as clinically useful. Moreover, traditional biomarkers may not apply equally to both men and women or between other population strata [162, 163].

Biomarkers that are most promising are those that are associated with the pathophysiological mechanisms of the disease. Since vascular inflammation and oxidative stress are fundamental processes associated with cardiovascular disease, markers of such vascular injury may provide important insights not only into the pathogenesis but also early detection and tracking of vascular disease. As such there has been growing interest in identifying and validating novel biomarkers of vascular inflammation and oxidative stress. Whether these will prove to be useful indices in the clinic awaits confirmation.

Acknowledgements Work from the author's laboratory was supported by grants 44018, from the Canadian Institutes of Health Research (CIHR), and grants from the British Heart Foundation (BHF). RMT is supported through a BHF Chair, PW through a BHF Fellowship, MD through a Marie Curie ITN (RADOX) and ACM through a Leadership Fellowship from the University of Glasgow.

References

1. Shimokawa H (2014) 2014 Williams Harvey Lecture: importance of coronary vasomotion abnormalities-from bench to bedside. Eur Heart J 35:3180–3193. doi:10.1093/eurheartj/ehu427
2. Savoia C, Burger D, Nishigaki N et al (2011) Angiotensin II and the vascular phenotype in hypertension. Expert Rev Mol Med 13:e11
3. Chaudhari N, Talwar P, Parimisetty A et al (2014) A molecular web: endoplasmic reticulum stress, inflammation, and oxidative stress. Front Cell Neurosci 8:213
4. Harrison DG, Widder J, Grumbach I et al (2006) Endothelial mechanotransduction, nitric oxide and vascular inflammation. J Intern Med 259(4):351–363
5. De Ciuceis C, Amiri F, Brassard P et al (2005) Reduced vascular remodeling, endothelial dysfunction, and oxidative stress in resistance arteries of angiotensin II-infused macrophage colony-stimulating factor-deficient mice: evidence for a role in inflammation in angiotensin-induced vascular injury. Arterioscler Thromb Vasc Biol 25:2106–2113
6. Tano JY, Schleifenbaum J, Gollasch M (2014) Perivascular adipose tissue, potassium channels, and vascular dysfunction. Arterioscler Thromb Vasc Biol 34(9):1827–1830
7. Sedeek M, Montezano AC, Hebert RL et al (2012) Oxidative stress, Nox isoforms and complications of diabetes–potential targets for novel therapies. J Cardiovasc Transl Res 5(4):509–518
8. Usui F, Shirasuna K, Kimura H et al (2015) Inflammasome activation by mitochondrial oxidative stress in macrophages leads to the development of angiotensin II-induced aortic aneurysm. Arterioscler Thromb Vasc Biol 35:127–136. doi:10.1161/ATVBAHA.114.303763
9. Wang Y, Wang GZ, Rabinovitch PS, Tabas I (2014) Macrophage mitochondrial oxidative stress promotes atherosclerosis and nuclear factor-κB-mediated inflammation in macrophages. Circ Res 114(3):421–433
10. Paneni F, Costantino S, Cosentino F (2014) Molecular mechanisms of vascular dysfunction and cardiovascular biomarkers in type 2 diabetes. Cardiovasc Diagn Ther 4(4):324–332
11. Signorelli SS, Fiore V, Malaponte G (2014) Inflammation and peripheral arterial disease: the value of circulating biomarkers. Int J Mol Med 33(4):777–783
12. Koenig W (2013) High-sensitivity C-reactive protein and atherosclerotic disease: from improved risk prediction to risk-guided therapy. Int J Cardiol 168(6):5126–5134
13. Galano JM, Mas E, Barden A et al (2013) Isoprostanes and neuroprostanes: total synthesis, biological activity and biomarkers of oxidative stress in humans. Prostaglandins Other Lipid Mediat 107:95–102
14. Biomarkers Definitions Working Group (2001) Biomarkers and surrogate endpoints: preferred definitions and conceptual framework. Clin Pharmacol Ther 69(3):89–95
15. Wang TJ (2011) Assessing the role of circulating, genetic, and imaging biomarkers in cardiovascular risk prediction. Circulation 123:551–565
16. Weber M, Hamm C (2006) Role of B-type natriuretic peptide (BNP) and NT-proBNP in clinical routine. Heart 92:843–849
17. Ho E, Karimi Galougahi K, Liu CC et al (2013) Biological markers of oxidative stress: applications to cardiovascular research and practice. Redox Biol 1(1):483–491
18. Rodrigo R, Libuy M, Feliú F, Hasson D (2013) Oxidative stress-related biomarkers in essential hypertension and ischemia-reperfusion myocardial damage. Dis Markers 35(6):773–790

19. Sherwood MW, Kristin Newby L (2014) High-sensitivity troponin assays: evidence, indications, and reasonable use. J Am Heart Assoc 3(1):e000403
20. Viel EC, Lemarié CA, Benkirane K et al (2010) Immune regulation and vascular inflammation in genetic hypertension. Am J Physiol Heart Circ Physiol 298:H938–H944
21. Sadat U, Jaffer FA, van Zandvoort MA et al (2014) Inflammation and neovascularization intertwined in atherosclerosis: imaging of structural and molecular imaging targets. Circulation 130(9):786–794
22. von Hundelshausen P, Schmitt MM (2014) Platelets and their chemokines in atherosclerosis-clinical applications. Front Physiol 5:294
23. Tuttolomondo A, Di Raimondo D, Pecoraro R et al (2012) Atherosclerosis as an inflammatory disease. Curr Pharm Des 18(28):4266–4288
24. Pitocco D, Tesauro M, Alessandro R et al (2013) Oxidative stress in diabetes: implications for vascular and other complications. Int J Mol Sci 14(11):21525–21550
25. Schiffrin EL (2010) T Lymphocytes: a role in hypertension? Curr Opin Nephrol Hypertens 19:181–186
26. Guzik TJ, Hoch NE, Brown KA (2007) Role of T cell in the genesis of angiotensin II induced hypertension and vascular dysfunction. J Exp Med 204:2449–2460
27. Marvar PJ, Thabet SR, Guzik TJ et al (2010) Central and peripheral mechanisms of T-lymphocyte activation and vascular inflammation produced by angiotensin II-induced hypertension. Circ Res 107(2):263–270
28. Barhoumi T, Kasal DAB, Li MW et al (2011) T regulatory lymphocytes prevent angiotensin II-induced hypertension and vascular injury. Hypertension 57:469–476
29. Droge W (2002) Free radicals in the physiological control of cell function. Physiol Rev 82(1):47–95
30. Brandes RP, Weissmann N, Schröder K (2014) Nox family NADPH oxidases: molecular mechanisms of activation. Free Radic Biol Med 76C:208–226
31. Montezano AC, Touyz RM (2014) Reactive oxygen species, vascular Noxs, and hypertension: focus on translational and clinical research. Antioxid Redox Signal 20(1):164–182
32. Lassègue B, San Martín A, Griendling KK (2012) Biochemistry, physiology, and pathophysiology of NADPH oxidases in the cardiovascular system. Circ Res 110(10):1364–1390
33. Liu J, Ormsby A, Oja-Tebbe N, Pagano PJ (2004) Gene transfer of NAD(P)H oxidase inhibitor to the vascular adventitia attenuates medial smooth muscle hypertrophy. Circ Res 95(6):587–594
34. Mochin MT, Underwood KF, Cooper B et al (2014) Hyperglycemia and redox status regulate RUNX2 DNA-binding and an angiogenic phenotype in endothelial cells. Microvasc Res 97C:55–64
35. Ali ZA, de Jesus Perez V, Yuan K et al (2014) Oxido-reductive regulation of vascular remodeling by receptor tyrosine kinase ROS1. J Clin Invest 124:5159–5174. pii:77484
36. Chen J, Xu L, Huang C (2014) DHEA inhibits vascular remodeling following arterial injury: a possible role in suppression of inflammation and oxidative stress derived from vascular smooth muscle cells. Mol Cell Biochem 388(1–2):75–84
37. Nguyen Dinh Cat A, Montezano AC, Burger D, Touyz RM (2013) Angiotensin II, NADPH oxidase, and redox signaling in the vasculature. Antioxid Redox Signal 19(10):1110–1120
38. Al Ghouleh I, Khoo NK, Knaus UG et al (2011) Oxidases and peroxidases in cardiovascular and lung disease: new concepts in reactive oxygen species signaling. Free Radic Biol Med 51(7):1271–1288
39. Touyz RM (2005) Reactive oxygen species as mediators of calcium signalling by angiotensin II: implications in vascular physiology and pathophysiology. Antioxid Redox Signal 7(9–10):1302–1314
40. Bruder-Nascimento T, Callera GE, Montezano AC et al (2015) Vascular injury in diabetic db/db mice is ameliorated by atorvastatin: role of Rac1/2-sensitive Nox-dependent pathways. Clin Sci (Lond) 128:411–423. doi:10.1042/cs20140456
41. Heneberg P (2014) Reactive nitrogen species and hydrogen sulfide as regulators of protein tyrosine phosphatase activity. Antioxid Redox Signal 20(14):2191–2209

42. Tabet F, Savoia C, Schiffrin EL, Touyz RM (2004) Differential calcium regulation by hydrogen peroxide and superoxide in vascular smooth muscle cells from spontaneously hypertensive rats. J Cardiovasc Pharmacol 44(2):200–208
43. Pastore A, Piemonte F (2013) Protein glutathionylation in cardiovascular diseases. Int J Mol Sci 14(10):20845–20876
44. Iqbal A, Paviani V, Moretti AI et al (2014) Oxidation, inactivation and aggregation of protein disulfide isomerase promoted by the bicarbonate-dependent peroxidase activity of human superoxide dismutase. Arch Biochem Biophys 557:72–81
45. Touyz RM, Briones AM (2011) Reactive oxygen species and vascular biology: implications in human hypertension. Hypertens Res 34(1):5–14
46. Kleikers PW, Wingler K, Hermans JJ et al (2012) NADPH oxidases as a source of oxidative stress and molecular target in ischemia/reperfusion injury. J Mol Med (Berl) 90(12):1391–1406
47. Maghzal GJ, Krause KH, Stocker R, Jaquet V (2012) Detection of reactive oxygen species derived from the family of NOX NADPH oxidases. Free Radic Biol Med 53(10):1903–1918
48. Kaludercic N, Deshwal S, Di Lisa F (2014) Reactive oxygen species and redox compartmentalization. Front Physiol 5:285
49. McNeill E, Channon KM (2012) The role of tetrahydrobiopterin in inflammation and cardiovascular disease. Thromb Haemost 108(5):832–839
50. Lassegue B, Clempus RE (2003) Vascular NAD(P)H oxidases: specific features, expression, and regulation. Am J Physiol Regul Integr Comp Physiol 285:R277–R297
51. Kietadisorn R, Juni RP, Moens AL (2012) Tackling endothelial dysfunction by modulating NOS uncoupling: new insights into its pathogenesis and therapeutic possibilities. Am J Physiol Endocrinol Metab 302(5):E481–E495
52. Cai H, Harrison DG (2000) Endothelial dysfunction in cardiovascular diseases: the role of oxidant stress. Circ Res 87:840–844
53. Zhang YH, Casadei B (2012) Sub-cellular targeting of constitutive NOS in health and disease. J Mol Cell Cardiol 52(2):341–350
54. Nagababu E, Rifkind JM (2010) Measurement of plasma nitrite by chemiluminescence. Methods Mol Biol 610:41–49
55. Bouras G, Deftereos S, Tousoulis D et al (2013) Asymmetric Dimethylarginine (ADMA): a promising biomarker for cardiovascular disease? Curr Top Med Chem 13(2):180–200
56. Juonala M (2007) Brachial artery flow-mediated dilation and asymmetrical dimethylarginine in the cardiovascular risk in young Finns study. Circulation 116(12):1367–1373
57. Paiva H (2010) Levels of asymmetrical dimethylarginine are predictive of brachial artery flow-mediated dilation 6 years later. The Cardiovascular Risk in Young Finns Study. Atherosclerosis 212(2):512–515
58. Wolin MS, Gupte SA, Neo BH et al (2010) Oxidant-redox regulation of pulmonary vascular responses to hypoxia and nitric oxide-cGMP signaling. Cardiol Rev 18(2):89–93
59. O'Donnell VB (1997) Nitric oxide inhibition of lipid peroxidation: kinetics of reaction with lipid peroxyl radicals and comparison with alpha-tocopherol. Biochemistry 36(49):15216–15223
60. Roberts LJ, Morrow JD (2000) Measurement of F(2)-isoprostanes as an index of oxidative stress in vivo. Free Radic Biol Med 28(4):505–513
61. Armstrong D, Browne R (1994) The analysis of free radicals, lipid peroxides, antioxidant enzymes and compounds related to oxidative stress as applied to the clinical chemistry laboratory. Adv Exp Med Biol 366:43–58
62. Heitzer T, Schlinzig T, Krohn K et al (2001) Endothelial dysfunction, oxidative stress, and risk of cardiovascular events in patients with coronary artery disease. Circulation 104(22):2673–2678
63. Annuk M, Zilmer M, Lind L et al (2001) Oxidative stress and endothelial function in chronic renal failure. J Am Soc Nephrol 12(12):2747–2752
64. Annuk M, Zilmer M, Fellstrom B (2003) Endothelium-dependent vasodilation and oxidative stress in chronic renal failure: impact on cardiovascular disease. Kidney Int Suppl 84:S50–S53
65. Guarneri M (2010) Flow mediated dilation, endothelial and inflammatory biomarkers in hypertensives with chronic kidney disease. J Hypertens 28:e118

66. Recio-Mayoral A, Banerjee D, Streather C, Kaski JC (2011) Endothelial dysfunction, inflammation and atherosclerosis in chronic kidney disease – a cross-sectional study of predialysis, dialysis and kidney-transplantation patients. Atherosclerosis 216:446–451

67. Yeun JY, Levine RA, Mantadilok V, Kaysen GA (2000) C-Reactive protein predicts all-cause and cardiovascular mortality in hemodialysis patients. Am J Kidney Dis 35(3):469–476

68. Ferroni P, Guadagni F (2008) Soluble CD40L and its role in essential hypertension: diagnostic and therapeutic implications. Cardiovasc Hematol Disord Drug Targets 8(3):194–202

69. Goldberg RB (2009) Cytokine and cytokine-like inflammation markers, endothelial dysfunction, and imbalanced coagulation in development of diabetes and its complications. J Clin Endocrinol Metab 94(9):3171–3182

70. Binder BR, Christ G, Gruber F et al (2002) Plasminogen activator inhibitor 1: physiological and pathophysiological roles. News Physiol Sci 17:56–61

71. Yang P, Liu YF, Yang L et al (2010) Mechanism and clinical significance of the prothrombotic state in patients with essential hypertension. Clin Cardiol 33(6):E81–E86

72. Paulinska P, Spiel A, Jilma B (2009) Role of von Willebrand factor in vascular disease. Hamostaseologie 29(1):32–38

73. Dignat-George F, Boulanger CM (2011) The many faces of endothelial microparticles. Arterioscler Thromb Vasc Biol 31(1):27–33

74. Beyer C, Pisetsky DS (2010) The role of microparticles in the pathogenesis of rheumatic diseases. Nat Rev Rheumatol 6(1):21–29

75. Jy W, Horstman LL, Jimenez JJ et al (2004) Measuring circulating cell-derived microparticles. J Thromb Haemost 2(10):1842–1851

76. Lacroix R, Robert S, Poncelet P, Dignat-George F (2010) Overcoming limitations of microparticle measurement by flow cytometry. Semin Thromb Hemost 36(8):807–818

77. Burger D, Montezano AC, Nishigaki N et al (2011) Endothelial microparticle formation by angiotensin II is mediated via AT1R/NADPH Oxidase/Rho kinase pathways targeted to lipid rafts. Arterioscler Thromb Vasc Biol 31:1898–1907

78. Burger D, Schock S, Thompson CS et al (2013) Microparticles: biomarkers and beyond. Clin Sci (Lond) 124(7):423–441

79. Burger D, Touyz RM (2012) Cellular biomarkers of endothelial health: microparticles, endothelial progenitor cells, and circulating endothelial cells. J Am Soc Hypertens 6(2):85–99

80. Burger D, Kwart DG, Montezano AC et al (2012) Microparticles induce cell cycle arrest through redox-sensitive processes in endothelial cells: implications in vascular senescence. J Am Heart Assoc 1(3):e001842

81. Leroyer AS, Anfosso F, Lacroix R et al (2010) Endothelial-derived microparticles: biological conveyors at the crossroad of inflammation, thrombosis and angiogenesis. Thromb Haemost 104(3):456–463

82. Shantsila E, Kamphuisen PW, Lip GY (2010) Circulating microparticles in cardiovascular disease: implications for atherogenesis and atherothrombosis. J Thromb Haemost 8(11):2358–2368

83. Boulanger CM, Amabile N, Tedgui A (2006) Circulating microparticles: a potential prognostic marker for atherosclerotic vascular disease. Hypertension 48(2):180–186

84. Azevedo LC, Pedro MA, Laurindo FR (2007) Circulating microparticles as therapeutic targets in cardiovascular diseases. Recent Pat Cardiovasc Drug Discov 2(1):41–51

85. Ridker PM, Lüscher TF (2014) Anti-inflammatory therapies for cardiovascular disease. Eur Heart J 35(27):1782–1791

86. Kaptoge S, Di AE, Pennells L, Wood AM (2012) C-reactive protein, fibrinogen, and cardiovascular disease prediction. N Engl J Med 367:1310–1320

87. Gillett MJ (2009) International Expert Committee report on the role of the A1C assay in the diagnosis of diabetes. Diabetes Care 32:1327–1334

88. Ridker PM (2003) Clinical application of C-reactive protein for cardiovascular disease detection and prevention. Circulation 107:363–369

89. Kaptoge S, Di Angelantonio E, Lowe G et al (2010) C-reactive protein concentration and risk of coronary heart disease, stroke, and mortality: an individual participant meta-analysis. Emerging Risk Factors Collaboration. Lancet 375(9709):132–140

90. Meisinger C, Heier M, von Scheidt W, Kuch B (2010) Admission C-reactive protein and short- as well as long-term mortality in diabetic versus non-diabetic patients with incident myocardial infarction. MONICA/KORA Myocardial Infarction Registry. Clin Res Cardiol 99(12):817–823

91. Miyazaki T, Chiuve S, Sacks FM et al (2014) Plasma pentraxin 3 levels do not predict coronary events but reflect metabolic disorders in patients with coronary artery disease in the CARE trial. PLoS One 9(4):e94073

92. Dubin R, Li Y, Ix JH et al (2012) Associations of pentraxin-3 with cardiovascular events, incident heart failure, and mortality among persons with coronary heart disease: data from the Heart and Soul Study. Am Heart J 163(2):274–279

93. Xanthakis V, Enserro DM, Murabito JM et al (2014) Ideal cardiovascular health: associations with biomarkers and subclinical disease and impact on incidence of cardiovascular disease in the Framingham offspring study. Circulation 130(19):1676–1683

94. Keller T, Zeller T, Peetz D et al (2009) Sensitive troponin I assay in early diagnosis of acute myocardial infarction. N Engl J Med 361:868–877

95. Kotzé RC, Ariëns RA, de Lange Z, Pieters M (2014) CVD risk factors are related to plasma fibrin clot properties independent of total and or γ' fibrinogen concentration. Thromb Res 134:963–969. pii:S0049-3848(14)00454-X

96. Tecchio C, Micheletti A, Cassatella MA (2014) Neutrophil-derived cytokines: facts beyond expression. Front Immunol 5:508

97. Kaptoge S, Seshasai SR, Gao P et al (2014) Inflammatory cytokines and risk of coronary heart disease: new prospective study and updated meta-analysis. Eur Heart J 35(9):578–589

98. Su D, Li Z, Li X et al (2013) Association between serum interleukin-6 concentration and mortality in patients with coronary artery disease. Mediators Inflamm 2013:726178

99. Murdaca G, Spanò F, Cagnati P, Puppo F (2013) Free radicals and endothelial dysfunction: potential positive effects of TNF-α inhibitors. Redox Rep 18(3):95–99

100. Tam LS, Kitas GD, González-Gay MA (2014) Can suppression of inflammation by anti-TNF prevent progression of subclinical atherosclerosis in inflammatory arthritis? Rheumatology (Oxford) 53(6):1108–1119

101. Garlanda C, Dinarello CA, Mantovani A (2013) The interleukin-1 family: back to the future. Immunity 39(6):1003–1018

102. Dinarello CA, van der Meer JW (2013) Treating inflammation by blocking interleukin-1 in humans. Semin Immunol 25(6):469–484

103. Garbers C, Scheller J (2013) Interleukin-6 and interleukin-11: same same but different. Biol Chem 394(9):1145–1161

104. Bustamante A, Sobrino T, Giralt D et al (2014) Prognostic value of blood interleukin-6 in the prediction of functional outcome after stroke: a systematic review and meta-analysis. J Neuroimmunol 274(1–2):215–224

105. Trott DW, Harrison DG (2014) The immune system in hypertension. Adv Physiol Educ 38(1):20–24

106. Gomolak JR, Didion SP (2014) Angiotensin II-induced endothelial dysfunction is temporally linked with increases in interleukin-6 and vascular macrophage accumulation. Front Physiol 5:396

107. Spranger J, Kroke A, Möhlig M et al (2003) Inflammatory cytokines and the risk to develop type 2 diabetes: results of the prospective population-based European Prospective Investigation into Cancer and Nutrition (EPIC)-Potsdam Study. Diabetes 52(3):812–817

108. Lowe G, Woodward M, Hillis G et al (2014) Circulating inflammatory markers and the risk of vascular complications and mortality in people with type 2 diabetes and cardiovascular disease or risk factors: the ADVANCE study. Diabetes 63(3):1115–1123

109. Kawai VK, Chung CP, Solus JF et al (2014) The ability of the 2013 ACC/AHA cardiovascular risk score to identify rheumatoid arthritis patients with high coronary artery calcification scores. Arthritis Rheumatol. doi:10.1002/art.38944

110. Puttevils D, De Vusser P, Geusens P, Dens J (2014) Increased cardiovascular risk in patients with rheumatoid arthritis: an overview. Acta Cardiol 69(2):111–118

111. Damjanov N, Nurmohamed MT, Szekanecz Z (2014) Biologics, cardiovascular effects and cancer. BMC Med 12:48
112. Greenberg JD, Kremer JM, Curtis JR, CORRONA Investigators (2011) Tumour necrosis factor antagonist use and associated risk reduction of cardiovascular events among patients with rheumatoid arthritis. Ann Rheum Dis 70(4):576–582
113. Desai RJ, Rao JK, Hansen RA et al (2014) Tumor necrosis factor-α inhibitor treatment and the risk of incident cardiovascular events in patients with early rheumatoid arthritis: a nested case-control study. J Rheumatol 41(11):2129–2136
114. Niki E (2014) Biomarkers of lipid peroxidation in clinical material. Biochim Biophys Acta 1840(2):809–817
115. Del Rio D, Stewart AJ, Pellegrini N (2005) A review of recent studies on malondialdehyde as toxic molecule and biological marker of oxidative stress. Nutr Metab Cardiovasc Dis 15(4):316–328
116. Yagi K (1998) Simple assay for the level of total lipid peroxides in serum or plasma. Methods Mol Biol 108:101–106
117. White M, Ducharme A, Ibrahim R et al (2006) Increased systemic inflammation and oxidative stress in patients with worsening congestive heart failure: improvement after short-term inotropic support. Clin Sci (Lond) 110(4):483–489
118. White M, Cantin B, Haddad H et al (2013) Cardiac signaling molecules and plasma biomarkers after cardiac transplantation: impact of tacrolimus versus cyclosporine. J Heart Lung Transplant 32(12):1222–1232
119. Kurlak LO, Green A, Loughna P et al (2014) Oxidative stress markers in hypertensive states of pregnancy: preterm and term disease. Front Physiol 5:310
120. da Cruz AC, Petronilho F, Heluany CC et al (2014) Oxidative stress and aging: correlation with clinical parameters. Aging Clin Exp Res 26(1):7–12
121. Lee WC, Wong HY, Chai YY et al (2012) Lipid peroxidation dysregulation in ischemic stroke: plasma 4-HNE as a potential biomarker? Biochem Biophys Res Commun 425(4):842–847
122. Tanaka S, Miki T, Sha S et al (2011) Serum levels of thiobarbituric acid-reactive substances are associated with risk of coronary heart disease. J Atheroscler Thromb 18(7):584–591
123. Salonen JT, Nyyssonen K, Salonen R et al (1997) Lipoprotein oxidation and progression of carotid atherosclerosis. Circulation 95:840–845
124. Zhang ZJ (2013) Systematic review on the association between F2-isoprostanes and cardiovascular disease. Ann Clin Biochem 50(Pt 2):108–114
125. Lee R, Margaritis M, Channon KM, Antoniades C (2012) Evaluating oxidative stress in human cardiovascular disease: methodological aspects and considerations. Curr Med Chem 19(16):2504–2520
126. Campos C, Guzmán R, López-Fernández E, Casado Á (2011) Urinary biomarkers of oxidative/nitrosative stress in healthy smokers. Inhal Toxicol 23(3):148–156
127. Morrow JD, Frei B, Longmire AW et al (1995) Increase in circulating products of lipid peroxidation (F2-isoprostanes) in smokers. Smoking as a cause of oxidative damage. N Engl J Med 332(18):1198–1203
128. Davies SS, Roberts LJ 2nd (2011) F2-isoprostanes as an indicator and risk factor for coronary heart disease. Free Radic Biol Med 50(5):559–566
129. Basu S (2010) Bioactive eicosanoids: role of prostaglandin F(2α) and F$_2$-isoprostanes in inflammation and oxidative stress related pathology. Mol Cells 30(5):383–391
130. Tsimikas S (2006) Oxidative biomarkers in the diagnosis and prognosis of cardiovascular disease. Am J Cardiol 98(11A):9P–17P
131. Pignatelli P, Pastori D, Carnevale R et al (2014) Serum NOX2 and urinary isoprostanes predict vascular events in patients with atrial fibrillation. Thromb Haemost. doi:10.1160/TH14-07-0571
132. Spickett CM (2013) The lipid peroxidation product 4-hydroxy-2-nonenal: advances in chemistry and analysis. Redox Biol 1(1):145–152
133. Asselin C, Shi Y, Clément R et al (2007) Higher circulating 4-hydroxynonenal-protein thioether adducts correlate with more severe diastolic dysfunction in spontaneously hypertensive rats. Redox Rep 12(1):68–72

134. Mali VR, Ning R, Chen J et al (2014) Impairment of aldehyde dehydrogenase-2 by 4-hydroxy-2-nonenal adduct formation and cardiomyocyte hypertrophy in mice fed a high-fat diet and injected with low-dose streptozotocin. Exp Biol Med 239(5):610–618

135. Zhang Y, Sano M, Shinmura K et al (2010) 4-hydroxy-2-nonenal protects against cardiac ischemia-reperfusion injury via the Nrf2-dependent pathway. J Mol Cell Cardiol 49(4): 576–586

136. Usberti M, Gerardi GM, Gazzotti RM et al (2002) Oxidative stress and cardiovascular disease in dialyzed patients. Nephron 91(1):25–33

137. Gerardi G, Usberti M, Martini G et al (2002) Plasma total antioxidant capacity in hemodialyzed patients and its relationships to other biomarkers of oxidative stress and lipid peroxidation. Clin Chem Lab Med 40(2):104–110

138. Fraga CG, Oteiza PI, Galleano M (2014) In vitro measurements and interpretation of total antioxidant capacity. Biochim Biophys Acta 1840(2):931–934

139. Pinchuk I, Shoval H, Dotan Y, Lichtenberg D (2012) Evaluation of antioxidants: scope, limitations and relevance of assays. Chem Phys Lipids 165(6):638–647

140. Lotito SB, Frei B (2006) Consumption of flavonoid-rich foods and increased plasma antioxidant capacity in humans: cause, consequence, or epiphenomenon? Free Radic Biol Med 41(12):1727–1746

141. Hollman PC, Cassidy A, Comte B et al (2011) The biological relevance of direct antioxidant effects of polyphenols for cardiovascular health in humans is not established. J Nutr 141(5): 989S–1009S

142. Wang Y, Chun OK, Song WO (2013) Plasma and dietary antioxidant status as cardiovascular disease risk factors: a review of human studies. Nutrients 5(8):2969–3004

143. Bartosz G (2010) Non-enzymatic antioxidant capacity assays: limitations of use in biomedicine. Free Radic Res 44(7):711–720

144. Gedikli O, Ozturk S, Yilmaz H et al (2009) Low total antioxidative capacity levels are associated with augmentation index but not pulse-wave velocity. Heart Vessels 24(5):366–370

145. Dean RT, Fu S, Stocker R, Davies MJ (1997) Biochemistry and pathology of radical-mediated protein oxidation. Biochem J 324(Pt 1):1–18

146. Shacter E (2000) Quantification and significance of protein oxidation in biological samples. Drug Metab Rev 32(3–4):307–326

147. Cai Z, Yan LJ (2013) Protein oxidative modifications: beneficial roles in disease and health. J Biochem Pharmacol Res 1(1):15–26

148. Dalle-Donne I, Giustarini D, Colombo R, Rossi R, Milzani A (2003) Protein carbonylation in human diseases. Trends Mol Med 9:169–176

149. Kojer K, Riemer J (2014) Balancing oxidative protein folding: the influences of reducing pathways on disulfide bond formation. Biochim Biophys Acta 1844(8):1383–1390

150. Rhee SG, Jeong W, Chang TS, Woo HA (2007) Sulfiredoxin, the cysteine sulfinic acid reductase specific to 2-Cys peroxiredoxin: its discovery, mechanism of action, and biological significance. Kidney Int Suppl 106:S3–S8

151. Arai H (2014) Oxidative modification of lipoproteins. Subcell Biochem 77:103–114

152. Collins AR (2005) Assays for oxidative stress and antioxidant status: applications to research into the biological effectiveness of polyphenols. Am J Clin Nutr 81(1 Suppl):261S–267S

153. Haque A, Andersen JN, Salmeen A et al (2011) Conformation-sensing antibodies stabilize the oxidized form of PTP1B and inhibit its phosphatase activity. Cell 147(1):185–198

154. Nelson KJ, Klomsiri C, Codreanu SG et al (2010) Use of dimedone-based chemical probes for sulfenic acid detection methods to visualize and identify labeled proteins. Methods Enzymol 473:95–115

155. Paulsen CE, Truong TH, Garcia FJ et al (2012) Peroxide-dependent sulfenylation of the EGFR catalytic site enhances kinase activity. Nat Chem Biol 8(1):57–64

156. Ckless K (2014) Redox proteomics: from bench to bedside. Adv Exp Med Biol 806:301–317

157. Groitl B, Jakob U (2014) Thiol-based redox switches. Biochim Biophys Acta 1844(8): 1335–1343

158. Becatti M, Marcucci R, Bruschi G et al (2014) Oxidative modification of fibrinogen is associated with altered function and structure in the subacute phase of myocardial infarction. Arterioscler Thromb Vasc Biol 34(7):1355–1361

159. Goff DC Jr, Lloyd-Jones DM, Bennett G, American College of Cardiology/American Heart Association Task Force on Practice Guidelines et al (2014) 2013 ACC/AHA guideline on the assessment of cardiovascular risk: a report of the American College of Cardiology/American Heart Association Task Force on Practice Guidelines. Circulation 129(25 Suppl 2):S49–S73

160. Davies KJ, Thapar A, Kasivisvanathan V et al (2013) Review of trans-atlantic cardiovascular best medical therapy guidelines – recommendations for asymptomatic carotid atherosclerosis. Curr Vasc Pharmacol 11(4):514–523

161. Davidson MH, Corson MA, Alberts MJ et al (2008) Consensus panel recommendation for incorporating lipoprotein-associated phospholipase A2 testing into cardiovascular disease risk assessment guidelines. Am J Cardiol 101(12A):51F–57F

162. Paynter NP, Everett BM, Cook NR (2014) Cardiovascular disease risk prediction in women: is there a role for novel biomarkers? Clin Chem 60(1):88–97

163. Abbasi A, Corpeleijn E, Meijer E et al (2012) Sex differences in the association between plasma copeptin and incident type 2 diabetes: the Prevention of Renal and Vascular Endstage Disease (PREVEND) study. Diabetologia 55(7):1963–1970

Neurohormonal Interactions

10

Gino Seravalle and Guido Grassi

Cardiovascular homeostasis represents the mechanism through which organ perfusion, metabolic balance, and thermoregulation are modulated to provide the body's requirements. This is obtained with complex interactions among local, humoral, and neural factors capable to modify cardiac and vascular function according to the changing requirements of daily life. We will describe the different factors involved in the homeostatic control of the cardiovascular system starting from the neural mechanisms, passing through the several humoral mechanisms and, last but not least, the local factors at the endothelial levels.

10.1 Neuroregulatory Mechanisms

The central nervous system (CNS) plays an important role in the regulation of the cardiovascular system [1, 2]. By controlling both peripheral autonomic nervous system activity and the release of circulating hormonal factors, the CNS acutely modifies blood pressure and heart rate, thus facilitating cardiovascular homeostasis and appropriate responses to the environment. The sympathetic component of the autonomic nervous system (SNS) is known to play the major

G. Seravalle (✉)
Cardiology, IRCCS Ospedale S. Luca, Istituto Auxologico Italiano,
Piazza Brescia 20, Milan 20149, Italy
e-mail: g_seravalle@yahoo.com

G. Grassi
Clinica Medica, Ospedale S. Gerardo dei Tintori, University Milano-Bicocca,
Via Pergolesi 33, Monza 20052, Italy
e-mail: guido.grassi@unimib.it

© Springer International Publishing Switzerland 2015
A. Berbari, G. Mancia (eds.), *Arterial Disorders:*
Definition, Clinical Manifestations, Mechanisms and Therapeutic Approaches,
DOI 10.1007/978-3-319-14556-3_10

role in cardiovascular homeostasis [3, 4]. SNS is the effector of neurogenic control of vascular tone inducing vasoconstriction of small resistance arteries. It is mainly involved in short-term regulation of vasomotor tone allowing fast adaptation to different physiological conditions by means of autonomic reflexes (baro- and chemoreflexes) that, acting as a feedback mechanism, maintain cardiovascular homeostasis [3, 5]. A role of the SNS in long-term blood pressure control has also been established [6, 7].

Recent evidences suggest that sympathetic activity and vascular function could be linked in a more complex fashion. The same pathways are involved in autonomic regulation as well as in vascular function regulation, suggesting that vascular homeostasis is maintained through pathways activated by the same signaling, allowing an integrated and multidistrict response [8–11]. SNS may also directly modulate functional and mechanical properties of large arteries. This is suggested by the evidence that markers of vascular function are inversely related to sympathetic discharge and it is in line with the induction of endothelial dysfunction by sympathoexcitatory stimuli [12–14]. Adrenergic activation is present in several cardiovascular diseases, inducing chronic changes in vascular function and structure, i.e., vascular remodeling [7]. Sympathetic activity may induce these alterations through several mechanisms: inducing peripheral vasoconstriction; potentiating cardiac contraction; reducing venous capacitance; affecting renal sodium and water excretion, through baroreflex dysfunction; and altering insulin and glucose metabolism [6, 15].

10.2   Humoral Regulation

The modulation of vascular contraction and fluid dynamics is accomplished at least in part through endo-, para-, auto-, intracrine acting hormones which, as a part of a complex regulatory system, are more or less quickly released or inhibited by changes in volume and/or blood pressure and other conditions capable of maintaining homeostasis. Several vasopressor and depressor hormones have been identified and their physiological role known (Table 10.1).

Table 10.1 Hormones and local factors involved in vascular function

Vasoconstriction	Vasodilation
Angiotensin II	Natriuretic peptides
Arginine-vasopressin	Kinin-kallikrein system
Catecholamines	Medullipine system
Endothelin	Adrenomedullin
	Prostaglandins
	Estrogens
	Insulin
	Nitric Oxide

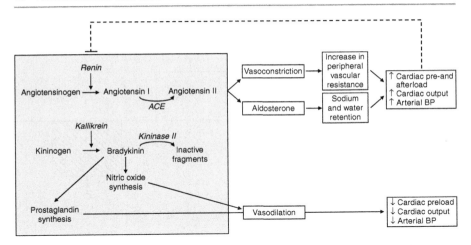

Fig. 10.1 Effects of the renin-angiotensin-aldosterone system and the renal kinin system and their interactions. *ACE* angiotensin converting enzyme, *BP* blood pressure, *dashed line* indicates the inhibition of renin secretion through negative feedback

10.2.1 Renin-Angiotensin System

The systemic renin-angiotensin system (RAS) is central to the regulation of fluid balance. Hyponatremia, hypovolemia, hypotension, and adrenergic stimuli activate the production and release of renin, which enzymatically induce the production of angiotensin I (inactive) that is converted to the vasoactive angiotensin II (Ang II) by a nonspecific converting enzyme (ACE) (Fig. 10.1) [16]. Ang II brings about a constriction of the arteriolar vascular smooth musculature and a release of aldosterone from the adrenal cortex with a resultant increase in tubular sodium and water reabsorption. Since hypervolemia, hypernatremia, and increases in blood pressure and Ang II concentrations, under physiological conditions, supplant renin activation through a negative feedback mechanism, this system may represent a regulatory circuit serving fluid and blood pressure homeostasis. Ang II is able to potentiate SNS activity at different levels [8]. Experimental studies have shown that intracerebral infusion of Ang II was able to induce hypertension, systemic vasoconstriction, and baroreflex reset towards higher blood pressure levels [17]. It has been also demonstrated that vascular smooth muscle nicotinamide dinucleotide phosphate (NADPH) oxidase is activated by Ang II and this increases vascular reactive oxygen species (ROS) levels [18]. More recently, it has been shown that a similar phenomenon occurs within the central nervous system where Ang II upregulates NADPH oxidase activating type 1 (AT1) receptors in neuroanatomical areas implicated in central sympathetic regulation such as the rostroventrolateral medulla (RVLM) in the bulbar area, the circumventricular organs, and the paraventricular nuclei [19–21]. At the peripheral level, Ang II facilitates neural transmission within sympathetic ganglia; favors norepinephrine release by sympathetic nerve terminals, acting on presynaptic receptors; and enhances α-mediated vasoconstriction in arterioles [8, 17, 22–25] (Fig. 10.2). Ang II can stimulate the synthesis of the

Fig. 10.2 Changes in coronary hemodynamics and systemic blood pressure induced by diving during the intracoronary infusion of saline and angiotensin II (Data from Saino et al. [25])

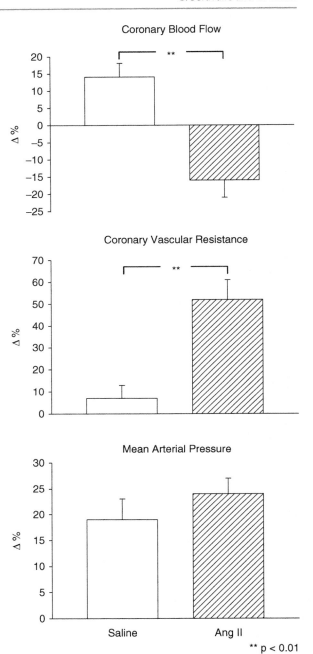

constitutive enzyme nitric oxide synthase (eNOS) and enhance the production of NO [26, 27]. In the renal circulation, this Ang II-NO interaction may protect the preglomerular vessels from the constrictor effect of Ang II [28]. In patients with coronary artery disease, ACE inhibitors attenuate sympathetic coronary vasoconstriction, not only when the drugs are systematically administered [29], but also when small doses of these compounds are infused at the level of the coronary circulation [30]. This finding suggests that not only systemic but also the local renin-angiotensin system is important for preserving cardiovascular homeostasis via an interaction with endothelial factors.

10.2.2 Endothelin

Endothelin-1 (ET-1) is a vasoconstrictor peptide produced by endothelial cells with an important role in regulation of vascular tone [31]. The role of the ET system in cardiovascular homeostasis is not limited to its direct vascular effects but also involves the neural regulation of vasomotor tone [32]. ET-1 can stimulate central and peripheral SNS activity through ET_A receptors [33, 34]. The mechanism of ET-mediated vasoconstriction involves binding to specific receptors on vascular smooth muscle and direct activation of voltage-operated calcium channels in vascular smooth muscle membrane. Two distinct ET receptors have been identified. The ET_A receptor is expressed in vascular smooth muscle cells, whereas the ET_B receptor has been localized to the endothelial and smooth muscle cells. The ET_B receptor may have a dual vasoconstrictive and vasodilatory effect. While in vivo selective ET_A receptor antagonists causes forearm vasodilatation in resistance vessels due mostly to increased NO generation, stimulation of ET_A receptors triggers acute vasoconstriction of large conduit arteries [33]. The ET_B receptor antagonism causes local vasoconstriction, indicating that these receptors in blood vessels respond to ET-1 majorly causing vasodilation [34]. While intracerebral administration of ET-1 can increase BP and SNS activity mainly through ET_A receptors both in hypertensives and normotensives, the administration of an ET_A receptor antagonist determines the opposite effect only in hypertensives, suggesting a specific sympathoexcitatory role for the endogenous ET system in this condition [35, 36]. The increased ET-1 vascular tone observed in essential hypertension seems to be a consequence of reduced NO availability, due to the complex interactions between endothelium-derived substances [37]. At the peripheral autonomic nervous system level, ET-1 can act in carotid bodies and in cervical superior and nodose ganglia, influencing baroreflex and chemoreflex regulation. ET-1 is also released by postganglionic sympathetic neurons, modulating catecholamine release and vascular tone, and stimulates catecholamine release from adrenal gland [38].

10.2.3 Arginine-Vasopressin

The peptide hormone arginine-vasopressin or antidiuretic hormone (ADH) is produced in the hypothalamus and stored in the neurohypophysis. The hormone release is induced by hyperosmolarity and volume decrease and causes a rise in iso-osmotic reabsorption of primary urine in the distal tubule and collecting duct of the kidney. It has also been proven in isolated vascular preparations that vasopressin has a strong vasoconstrictor effect [39].

10.2.4 Natriuretic Peptides

The atrial-, brain-, and C-type natriuretic peptides (ANP, BNP, CNP) are a family, structurally similar, with natriuretic and diuretic properties.

ANP, formed and stored in the atrium and released into the plasma through atrial stretching, is a circulatory peptide hormone which may be involved in the regulation of sodium homeostasis and blood pressure [40]. Under physiological conditions, it is possible to detect relatively constant ANP plasma levels which, considering the high clearance rate of this hormone, suggests a continuous and relatively high production rate. In the 1990s, several papers have shown a complex interaction between this substance and the major reflex mechanisms responsible for cardiovascular homeostasis. Animal studies have shown that the reduction in blood pressure that follows the administration of natriuretic peptides is not accompanied by the expected tachycardia [41], which suggests that these substances may produce an activation of the arterial and/or cardiopulmonary baroreflexes. Direct demonstration of ANP-induced potentiation of the baroreceptor-heart rate reflex has been provided in conscious normotensive rats [42]. Thoren et al. [43] have also shown the link with cardiopulmonary reflex activation providing that these peptides were able to stimulate vagal inhibitory fibers in the cardiopulmonary region.

BNP is found predominantly in the ventricles and atria of the heart [44]. Infusion of BNP, as well as ANP, is able to induce natriuresis and diuresis. Increased plasma levels of this peptide hormone, along with higher intravascular volume and increased ventricular pressure, have been observed in several pathophysiological conditions like congestive heart failure, pulmonary hypertension, arterial hypertension, cerebrovascular diseases, liver dysfunction, and chronic kidney disease [45–49]. A role of cardiac natriuretic peptides has been recently shown also in inflammation and rheumatic diseases [50, 51].

In contrast to ANP and BNP, whose primary target organ is the kidney, C-type natriuretic peptide appears primarily to be a paracrine hormone involved in the regulation of vascular tone. CNP is formed from and secreted by vascular endothelium and has been detected in various areas of the brain. It has been proposed to mediate vascular relaxation by causing endothelium-dependent hyperpolarization. To study this in porcine coronary arteries, the endothelium-dependent relaxation and hyperpolarization of CNP and bradykinin were compared. In contrast to bradykinin, CNP induced endothelium-independent and weaker relaxation and hyperpolarization of coronary artery vascular smooth muscle, suggesting that it is an unlikely mediator of endothelium-dependent hyperpolarization of porcine coronary arteries [52].

10.2.5 The Kinin-Kallikrein System and Prostaglandins

Kinins are generated from precursor known as kininogens by enzymes such as tissue and plasma kallikrein (Fig. 10.1). Some of the effects of kinins are mediated via autocoids such as eicosanoids, NO, endothelium-derived hyperpolarizing factor (EDHF), and/or tissue plasminogen activator (tPA). Kinins, acting via NO, help protect against cardiac ischemia contributing to the vascular protective effect of ACE inhibitors during neointima formation and help reduce infarct size following preconditioning or treatment with ACE inhibitors. This mechanism is also useful in heart failure secondary to ischemic heart diseases. In the kidney, kinins are essential for proper regulation of papillary blood flow and water and sodium excretion. Kinins are involved in the acute antihypertensive effects of ACE inhibitors but not their chronic effects (save for mineralocorticoid-salt-induced hypertension). Kinins appear to play a role in the pathogenesis of inflammatory diseases such as arthritis and skin inflammation; they act as mediators of inflammation by promoting maturations of dendritic cells, which activate the body's adaptive immune system and stimulate mechanisms that promote inflammation. Several prostaglandin derivates (prostacyclin, PGE_2), whose synthesis can be stimulated by kinins, are likewise classified as vasoactive, dilatory tissue hormones [53–55].

10.2.6 Medullipin System

Medullipin is a substance formed and released in the renal medulla and converted in the liver to the vasodilatory, blood pressure-decreasing, circulating hormone medullipin II. It lowers intrarenal vascular resistance and increases renal plasma flow, the glomerular filtration rate, diuresis, and natriuresis [56].

10.2.7 Adrenomedullin

Endogenous adrenomedullin is an autocrine or paracrine factor in cardiovascular and renal regulation. This newly identified peptide is widely distributed in human tissue. Adrenomedullin is a potent vasodilator in vivo in both human and animal arteries and, at least in vitro, inhibits cell proliferation and migration as well as ET-1 and Ang II production and oxidative stress. Adrenomedullin exerts cardiovascular protective actions, such as decreasing blood pressure, reducing intima hyperplasia, and is involved in the regulation of in situ vascular proliferations and vascular remodeling, as well as vascular tone. In the kidney, adrenomedullin elicits a dose-dependent increase in renal blood flow, glomerular filtration rates, and urinary sodium excretion. Thus, adrenomedullin plays a role in the physiological regulation of renal hemodynamic and in pathological condition such as salt-sensitive hypertension [57, 58].

10.2.8 Estrogens

Both endothelial and vascular smooth muscle cells possess estrogen receptors. Estrogens regulate the transcription of numerous genes, and its cellular actions are mediated through the translation of specific mNA transcripts and synthesis of proteins. It stimulates the native synthesis of NO in the blood vessels, heart, and skeletal muscles [59, 60]. Estrogens enhance the binding activity of the transcription factor Spl, whose function is essential for eNOS transcription. Even modest increases in eNOS expression may display protective effects against cardiovascular disease [61]. Other potential protective mechanisms of estrogen are represented by the suppression of a prostaglandin H synthase-dependent vasoconstriction [62] and the inhibition of cyclooxygenase-dependent production of oxidative stress [63]. In perimenopausal women, estrogen supplementation reduces arterial blood pressure and enhances basal NO release in forearm resistance arteries [64].

10.2.9 Insulin

Insulin is synthetized and secreted by the pancreas. Although the liver is the main source of circulating IGF-I levels, it is formed in endothelial and vascular smooth muscle cells. The net effects of insulin on the vasculature are determined by different cellular signaling pathways that are activated by stimulation of the insulin receptor (IR) (Fig. 10.3) [65, 66]. Insulin metabolic signaling results in vasodilation via increased NO production and increases in bioavailable NO. However in conditions of insulin resistance, it promotes vasoconstriction and vascular proliferation. Binding of insulin to IR triggers its phosphorylation and activation via an intrinsic kinase activity, leading to tyrosine phosphorylation of the insulin receptor substrate (IRS) proteins. The activation of the PI3K-Akt pathway induces phosphorylation of eNOS and production of NO, modulated in a Ca^{2+}/calmodulin-sensitive manner, with consequent decrease in vascular tone and vascular smooth muscle cell (VSMC) proliferation and reduction in adhesion of inflammatory cells and platelet aggregation to endothelium [67]. Insulin also promotes, with different eNOS phosphorylation, the production of reactive oxygen species (ROS) and modulates the production of prostaglandins and endothelium-derived hyperpolarizing factors. In addition to vasodilation, insulin can promote vasoconstriction. Under some circumstances, insulin activates the mitogen-activated protein kinase (MAPK) cascade that coordinates insulin vasoconstriction and growth-promoting effects [66]. These effects are mediated in part by the increased production of ET-1 and the activation of signaling through the vascular tissue RAAS [65, 66]. ET-1, via ET_A receptors, causes vasoconstriction, increases oxidative stress, and promotes cell growth and mitogenesis in VSMCs [33]. Similar deleterious effects are seen with the activation of vascular

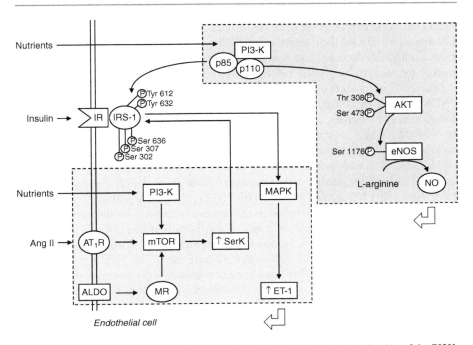

Fig. 10.3 Insulin effects on endothelial cells. Stimulation of IR results in activation of the PI3K-Akt pathway, eNOS phosphorylation, and vasodilation. Insulin resistance induced by RAAS activation and excess nutrients causes increased serine phosphorylation of insulin receptor substrate and metabolic signaling with uninhibited activation of mitogenic and growth pathways. *ALDO* aldosterone, *Ang II* angiotensin II, *ATIR* angiotensin II type 1 receptor, *eNOS* endothelial NO synthase, *ET-1* endothelin 1, *IR* insulin receptor, *mTOR* mammalian target of rapamycin, *MR* mineralcorticoid receptor, *MAPK* mitogen-activated protein kinase, *NO* nitric oxide, *PI3K* phosphatidylinositol 3 kinase, *p* phosporylation, *Akt* protein kinase B, *Ser* serine, *SerK* serine kinase, *thr* threonine, *Tyr* tyrosine (With permission from Muniyappa and Yavuz [66])

tissue RAAS [66]. Insulin plays a modulatory role on skeletal muscle vasculature by increasing blood flow and regulating its own delivery during increased metabolic demands [68]. The mechanism is dependent on an intact endothelium and involves activation of the α-adrenergic receptors to restrict the vasodilation to actively contracting areas of the muscle. Once the terminal arterioles are maximally dilated, adequate skeletal muscle capillary recruitment is needed. An impaired capillary recruitment is present in clinical conditions characterized by insulin resistance such as obesity and type 2 diabetes mellitus [68, 69].

10.3 Endothelial Factors

NO is produced from the amino acid L-arginine by the enzyme NO synthase (NOS) which is present in three isoforms [70]: neuronal NOS (nNOS) is expressed in neurons in central and peripheral nervous system and also in macrophages and endothelial cells where it plays a role in regulation of basal vascular tone [71]; inducible

NOS (iNOS) is expressed in different cellular types and its activity is induced by inflammatory stimuli [70]; endothelial NOS (eNOS) is a constitutive enzyme isoform found in endothelial and neural cells. NO release from endothelium is determined by receptor-mediated mechanisms (acetylcholine, bradykinin, serotonin, substance P, adenosine diphosphate) and by mechanical stimuli (shear stress) [72]. eNOS expression is negatively influenced by hypoxia, tumor necrosis factor-α, inflammatory cytokines, and by false substrates such as N-monomethyl-L-arginine (L-NMMA), which are commonly used to test the degree of endothelium-dependent vasodilation [70]. Asymmetric dimethylarginine (ADMA), a naturally occurring amino acid, is an endogenous inhibitor of eNOS, which can cause endothelial dysfunction and is associated with increased cardiovascular risk [72]. Several evidences have shown that NO acts as a sympathoinhibitory substance within the central nervous system [9]. It is well established that acute or chronic administration of exogenous NOS inhibitors are able to induce vasoconstriction and favor blood pressure raising [73]. This effect could be due to the impairment of NO basal vascular tone and endothelium-mediated vasodilation but above all by the SNS activation. This was found by Sakuma et al. [74] that after an acute intravenous administration of the NOS inhibitor L-NMMA, recorded an increase in BP, in norepinephrine values and in renal sympathetic nerve activity. They have also found a further increment of these responses after baroreceptor deafferentation while a disappearance was observed after cervical spine section, suggesting that L-NMMA pressor effects are mostly due to its effect on SNS. These results are supported by the evidence that ganglionic blockade and sympathectomy suppress BP and heart rate increase induced by another NOS inhibitor such as L-NAME [75, 76]. NO modulation is also particularly relevant in RVLM, the main bulbar area of integration of excitatory autonomic efferent fibers involved in cardiovascular regulation, and in hypothalamic paraventricular nuclei. Microinjection of NOS inhibitors at this level causes renal SNA and BP increase, while NO donors exhibit opposite effects [77, 78].

NO seems to play a role in the pathophysiology of diseases characterized by increased sympathetic discharge. A reduced activity of the intracerebral NO-pathway has been found in renovascular hypertension and heart failure [11, 79].

As regards to the neurogenic control of vascular function, it has been shown that sympathetically induced vasoconstriction may increase shear stress on the vascular wall with consequent increase in NO release from vascular endothelial cells favoring norepinephrine neuronal reuptake in sympathetic nerve terminals [80, 81].

Some other functions deserve to be mentioned. First, NOS may catalyze formation of hydrogen peroxide (H_2O_2) that is a potent vasodilator, but prolonged increased concentrations may be harmful to endothelial and vascular smooth muscle cells, leading to a shift in the balance between the production of protective NO and deleterious O_2^- [82]. O_2^- from the adventitia of the blood vessel can also inactivate NO [83]. It has been shown that oxygen-derived free radicals induced by low-density lipoproteins, Ang II, and pulsatile stretch in artery smooth muscle cells have been implicated in the pathogenesis of atherosclerosis and vascular restenosis in humans [84]. Second, NO has also the role to maintain a balance in the kidney between oxygen consumption and sodium reabsorption [85]. Third, NO released from the vascular endothelium plays an important role in the regulation of tissue mitochondrial respiration in skeletal muscle and in the regulation of cardiac contractile function [86, 87]. Fourth, in healthy adults, the pulmonary vascular resistance is maintained in part through the continuous local production of NO [88].

References

1. Wyss JM, Oparil S, Chen YF (1990) The role of the central nervous system in hypertension. In: Laragh JH, Brenner BM (eds) Hypertension: pathophysiology, diagnosis and management, 3rd edn. Raven Press, New York, pp 679–701
2. Goldstein DS, Kopin IJ (1990) The autonomic nervous system and catecholamines in normal blood pressure control and in hypertension. In: Laragh JH, Brenner BM (eds) Hypertension: pathophysiology, diagnosis and management, 3rd edn. Raven Press, New York, pp 711–747
3. Chalmers J, Arnolda L, Llewellyn-Smith I et al (1997) Central neural control of the cardiovascular system. In: Zanchetti A, Mancia G (eds) Handbook of hypertension, vol 17, Pathophysiology of hypertension. Elsevier, Amsterdam, pp 524–567
4. Wallin BG, Charkoudian N (2007) Sympathetic neural control of integrated cardiovascular function: insights from measurement of human sympathetic nerve activity. Muscle Nerve 36:595–614
5. Mancia G, Grassi G, Ferrari AU (1997) Reflex control of the circulation in experimental and human hypertension. In: Zanchetti A, Mancia G (eds) Handbook of hypertension, vol 17, Pathophysiology of hypertension. Elsevier, Amsterdam, pp 568–601
6. Fink GD, Arthur C (2009) Corcoran memorial lecture. Sympathetic activity, vascular capacitance, and long-term regulation of arterial pressure. Hypertension 53:307–312
7. Grassi G (2009) Assessment of sympathetic cardiovascular drive in human hypertension: achievements and perspectives. Hypertension 54:690–697
8. Grassi G (2001) Renin-angiotensin-sympathetic crosstalk in hypertension: reappraising the relevance of peripheral interactions. J Hypertens 19:1713–1716
9. Patel KP, Li YF, Hirooka Y (2001) Role of nitric oxide in central sympathetic outflow. Exp Biol Med 226:814–824
10. Bruno RM, Sudano I, Ghiadoni L et al (2011) Interactions between sympathetic nervous system and endogenous endothelin in patients with essential hypertension. Hypertension 57:79–84
11. Hirooka Y, Kishi T, Sakai K et al (2011) Imbalance of central nitric oxide and reactive oxygen species in the regulation of sympathetic activity and neural mechanisms of hypertension. Am J Physiol Regul Integr Comp Physiol 300:R818–R826
12. Sverrisdottir YB, Jansson LM, Hagg U, Gan LM (2010) Muscle sympathetic nerve activity is related to a surrogate marker of endothelial function in healthy individuals. PLos One 5:e9257. doi:10.1371/journal.pone.0009257
13. Swierblewska E, Hering D, Kara T et al (2010) An independent relationship between muscle sympathetic nerve activity and pulse wave velocity in normal humans. J Hypertens 28:979–984
14. Padilla J, Young CN, Simmons GH et al (2010) Increased muscle sympathetic nerve activity acutely alters conduit artery shear rate patterns. Am J Physiol Heart Circ Physiol 298:H1128–H1135
15. Lembo G, Napoli R, Capaldo B et al (1992) Abnormal sympathetic overactivity evoked by insulin in the skeletal muscle of patients with essential hypertension. J Clin Invest 90:24–29
16. MacGregor GA, Markandu ND, Roulston JE, Jones JC (1981) Maintenance of blood pressure by the renin-angiotensin system in normal man. Nature 291:329–331
17. Reid IA (1992) Interactions between Ang II, sympathetic nervous system, and baroreceptor reflexes in regulation of blood pressure. Am J Physiol 262:E763–E778

18. Griendling KK, Minieri CA, Ollerenshaw JD, Alexander RW (1994) Angiotensin II stimulates NADH and NADPH oxidase activity in cultured vascular smooth muscle cells. Circ Res 74:1141–1148
19. Carlson SH, Wyss JM (2008) Neurohormonal regulation of the sympathetic nervous system: new insights into central mechanisms of action. Curr Hypertens Rep 10:233–240
20. Gao L, Wang W, Li YL et al (2005) Sympathoexcitation by central Ang II: roles for AT1 receptor upregulation and NAD(P)H oxidase in RVLM. Am J Physiol Heart Circ Physiol 288: H2271–H2279
21. Li YF, Wang W, Mayhan WG, Patel KP (2006) Angiotensin-mediated increase in renal sympathetic nerve discharge within the PVN: role of nitric oxide. Am J Physiol Regul Integr Comp Physiol 290:R1035–R1043
22. Reit E (1972) Actions of angiotensin on the adrenal medulla and autonomic ganglia. Fed Proc 31:1338–1343
23. Starke K (1977) Regulation of noradrenaline release by presynaptic receptor system. Rev Physiol Biochem Pharmacol 77:1–124
24. Taddei S, Virdis A, Mattei P et al (1995) Angiotensin II and sympathetic activity in sodium-restricted essential hypertension. Hypertension 25:595–601
25. Saino A, Pomidossi G, Perondi R et al (1997) Intracoronary angiotensin II potentiates coronary sympathetic vasoconstriction in humans. Circulation 96:148–153
26. Taddei S, Grassi G (2005) Angiotensin II as the link between nitric oxide and neuroadrenergic function. J Hypertens 23:935–937
27. van der Linde NAJ, Boomsma F, van der Meiracker AH (2005) Role of the nitric oxide in modulating systemic pressor responses to different vasoconstrictors in man. J Hypertens 23:1009–1015
28. Hennington BS, Zhang H, Miller MT et al (1998) Angiotensin II stimulates synthesis of endothelial nitric oxide synthase. Hypertension 31:283–288
29. Perondi R, Saino A, Tio RA et al (1992) ACE inhibition attenuates sympathetic coronary vasoconstriction in patients with coronary artery disease. Circulation 85:2004–2013
30. Saino A, Pomidossi G, Perondi R et al (2000) Modulation of sympathetic coronary vasoconstriction by cardiac renin-angiotensin system in human coronary artery disease. Circulation 101:2277–2283
31. Dhaun N, Goddard J, Kohan DE et al (2008) Role of endothelin-1 in clinical hypertension: 20 years on. Hypertension 52:452–459
32. Mosqueda-Garcia R, Inagami T, Appalsamy M et al (1993) Endothelin as a neuro peptide. Cardiovascular effects in the brainstem of normotensive rats. Circ Res 72:20–35
33. Spieker LE, Luscher TF, Noll G (2003) ETA receptors mediated vasoconstriction of large conduit arteries during reduced flow in humans. J Cardiovasc Pharmacol 42:315–318
34. Verhaar MC, Strachan FE, Newby DE et al (1998) Endothelin-A receptor antagonist-mediated vasodilation is attenuated by inhibition of nitric oxide synthesis and by endothelin-B receptor blockade. Circulation 97:752–756
35. Gulati A, Rebello S, Kumar A (1997) Role of sympathetic nervous system in cardiovascular effects of centrally administered endothelin-1 in rats. Am J Physiol 273:H1177–H1186
36. Nakamura K, Sasaki S, Moriguchi J et al (1999) Central effects of endothelin and its antagonists on sympathetic and cardiovascular regulation in SHR-SP. J Cardiovasc Pharmacol 33:876–882
37. Taddei S, Virdis A, Ghiadoni L et al (1999) Vasoconstriction to endogenous endothelin-1 is increased in the peripheral circulation of patients with essential hypertension. Circulation 100:1680–1683
38. Mortensen LH (1999) Endothelin and the central and peripheral nervous systems: a decade of endothelin research. Clin Exp Pharmacol Physiol 26:980–984
39. Mohr E, Richter D (1994) Vasopressin in the regulation of body functions. J Hypertens 12:577–584
40. Inagami T (1994) Atrial natriuretic factor as a volume regulator. J Clin Pharmacol 34: 424–426

41. Ackerman W, Irizawa TG, Milojevic S, Sonnemberg H (1984) Cardiovascular effects of atrial extracts in anesthetized rats. Can J Physiol Pharmacol 62:819–826

42. Ferrari AU, Daffonchio A, Sala C et al (1990) Atrial natriuretic factor and arterial baroreceptor reflexes in unanesthetized rats. Hypertension 15:162–167

43. Thoren P, Mark AL, Morgan D et al (1986) Activation of vagal depressor reflexes by atriopeptins inhibits renal sympathetic nerve activity. Am J Physiol 251:H1252–H1259

44. Cheung BM, Brown MJ (1994) Plasma brain natriuretic peptide in essential hypertension. J Hypertens 12:449–454

45. Sergeeva IA, Christoffels VM (2013) Regulation of expression of atrial and brain natriuretic peptides biomarkers for heart development and disease. Biochem Biophys Acta 1832: 2403–2413

46. Seeger W, Adir Y, Barbera JA et al (2013) Pulmonary hypertension in chronic lung diseases. J Am Coll Cardiol 62:D109–D116

47. Mishra RK, Beatty AL, Jaganath R et al (2014) B-type natriuretic peptides for the prediction of cardiovascular events in patients with stable coronary heart disease: the heart and soul study. J Am Heart Assoc 3:e000907. doi:10.1161/JAHA.114.000907

48. Bentsson J, Zia E, Borne Y et al (2014) Plasma natriuretic peptides and incidence of subtypes of ischemic stroke. Cardiovasc Dis 37:444–450

49. Henriksen JH, Gotze IP, Fuglsang S et al (2003) Increased circulating pro-brain natriuretic peptide (pro-BNP) and brain natriuretic peptide (BNP) in patients with cirrhosis: relation to cardiovascular dysfunction and severity of disease. Gut 52:1511–1517

50. de Bold AJ (2009) Cardiac natriuretic peptides gene expression and secretion on inflammation. J Investig Med 57:29–32

51. Dimitroulas T, Giannakoulas G, Karvounis H et al (2012) B-type natriuretic peptide in rheumatic diseases: a cardiac biomarker or a sophisticated acute phase reactant? Autoimmun Rev 11:837–843

52. Barton M, Beny JL, d'Uscio LV et al (1998) Endothelium independent relaxation and hyperpolarization to C-type natriuretic peptide in porcine coronary arteries. J Cardiovasc Pharmacol 31:377–383

53. Regoli D, Plante GE, Gobell F Jr (2012) Impact of kinins in the treatment of cardiovascular diseases. Pharmacol Ther 135:94–111

54. Kayashima Y, Smithies O, Kakoki M (2012) The kallikrein-kinin system and oxidative stress. Curr Opin Nephrol Hypertens 21:92–96

55. Rhaleb NE, Yang XP, Carretero OA (2011) The kallikrein-kinin system as a regulator of cardiovascular and renal function. Compr Physiol 1:971–993

56. Gothberg G (1994) Physiology of the renomedullary depressor system. J Hypertens 12: S57–S64

57. Samson WK (1999) Adrenomedullin and the control of fluid and electrolyte homeostasis. Annu Rev Physiol 61:363–389

58. Holmes D, Campbell M, Harbinson M, Bell D (2013) Protective effects of intermedin on cardiovascular, pulmonary and renal diseases: comparison with adrenomedullin and CGRP. Curr Protein Pept Sci 14:294–329

59. Rubanyi GM, Johns A, Kauser K (2002) Effects of estrogen on endothelial function and angiogenesis. Vasc Pharmacol 38:89–98

60. Chambliss KL, Shaul PW (2002) Estrogen modulation of endothelial nitric oxide synthase. Endocr Rev 23:665–686

61. Kleinert H, Wallerath T, Euchenhofer C et al (1998) Estrogens increase transcription of the human endothelial NO synthase gene: analysis of the transcription factors involved. Hypertension 31:582–588

62. Davidge ST, Zhang Y (1998) Estrogen replacement suppresses a prostaglandin H synthase-dependent vasoconstrictor in rat mesenteric arteries. Circ Res 83:388–395

63. Virdis A, Ghiadoni L, Pinto S, Lombardo M, Petraglia F, Gennazzani A, Buralli S, Taddei S, Salvetti A (2000) Mechanisms responsible for endothelial dysfunction associated with acute estrogen deprivation in normotensive women. Circulation 101:2258–2263

64. Tolbert T, Oparil S (2001) Cardiovascular effects of estrogen. Am J Hypertens 14:186S–193S
65. Muniyappa R, Montagnani M, Koh KK, Quon MJ (2007) Cardiovascular action of insulin. Endocr Rev 28:463–491
66. Muniyappa R, Yavuz S (2012) Metabolic actions of angiotensin II and insulin: a microvascular endothelial balancing act. Mol Cell Endocrinol 378:59–69
67. Michel JB, Feron O, Sacks D, Michel T (1997) Reciprocal regulation of endothelial nitric-oxide synthase by Ca2+-calmodulin and caveolin. J Biol Chem 272:15583–15586
68. Barrett EJ, Wang H, Upchurch CT, Liu Z (2011) Insulin regulates its own delivery to skeletal muscle by fed-forward actions on the vasculature. Am J Physiol Endocrinol Metab 301: E252–E263
69. Womack L, Peters D, Barrett EJ et al (2009) Abnormal skeletal muscle capillary recruitment during exercise in patients with type 2 diabetes mellitus and microvascular complications. J Am Coll Cardiol 53:2175–2183
70. Luscher TF, Vanhoutte PM (1990) The endothelium: modulator of cardiovascular function. CRC Press, Florida
71. Seddon MD, Chowienczyk PJ, Brett SE et al (2008) Neuronal nitric oxide synthase regulates basal microvascular tone in humans in vivo. Circulation 117:1991–1996
72. Bruno RM, Taddei S (2011) Nitric oxide. In: Mooren FC, Skinner JS (eds) Encyclopedia of exercise medicine in health and disease. Springer, Berlin, pp 645–648
73. Huang M, Leblanc ML, Hester RL (1994) Systemic and regional hemodynamics after nitric oxide synthase inhibition: role of a neurogenic mechanism. Am J Physiol 267:R84–R88
74. Sakuma I, Togashi H, Yoshioka M et al (1992) NG-methyl-L-arginine, an inhibitor of L-arginine-derived nitric oxide synthesis, stimulates renal sympathetic nerve activity in vivo. A role for nitric oxide in the central regulation of sympathetic tone? Circ Res 7:607–611
75. Cunha RS, Cabral M, Vasquez EC (1993) Evidence that the autonomic nervous system plays a major role in the L-NAME-induced hypertension in conscious rats. Am J Hypertens 6:806–809
76. Sander M, Hansen PG, Victor RG (1995) Sympathetically mediated hypertension caused by chronic inhibition of nitric oxide. Hypertension 26:691–695
77. Zanzinger J, Czachurski J, Seller H (1995) Inhibition of basal and reflex-mediated sympathetic activity in the RVLM by nitric oxide. Am J Physiol 268:R958–R962
78. Zhang K, Mayhan WG, Patel KP (1997) Nitric oxide within the paraventricular nucleus mediates changes in renal sympathetic nerve activity. Am J Physiol 273:R864–R872
79. Zucker IH (2006) Novel mechanisms of sympathetic regulation in chronic heart failure. Hypertension 48:1005–1011
80. Toda N, Okamura T (2003) The pharmacology of nitric oxide in the peripheral nervous system of blood vessels. Pharmacol Rev 55:271–324
81. Simaan J, Sabra R (2011) In vivo evidence of a role for nitric oxide in regulating the activity of the norepinephrine transporter. Eur J Pharmacol 671:102–106
82. Cosentino F, Luscher TF (1998) Tetrahydrobiopterin and endothelial function. Eur Heart J 19:G3–G8
83. Wang HD, Pagano PJ, Du Y et al (1998) Superoxide anion from the adventitia of the rat thoracic aorta inactivates nitric oxide. Circ Res 82:810–818
84. Hishikawa K, Oemar BS, Yang Z, Luscher TF (1997) Pulsatile stretch stimulates superoxide production and activates nuclear factor kB in human coronary smooth muscle. Circ Res 81:797–801
85. Laycock SK, Vogel T, Forfia PR et al (1998) Role of nitric oxide in the control of renal oxygen consumption and the regulation of chemical work in the kidney. Circ Res 82:1263–1271
86. Shen W, Hintze TH, Wolin MS (1995) Nitric oxide. An important signaling mechanism between vascular endothelium and parenchymal cells in the regulation of oxygen consumption. Circulation 92:3505–3512
87. Kelly RA, Balligand JL, Smith TW (1996) Nitric oxide and cardiac function. Circ Res 79:363–380
88. Cooper CJ, Landzberg MJ, Anderson TJ et al (1996) Role of nitric oxide in the local regulation of pulmonary vascular resistance in humans. Circulation 93:266–271

Arterial Interactions with Mineral and Bone Disorders

11

Gérard M. London

Associated with deleterious changes in the structure and function damage to large arteries is a major risk factor contributing to the cardiovascular complications in hypertension, diabetes, chronic kidney disease, and chronic inflammatory diseases [1–3]. In many circumstances, these changes are in many aspects similar to those occurring with aging, with this age-related process accelerated and intensified in diabetes and chronic kidney disease (CKD) [4, 5]. Although atherosclerosis and plaque-associated occlusive lesions are the frequent underlying causes of these complications, the spectrum of arterial alterations is broader, including remodeling of large arteries and stiffening of arterial walls, with consequences that differ from those due to atherosclerotic plaques burden [6, 7]. Arterial stiffening is related to intrinsic changes in biophysical and geometric characteristics of arteries with increased calcium content and arterial calcifications (AC) as one of the most frequent consequences of arterial damage associated with deleterious changes in the structure and function of the arterial system [7–10]. AC are frequently associated with mineral and bone disorders which play an important pathophysiological role in the pathogenesis and progression of arterial damage [11–16]. Many studies showed that the extents of calcifications are associated with subsequent cardiovascular mortality and morbidity beyond established conventional risk factors [17–20].

G.M. London, MD
Service d'Hémodialyse, Hôpital F.H. Manhès,
8, rue Roger Clavier, 91712 Fleury-Mérogis, France
e-mail: glondon@club-internet.fr

© Springer International Publishing Switzerland 2015
A. Berbari, G. Mancia (eds.), *Arterial Disorders:*
Definition, Clinical Manifestations, Mechanisms and Therapeutic Approaches,
DOI 10.1007/978-3-319-14556-3_11

11.1   Arterial Calcifications and Mineral and Bone Disorders

AC develop in two distinct sites: the intima and media layers of the large and medium-sized arterial wall. These two forms are frequently associated. Intima plaque calcification occurs in the context of common atherosclerosis and progresses in parallel with the plaque evolution. Calcium accumulation in the media (Mönckeberg's sclerosis or mediacalcosis) of arteries is observed with high frequency with aging, diabetes, and CKD [4, 5, 10, 11]. For a long time, it was thought that these calcifications resulted from passive deposition of calcium salts as the consequence of extracellular fluid volume oversaturation with a high calcium–phosphate product. Experimental and clinical studies indicate that cardiovascular calcifications are an active process that is regulated by a variety of genes and proteins involved in mineral and bone metabolism. AC is a process akin to bone formation, regulated by an equilibrium between factors promoting or inhibiting calcification [21–23]. Emerging evidence indicates that senescence, diabetes, inflammation, dyslipidemia, oxidative stress, estrogen deficiency, and vitamin D and K deficiencies could provide stimuli for osteogenic phenotype expression process involving differentiation of contractile vascular smooth muscle cells, pericytes, and calcifying vascular cells into phenotypically distinct, "osteoblast-like" cells with secretory phenotype [24–31].

Aging is the most typical condition associated with the development of vascular calcifications. VSMC senescence is associated with the switch to a secretory phenotype (senescence-associated secretory phenotype, SASP) that initiates osteoblastic transition with calcifications and artery-wall remodeling [32, 33]. SASP is linked to low-grade arterial inflammation with production of proinflammatory cytokines (IL-1, TNF-α) and oxidative stress all factors leading to NF-κB activation [34]. NF-κB activity, inflammation, and excessive production of reactive oxygen species (ROS) are associated with several features of the progeroid syndrome, such as accumulation of prelamin A [35], low telomerase activity and telomere shortening [36], and DNA damage [37], all conditions being associated with the development of an osteogenic program by activation of BMP 2/4 and Wnt/β-catenin signals (Fig. 11.1).

Molecular imaging in vivo has demonstrated inflammation-associated osteogenesis in early stages of atherosclerosis [38], confirming the role of inflammation in triggering the metabolic cascade leading to the transformation of VSMC into an osteogenic phenotype. Macrophage activation releases proinflammatory cytokines (such as IL-6 and TNFα) and proteolytic enzymes (metalloproteinases MMP 2, MMP 9, and cathepsin S) whose release is associated with osteochondrocytic VSMC transdifferentiation [23, 38]. IL-6 and TNFα are the first steps for the activation of BMP2:BMP4 and Msx2 which promote calcification by activating paracrine Wnt signals and nuclear activation and localization of β-catenin, an indispensable coregulator of expression of Runx2, osterix, and Sox9 which are all transcription factors associated with the osteochondrogenic phenotype conversion of VSMC and pericytes [23, 38–40]. The second aspect of inflammation-related calcification is the proteolytic activation of elastolysis and degradation of extracellular matrix. The fragmentation of elastic lamellae and release of biologically active elastin-derived peptides also promote VSMC dedifferentiation and calcium deposition [41].

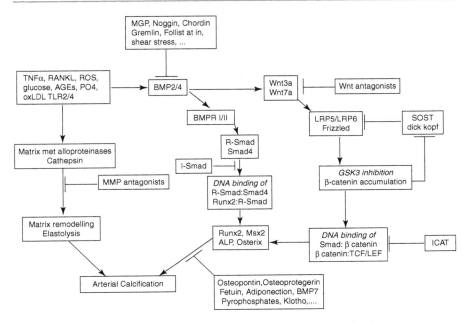

Fig. 11.1   Osteochondrogenic BMP- Msx2-Wnt signaling in arterial calcifications

In the presence of normal serum, VSMC do not calcify. Serum inhibits spontaneous calcium and phosphate precipitation in solution [42], indicating that systemic calcification inhibitors are present in the serum. VSMC which constitutively express potent local or systemic inhibitors of calcification [21], such as matrix GLA protein [43], may limit AC by binding to bone morphogenic proteins [44]. Osteopontin and osteoprotegerin are potent inhibitors of AC in vivo, and inactivation of their genes enhances the calcification process [45, 46]. Fetuin-A (AHSG or α_2 HS glycoprotein) is a potent circulating AC inhibitor that is abundant in the plasma [47]. Pyrophosphate is another potent inhibitor. In vitro, phosphate-stimulated apatite production can be completely prevented by adding pyrophosphates that antagonize the cellular sodium–phosphate cotransport system [48].

While in the general populations the presence of cardiovascular calcifications could be observed in the absence of overt mineral metabolism disorders in several clinical conditions such as CKD/ESRD, the associations between vascular calcifications are associated with deterioration of mineral and bone metabolism caused by changes in serum phosphorus and calcium and disruption of endocrine and humoral pathways including parathyroid hormone (PTH), calcitriol, FGF-23/Klotho, and vitamin D. In vitro, calcium and phosphate promote both synergistically and independently VSMC calcification [28, 49]. Recent findings indicate that hyperphosphatemia, through activation of mitochondrial respiration, stimulates the production of ROS with final activation of NF-κB, enhancing Runx2 (Cbfa1) activation [50].

Hyperphosphatemia is tightly related to disruption of Klothe-FGF23 axis [51, 52]. Several experimental models and clinical conditions such as CKD are characterized by increased FGF23 and decreased Klotho activity [53, 54]. In animal models, Klotho and FGF23 knockout animals are characterized by short life span, accelerated aging phenotype, extensive arterial calcifications, osteoporosis, and hyperphosphatemia [52, 55, 56]. Suppression of phosphate from the diet or knockout of gene for Pit1 and sodium-dependent phosphate uptake restores normal life span and phenotype [52, 55]. Klotho deficiency increases expression of Pit1 and expression of Runx2 associated with secretory osteogenic phenotype of VSMC [53]. In animal models, FGF23 is not directly associated with vascular calcifications since neutralization of FGF23 with specific antibodies results in extensive arterial calcifications and premature death of animals [57].

Decreased Klotho expression and increased FGF23 precede the elevation of parathormone (PTH) secretion also responsible for mineral and bone homeostasis [58]. Chronic elevation of PTH upregulates RANKL and downregulates OPG gene expression and enhances the RANKL–OPG ratio, RANK–RANKL–OPG (receptor activator of nuclear factor (NF)-κB–receptor activator of NF-κB ligand–osteoprotegerin) signaling pathway, and the RANKL–OPG ratio [59–61]. Once bound to RANK, RANKL activates the alternative NF-κB pathway and initiates production of inflammatory cytokines and activates MSx2/Runx2 pathway. Results of a recent study demonstrated that RANKL increased VSMC calcification directly through BMP4 upregulation, providing autocrine stimulus and activation of Wnt signaling [62]. The arterial calcifications observed with increased PTH secretion are attributed to RANKL-mediated bone resorption by osteoclast-associated excessive calcium and phosphate releases.

11.2   Bone–Vascular Cross-Talk

There is growing clinical and experimental evidence linking bone pathology and different functional and structural characteristics of cardiovascular system. Several population-based longitudinal studies demonstrated associations between osteoporosis and AC or arterial stiffness, as well as an association between the progression of aortic calcifications and decreased bone mineral density [14–17, 63–65]. The mechanisms accounting for these associations are not well understood. Several possibilities should be considered: (1) common risk factors for osteoporosis or bone remodeling and vascular calcifications, (2) role of primary vascular pathologies on bone function and remodeling, and/or (3) the participation of bone cells in vascular remodeling.

11.2.1 Common Factors

Clinical data show that osteoporosis and vascular calcifications are influenced by several common risk factors, such as age, menopausal status, diabetes, dyslipidemia with inflammation, and oxidative stress as the final common mechanisms [27, 66–69].

Aging is associated with bone loss and with development of vascular calcifications especially in postmenopausal women [66, 67]. Nevertheless, this bone–vascular association remained significant after adjustment for age suggesting a biologically linked phenomenon [14, 16, 65]. Aging is the most typical condition associated with the development of vascular calcifications. VSMC senescence is associated with the switch to a secretory phenotype (senescence-associated secretory phenotype, SASP) linked to low-grade arterial inflammation with production of proinflammatory cytokines associated with AC by activation of BMP 2/4 and Wnt/β-catenin signals [32, 33]. Direct evidence that inflammation was the factor linking bone remodeling and arterial calcifications was recently provided by Hjortnaes et al. who, using near-infrared fluorescence molecular imaging, showed that arterial and aortic valve calcifications inversely were correlated with osteoporotic bone remodeling [69]. Chronic inflammation is also associated with unbalanced bone formation and bone resorption [70].

Normal bone remodeling is characterized by a balance between osteoclast bone resorption and osteoblast bone matrix deposition. This balance is disrupted in osteoporosis and is influenced by the RANKL–OPG equilibrium. The discovery that OPG-deficient mice develop severe arterial calcifications concomitantly with severe osteoporosis, cortical and trabecular bone porosity, and their high fracture rate provided robust evidence pointing to the RANKL–OPG disequilibrium as a possible common factor linking osteoporosis and arterial calcifications [71]. RANKL activates the alternative NF-κB pathway and initiates production of inflammatory cytokines and arterial calcifications in parallel with RANKL-mediated bone resorption by osteoclasts whose apoptosis is suppressed osteoclast apoptosis. The association between arterial calcification and osteoporosis is most typically observed in postmenopausal women. It could largely reflect estrogen deficiency since estrogen inhibits RANKL-signaling and induces osteoblast OPG expression [72].

Osteopenia, poor fracture healing, arterial calcifications, and higher risk of hip fractures are frequently found simultaneously in patients with diabetes mellitus [73]. Increased AGE accumulation could be the common factor linking bone and arterial pathologies in diabetes. Endogenous ligands for AGE receptors (RAGE) trigger activation of transcription factor NF-κB and ROS signaling, leading to the production of proinflammatory cytokines and activation of VSMC osteogenic BMP/Wnt signaling through Runx2 upregulation inducing AC [74]. In vitro, through their accumulation in diabetes, AGEs stimulate osteoblast apoptosis and modify osteoclast activity by delaying bone regeneration and contributing to defective bone formation [75, 76].

11.2.2 Arterial Disorders and Bone Alterations

Atherosclerosis also affects bone circulation and impaired bone perfusion. With aging, bone arteries and arterioles are subjected to arteriosclerosis, with reduced bone marrow blood supply that renders the marrow ischemic and diminishes the cortex blood supply, which is replaced by the periosteal circulation [77]. That a link between compromised intraosseous circulation and consequent osteoporosis might exist is also suggested by the observation associating decreased bone mineral density and peripheral artery disease [78]. Intraosseous angiogenesis and bone remodeling are regulated by similar cytokines and growth factors, and bone formation–resorption and blood supply are tightly associated [79]. Some results showed that, in healthy women, bone perfusion indices were lower in subjects with osteoporosis than those with osteopenia or normal bone–mineral density [79, 80].

11.2.3 Bone Functions and Arterial Alterations

Several experimental findings support that bone and osteoblast physiology are involved in the control of fat-tissue metabolism and adipokine release, energy expenditure, and insulin secretion and sensitivity, all factors directly affecting cardiovascular function and health. Lee et al. [81] showed that osteoblasts exert endocrine regulation on energy metabolism, with osteocalcin (OCN) playing an important role. Uncarboxylated osteocalcin can regulate the expression of insulin genes and β-cell proliferation and adiponectin (ADPN) release and expression by adipocytes [81, 82]. In CKD patients, serum OCN was positively associated with serum ADPN [83]. ADPN is anti-inflammatory, suppresses atherosclerosis, increases insulin secretion and sensitivity, and activates osteoblastogenesis [84]. Moreover, ADPN regulates arterial calcifications [85], and an inverse relationship was observed between ADPN and the progression of coronary calcifications [86]. In ESRD patients, cardiovascular calcifications are frequently observed in the presence of low bone volume and adynamic bone disease, characterized by decreased osteoblast numbers/activity [15, 87] suggesting that bone cells could influence vascular function and calcification. In a recent study in ESRD patients, it has been shown that peripheral artery disease with extensive calcifications is associated with low osteoblastic activity characterized by pronounced osteoblast resistance to PTH [87].

In conclusion, the results of cross-sectional studies on general populations and several clinical conditions showed an association between atherosclerosis/arteriosclerosis and arterial calcifications. The two types of calcifications, i.e., intimal and medial, have a different impact on arterial functions. The intimal calcification as a part of advanced atherosclerosis results in the development of plaques and arterial lumen decrease or occlusion and ischemic lesions downstream. Medial calcifications result in the stiffening of arterial walls with increased systolic and decreased diastolic pressures. Arterial changes occur in relation with mineral and bone disorders, including osteoporosis, low bone volume, and high or low bone activity. The pathophysiology and biological links between bone and arterial abnormalities suggest the existence of bone-vascular cross-talk and common regulatory factors shared by vascular and bone systems.

This leads to cardiac pressure overload, left ventricular hypertrophy, and decreased myocardial perfusion. The two types of calcifications are associated with increased mortality.

References

1. Briet M, Boutouyrie P, Laurent S, London GM (2012) Arterial stiffness and pulse pressure in CKD and ESRD. Kidney Int 82:383–400
2. Hayden MR, Tyagi SC, Kolb L et al (2005) Vascular ossification – calcification in metabolic syndrome, type 2 diabetes mellitus, chronic kidney disease, and calciphylaxis – calcific uremic arteriolopathy: the emerging role of sodium thiosulfate. Cardiovasc Diabetol 4:1–22
3. London GM, Drüeke TB (1997) Atherosclerosis and arteriosclerosis in chronic renal failure. Kidney Int 51:1678–1695
4. Lindner A, Charra B, Sherrard D, Scribner BM (1974) Accelerated atherosclerosis in prolonged maintenance hemodialysis. N Engl J Med 290:697–702
5. Longenecker JC, Coresh J, Powe NR et al (2002) Traditional cardiovascular disease risk factors in dialysis patients compared with the general population: the CHOICE Study. J Am Soc Nephrol 13:1918–1927
6. O'Rourke MF (1995) Mechanical principles in arterial disease. Hypertension 26:2–9
7. Guérin AP, London GM, Marchais SJ, Métivier F (2000) Arterial stiffening and vascular calcifications in end-stage renal disease. Nephrol Dial Transplant 15:1014–1021
8. Braun J, Oldendorf M, Moshage W et al (1996) Electron beam computed tomography in the evaluation of cardiac calcifications in chronic dialysis patients. Am J Kidney Dis 27:394–401
9. Goodman WG, Goldin J, Kuizon BD et al (2000) Coronary artery calcification in young adults with end-stage renal disease who are undergoing dialysis. N Engl J Med 342:1478–1483
10. Ibels LS, Alfrey AL, Huffer WE et al (1979) Arterial calcification and pathology in uremic patients undergoing dialysis. Am J Med 66:790–796
11. Block GA, Klassen PS, Lazarus JM et al (2004) Mineral metabolism, mortality, and morbidity in maintenance hemodialysis. J Am Soc Nephrol 15:2208–2218
12. Jono S, McKee MD, Murry CE et al (2000) Phosphate regulation of vascular smooth muscle cell calcification. Circ Res 87:E10–E17
13. Yang H, Curinga G, Giachelli CM (2004) Elevated extracellular calcium levels induce smooth muscle cell matrix mineralization in vitro. Kidney Int 66:2293–2299
14. Hak AE, Pols HA, van Hemert AM et al (2000) Progression of aortic calcification is associated with metacarpal bone loss during menopause: a population-based longitudinal study. Arterioscler Thromb Vasc Biol 20:1926–1931
15. London GM, Marty C, Marchais SJ et al (2004) Arterial calcifications and bone histomorphometry in end-stage renal disease. J Am Soc Nephrol 15:1943–1951
16. Schulz E, Arfai K, Liu X et al (2004) Aortic calcification and the risk of osteoporosis and fractures. J Clin Endocrinol Metab 89:4246–4253
17. Wilson PWF, Kauppila LI, O'Donnell CJ et al (2001) Abdominal aortic calcific deposits are an important predictor of vascular morbidity and mortality. Circulation 103:1529–1534
18. Sangiorgi G, Rumberger JA, Severson A et al (1998) Arterial calcification and not lumen stenosis is highly correlated with atherosclerotic plaque burden in humans: a histologic study of 723 coronary artery segments using nondecalcifying methodology. J Am Coll Cardiol 31:126–133
19. Detrano R, Hsiai T, Wang S et al (1996) Prognostic value of coronary calcification and angiographic stenoses in patients undergoing coronary angiography. J Am Coll Cardiol 27:285–290
20. Blacher J, Guérin AP, Pannier B et al (2001) Arterial calcifications, arterial stiffness, and cardiovascular risk in end-stage renal disease. Hypertension 38:938–942
21. Schoppet M, Shroff RC, Hofbauer LC, Shanahan CM (2008) Exploring the biology of vascular calcification in chronic kidney disease: what's circulating? Kidney Int 73:384–390
22. Demer LL, Tintut Y (2008) Vascular calcification: pathobiology of multifaceted disease. Circulation 117:2938–2948
23. Bostrom KI, Rajamannan NM, Towler DA (2011) The regulation of valvular and vascular sclerosis by osteogenic morphogens. Circ Res 109:564–577
24. Jono S, Nishizawa Y, Shioi A, Morii H (1998) 1,25-Dihydroxyvitamin D3 increases in vitro vascular calcification by modulating secretion of endogenous parathyroid-hormone-related peptide. Circulation 98:1302–1306

25. Steitz SA, Speer ME, Curinga G et al (2001) Smooth muscle cell phenotypic transition associated with calcification. Upregulation of Cbfa1 and downregulation of smooth muscle lineage markers. Circ Res 89:1147–1154
26. Tintut Y, Patel J, Parhami F, Demer LL (2000) Tumor necrosis factor-alpha promotes in vitro calcification of vascular cells via cAMP pathway. Circulation 102:2636–2642
27. Parhami F, Garfinkel A, Demer LL (2000) Role of lipids in osteoporosis. Arterioscler Thromb Vasc Biol 20:2346–2348
28. Reynolds JL, Joannides AJ, Skepper JN et al (2004) Human vascular smooth muscle cells undergo vesicle-mediated calcification in response to changes in extracellular calcium and phosphate concentrations: a potential mechanism for accelerated vascular calcification in ESRD. J Am Soc Nephrol 15:2857–2867
29. Braam LA, Hoeks APG, Brouns F et al (2004) Beneficial effects of vitamins D and K on the elastic properties of the vessel wall in postmenopausal women: a follow-up study. Thromb Haemost 91:373–380
30. Shao J-S, Cai J, Towler DA (2006) Molecular mechanisms of vascular calcification: lessons learned from the aorta. Arterioscler Thromb Vasc Biol 26:1423–1430
31. Shao JS, Sadhu J, Towler DA (2010) Inflammation and the osteogenic regulation of vascular calcification. A review and perspective. Hypertension 55:579–592
32. Wang M, Monticone RE, Lakatta EG (2010) Arterial aging: a journey into subclinical arterial disease. Curr Opin Nephrol Hypertens 19:201–207
33. Nakano-Kurimoto R, Ikeda K, Uraoka M et al (2009) Replicative senescence of vascular smooth muscle cells enhances the calcification through initiating the osteoblastic transition. Am J Physiol Heart Physiol 297:H1673–H1684
34. Newgard CB, Sharpless NE (2013) Coming of age: molecular drivers of aging and therapeutic opportunities. J Clin Invest 123:946–950
35. Ragnauth CD, Warren DT, Yiwen Liu Y et al (2010) Prelamin A acts to accelerate smooth muscle cell senescence and is a novel biomarker of human vascular aging. Circulation 121:2200–2210
36. Carrero JJ, Stenvinkel P, Fellstro¨m B et al (2008) Telomere attrition is associated with inflammation, low fetuin-A levels and high mortality in prevalent haemodialysis patients. J Intern Med 263:302–312
37. Tistra JS, Robinson AR, Wang L et al (2012) NF-κB inhibition delays DNA damage-induced senescence and aging in mice. J Clin Invest 122:2601–2612
38. Aikawa E, Nahrendor M, Figueiredo J-L et al (2007) Osteogenesis associates with inflammation in early-stage atherosclerosis evaluated by molecular imaging in vivo. Circulation 116:2841–2850
39. Shao J-S, Cheng S-L, Joyce M et al (2005) Msx2 promotes cardiovascular calcification by activating paracrine Wnt signals. J Clin Invest 115:1210–1220
40. Al-Aly Z, Shao J-S, Lai C-F et al (2007) Aortic Msx2-Wnt calcification cascade is regulated by TNF-α-dependent signals in diabetic ldlr −/− mice. Arterioscler Thromb Vasc Biol 27:2589–2596
41. Aikawa E, Aikawa M, Libby P et al (2009) Arterial and aortic valve calcification abolished by elastolytic cathepsin deficiency in chronic renal disease. Circulation 119:1785–1794
42. Moe SM, Duan D, Doehle BP et al (2003) Uremia induces the osteoblast differentiation factor Cbfa1 in human blood vessels. Kidney Int 63:1003–1011
43. Luo G, Ducy P, McKee MD et al (1997) Spontaneous calcification of arteries and cartilage in mice lacking matrix GLA protein. Nature 386:78–81
44. Sweatt A, Sane DC, Hutson SM et al (2003) Matrix Gla protein (MGP) and bone morphogenetic protein-2 in aortic calcified lesions of aging rats. J Thromb Haemost 1:178–185
45. Speer MY, McKee MD, Guldberg RE et al (2002) Inactivation of osteopontin gene enhances vascular calcification of matrix Gla protein-deficient mice : evidence for osteopontin as an inducible inhibitor of vascular calcification in vivo. J Exp Med 196:1047–1055
46. Price PA, June HH, Buckley JR et al (2001) Osteoprotegerin inhibits artery calcification induced by warfarin and by vitamin D. Arterioscler Thromb Vasc Biol 21:1610–1616

47. Schafer C, Heiss A, Schwarz A et al (2003) The serum protein alpha 2-Heremans–Schmid glycoprotein/fetuin-A is a systemically acting inhibitor of ectopic calcification. J Clin Invest 112:357–366
48. Lomashvili K, Cobbs S, Hennigar RA et al (2004) Phosphate-induced vascular calcification: role of pyrophosphate and osteopontin. J Am Soc Nephrol 15:1392–1401
49. Shanahan C, Crouthamel MH, Kapustin A et al (2011) Arterial calcification in chronic kidney disease: key role for calcium and phosphate. Circ Res 109:697–711
50. Zhao M-M, Xu M-J, Cai Y et al (2011) Mitochondrial reactive oxygen species promote p65 nuclear translocation mediating high-phosphate induced vascular calcification in vitro and in vivo. Kidney Int 79:1071–1079
51. Quarles LD (2008) Endocrine function of bone in mineral regulation. J Clin Invest 118:3820–3828
52. Stubbs JR, Liu S, Tang W et al (2007) Role of hyperphosphatemia and 1,25-dihydroxy vitamin D in vascular calcifications and mortality in fibroblast growth factor 23 null mice. J Am Soc Nephrol 18:2116–2124
53. Hu MC, Shi M, Zhang J et al (2011) Klotho deficiency causes vascular calcification in chronic kidney disease. J Am Soc Nephrol 22:124–136
54. Lim K, Lu T-S, Molostvov G et al (2012) Klotho deficiency potentiates the development of human artery calcification and mediates resistance to fibroblast growth factor 23. Circulation 125:2243–2255
55. Ohnishi M, Razzaque MS (2010) Dietary and genetic evidence for phosphate toxicity accelerating mammalian aging. FASAB J 24:3562–3571
56. Kuro-O M (2009) Klotho and aging. Biochem Biophys Acta 1790:1049–1058
57. Shalhoub V, Shatzen EM, Ward SC et al (2012) FGF23 neutralization improves chronic kidney disease-associated hyperparathyroidism yet increases mortality. J Clin Invest 122:2543–2553
58. Isakova T, Wahl P, Vargas GS et al (2011) Fibroblast growth factor 23 is elevated before parathyroid hormone and phosphate in chronic kidney disease. Kidney Int 79:1370–1378
59. Huang JC, Sakata T, Pfleger LL et al (2004) PTH differentially regulates expression of RANKL and OPG. J Bone Miner Res 19:234–244
60. Hofbauer LC, Schoppet M (2004) Clinical implications of the osteoprotegerin/RANKL/RANK system for bone and vascular diseases. JAMA 292:490–495
61. Collin-Osdoby P (2004) Regulation of vascular calcification by osteoclast regulatory factors RANKL and osteoprotegerin. Circ Res 95:1046–1057
62. Panizo S, Cardus A, Encinas M et al (2009) RANKL increases vascular smooth muscle cell calcification through a RANK-BMP4 dependent pathway. Circ Res 104:1041–1048
63. Raggi P, Bellasi A, Ferramosca E et al (2007) Pulse wave velocity is inversely related to vertebral bone density in hemodialysis patients. Hypertension 49:1278–1284
64. Toussaint ND, Lau KK, Strauss BJ et al (2008) Association between vascular calcification, arterial stiffness and bone mineral density in chronic kidney disease. Nephrol Dial Transplant 23:586–593
65. Kiel DP, Kauppila LI, Cuples LA et al (2001) Bone loss and progression of abdominal aortic calcification over a 25 year period: the Framingham Heart Study. Calcif Tissue Int 68:271–276
66. Tanko LB, Christiansen C, Cox DA et al (2005) Relationship between osteoporosis and cardiovascular disease in postmenopausal women. J Bone Miner Res 20:1912–1920
67. Hamerman D (2005) Osteoporosis and atherosclerosis: biological linkage and the emergence of dual-purpose therapies. Q J Med 98:467–484
68. Doherty TM, Asotra K, Fitzpatrick LA et al (2003) Calcification in atherosclerosis: bone biology and chronic inflammation at the arterial crossroads. Proc Natl Acad Sci U S A 100:11201–11206
69. Hjortnaes J, Butcher J, Figueiredo J-L et al (2010) Arterial and aortic valve calcification inversely correlates with osteoporotic bone remodelling: a role for inflammation. Eur Heart J 31:1975–1984
70. Koh JM, Khang YH, Jung CH et al (2005) Higher circulating hsCRP levels are associated with lower bone mineral density in healthy pre- and postmenopausal women: evidence for a link between systemic inflammation and osteoporosis. Osteoporos Int 16:1263–1271

71. Bucay N, Sarosi I, Dunstan CR et al (1998) Osteoprotegerin-deficient mice develop early onset osteoporosis and arterial calcification. Genes Dev 12:1260–1268
72. Osako MK, Nakagami H, Koibuchi N et al (2010) Estrogen inhibits vascular calcification via vascular RANKL system: common mechanism of osteoporosis and vascular calcification. Circ Res 107:466–475
73. Hofbauer LC, Bueck CC, Singh SK, Dobnig H (2007) Osteoporosis in patients with diabetes mellitus. J Bone Miner Res 22:1317–1328
74. Tanikawa T, Okaya Y, Tanikawa R, Tanaka Y (2009) Advanced glycation end products induce calcification of vascular smooth muscle cells through RAGE/p38 MAPK and upregulation of Runx2. J Vasc Res 46:572–580
75. Alikhani M, Alikhani Z, Boyd C et al (2007) Advanced glycation end-products stimulate osteoblast apoptosis via MAP kinase and cytosolic apoptotic pathway. Bone 40:345–353
76. Valcourt U, Merle B, Gineyts E et al (2007) Non-enzymatic glycation of bone collagen modifies osteoclastic activity and differentiation. J Biol Chem 282:5691–5703
77. Bridgeman G, Brookes M (1996) Blood supply to the human femoral diaphysis in youth and senescence. J Anat 188:611–621
78. Laroche M (2002) Intraosseous circulation from physiology to disease. Joint Bone Spine 69:262–269
79. Alagiakrishnan K, Juby A, Hanley D et al (2008) Role of vascular factors in osteoporosis. J Gerontol 4:362–366
80. Griffith JF, Yeung DK, Tsang PH et al (2008) Compromised bone marrow perfusion in osteoporosis. J Bone Miner Res 23:1068–1075
81. Lee NK, Sowa H, Hinoi E et al (2007) Endocrine regulation of energy metabolism by the skeleton. Cell 130:456–469
82. Ferron M, Wei J, Yoshizawa T et al (2010) Insulin signaling in osteoblasts integrates bone remodeling and energy metabolism. Cell 142:296–308
83. Bacchetta J, Boutroy S, Guebre-Egziabher F et al (2009) The relationship between adipokines, osteocalcin and bone quality in chronic kidney disease. Nephrol Dial Transplant 24:3120–3125
84. Oshima K, Nampei A, Matsuda M et al (2005) Adiponectin increases bone mass by suppressing osteoclasts and activating osteoblasts. Biochem Biophys Res Commun 331:520–526
85. Luo XH, Zhao LL, Yuan LQ et al (2009) Development of arterial calcification in adiponectin-deficient mice: adiponectin regulates arterial calcification. J Bone Miner Res 24:1461–1468
86. Maahs DM, Ogden LG, Kinney GL et al (2005) Low plasma adiponectin levels predict progression of coronary artery calcification. Circulation 111:747–753
87. London GM, Marchais SJ, Guérin AP, de Vernejoul MCh (2015) Ankle–brachial index and bone turnover in patients on dialysis. J Am Soc Nephrol 26:476–483

Endothelial Function in Health and Disease

Arno Greyling, Maria T. Hopman, and Dick H.J. Thijssen

12.1   Introduction

It has been said that one is as old as one's arteries. In view of the supreme importance of endothelium in arterial function I would like to modify, or rather simplify, this statement by saying the one is as old as one's endothelium. [1]

Dr. Rudolf Altschul prefaced his book 'Endothelium: Its Development, Morphology, Function and Pathology' with this statement. Embedded in our current knowledge, this statement seems like an open door. However, it was made in 1954, a time during which relatively little was known on the subject. This contrasts with contemporary interest in the endothelium, supported by the publication of approximately 10,000 publications by 2014.

Since the discovery of the endothelium by Friedrich von Recklinghausen in mid-1800, appreciation of the morphology and functions of the endothelium saw slow progress. Notable milestones include the definition of Starling's 'Law of capillary exchange' which established the endothelium as a selectively permeable barrier [2] and the use of electron microscopy which enabled assessment of the endothelium's ultrastructure. Only recently has it been found that the endothelium produces

A. Greyling • M.T. Hopman
Department of Physiology, Radboud University Medical Centre,
PO Box 9101, Geert Grooteplein Zuid 30, Nijmegen 6525 GA, The Netherlands
e-mail: Arno.Greyling@radboudumc.nl; Maria.Hopman@radboudumc.nl

D.H.J. Thijssen (✉)
Department of Physiology, Radboud University Medical Centre,
PO Box 9101, Geert Grooteplein Zuid 30, Nijmegen 6525 GA, The Netherlands

Research Institute for Sport and Exercise Sciences, Liverpool John Moores
University, Liverpool, UK
e-mail: Dick.Thijssen@radboudumc.nl

© Springer International Publishing Switzerland 2015
A. Berbari, G. Mancia (eds.), *Arterial Disorders:*
Definition, Clinical Manifestations, Mechanisms and Therapeutic Approaches,
DOI 10.1007/978-3-319-14556-3_12

vasoactive substances, such as prostacyclin in 1976 [3] and followed by the Nobel Prize winning work from Robert Furchgott who discovered the endothelium's ability to produce nitric oxide in 1980 [4].

We now know that the deceptively simple appearance of this single layer of cells belies the fact that it is 'the largest endocrine gland in the body' [5] with myriad of complex functions that play an integral part in vascular homeostasis. This chapter will focus on the (patho)physiological role of the vascular endothelium.

12.2 Physiological Functions of the Endothelium

The endothelium forms a barrier between blood-borne cells and macro-molecules and the underlying artery wall. Its permeability and integrity is regulated by transcellular (through endothelial cells) and paracellular (between endothelial cells) passage mechanisms. Transcellular transport takes place via transport vesicles (e.g. caveolae and vesiculo-vacuolar organelles) and is the primary means by which albumin, lipids, steroid hormones and fat-soluble vitamins cross the endothelium. Transport vesicles can also fuse into channels that traverse single cells, allowing the passage of leukocytes and solutes [6]. Furthermore, specialised fenestrae are present that control transcellular permeability to water and solutes. Paracellular transport occurs through the coordinated opening and closure of endothelial cell-cell junctions. Endothelial cell junctions also regulate contact-induced inhibition of cell growth, apoptosis, gene expression and new vessel formation [7]. The importance of controlling permeability is highlighted by the observation that increases in the permeability of the endothelium, which is linked to endothelium dysfunction and aids in the formation and progression of atherosclerosis [8].

In addition to the 'barrier function', the endothelium controls maintenance of vascular homeostasis. Through the autocrine secretion of substances, it exerts bidirectional control to form a finely balanced interdependent system [9] (Fig. 12.1). The most important functions of the endothelium include (1) regulation of vascular tone, (2) control of thrombosis and haemostasis, (3) immune and inflammatory responses and (4) facilitation of vascular growth, repair and remodelling. These functions of the endothelium are discussed below.

12.2.1 Regulation of Vascular Tone

12.2.1.1 Nitric Oxide

The endothelium regulates vascular tone through the rapid synthesis of vasodilators and vasoconstrictors (Fig. 12.1). Nitric oxide (NO) is an important and powerful vasodilator which is produced by the endothelium as a soluble gas with a short half-life (6–30 s in the artery wall and a few seconds in the blood). Its production involves a two-step oxidation of L-arginine to L-citrulline, with concomitant production of NO. This reaction is catalysed by NO-synthases (NOS) with the aid of cofactors, including tetrahydrobiopterin and nicotinamide adenine dinucleotide phosphate

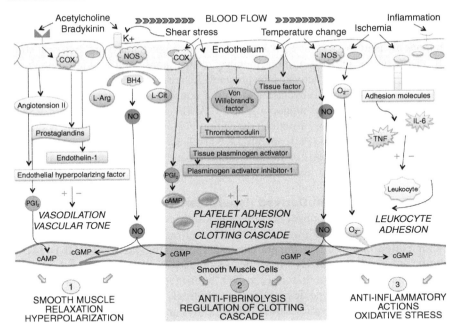

Fig. 12.1 The endothelium is responsible for a number of physiological functions, including (1) regulation of vascular tone, (2) control of blood fluidity and coagulation, and (3) regulation of inflammatory processes. *cAMP* cyclic adenosine monophosphate, *cGMP* cyclic guanosine monophosphate, *COX* cyclooxygenase, *BH4* tetrahydrobiopterin, *IL* interleukin, *TNF* tumour necrosis factor, l-*arg* L-arginine, l-*cit* L-citrulline, *NO* nitric oxide, *NOS* nitric oxide synthase, *O2*–superoxide (With permission from Marti et al. [9])

(NADPH) (Fig. 12.1). The NOS family plays a central role in the production of NO and consists of three different isoforms named after the tissues in which they were first identified: the neuronal (nNOS), inducible (iNOS) and endothelial (eNOS) isoforms. Many tissues can express more than one isoform, and all three may be constitutive or inducible [10]. Nonetheless, eNOS is the predominant form in endothelial cells and is the main source of endothelium-derived NO. eNOS is constitutively expressed and continuously produces small amounts of NO. eNOS can be stimulated by various hormones as well as haemodynamic factors. These stimuli induce an increase in intercellular Ca^{2+} that displaces the inhibitor caveolin from calmodulin to activate eNOS.

After production, NO diffuses to vascular smooth muscle cells (VSMCs) and activates guanylate cyclase, causing an increase in intracellular cyclic guanosine monophosphate (cGMP). This action leads to relaxation of the VSMCs and subsequent vasodilation. The importance of NO is supported by experimental work where inactivation of eNOS results in vasoconstriction and elevation in arterial blood pressure [11]. NO also exerts inhibitory effects on platelet aggregation, leukocyte adhesion and VSMC migration and proliferation, highlighting the importance of this hormone for vascular homeostasis [10].

12.2.1.2 Prostacyclin

The endothelium produces a family of prostaglandins through the catabolism of arachidonic acid by cyclooxygenases in response to mechanical and humoral stimuli. Prostacyclin (PGI_2) is a major member of this family and acts as a paracrine-signalling molecule and activates the prostacyclin receptors on VSMC and platelets. This stimulates adenylate cyclase and with a consequent increase in intracellular levels of cyclic adenosine monophosphate (cAMP), ultimately resulting in VSMC relaxation and inhibition of platelet activation [12]. The action of PGI_2 is closely related to that of NO since PGI_2 potentiates NO release (and vice versa). Nonetheless, PGI_2 seems less important for vascular control than NO, but plays a central role in the coagulation pathway (see Sect. 12.2.2).

12.2.1.3 Endothelium-Derived Hyperpolarizing Factor

Some of the endothelium-dependent vasodilation has generally been associated with hyperpolarization of the VSMCs and referred to a non-characterised factor called endothelium-dependent hyperpolarizing factor (EDHF) [13]. A number of candidate EDHFs have been suggested, including arachidonic acid metabolites, gaseous mediators (e.g. NO, hydrogen sulfide and carbon monoxide), reactive oxygen species, vasoactive peptides, potassium ions and adenosine. Irrespective of its exact nature, EDHF plays an important role in regulating vascular tone.

12.2.1.4 Endothelin

Endothelins are a family of potent vasoconstrictor peptides. Endothelin-1 (ET-1) is the predominant isoform and is primarily secreted by the endothelium in response to a variety of humoral and physical stimuli. After the production of ET-1 by the endothelium, it binds to the ET_A and ET_B receptors on VSMCs resulting in a sustained vasoconstriction. Endothelial cells also express ET_B receptors whose stimulation results in the release of NO and PGI2, leading to vasodilation (and therefore serves as a feedback mechanism to partially oppose the vasoconstrictive effects of VSMC-located $ET_{A/B}$-receptors). ET-1 also induces VSMC proliferation and growth in a dose-dependent manner, suggesting an important role for ET-1 to contribute to the atherosclerotic process [14].

12.2.1.5 Angiotensin

After cleavage of angiotensinogen to angiotensin (Ang) I via renin, this peptide is cleaved by the angiotensin-converting enzyme (produced by pulmonary and systemic vascular endothelium) into Ang II. The smooth muscle cell-localised AT1 receptor subtype mediates the predominant action of Ang II: vasoconstriction. These vasoactive actions are partly counteracted by the AT2 receptor, which causes vasodilatation [15]. Besides the vasoactive effects, Ang II leads to proliferation and growth of the VSMCs through activation of the AT1 receptor. Similarly to ET-1, the vasoconstrictive effects of AT1 are, at least partly, counterbalanced by a negative feedback loop in the vascular wall.

12.2.1.6 Thromboxane A$_2$

Thromboxane A$_2$ (TXA$_2$) is an end product of arachidonic acid metabolism and is produced by TXA$_2$ synthase. TXA$_2$ is primarily produced by platelets, but also by the endothelium. The primary physiological role of TXA$_2$ is platelet aggregation, but it has also been demonstrated to contribute to vasoconstriction [16].

12.2.1.7 Prostaglandin H$_2$

In contrast to most members of the prostaglandin family, prostaglandin H$_2$ (PGH$_2$) is a vasoconstrictor substance. PGH$_2$ is closely related to TXA$_2$ as both are formed during arachidonic acid metabolism. Furthermore, PGH$_2$ is the precursor of TXA$_2$ and exerts its vascular effects through the same receptors [17].

12.2.2 Control of Blood Fluidity and Coagulation

The endothelium actively maintains an anticoagulant and antithrombotic surface through several mechanisms (Fig. 12.1). First, the endothelium keeps circulating platelets in a quiescent state, mainly through release of NO and PGI$_2$ which synergistically increase cAMP content in platelets to repress activation and aggregation. Endothelial expression of ectonucleotidases also contributes to this process by converting ADP (a powerful trigger of platelet activation) to AMP and then adenosine. If platelet aggregation occurs, the release of serotonin and ADP from aggregating platelets will stimulate NO and PGI2 production to inhibit platelet aggregation and limit thrombus formation. Furthermore, vasodilation in response to NO and PGI$_2$ serve to mechanically impede the progression of the coagulation process [18].

Secondly, endothelial cells promote the activity of anticoagulant pathways (Fig. 12.2). Anticoagulation is achieved through expression of thrombomodulin which interacts with thrombin, forming a complex that prevents activation of platelets or the conversion of fibrinogen to fibrin, a key step in the coagulation cascade. This complex also activates protein C, which works in combination with protein S to inactivate two essential cofactors for blood coagulation, VIIIa and Va. The endothelial surface layer (glycocalyx) contains heparan sulfate proteoglycans which binds and activates antithrombin III to inactivate thrombin and factors IXa, Xa and XIa. Finally, endothelial cells regulate initiation of coagulation by inhibiting the activation of factor X [19]. In addition to the strong anticoagulation effects, the endothelium can also contribute to coagulation. Endothelial expression of tissue factor (TF) enhances the activity of factor VII, which ultimately activates thrombin to facilitate activation of platelets and release of the von Willebrand factor (vWF) to further promote platelet aggregation.

A third step in the coagulation pathway is the ability of the endothelium to influence fibrinolysis (Fig. 12.2) by the production of tissue-type plasminogen activator (t-PA) and urokinase-type plasminogen activator (uPA). These factors activate the liver-derived plasminogen into plasmin which then degrades fibrin. It is important to note that this activity is inhibited through the (endothelial) production of plasminogen activator inhibitor (PAI)-1 [19].

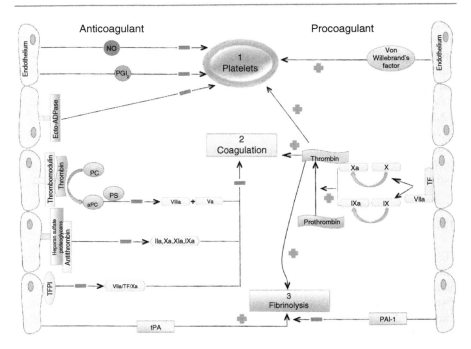

Fig. 12.2 Anticoagulant and procoagulant properties of the endothelium. The endothelium maintains blood fluidity through a balance between factors that either inhibit (*left*) or promote (*right*) (*1*) platelet activation, aggregation, and (*2*) coagulation, and inhibit (*left*) or promote (*right*) (*3*) fibrinolysis. *NO* nitric oxide, *PGI2* prostacyclin, *PC* protein C, *PS* protein S, *TF* tissue factor, *TFPI* tissue factor pathway inhibitor, *tPA* tissue-type plasminogen activator, *PAI-1* plasminogen activator inhibitor 1

12.2.3 Inflammatory Responses

Under noninflammatory conditions, interaction of endothelial cells with leukocytes is suppressed by inhibiting the endothelium-dependent production of adhesion molecules (Fig. 12.1). Also NO production inhibits the fusion of Weibel-Palade bodies with the surface of the endothelial cell and leukocyte activation. However, during inflammation, a rapid response to infectious microbes or injured tissues occurs, involving local recruitment and activation of leukocytes. The purpose of the inflammatory response is to kill microbes and remove cellular debris. Endothelial cell activation in response to inflammation can be divided into rapid responses (type I) and slower responses (type II).

Type I responses are rapid (<10–20 min), transient and independent of protein synthesis. These responses generally initiate a signalling cascade that increases intracellular Ca^{2+} levels to serve a number of purposes. First, this response facilitates increased NO and PGI_2 production, contributing to an increased blood flow and delivery of leukocytes. Secondly, increased Ca^{2+} levels enhance survival and migration of invading leukocytes and cause contraction of endothelial cells, which opens gaps between adjacent endothelial cells and increase permeability for leukocytes. Finally, expression of P-selectin and platelet-activating factor (PAF) is initiated which promotes the binding and activation of leukocytes [20].

Type II activation of endothelial cells involves a more persistent form of activation. During sustained inflammation, leukocytes produce inflammatory cytokines (e.g. tumour necrosis factor-α (TNF-α) and interleukin-1 (IL-1)) which results in the increased transcription of genes responsible for expression of a pro-adhesive and prothrombotic endothelial cell phenotype (IL-8 and adhesion molecules). Increased expression of these factors contributes to further leukocyte migration, adhesion and extravasation into the inflamed tissue. Inflammatory cytokines also induce leakage of plasma proteins into the affected tissue. Since these responses require transcription and translation of new proteins, type II activation is slower in onset but has more sustained effects than type I activation (i.e. hours–days). Accordingly, endothelial cells contribute to restoration of normal tissue architecture or form a connective tissue scar in response to inflammation [21].

12.2.4 Facilitation of Remodelling, Growth and Repair

Remodelling or adaptation of the vasculature refers to a basic compensatory response intended to maintain the functional integrity of the vessel in the presence of (potentially harmful) haemodynamic, metabolic and inflammatory stimuli. Sustained exposure to such stimuli, especially in conjunction with CVD risk factors, eventually transforms the initial (protective) response into a self-perpetuating and pathogenic process that contributes to the development of atherosclerosis (Fig. 12.3) [22].

12.2.4.1 Remodelling

Straight portions of arteries are associated with laminar shear, which produces an atheroprotective genotype that mitigates the effects of risk factors. However, at flow dividers, disturbed flow impedes such atheroprotective functions and initiates increased expression of proatherogenic genes/proteins and (chronic) inflammatory responses. As a lesion forms and grows, matrix remodelling takes place, paving the way for abluminal expansion or outward growth of the growing atheroma that preserves the lumen of the artery and maintains blood flow. Ultimately, plaque growth can outstrip this compensatory enlargement of the artery wall, allowing the atheroma to encroach on the lumen and cause stenosis (Fig. 12.3). Smaller arterioles resist the atherosclerotic lesion formation. However, due to increases in pressure, these smaller vessels develop medial hypertrophy and intimal thickening, which sustains and aggravates hypertension [22].

Endothelial cells play a pivotal role in the process of remodelling. For example, early animal studies found that the presence of the endothelium is essential for arteries to adapt in luminal size [23]. When the endothelium is removed from an artery, exposure to elevations in shear stress does not induce a change in diameter. The adaptive response is therefore dependent on the endothelium, and more specifically,

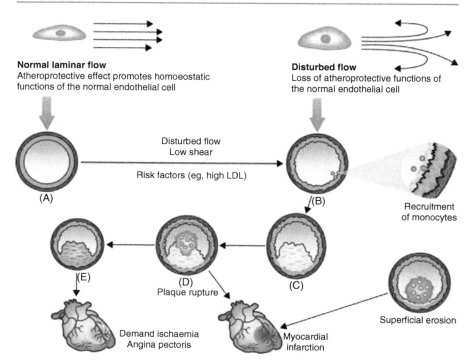

Fig. 12.3 Arterial remodelling influences the clinical consequences of atherosclerosis. Normal laminar shear stress maintains normal arterial calibre and properties (*A*). Disturbed flow characterised by a non-laminar, oscillatory flow promotes the upregulation of proatherogenic genes and recruitment of monocytes, as depicted to the right in the enlarged nascent plaque (*B*). Monocyte/macrophage accumulation yields a thin-capped, lipid-rich inflamed plaque (*C*), which can rupture and cause a thrombus (*D*), leading to myocardial infarction (*central bottom*). Alternatively, the plaque in (*E*) can undergo constrictive remodelling to promote flow-limiting stenosis that can cause demand ischaemia and angina pectoris. Less commonly, superficial erosion (*bottom right*) can cause myocardial infarction (With permission from Heusch et al. [22])

dependent on gene expression of eNOS and suppression of the bioavailability of ET-1 [24]. Also, immediate changes in vessel diameter in response to elevations in shear stress are dependent on an intact endothelium that releases vasoactive substances [25], highlighting the importance of the endothelium to respond (acutely and chronically) to changes in shear.

12.2.4.2 Repair

During the past decade, evidence supported the presence of repair mechanisms of damaged or 'old' endothelial cells by bone marrow-derived cells: endothelial progenitor cells (EPCs). These immature cells have the capacity to maintain endothelial integrity and function by differentiating into mature endothelial cells, replacing damaged endothelial cells and initiating neovascularisation [26]. Vascular injury mobilises circulating EPCs, which localise at the site of damage where they divide, proliferate and adhere to the sub-endothelium promoting growth of new endothelium. Endothelial injury causes a cytokine-mediated release of stromal-derived factor-1 (SDF-1) which, in turn, determines recruitment and proliferation of EPCs. Intact NO bioavailability is linked to efficient mobilisation and functionality of EPCs, which may explain why the number of CVD risk factors is inversely related to the number and migratory activity of circulating EPCs. Impairment in the ability and/or efficacy of repair mechanisms of the endothelium logically follows the presence of CVD risk factors and progression of atherosclerosis [27].

12.3 Haemodynamic Forces Affecting the Endothelium

12.3.1 Shear Stress

Blood imparts a tangential frictional force on the endothelial surface, typically referred to as shear stress (SS). Endothelial cells' ability to detect SS and other haemodynamic forces is mediated by different sensing mechanisms, including ion channels, caveolae, G-protein-coupled receptors, tyrosine kinase receptors, cell adhesion molecules, glycocalyx, primary cilia and the cell cytoskeleton and the lipid bilayer of the cell membrane [28]. Mechanoactivation of the signalling pathways results in the activation of transcription factors, leading to modulation of gene expressions in endothelial cells. Importantly, responses to SS are not simply linked to the absolute level of SS, but also the type of SS (i.e. laminar or oscillatory).

Straight portions of arteries are exposed to a steady, laminar SS. Sustained elevation of such types of SS generates an atheroprotective phenotype. This is highlighted by the expression of approximately 3,000 cultured endothelial cell genes after exposure to elevations in laminar SS [29]. Gene expressions that are upregulated by laminar SS involve growth factors (e.g. FGF, TGF-β), vasodilators (e.g. NO, PGI_2), antithrombotic components (e.g. TPA, thrombomodulin, COX-2) and endogenous antioxidants, whilst downregulation is observed in adhesion molecules (e.g. VCAM-1), vasoconstrictors (e.g. ET-1) and coagulation factors (e.g. PAI-1) [28]. Conversely, regions of disturbed blood SS (e.g. branch points, curvatures, poststenotic regions), typically include periods of reciprocating flow reversal that create oscillating wall SS. Experiments suggest that oscillating SS patterns produce a proatherogenic endothelial cell phenotype, characterised with decreased eNOS mRNA and increased VCAM-1, ICAM-1, MCP-1, ET-1 and NADPH oxidase 4 [28, 30].

The impact of elevation in SS is well established from animal and human experiments. Subjects exposed to 8-week repeated exposure to elevated SS via handgrip training demonstrate improvement in vascular function and structure, whilst such adaptations were not present when the exercise-induced elevation in SS was artificially attenuated [31]. Furthermore, the detrimental effect of oscillatory SS is confirmed in humans in vivo as this leads to a dose-dependent decline in endothelial function [32]. These observations highlight the importance of the magnitude *and* pattern of SS for endothelial function and vascular structure.

12.3.2 Transmural Pressure and Cyclic Strain

Elevations in blood pressure exposes endothelial cells to an increased transmural force and increased cyclic strain, both of which are signals that can alter endothelial cell phenotype. High transmural pressure directly affects endothelial cell NO production [33]. Both in vitro and in vivo experiments in animals and humans demonstrate that exposure of arteries to short-term increases in transmural pressure depresses endothelium-dependent vasodilation by activating ROS-dependent mechanisms. More specifically, elevation in transmural pressure increases intracellular Ca^{2+} concentrations and protein kinase C activation, which ultimately results in NADPH oxidase activation and causes an increase in ROS production [34]. The increased oxidative stress contributes to a proatherogenic phenotype of endothelial cells and, consequently, contributes to the atherosclerotic process [34].

Elevation in pressure across the cardiac cycle also produces an increase in the rhythmic stretching (cyclic strain) of the vessel. Data obtained from in vitro cell culture preparations suggest that cyclic strain produced an antiatherogenic endothelial cell phenotype [35]. However, more recent data obtained from an isolated vessel preparation suggest a proatherogenic phenotype and increased ROS production [36]. Although speculative, the discrepancies in results between whole vessel preparations versus endothelial and smooth muscle cell culture may reflect the importance of crosstalk between endothelial and VSMCs. Research using co-cultured endothelial and VSMCs is required to determine the ultimate importance of cyclic strain on the phenotype of the endothelium.

12.4 CVD Risk Factors Affecting the Endothelium

Loss of the delicate balance of the various functions of the endothelium leads to a dysfunctional state in which the vasoconstricting, prothrombotic and proliferative characteristics of the endothelium predominate, ultimately facilitating the process of atherosclerosis. Below, we describe how important cardiovascular risk factors influence this balance.

12.4.1 Dyslipidaemia

Dyslipidaemia relates to excessive levels of low-density lipoproteins (LDL) and/or low levels of high-density lipoproteins (HDL). High levels of LDL, and especially oxidised LDL, inhibit eNOS activity through inactivation of eNOS and 'eNOS uncoupling'. This latter process is initiated by superoxide, which reacts with NO to form peroxynitrite. Peroxynitrite then oxidises the eNOS-cofactor tetrahydrobiopterin, which causes the generation of superoxide [37]. This process reduces NO production and potentiates the pre-existing oxidative stress. Conversely, high levels of HDL protect the endothelium through the prevention of LDL-induced eNOS uncoupling and upregulation of eNOS mRNA and protein levels, anti-inflammatory effects through inhibition of NF-κB, as well as antithrombotic activity [38].

12.4.2 Diabetes

Hyperglycaemia, a common feature in diabetes type 1 and 2, induces reduced NO bioavailability as a result of oxidative stress and eNOS uncoupling. Hyperglycaemia increases synthesis of vasoconstrictor prostanoids (e.g. PGH2, TXA) [39], causing an immediate decline in endothelial function. Another pathway by which diabetes impacts the endothelium is production of insulin, which normally acts as a vasodilator and stimulates endothelial NO production to facilitate glucose uptake in the muscle. In diabetes, this signalling pathway is inhibited, possibly via excess production of free fatty acids and inflammatory cytokines from adipose tissue [39] (especially in type 2 diabetes).

12.4.3 Hypertension

In addition to the effects of elevation in transmural pressure (Sect. 12.3.2), Ang II plays a major role in hypertension through profound vasoconstriction, increased renal sodium absorption and elevated pressor responses. This high blood pressure stimulates oxidative stress by enhancing NADPH oxidase activity, increasing media stress and stimulation of mechanoreceptors. Ang II also influences remodelling of the vessel wall by stimulating Ca^{2+} release leading to vasoconstriction that may become embedded as deposition of extracellular matrix occurs. In addition, Ang II enhances all stages of the inflammatory response [40]. These effects of Ang II establish a vicious cycle where hypertension begets hypertension through its adverse effects on the endothelium and vascular structure.

12.4.4 Obesity

Obesity is independently associated with endothelial dysfunction [41]. Visceral adipose tissue acts as an endocrine organ and is capable of producing proinflammatory adipokines (e.g. leptin, resistin and adiponectin). Leptin induces oxidative stress in endothelial cells and stimulates the secretion of the proinflammatory cytokines TNF-α and IL-6 causing a state of chronic low-grade inflammation. Resistin inhibits glucose uptake in skeletal muscle cells and stimulates ET-1 production. Conversely, obesity is typically characterised by a reduced production and activity of adiponectin [42]. Adiponectin has antiatherogenic properties and stimulates insulin sensitivity, reduces the expression of adhesion molecules, inhibits the transformation of macrophages into foam cells and reduces VSMC proliferation. Furthermore, obesity is associated with increased plasma levels of free fatty acids which may contribute to endothelial dysfunction [41].

12.5 Concluding Remarks

The endothelium is the central regulator of vascular homeostasis. Changes in endothelial cell phenotype support vessel repair, remodelling and resolution of infection or inflammation. Whilst these alterations are usually transient, prolonged exposure to harmful stimuli activates various processes that ultimately lead to endothelial dysfunction. This process, characterised by reduced NO bioavailability, represents a critical step in the atherosclerosis process and is present long before overt pathophysiological changes occur. Therefore, the endothelium remains an attractive target for (1) early prediction of future CVD and (2) therapies preventing CVD.

References

1. Altschul R (1954) Endothelium: its development, morphology, function, and pathology. Macmillan, New York
2. Starling EH (1896) On the absorption of fluids from the connective tissue spaces. J Physiol 19(4):312–326
3. Moncada S, Gryglewski R, Bunting S, Vane JR (1976) An enzyme isolated from arteries transforms prostaglandin endoperoxides to an unstable substance that inhibits platelet aggregation. Nature 263(5579):663–665
4. Furchgott RF, Zawadzki JV (1980) The obligatory role of endothelial cells in the relaxation of arterial smooth muscle by acetylcholine. Nature 288(5789):373–376
5. Anggard EE (1990) The endothelium–the body's largest endocrine gland? J Endocrinol 127(3):371–375
6. Simionescu M (2007) Implications of early structural-functional changes in the endothelium for vascular disease. Arterioscler Thromb Vasc Biol 27(2):266–274
7. Lampugnani MG (2012) Endothelial cell-to-cell junctions: adhesion and signaling in physiology and pathology. Cold Spring Harb Perspect Med 2(10) pii: a006528
8. Hirase T, Node K (2012) Endothelial dysfunction as a cellular mechanism for vascular failure. Am J Physiol Heart Circ Physiol 302(3):H499–H505
9. Marti CN, Gheorghiade M, Kalogeropoulos AP et al (2012) Endothelial dysfunction, arterial stiffness, and heart failure. J Am Coll Cardiol 60(16):1455–1469
10. Li H, Forstermann U (2000) Nitric oxide in the pathogenesis of vascular disease. J Pathol 190(3):244–254
11. Vallance P, Collier J, Moncada S (1989) Effects of endothelium-derived nitric oxide on peripheral arteriolar tone in man. Lancet 2(8670):997–1000
12. Coleman RA, Smith WL, Narumiya S (1994) International Union of Pharmacology classification of prostanoid receptors: properties, distribution, and structure of the receptors and their subtypes. Pharmacol Rev 46(2):205–229
13. Feletou M, Vanhoutte PM (2007) Endothelium-dependent hyperpolarizations: past beliefs and present facts. Ann Med 39(7):495–516
14. Haynes WG, Webb DJ (1998) Endothelin as a regulator of cardiovascular function in health and disease. J Hypertens 16(8):1081–1098
15. Hernandez Schulman I, Zhou MS, Raij L (2007) Cross-talk between angiotensin II receptor types 1 and 2: potential role in vascular remodeling in humans. Hypertension 49(2):270–271
16. Oates JA, FitzGerald GA, Branch RA et al (1988) Clinical implications of prostaglandin and thromboxane A2 formation. N Engl J Med 319(11):689–698
17. Davidge ST (2001) Prostaglandin H synthase and vascular function. Circ Res 89(8):650–660
18. Wu KK, Thiagarajan P (1996) Role of endothelium in thrombosis and hemostasis. Annu Rev Med 47:315–331

19. van Hinsbergh VWM (2012) Endothelium–role in regulation of coagulation and inflammation. Semin Immunopathol 34(1):93–106
20. Wojta J (2011) Sites of injury: the endothelium. In: Podesser BK, Chambers DJ (eds) New solutions for the heart. Springer, Vienna, pp 57–69
21. Pober JS, Sessa WC (2007) Evolving functions of endothelial cells in inflammation. Nat Rev Immunol 7(10):803–815
22. Heusch G, Libby P, Gersh B et al (2014) Cardiovascular remodelling in coronary artery disease and heart failure. Lancet 383(9932):1933–1943
23. Langille BL, O'Donnell F (1986) Reductions in arterial diameter produced by chronic decreases in blood flow are endothelium-dependent. Science 231(4736):405–407
24. Nadaud S, Philippe M, Arnal JF et al (1996) Sustained increase in aortic endothelial nitric oxide synthase expression in vivo in a model of chronic high blood flow. Circ Res 79(4):857–863
25. Dawson EA, Rathore S, Cable NT et al (2010) Impact of catheter insertion using the radial approach on vasodilatation in humans. Clin Sci (Lond) 118(10):633–640
26. Asahara T, Murohara T, Sullivan A et al (1997) Isolation of putative progenitor endothelial cells for angiogenesis. Science 275(5302):964–967
27. Leone AM, Valgimigli M, Giannico MB et al (2009) From bone marrow to the arterial wall: the ongoing tale of endothelial progenitor cells. Eur Heart J 30(8):890–899
28. Johnson BD, Mather KJ, Wallace JP (2011) Mechanotransduction of shear in the endothelium: basic studies and clinical implications. Vasc Med 16(5):365–377
29. Himburg HA, Dowd SE, Friedman MH (2007) Frequency-dependent response of the vascular endothelium to pulsatile shear stress. Am J Physiol Heart Circ Physiol 293(1):H645–H653
30. Chiu JJ, Chien S (2011) Effects of disturbed flow on vascular endothelium: pathophysiological basis and clinical perspectives. Physiol Rev 91(1):327–387
31. Tinken TM, Thijssen DH, Hopkins N et al (2009) Impact of shear rate modulation on vascular function in humans. Hypertension 54(2):278–285
32. Thijssen DH, Dawson EA, Tinken TM et al (2009) Retrograde flow and shear rate acutely impair endothelial function in humans. Hypertension 53(6):986–992
33. Hishikawa K, Nakaki T, Suzuki H et al (1992) Transmural pressure inhibits nitric oxide release from human endothelial cells. Eur J Pharmacol 215(2–3):329–331
34. Csiszar A, Lehoux S, Ungvari Z (2009) Hemodynamic forces, vascular oxidative stress, and regulation of BMP-2/4 expression. Antioxid Redox Signal 11(7):1683–1697
35. Awolesi MA, Sessa WC, Sumpio BE (1995) Cyclic strain upregulates nitric oxide synthase in cultured bovine aortic endothelial cells. J Clin Invest 96(3):1449–1454
36. Thacher T, Gambillara V, da Silva RF et al (2010) Reduced cyclic stretch, endothelial dysfunction, and oxidative stress: an ex vivo model. Cardiovasc Pathol 19(4):e91–e98
37. Li H, Forstermann U (2013) Uncoupling of endothelial NO synthase in atherosclerosis and vascular disease. Curr Opin Pharmacol 13(2):161–167
38. Campbell S, Genest J (2013) HDL-C: clinical equipoise and vascular endothelial function. Expert Rev Cardiovasc Ther 11(3):343–353
39. Sena CM, Pereira AM, Seica R (2013) Endothelial dysfunction – a major mediator of diabetic vascular disease. Biochim Biophys Acta 1832(12):2216–2231
40. Schiffrin EL (2012) Vascular remodeling in hypertension: mechanisms and treatment. Hypertension 59(2):367–374
41. Campia U, Tesauro M, Cardillo C (2012) Human obesity and endothelium-dependent responsiveness. Br J Pharmacol 165(3):561–573
42. Virdis A, Neves MF, Duranti E et al (2013) Microvascular endothelial dysfunction in obesity and hypertension. Curr Pharm Des 19(13):2382–2389

Pharmacologic and Environmental Factors: Coffee, Smoking, and Sodium

13

Charalambos Vlachopoulos, Panagiota Pietri, and Dimitrios Tousoulis

Given the prognostic role of arterial stiffness and central hemodynamics [1–4], a large body of research has focused on the recognition of lifestyle interventions that may either worsen arterial function, and thus, they should be prohibited or at least discouraged, or exert favorable effects, and, consequently, they should be encouraged.

Active smoking has shown a detrimental effect on arterial stiffness either in the acute or chronic phase, while passive smoking is not less innocent. Quitting smoking is related to an improvement in the arterial elastic properties. The effect of pharmaceutical aids for smoking cessation, such as varenicline, needs further investigation, while electronic cigarette is an issue of concern that should be further evaluated.

Among elements of nutrition, dietary foods and beverages, salt increases blood pressure (BP) and, consequently, arterial stiffness. The unfavorable effect of salt on arterial stiffness may be exerted through BP-independent mechanisms as well, while genetic predisposition to salt-induced vascular damage has also been proposed. Salt restriction is accompanied by a decrease in aortic stiffness, but the recommended daily consumption has to be better defined since recent data raise skepticism related to an existence of a J-curve between salt intake and cardiovascular events. Regarding coffee, we should stress that the latter and caffeine are not interchangeable terms, and results of studies should be interpreted in the context of the particular beverage/substance investigated. Generally, caffeine increases aortic stiffness, whereas when ingested in coffee, this effect seems to be ameliorated. Nevertheless, chronic coffee consumption increases aortic stiffness. On the other hand, beverages with substantiated beneficial effects on arterial function are those that are rich in flavonoids. Indeed, consumption of foods rich in polyphenols, such

C. Vlachopoulos, MD (✉) • P. Pietri • D. Tousoulis
Hypertension Unit and Peripheral Vessels Unit, 1st Department of Cardiology,
Hippokration Hospital, Athens Medical School, Profiti Elia 24, Athens 14575, Greece
e-mail: cvlachop@otenet.gr

© Springer International Publishing Switzerland 2015
A. Berbari, G. Mancia (eds.), *Arterial Disorders:*
Definition, Clinical Manifestations, Mechanisms and Therapeutic Approaches,
DOI 10.1007/978-3-319-14556-3_13

as cocoa and wine, all in moderate doses, is becoming synonymous to vascular health in popular culture due mainly to antioxidant and anti-inflammatory properties of polyphenols. Also vegetables rich in these compounds, such as tomatoes, have shown beneficial effects on endothelial function.

In the present chapter, we discuss data for the relationship of arterial properties and three environmental/dietary compounds to which most people are exposed: smoking, caffeine/coffee, and salt. Possible underlying mechanisms are identified, and current recommendations on their daily consumption (if applicable) are reported.

13.1 Smoking

Smoking is an independent risk factor for cardiovascular disease (CVD), while it remains the leading preventable cause of death worldwide. Although the association of smoking with CVD is undoubted, the underlying mechanisms for this association are not yet fully explored. Endothelial dysfunction, inflammation, sympathetic activation, oxidative stress, prothrombotic enhancement, and lipid modification are among the potential pathophysiological links between smoking and CVD [5]. Importantly, arterial stiffening is implicated in the complex interplay between smoking and CVD.

Active smoking has a detrimental effect on arterial stiffness and wave reflections that is exerted both acutely and chronically [6]. Acute smoking, apart from transiently increasing BP and heart rate, increases arterial stiffness and indices of wave reflections in smokers [7–12], nonsmokers [10] (Fig. 13.1), and hypertensive patients [13]. The maximal adverse effect of cigarette smoking seems to take place in the first 5–10 min [8–13]. The acute effect of smoking seems to be not nicotine dose

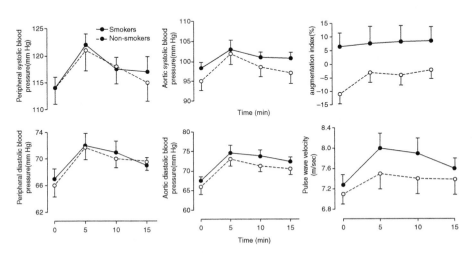

Fig. 13.1 Changes in brachial and aortic blood pressures, corrected augmentation index, and pulse wave velocity at 5, 10, and 15 min after smoking one cigarette in healthy smokers and non-smokers. All parameters increased in both groups. Data are presented as mean ± SEM (Reproduced with permission from Mahmud and Feely [10])

dependent since data have shown that light cigarette smoking has the same unfavorable effect on endothelial function and aortic distensibility as the regular cigarette smoking [14]. Cigar smoking is not innocent either, since arterial stiffness increases for at least 1 h after smoking one cigar [11]. Importantly, the combined consumption of smoking and coffee has a synergistic effect on aortic stiffness [15], whereas red wine decreases wave reflections in uncomplicated habitual smokers [16].

The *chronic* effect of smoking seems to be analogous to that of the acute effect [15, 17–20]. The impact on arterial stiffness appears to be unrelated to the intensity and duration of smoking since small quantities of smoking are able to produce its deleterious effects. The effect of smoking on aortic stiffness may be both BP dependent and BP independent [8]. Interestingly, studies have shown that augmentation index (AIx) and central pressures are higher and pulse pressure is reduced in current and former smokers as compared to never smokers for the same brachial BP levels [10, 19, 21]. The long-term effect of cigarette smoking on the incidence of hypertension has not been elucidated. In two large population studies, current cigarette smoking was independently, yet modestly, associated with an elevated risk of developing hypertension [22, 23]. However, other studies have reported lower BP levels among smokers [24] and increases in BP after smoking cessation [25]. The mildly lower BP in smokers can be attributed to lower body weight [26]. Interestingly, a recent study showed that aerobic exercise may mitigate the harmful effects of smoking since brachial-ankle pulse wave velocity (PWV) values were not different between physically active nonsmokers and physically active smokers [27].

Passive smoking is a well-established risk factor for coronary heart disease [28] with similar detrimental effects on the cardiovascular system to those of active smoking. Passive smoking has immediate and substantial effects on aortic stiffness in smokers [29–31]. These effects are mediated through a nicotine-dependent pathway, impairment of microvascular function, and increase of asymmetrical dimethylarginine [31]. Importantly, data have shown that parental smoking is associated with the development of several cardiovascular risk factors in their children, whereas the exposure to smoking in childhood is associated with impaired endothelial function later in life [32].

Regarding mechanisms and considering that endothelium-derived nitric oxide regulates arterial elasticity [33], smoking-induced endothelial dysfunction may serve as one of the substrates for the increased aortic stiffness. Cigarette smoking is related to increased endothelin-1, angiotensin II, and thromboxane resulting in vasoconstriction and endothelial dysfunction [34]. Smokers have reduced flow-mediated dilatation [35], whereas sildenafil, a specific type 5 phosphodiesterase inhibitor with vasodilatory effects, abolishes the decrease in FMD of the brachial artery induced by acute smoking [36]. Airflow limitation is associated with higher arterial stiffness. Interestingly, brachial-ankle PWV was an independent determinant of airflow limitation in current and past smokers but not in never smokers with airflow limitation, putting forward an etiological role of smoking in this association [37].

The effect of *smoking cessation* on arterial stiffness and wave reflections has also been investigated. Arterial stiffness is continuously decreasing along with the duration of smoking cessation. Values of carotid-femoral PWV, AIx, and transit time equal those of nonsmokers after a decade of smoking cessation [29] (Fig. 13.2). Nevertheless, the effect of smoking cessation is more rapidly evident on wave

Fig. 13.2 Pulse wave velocity, augmentation index, and transit time of current smokers, never smokers, and ex-smokers (Reproduced with permission from Jatoi et al. [19])

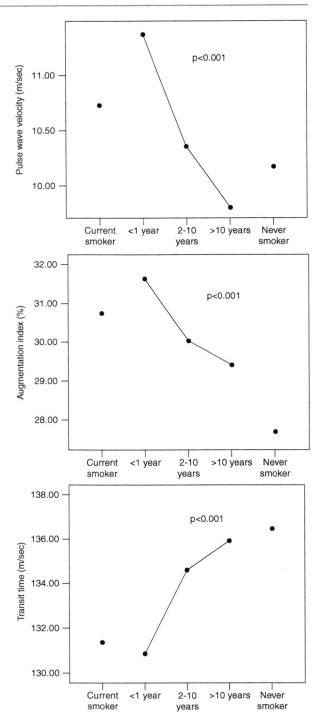

reflections than aortic stiffness. In intervention studies, cessation of smoking for 4 weeks resulted in a decrease in AIx [18], while 6 months of smoking cessation was associated with clear improvement of AIx and corrected heart rate, aortic pressure, and aortic PWV, and with a reduction of daytime BP [20]. In a study using nicotine replacement therapy, improvement of AIx was evident at a short time frame, while at the same time course, no improvement of PWV was demonstrated [38]. Patients who achieved smoking cessation with varenicline (a partial agonist of a4–b2 nicotine acetylcholine receptors) treatment showed significant improvement in central hemodynamics and brachial-ankle PWV, whereas these parameters showed no significant change in those who failed to quit smoking under the same treatment, thus highlighting the beneficial effect of smoking cessation per se on vascular function [39]. Electronic cigarettes are being advocated as tools for smoking cessation with rapidly increasing use. These cigarettes are battery-powered devices that have cartridges or refillable tanks containing a liquid mixture composed primarily of propylene glycol and/or glycerol and nicotine, as well as flavorings and other chemicals. No firm evidence exists on the effect of such an intervention on aortic stiffness and total cardiovascular health, thus no definite recommendations can be made [40].

13.2 Diet and Nutrition

13.2.1 Coffee and Caffeine

Coffee is a complex mixture of compounds that may have variable effects on the cardiovascular system. However, the effects of coffee are often confused with the effects of caffeine. Caffeine is a methylated xanthine derivative consumed in coffee, tea, and soft drinks, and it is the most widely used pharmacologically active substance. It should be noted that coffee and caffeine are not interchangeable terms, and results of studies should be interpreted in the context of the particular beverage/substance investigated. Data on the association of coffee consumption with cardiovascular risk are controversial; they are equivocally varying from a positive to a neutral or to even a J- or a U-shaped association [41]. In a recent large study, based upon self-reported drinking habits, two or more cups of coffee per day seemed to reduce all-cause mortality in women (but not in men), primarily due to a reduction in cardiovascular mortality [41]. Similar findings were noted with decaffeinated coffee, suggesting a beneficial effect from a component other than caffeine. The latter appears to be not innocent. Interestingly, regular caffeine intake increases BP, but when ingested through coffee, the BP effect of caffeine is small [42]. The rate of caffeine metabolism through genetic predisposition may be an important determinant of the effect of coffee intake on coronary heart disease risk and account for these discrepancies in outcomes of studies.

Many studies indicate that caffeine intake, in the form of a tablet or in coffee, exerts an acute detrimental effect on aortic stiffness and indices of wave reflections, both in normal subjects and in hypertensive subjects [15, 43–47]. The ingestion of

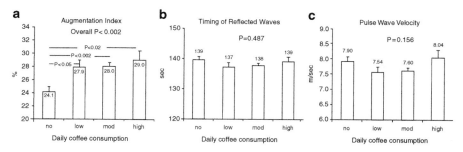

Fig. 13.3 Augmentation index, timing of reflected waves, and pulse wave velocity in different groups of daily coffee consumption (low, <200 ml/day; moderate, 200–450 ml/day; and high, >450 ml/day (Reproduced with permission from Vlachopoulos et al. [48])

Fig. 13.4 Acute pulse wave velocity responses to caffeine, caffeine plus smoking, or smoking alone. Note the synergistic effect when caffeine and smoking are combined (Reproduced with permission from Vlachopoulos et al. [15])

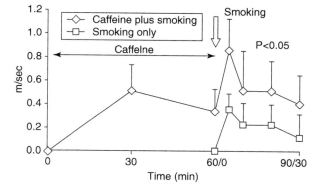

caffeine results in a sustained impairment of arterial stiffness, which lasts longer in hypertensive subjects (at least 3 h) compared with normotensives. Interestingly, the unfavorable effect of caffeine is more evident in central hemodynamics than in peripheral pressure [48] (Fig. 13.3), and coffee increases arterial stiffness to a lesser degree than its contained caffeine [49].

Chronic coffee consumption is associated with increased aortic stiffness and wave reflections in healthy normotensives, whereas in hypertensive patients, wave reflections, but not aortic stiffness, are increased [50]. The latter implies that the stiffening effect of coffee in the aorta is probably less prominent in the already stiff aortas of hypertensive patients than in normal aortas.

The caffeine-induced effect on arterial stiffness is probably related to vasoconstriction due to an increase in sympathetic activity and circulating catecholamine concentrations mediated by central nervous system stimulation and antagonism of endogenous adenosine.

Coffee consumption is very frequently combined with smoking. Interestingly enough, the combination of acute caffeine intake/chronic coffee consumption and smoking has a synergistic detrimental effect on carotid-femoral PWV and aortic AIx [15] (Fig. 13.4). Clinical evidence shows that coffee drinking is unrelated to coronary artery disease risk in never smokers, but in ex-smokers and current baseline smokers, daily coffee intake is associated with higher coronary artery disease risk [51].

13.2.2 Salt

therefore, if large amounts of salt are taken,
     the pulse will stiffen and harden.
     Huang Ti Nei Ching Su Wein, Chinese physician
     (1700 BC)

   Salt intake is associated with increased BP, and studies have shown a relationship between high salt consumption and increased arterial stiffness. Considering the adverse prognostic role of arterial stiffness, the latter might serve as a potential mechanism, apart from the BP per se, through which salt might be associated with increased cardiovascular risk.

   In a seminal study of two Chinese populations, the age-associated increase in carotid-femoral PWV was blunted in the population with a lower salt intake [52]. In insulin-dependent diabetic patients, high sodium intake was associated with decreased femoral arterial distensibility compared to nondiabetic subjects [53]; interestingly, a plausible concept suggests that BP in insulin-dependent diabetes is sodium sensitive and a high sodium intake may be a factor that predisposes to the development of diabetic vascular disease. Although an adverse effect of high salt intake on arterial stiffness is evident in most of the studies, the effect on wave reflections is less clear. Central hemodynamics including central pulse pressure, augmented aortic pressure, and AIx have been independently associated with estimated 24-h sodium excretion, whereas an inverse association was demonstrated between sodium excretion and pulse pressure amplification [54]. However, contrary to these observations, a recent study showed that increase in urinary sodium concentration was independently but inversely associated with central AIx; to further blur the picture, no relationship was established between carotid-femoral PWV and urinary sodium concentrations. Nevertheless, these findings require additional investigation concerning possible mechanistic changes in renal microcirculation after high sodium intake that may explain a possible disassociation between salt intake, aortic stiffness, and wave reflections [55].

   Regarding intervention, beneficial effects of low-sodium diet on arterial stiffness have been demonstrated. In older adults with systolic hypertension, sodium restriction led to a rapid increase in large artery compliance, while the accompanying lowering of systolic BP suggests that this improvement in elastic properties may be a key mechanism for the rapid normalization of systolic BP by sodium restriction in such patients [56] (Fig. 13.5). Furthermore, a modest reduction in salt intake for 6 weeks reduced carotid-femoral PWV in mild hypertensives [57]. However, subgroup analysis indicated that the effect was significant only in blacks despite the fact that these subjects achieved a smaller reduction in salt intake and a similar fall in BP compared to whites and Asians, a finding suggesting that the favorable effects of low-sodium diet are more pronounced in salt-sensitive patients. In addition, DASH diet is associated with decreased carotid-femoral PWV [58].

   The effect of salt intake on the large arteries may be exerted either through BP-dependent or BP-independent mechanisms. Sodium chloride increases BP, an effect that is due to either an increase in blood volume or an increase in vascular resistance. According to the first observations by Guyton et al. [59], the kidneys

Fig. 13.5 Carotid artery compliance and β-stiffness index at baseline (base), in each of the 4 weeks of the low-sodium condition (L1–L4) and during the 4 weeks of the normal-sodium condition (N1–N4). * Lower than baseline ($P < 0.05$). † Lower than any given normal week ($P < 0.05$). The improvement in compliance occurred rapidly, starting by the end of the first week of reduced sodium intake and reaching peak values after only 2 weeks of sodium restriction (Reproduced with permission from Gates et al. [56])

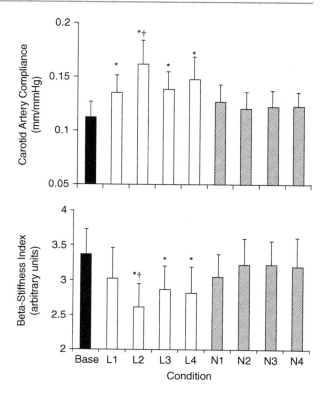

have a pivotal role in the pathogenesis of hypertension since the inability of the kidneys to excrete the excess sodium and promote natriuresis is a prerequisite for the BP increase. Sodium retention and the consequent volume expansion initially increase cardiac output. As a result of a process of local autoregulation, peripheral vascular resistance progressively rises so that the long-term sodium-induced BP increase is maintained by an increase in peripheral resistance rather than in cardiac output. Moreover, sodium chloride may also induce alterations in small arteries through endothelial dysfunction as data have shown in resistance arteries of sponta-neously hypertensive rats [60]. Furthermore, it also decreases NO synthase activity in rats [61] and enhances the production of endothelin-1 in salt-sensitive hyperten-sive patients [62]. Additionally, by increasing sympathetic activity, high salt intake may increase the muscular tone of small arteries [63].

A BP-independent relationship of salt intake with arterial stiffness is also likely. An experimental study in anesthetized Dahl rats which were fed either a low- or high-sodium diet for 5 weeks showed that the pressure-compliance curve of the carotid artery was shifted to the right compared with that of Dahl salt-resistant rats or even WKY rats [64]. This finding was evident regardless of the transmural BP. Interestingly, Benetos et al. have also shown that low-sodium diet was associ-ated with an increase in brachial artery diameter after 9 weeks in 20 hypertensive ambulatory patients, a result that was not related to BP fall [65]. On the contrary, no change in carotid artery diameter was observed, thus suggesting a different response of elastic- and muscular-type arteries to salt restriction.

Disassociation of sodium intake with BP changes and a prominent role of the genetic background are emerging. Indeed, data have shown that salt-sensitive hypertensive patients have increased arterial stiffness compared to salt-resistant individuals with the same BP levels, thus indicating that genetic predisposition to salt intake is a strong determinant of the salt-induced vascular changes [66]. In the previously mentioned study of Benetos et al. [64], results also suggest that sodium sensitivity, more than sodium intake, influenced the changes in the carotid artery mechanical properties. Other investigators have shown that in stroke-prone spontaneously hypertensive (SHR-SP) rats, carotid arterial thickness and collagen content were increased and BP was lower compared to SHR-SP rats fed with 1 % saline drinking water, further supporting the notion that genetic sensitivity to sodium, rather than BP itself, influences the changes in arterial structure [67].

Whatever the underlying mechanisms are, the association of arterial stiffness with salt intake is strong. However, although reduction in salt intake reduces arterial stiffness, there might be a threshold of salt consumption under which no further improvement of arterial stiffness is observed. Indeed, in a recent randomized trial in 29 overweight and obese normotensive individuals, no significant change in carotid-femoral PWV was demonstrated when salt intake was reduced from 9.2 to 3.8 g/day for 2 weeks, in spite of a significant improvement in endothelial function [68]. Such a finding raises skepticism about the appropriate recommended daily dose of salt intake. Indeed, associations may be rather complex. The relationship of sodium intake and BP is not linear with age. In a recent study including more than 100,000 adults from 18 countries, sodium intake and BP association was more pronounced not only in patients with hypertension but also in older subjects compared to younger ones [69]. Uncertainty also exists regarding the threshold for CV risk increase. There is evidence of a "J-shaped" relationship of sodium with cardiovascular outcomes. Individuals with low salt intake (less than 2.5 g/day), as well as those with high salt intake (more than 6.0 g/day), shared the same increased cardiovascular risk [70]. However, a more recent study showed that a high burden of deaths from cardiovascular causes was attributed to sodium consumption above a reference level of 2.0 g/day [71]. Until prospective randomized studies provide answers as to whether low or moderate salt consumption has the optimal cardiovascular benefit, the ESH guidelines argue in favor of salt restriction to 5–6 g/day, whereas AHA recommends reducing dietary sodium intake to lower than 1.5 g/day (1 g salt=400 mg of sodium) [72].

References

1. Vlachopoulos C, Aznaouridis K, Stefanadis C (2010) Prediction of cardiovascular events and all-cause mortality with arterial stiffness: a systematic review and meta-analysis. J Am Coll Cardiol 55:1318–1327
2. Vlachopoulos C, Aznaouridis K, O'Rourke MF et al (2010) Prediction of cardiovascular events and all-cause mortality with central haemodynamics: a systematic review and meta-analysis. Eur Heart J 31:1865–1871

3. Vlachopoulos C, Aznaouridis K, Stefanadis C (2014) Aortic stiffness for cardiovascular risk prediction: just measure it, just do it! J Am Coll Cardiol 63:647–649
4. Ben-Shlomo Y, Spears M, Boustred C et al (2014) Aortic pulse wave velocity improves cardiovascular event prediction: an individual participant meta-analysis of prospective observational data from 17,635 subjects. J Am Coll Cardiol 63:636–646
5. Siasos G, Tsigkou V, Kokkou E et al (2014) Smoking and atherosclerosis: mechanisms of disease and new therapeutic approaches. Curr Med Chem 21:1–13
6. Doonan RJ, Hausvater A, Scallan C et al (2010) The effect of smoking on arterial stiffness. Hypertens Res 33:398–410
7. Kool MJ, Hoeks AP, Struijker Boudier HA et al (1993) Short- and long-term effects of smoking on arterial wall properties in habitual smokers. J Am Coll Cardiol 22:1881–1886
8. Stefanadis C, Tsiamis E, Vlachopoulos C et al (1997) Unfavorable effect of smoking on the elastic properties of the human aorta. Circulation 95:31–38
9. Failla M, Grappiolo A, Carugo S et al (1997) Effects of cigarette smoking on carotid and radial artery distensibility. J Hypertens 15:1659–1664
10. Mahmud A, Feely J (2003) Effect of smoking on arterial stiffness and pulse pressure amplification. Hypertension 41:183–187
11. Vlachopoulos C, Alexopoulos N, Panagiotakos D et al (2004) Cigar smoking has an acute detrimental effect on arterial stiffness. Am J Hypertens 17:299–303
12. Lemogoum D, Van Bortel L, Leeman M et al (2006) Ethnic differences in arterial stiffness and wave reflections after cigarette smoking. J Hypertens 24:683–689
13. Rhee MY, Na SH, Kim YK et al (2007) Acute effects of cigarette smoking on arterial stiffness and blood pressure in male smokers with hypertension. Am J Hypertens 20:637–641
14. Ciftçi O, Günday M, Calişkan M et al (2013) Light cigarette smoking and vascular function. Acta Cardiol 68:255–261
15. Vlachopoulos C, Kosmopoulou F, Panagiotakos D et al (2004) Smoking and caffeine have a synergistic detrimental effect on aortic stiffness and wave reflections. J Am Coll Cardiol 44:1911–1917
16. Papamichael C, Karatzi K, Karatzis E et al (2006) Combined acute effects of red wine consumption and cigarette smoking on haemodynamics of young smokers. J Hypertens 24:1287–1292
17. van Trijp MJ, Bos WJ, Uiterwaal CS et al (2004) Determinants of AIx in young men: the ARYA study. Eur J Clin Invest 34:825–830
18. Rehill N, Beck CR, Yeo KR, Yeo WW (2006) The effect of chronic tobacco smoking on arterial stiffness. Br J Clin Pharmacol 61:767–773
19. Jatoi NA, Jerrard-Dunne P, Feely J, Mahmud A (2007) Impact of smoking and smoking cessation on arterial stiffness and aortic wave reflection in hypertension. Hypertension 49:981–985
20. Polónia J, Barbosa L, Silva JA, Rosas M (2009) Improvement of aortic reflection wave responses 6 months after stopping smoking: a prospective study. Blood Press Monit 14: 69–75
21. Minami J, Ishimitsu T, Ohrui M, Matsuoka H (2009) Association of smoking with aortic wave reflection and central systolic pressure and metabolic syndrome in normotensive Japanese men. Am J Hypertens 22:617–623
22. Primatesta P, Falaschetti E, Gupta S et al (2001) Association between smoking and blood pressure: evidence from the health survey for England. Hypertension 37:187–193
23. Bowman TS, Gaziano JM, Buring JE, Sesso HD (2007) A prospective study of cigarette smoking and risk of incident hypertension in women. J Am Coll Cardiol 50:2085–2092
24. Green MS, Jucha E, Luz Y (1986) Blood pressure in smokers and non-smokers: epidemiologic findings. Am Heart J 111(932–9):40
25. Lee D, Ha M, Kim J, Jacobs DR (2001) Effects of smoking cessation on changes in blood pressure and incidence of hypertension. Hypertension 37:194–198
26. Perkins KA, Epstein LH, Marks BL et al (1989) The effect of nicotine on energy expenditure during light physical activity. N Engl J Med 320:898–903
27. Park W, Miyachi M, Tanaka H (2014). Can aerobic exercise mitigate the effects of cigarette smoking on arterial stiffness? J Clin Hypertens 16:640–644

28. Carnoya J, Glantz SA (2005) Cardiovascular effects of secondhand smoke: nearly as large as smoking. Circulation 111:2684–2698
29. Stefanadis C, Vlachopoulos C, Tsiamis E et al (1998) Unfavorable effects of passive smoking on aortic function in men. Ann Intern Med 128:426–434
30. Mahmud A, Feely J (2004) Effects of passive smoking on blood pressure and aortic pressure waveform in healthy young adults–influence of gender. Br J Clin Pharmacol 57:37–43
31. Argacha JF, Adamopoulos D, Gujic M et al (2008) Acute effects of passive smoking on peripheral vascular function. Hypertension 51:1506–1511
32. Juonala M, Maqnussen CG, Raitakari OT (2013) Parental smoking produces long-term damage to vascular function in their children. Curr Opin Cardiol 28:569–574
33. Kinlay S, Creager M, Fukumoto M et al (2001) Endothelium-derived nitric oxide regulates arterial elasticity in human arteries in vivo. Hypertension 38:1049–1053
34. Milara J, Ortiz JL, Juan G et al (2010) Cigarette smoke exposure upregulates endothelin receptor B in human pulmonary artery endothelial cells: molecular and functional consequences. Br J Pharmacol 161:1599–1615
35. Gaenzer H, Neumayr G, Marschang P et al (2001) Flow-mediated vasodilation of the femoral and brachial artery induced by exercise in healthy non-smoking and smoking men. J Am Coll Cardiol 38:1313–1319
36. Vlachopoulos C, Tsekoura D, Alexopoulos N et al (2004) Type 5 phosphodiesterase inhibition by sildenafil abrogates acute smoking-induced endothelial dysfunction. Am J Hypertens 17:1040–1044
37. Tabara Y, Muro S, Takahashi Y, Nagahama Study Group (2014) Airflow limitation in smokers is associated with arterial stiffness: the Nagahama Study. Atherosclerosis 232:59–64
38. Roux A, Motreff P, Perriot J et al (2010) Early improvement in peripheral vascular tone following smoking cessation using nicotine replacement therapy: aortic wave reflection analysis. Cardiology 117:37–43
39. Takami T, Saito Y (2011) Effects of smoking cessation on central blood pressure and arterial stiffness. Vasc Health Risk Manag 7:633–638
40. Bhatnagar A, Whitsel L, Ribisl K et al; on behalf of the American Heart Association Advocacy Coordinating Committee, Council on Cardiovascular and Stroke Nursing, Council on Clinical Cardiology, and Council on Quality of Care and Outcomes Research. Electronic Cigarettes (2014) A policy statement from the American Heart Association. Circulation 130:1418–1436
41. Lopez-Garcia E, van Dam RM, Li TY et al (2008) The relationship of coffee consumption with mortality. Ann Intern Med 148:904–914
42. Noordzij M, Uiterwaal CS, Arends LR et al (2005) Blood pressure response to chronic intake of coffee and caffeine: a meta-analysis of randomized controlled trials. J Hypertens 23: 921–928
43. Vlachopoulos C, Hirata K, O'Rourke M (2001) Pressure-altering agents affect central aortic pressures more than is apparent from upper limb measurements in hypertensive patients: the role of arterial wave reflections. Hypertension 38:1456–1460
44. Mahmud A, Feely J (2001) Acute effect of caffeine on arterial stiffness and aortic pressure waveform. Hypertension 38:227–231
45. Vlachopoulos C, Hirata K, Stefanadis C et al (2003) Caffeine increases aortic stiffness in hypertensive patients. Am J Hypertens 16:63–66
46. Vlachopoulos C, Hirata K, O'Rourke MF (2003) Effect of caffeine on aortic elastic properties and wave reflection. J Hypertens 21:563–570
47. Waring WS, Goudsmit J, Marwick J et al (2003) Acute caffeine intake influences central more than peripheral blood pressure in young adults. Am J Hypertens 16:919–924
48. Vlachopoulos CV, Vyssoulis GG, Alexopoulos NA et al (2007) Effect of chronic coffee consumption on aortic stiffness and wave reflections in hypertensive patients. Eur J Clin Nutr 61:796–802
49. Ioakeimidis N, Vlachopoulos C, Alexopoulos N et al (2011) Coffee blunts the acute effect of caffeine on aortic stiffness and wave reflections after two weeks of daily consumption. Circulation 124:A12112 (abstr)

50. Papaioannou TG, Karatzi K, Karatzis E et al (2005) Acute effects of caffeine on arterial stiffness, wave reflections, and central aortic pressures. Am J Hypertens 18:129–136
51. Klatsky AL, Koplik S, Kipp H, Friedman GD (2008) The confounded relation of coffee drinking to coronary artery disease. Am J Cardiol 101:825–827
52. Avolio AP, Deng FQ, Li WQ et al (1985) Effects of aging on arterial distensibility in populations with high and low prevalence of hypertension: comparison between urban and rural communities in China. Circulation 71:202–210
53. Lambert J, Pijpers R, van Ittersum F et al (1997) Sodium, blood pressure and arterial distensibility in insulin-dependent diabetes mellitus. Hypertension 30:1162–1168
54. Park S, Park JB, Lakkata EG (2011). Association of central hemodynamics with estimated 24h-urinary sodium in patients with hypertension. J Hypertens 29:1502–1507
55. Liu Y-P, Thijs L, Kuznetsova T et al (2013) Central systolic augmentation indexes and urinary sodium in a white population. Am J Hypertens 26:95–103
56. Gates P, Tanaka H, Hiatt W, Seals D (2004) Dietary sodium restriction rapidly improves large elastic artery compliance in older adults with systolic hypertension. Hypertension 44:35–41
57. He F, Marciniak M, Visagie E et al (2009) Effect of modest salt reduction on blood pressure, urinary albumin, and pulse wave velocity in white, black and asian mild hypertensives. Hypertension 54:482–488
58. Blumenthal J, Babyak A, Sherwood A (2010) Effects of the DASH Diet alone and in combination with exercise and weight loss on blood pressure and cardiovascular biomarkers in men and women with high blood pressure: the ENCORE Study. Arch Intern Med 170:126–135
59. Guyton AC, Langston JB, Navar G (1964) Theory for renal autoregulation by feedback at the juxtaglomerular apparatus. Circ Res 14/15(Suppl I):I-187–I-197
60. Matrougui K, Schiavi P, Guez D, Henrion D (1998) High sodium intake decreases pressure-induced (myogenic) tone and flow-induced dilation in resistance arteries from hypertensive rats. Hypertension 32:176–179
61. Shultz PJ, Tolins JP (1993) Adaptation to increased dietary salt intake in the rat: role of endogenous nitric oxide. J Clin Invest 91:642–650
62. Ferri C, Bellini C, Mazzocchi C et al (1997) Elevated plasma and urinary endothelin-1 levels in human salt-sensitive hypertension. Clin Sci 93:35–41
63. Campese Vito M (1994) Salt sensitivity in hypertension: renal and cardiovascular implications. Hypertension 23:531–550
64. Benetos A, Bouaziz H, Albaladejo P et al (1995) Carotid artery mechanical properties of Dahl salt-sensitive rats. Hypertension 25:272–277
65. Benetos A, Yang-Yan X, Cuche J-L et al (1992) Arterial effects of salt restriction in hypertensive patients. A 9-week, randomised, double-blind, crossover study. J Hypertens 10:355–360
66. Draaijer P, Kool MJ, Maessen JM et al (1993) Vascular distensibility and compliance in salt-sensitive and salt-resistant borderline hypertension. J Hypertens 11:1199–1207
67. Levy B, Poitevin P, Duriez M et al (1997) Sodium, survival, and the mechanical properties of the carotid artery in stroke-prone hypertensive rats. J Hypertens 15:251–258
68. Dickinson KM, Keogh JB, Clifton PM (2009) Effects of a low-salt diet on flow-mediated dilatation in humans. Am J Clin Nutr 89:485–490
69. Mente A, O'Donnell M, Rangarajan S, PURE Investigators et al (2014) Association of urinary sodium and potassium excretion with blood pressure. N Engl J Med 371:601–611
70. Alderman MH, Cohen HW (2012) Dietary sodium intake and cardiovascular mortality: controversy resolved? Am J Hypertens 25:727–734
71. Mozaffarian D, Fahimi S, Singh G, Global Burden of Diseases Nutrition and Chronic Diseases Expert Group (NUTRICODE) et al (2014) Global sodium consumption and death from cardiovascular causes. N Engl J Med 371:624–634
72. Whelton P, Appel L, Sacco R et al (2012) Sodium, blood pressure and cardiovascular disease. Further evidence supporting the American Heart Association Sodium Reduction Recommendations. Circulation 126:2880–2889

Part IV

Systemic Arterial Disorders

Arterial Ageing

14

Peter M. Nilsson

The ageing of humans and its physiological consequences is regulated by both genetic factors, as selected by evolution, and environmental factors, for example, the influence of nutrition and caloric intake with its mitochondrial effects. Some of the mediating mechanisms have been characterised, but much is still unclear. As biological ageing is central to understand the development of many chronic disease conditions that increase in incidence with advancing chronological age, it is important to understand age-related mechanisms in order to find new ways to dissect the causality of disease and even to find new targets for preventive efforts. In the cardiovascular system, the development of disease is paralleled by age-associated changes, and these will be further discussed, with a focus on arterial ageing [1]. It is sometimes not easy to disentangle the pathological changes in the arterial tree from these changes that are age related in themselves, for example, related to atherosclerosis that increases in prevalence in large arteries with advancing age, at least in western populations.

14.1 Composition and Function of the Arterial Wall

The arterial wall consists of three distinct layers, from inside and out, the *tunica intima* (made up mainly by endothelial cells), *tunica media* (which is made up of smooth muscle cells and elastic tissue) and *tunica externa* (composed of connective tissue made up of collagen fibres). These layers are innervated by the autonomous

P.M. Nilsson, MD, PhD
Department of Clinical Sciences, Lund University, Skåne University Hospital,
Malmö 20502, Sweden
e-mail: Peter.Nilsson@med.lu.se

© Springer International Publishing Switzerland 2015
A. Berbari, G. Mancia (eds.), *Arterial Disorders:*
Definition, Clinical Manifestations, Mechanisms and Therapeutic Approaches,
DOI 10.1007/978-3-319-14556-3_14

nervous system and involved in the modification of arterial function following the propagation of the pulse wave from the heart with every heartbeat.

The endothelium is closest to the blood stream circulating in the arterial lumen and involved in regulating vasodilation and vasoconstriction by secretion of vasoactive substances such as nitric oxide (NO), endothelin and many more [2]. With ageing, the endothelial function starts to deteriorate, and less NO is produced by impaired induction of endothelial NO synthetase (eNOS). In addition the normal insulin sensitivity in the endothelial cells, associated with vasodilation by the hormone insulin in the postprandial state, is replaced by a gradual increase in endothelial insulin resistance [3]. This will lead to a loss of the vasodilatory capacity induced by insulin and therefore vasoconstriction and blood pressure elevation, another mechanism by which insulin resistance (resulting in hyperinsulinaemia) might lead to hypertension [4]. Furthermore, endothelial dysfunction is associated with reduced anticoagulant properties as well as increased adhesion molecule expression, chemokine and other cytokine release, promoting inflammation, in addition to reactive oxygen species (ROS) production from the endothelium. This leads to local inflammation with myofibroblast migration and proliferation inside the vessel, often linked to vascular remodelling. In addition perivascular inflammation can contribute to local vasoregulation. These factors taken together play important roles in the development of atherosclerosis, starting in the intima with fatty streaks and lipid deposits already at an early age in risk individuals [5], for example, with familiar hypercholesterolaemia.

The media of the artery consists of layers of elastic elements that are stretched by each pulse wave in systole and will be flexed back in diastole, thus contributing to a smooth forward propagation of the blood stream in both systole and diastole (so-called Windkessel effect). These elastic elements consist of elastin, a protein that is preformed in fetal life and decreases gradually during the lifespan. Another component is collagen as well as the smooth muscle cells causing contractions. The third, outward layer (tunica externa) is surrounded by perivascular fat in different amounts, with its own cytokine activities for local inflammation.

14.2   Age-Related Changes of Arterial Properties

During ageing the collagen content will become relatively increased, and cross-links will occur between collagen elements, also influenced and further enhanced by glycation of arterial wall proteins. The consequence of these two developments, a relative decrease in elastin and a corresponding relative increase in collagen (with cross-linkages and glycation), will contribute, together with impaired endothelial function, to a gradual stiffening of the large (elastic) arteries. This is in contrast to the medium-sized (muscular) arteries that will not undergo the same age-related changes. Therefore the aorta and the carotid arteries will show typical age-related increasing stiffness, while this is not the case for the brachial arteries. The changes of the femoral arteries are somewhat in between, with a notable stiffening taking place with ageing but not as pronounced as in the aorta. These arteries can also be affected by atherosclerosis, similar to what happens in the aorta and carotid arteries, but in contrast to the brachial artery that is not affected.

This gradual age-related stiffening of the large elastic arteries is named *arteriosclerosis* and occurs mainly in the media of the artery but is further facilitated by endothelial dysfunction. In addition, it is believed that haemodynamic stress; metabolic factors, most importantly hyperglycaemia; and chronic inflammation could contribute to this process. On the other hand, the development of *atherosclerosis* involves first of all the intima and later on also other layers of the artery, with well-described morphological changes [5]. The consequence could later on be incidence of cardiovascular disease events caused by atherosclerosis, for example, ischaemic heart disease (IHD), stroke or peripheral artery disease (PAD). These manifestations constitute the major public health problem in western societies and in a growing proportion of the population in developing countries according to the World Health Organization (WHO).

According to one hypothesis, arteriosclerosis starts very early in life and is influenced by fetal programming of the vasculature and its elastin content [6]. Later on the process of atherosclerosis starts and runs in parallel with arteriosclerosis. The clinical events are usually linked to atherosclerosis, based on its derived plaque formation and rupture, even if arterial stiffness has also been shown to be an independent predictor of future cardiovascular events and mortality, based on recent meta-analyses [7, 8]. In both conditions, oxidative stress, chronic inflammation and increased activity of the renin-angiotensin-aldosterone system (RAAS) seem to be of considerable importance.

14.3   How to Evaluate Arterial Function and Arterial Ageing?

The arterial function associated with ageing and the morphological changes in the arterial wall can be measured by use of different technical methods, from more simple to more sophisticated ones. Brachial blood pressure undergoes typical changes with ageing, at least in most populations. There is a constant increase in systolic blood pressure in both men and women, but a steeper relative increase in women at around the time of menopause. The diastolic blood pressure tends to increase until age 60–65 years and then flattens off or even decreases. This means that the pulse pressure will show an increasing trend from around 50 years, and this is a reflection of underlying arterial stiffness. Similar changes occur in the central circulation and are possible to measure indirectly by so-called pulse wave analysis (PWA) in the radial artery based on tonometry and an algorithm. A specific characteristic of the central blood pressure is that it tends to be lower than the peripheral blood pressure in younger subjects, and therefore a blood pressure amplification can be registered from the central to the peripheral blood pressure. This amplification is lost in midlife, and after that the central and peripheral pressures tend to be rather similar with few differences [9].

Of utmost importance to arterial ageing is the increase in pulse wave velocity (PWV) that occurs as a reflection of increasing arterial stiffness caused primarily by the morphological changes with relatively less elastin and more collagen (and cross-linkages) in the arterial media layer. In most cases PWV is measured directly along the aorta from the carotid to the femoral artery as c-f PWV [9]. In some circumstances it has also been proposed to measure PWV between the brachial artery and the femoral artery (b-f PWV) or the ankle arteries (b-a PWV), but this method involves muscular arteries (*art. brachialis*, *art. tibialis posterior*, *art. dorsalis pedis*) with less elastin content and is therefore less informative. However, in the Far East (Japan, China), cultural norms may preclude observers to measure stiffness in the groin via direct access to *art. femoralis*, that is why other more distal arterial alternatives are preferred. Based on a European study of several population-based cohorts, a group of about 1,400 healthy, normotensive subjects were used for definition of the age-specific normal range of c-f PWV [10]. Based on these data, a threshold for pathological c-f PWV and increased cardiovascular risk was first defined as >12 m/s [10], but after a revision in 2012 as >10 m/s [11]. This means that an increased c-f PWV is a marker of arterial stiffness affecting the large elastic arteries, and this biomarker has also been shown to predict not only cardiovascular morbidity and mortality but also total mortality in recent meta-analyses [7, 8].

14.4   The Concept of Early Vascular Ageing (EVA)

In recent years the interest in arterial stiffness has increased, as well as in the underlying *arteriosclerosis*, as a precursor to the more well-known and well-studied *atherosclerosis*, with its pathology influenced by genetics, high LDL cholesterol levels, smoking, hypertension, inflammation and overt type 2 diabetes [5]. In many cases it is believed that early life programming may cause a susceptibility for this increased tendency for arterial stiffening as well as other aspects of vascular tree, for example, the development of capillaries and the microcirculation. As this process is also related to ageing, it has been proposed that a process of early vascular ageing (EVA) is an early sign of arteriosclerosis (in the media) but linked also to early changes in the endothelial function (intima), haemodynamic changes and the influence of abnormal glucose metabolism and increased inflammation [12–14]. The difference between the concept of arterial ageing and EVA is that the latter also encompasses the smaller arteriolae and the microcirculation, based on the crosstalk between the macro- and microcirculation [14]. EVA is now being extensively studied in different population-based cohorts, both in Europe and in Latin America, but still no general definition has been agreed upon. One way to define EVA could be to use the outliers according to the normal range of c-f PWV, i.e. above the two standard deviations (SD) of the normal distribution of c-f PWV in the European reference group [10] (Fig. 14.1). Another way to describe EVA is based on statistical methods when arterial stiffness (c-f PWV), a central aspect of EVA, is used as the dependent variable in multiple regression analyses and a number of risk markers are used as independent variables, based on data from population-based studies. As the influence of haemodynamic changes and sympathetic nervous system (SNS) stimulation on the arterial tone is substantial, the data are normally adjusted for mean arterial pressure

Pulse wave velocity (m/s)

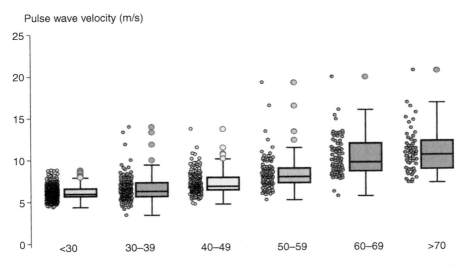

Fig. 14.1 Normal values for pulse wave velocity (c-f PWV): average according to age (1,455 healthy, normotensive subjects). *Boxes* contain 50 % of the data and *bars* contain the remainder (2 SD); *horizontal lines* indicate medians and the *circle* indicates outliers (From: The Reference Values for Arterial Stiffness' Collaboration [10])

(MAP) and heart rate (HR), the latter as a marker of SNS activity. Such investigations in a population-based study in Malmo, Sweden, have revealed that markers of glucose metabolism and dyslipidaemia (elevated triglycerides, low HDL cholesterol levels), as well as waist circumference (a marker of active abdominal fat tissue with inflammatory action), are significantly associated with arterial stiffness, but not LDL cholesterol, smoking or cystatin-C, a marker of impaired renal function [15]. The findings thus point to different clusters of cardiovascular risk factors involved in the development of arteriosclerosis and atherosclerosis, respectively.

Still there is a need to better define EVA in different age groups but also in relation to gender and ethnicity, as well as based on genetic studies for improved classification [16]. Some would argue that EVA is just a construct to cover one example of target organ damage (arterial stiffness) in subjects at high cardiovascular or metabolic risk and primarily influenced by haemodynamic changes and blood pressure levels. However, the modern genetics of hypertension and blood pressure regulation, based on a global study, could not show any marker on chromosome 13 [17], but exactly on this chromosome, a genetic locus (for the *COL4A1* gene, involved in collagen metabolism) was found for arterial stiffness in a study from Sardinia, Italy, with independent replication in another American cohort [18]. This shows that even if arterial stiffness (and EVA) is strongly influenced by the blood pressure load (MAP), HR and SNS activity, there could even exist some other important components (collagen protein synthesis, structure) and vascular risk factors (hyperglycaemia, dyslipidaemia, inflammation) independent of blood pressure regulation. If true, this opens up new possibilities to target these mechanisms of protein/collagen synthesis with new drugs to reduce arterial stiffness.

So far it has been shown that a prolonged control of hypertension will reverse early changes and have a long-term beneficial influence on arterial stiffness with decreasing c-f PWV levels over time, beyond the blood pressure control itself [19]. However, an ongoing randomised controlled study in France (SPARTE) aims to compare a treatment strategy for reduction of arterial stiffness (c-f PWV) by different means, including drugs that specifically influence the renin-angiotensin system, and another treatment strategy (control) to go for implementation of control of the conventional risk factors including blood pressure, as suggested in the guidelines [20]. SPARTE is supposed to continue for still a number of years until a sufficient number of cardiovascular end points have accumulated to show potential differences in outcomes between the treatment arms. Recruitment is ongoing.

14.5 Haemodynamic Effects of Vascular Ageing: Blood Pressure

As arterial stiffness is a characteristic of vascular ageing based on morphological changes in the arterial wall, there is also a need to better understand its haemodynamic consequence. A starting point is to try to list different characteristics of haemodynamic ageing and to try to understand the association with underlying morphological changes in the arteries (Table 14.1).

Well-known changes, as already alluded to, include an increase in brachial systolic blood pressure and a flattening off of the diastolic blood pressure to be followed by a decrease in diastolic blood pressure above the age of approximately 60–65 years. This will lead to increased risk of isolated systolic hypertension (ISH) and elevated pulse pressure, both conditions being associated with increased prospective risk of cardiovascular events [21]. The same holds true for corresponding

Table 14.1 Examples of haemodynamic ageing and its relationship to blood pressure (BP) and arterial stiffness

Age-related changes in brachial BP
Isolated systolic hypertension (ISH)
Elevated pulse pressure (PP)
Age-related changes in central BP
Increased central systolic BP and PP
Increased BP variability
Linked to arterial stiffness
Decreased heart rate variability (HRV)
Linked to arterial stiffness
Impaired endothelial function
Less vasodilation, linked to arterial stiffness
Impaired baroreceptor function, orthostatic hypotension
Linked to arterial stiffness
Microvascular disease in diabetes
Influenced by long-standing hyperglycaemia

changes in central systolic blood pressure and pulse pressure, because around the chronological age of 50 years, the blood pressure amplification between the central and peripheral circulation decreases, and thus central and brachial blood pressures tend to become more similar. These changes according to conventional blood pressure and central blood pressure recordings have previously been discussed in detail by Stanley Franklin et al. [21, 22]. For example, in participants from the Framingham Heart Study who were free of CVD events and antihypertensive therapy, in all 1,439, CVD events occurred between 1952 and 2001. In pooled logistic regression with the use of BP categories, combining SBP with DBP and PP with mean arterial pressure (MAP) improved model fit compared with individual BP components. Significant interactions were noted between SBP and DBP ($p = 0.02$) and between PP and MAP ($p = 0.01$) in multivariable models. The combination of PP + MAP (unlike SBP+DBP) had a continuous relation with cardiovascular risk and may provide greater insight into haemodynamics of altered arterial stiffness versus impaired peripheral resistance but is not superior to SBP+DBP in predicting CVD events [21]. This analysis is based on conventional blood pressure variables, but reflecting the age-related changes that more modern and sophisticated technologies can reveal.

14.6   Arterial Stiffness and Age-Related Haemodynamic Changes

Some other features of haemodynamic ageing are less well characterised, but all linked to arterial stiffness as an underlying contributing factor, and thereby also explaining most of the risk associated with these different features. One of them is increased blood pressure variability (BPV), linked to increased cardiovascular risk, i.e. for stroke [23]. Increased BPV can be evaluated on a visit-to-visit basis with weeks or months between visits but also based on shorter time intervals (days, hours, even beat-to-beat timing), as recently reviewed by Gianfranco Parati et al. [24]. An underlying feature is arterial stiffness, and it is reasonable to believe that this factor might explain most of the increased risk associated with increased BPV, even if also some mechanical changes could play a role based on changes in blood flow, shear stress or transmission of increased pulse wave energy to small arteries and the peripheral circulation [24].

In a corresponding way, it has been reported that a decrease in heart rate variability (HRV) is a marker of ageing and increased cardiovascular risk but also associated with increased arterial stiffness, for example, in patients with type 1 diabetes [25]. The decrease in heart rate variability is supposed to be influenced by an imbalance between the sympathetic and parasympathetic parts of the autonomous nervous system.

Furthermore, it is well known that episodes of orthostatic hypotension are associated with increased cardiovascular risk during follow-up, based on data from several epidemiological studies. Also here we notice underlying arterial stiffness as a common denominator, as shown in the Rotterdam study of elderly subjects [26]. The link could be the impaired stretching (compliance) of the carotid arterial wall close to the baroreceptor due to arterial stiffness and superimposed atherosclerosis, leading to impaired baroreceptor function in response to change of body position. This could contribute to the understanding of arterial stiffness being the true risk marker behind orthostatic reactions, often seen in aged subjects with, for example, diabetes of long duration. These orthostatic reactions should be separated from benign vasovagal reactions with orthostatic reactions in younger subjects.

It is conceivable to think that more widespread changes in innervation and the autonomous nervous system could contribute to the ageing of the neural system and thus linked to vascular ageing and decreased baroreceptor function as well as imbalance between sympathetic and parasympathetic activity. In one recent study, the relationship was tested between direct measures of sympathetic traffic and PWV in healthy humans [27]. The authors examined MSNA (microneurography), PWV (Complior® device), heart rate and blood pressure in 25 healthy male participants (mean age 43 years). It was reported that PWV correlated significantly with age ($r = 0.63$), SBP ($r = 0.43$) and MSNA ($r = 0.43$) but not with BMI, waist circumference, waist-to-hip ratio, heart rate, pulse pressure or DBP. Multiple linear regression analysis revealed that only age and MSNA were linked independently to PWV ($r^2 = 0.62$, $p < 0.001$), explaining 39 and 25 % of its variance, respectively. Individuals with excessive PWV had significantly greater MSNA than individuals with optimal PWV. Thus the relationship between MSNA and PWV is independent of age, BMI, waist circumference, waist-to-hip ratio, heart rate, pulse pressure or blood pressure [27]. This shows the contribution of neurophysiological ageing to vascular ageing.

In the arterial wall, there is a crosstalk between the sympathetic nervous system and the renin-angiotensin system that will further decrease elasticity and promote vascular ageing [28].

14.7   Cardiac-Arterial Coupling Influenced by Arterial Stiffness

Finally, it is self-evident that haemodynamic changes associated with ageing are not possible to describe without taking cardiac changes into account. In fact, there is a so-called cardiac-arterial coupling process that can be illustrated by echocardiography examinations [29]. In the end there is thus a crosstalk between cardiac function, as well as morphological changes, and the general circulation in the arterial tree. With increasing stiffening of the proximal thoracic aorta, the reflex wave from the periphery back to the central circulation and the heart can no longer be accommodated, even if the aorta root widens. Instead this pulse wave energy will impact on the heart with increased pressure waves and augmentation during systole leading to increased strain on the left ventricle, causing left ventricular hypertrophy (LVH), and a decreased perfusion pressure during diastole, leading to impaired blood flow in the coronary circulation. These two trends combined will increase the risk of morphological changes (LVH) in combination with coronary ischaemia, thus increasing the risk of CHD events. This is therefore a haemodynamic mechanism explaining some of the risk potential of arterial stiffness, as measured by increased PWV, for the development of CHD. It contributes to what has been called the cardiovascular ageing continuum by O'Rourke et al. [30].

14.8 Metabolic Syndrome and Arterial Stiffness

Even if it has been difficult to show a strong independent association between arterial stiffness and overt type 2 diabetes [31], there is evidence to show that hyperglycaemia as a continuous variable contributes to vascular ageing and arterial stiffness [32]. Diabetes mellitus was associated with c-f PWV in 52 % of studies in one meta-analysis, but the strength of the association was low [31]. Within the so-called metabolic syndrome (MetS), a number of risk factors tend to cluster, including hypertension, hyperglycaemia, dyslipidaemia (elevated triglyceride, decreased HDL cholesterol), increased waist circumference and underlying insulin resistance. Specific clusters of MetS components impact differentially on arterial stiffness (PWV). Recently, in several population-based studies participating in the MARE (Metabolic syndrome and Arteries REsearch) Consortium, the occurrence of specific clusters of MetS differed markedly across Europe and the USA. Based on data from 20,570 subjects included in nine cohorts representing eight different European countries and the USA in the MARE Consortium, MetS was defined in accordance with NCEP ATPIII criteria. PWV measured in each cohort was "normalised" to account for different acquisition methods. The results could show that MetS had an overall prevalence of 24.2 %. MetS accelerated the age-associated increase in PWV levels at any age and similarly in men and women. Therefore, different component clusters of MetS showed varying associations with arterial stiffness (PWV) across these nine cohorts [33].

Also in a local study from the Malmö Diet Cancer cohort, hyperglycaemia and dyslipidaemia showed independent associations with arterial stiffness in elderly subjects with mean age of 71 years [15].

14.9 Kidney Disease, Inflammation and Stiffness

It is well known that advanced chronic kidney disease is associated with vascular changes, as media sclerosis, and thus increasing arterial stiffness [34]. This is linked to oxidative stress and chronic inflammation [35, 36]. Uraemic toxins, particularly those associated with dysregulated mineral metabolism, can drive vascular smooth muscle cell damage and tissue changes that promote vascular calcification but may also promote DNA damage [36]. Epidemiological data suggest that some of these same risk factors in chronic kidney disease (CKD stages 1–5) associate with cardiovascular mortality in the aged general population. The advanced arterial changes in CKD thus resemble that of a fast progressing vascular ageing. This will further increase the overall cardiovascular risk that is very high in patients with CKD-5 and end-stage renal disease (ESRD).

14.10 Arterial Stiffness in the Elderly

The cardiovascular risk increases rapidly with advancing chronological age, based on arterial stiffness, advancing atherosclerosis and haemodynamic changes in the elderly [37, 38]. On the other hand, survival selection bias may influence the fact that some elderly subjects have survived in spite of advanced arterial stiffness. Epidemiological studies have thus shown that c-f PWV is a stronger risk marker in middle-aged as compared to elderly subjects [8]. No intervention studies exist so far to show the benefits of reducing arterial stiffness (PWV) in the elderly, as was already shown for control of hypertension in 80+-year-old subjects in the placebo-controlled HYVET trial [39].

Another aspect of great interest is the role of chronic inflammation and oxidative stress that are closely linked to the ageing process in general and therefore visible in elderly people [40]. If inflammation can be reduced, a reduction of arterial stiffness has been shown, for example, in patients with inflammatory bowel disease [41], a finding of great theoretical and practical importance. More studies should aim for control of inflammation to prevent cardiovascular disease, but still convincing human studies are lacking.

Arterial stiffness is also a reflection of biological and functional ageing in general. In the Whitehall II study in London, this has been investigated. Researchers aimed to analyse associations of arterial stiffness with age, subjective and objective measures of physical functioning and self-reported functional limitation [42]. Pulse wave velocity was measured by applanation tonometry among 5,392 men and women aged 55–78 years. Results showed that arterial stiffness was strongly associated with age (mean difference per decade: men, 1.37 m/s; women, 1.39 m/s). This association was robust to individual and combined adjustment for pulse pressure, mean arterial pressure, antihypertensive treatment and chronic disease. One SD higher stiffness was associated with lower walking speed and physical component summary score and poorer lung function adjusted for age, sex and ethnic group. Associations of stiffness with functional limitation were robust to multiple adjustments, including pulse pressure and chronic disease. The authors concluded that the concept of vascular ageing is reinforced by the observation that arterial stiffness is a robust correlate of physical functioning and functional limitation in early old age [42]. Why this is so merits further studies.

14.11 Future Perspectives

The development of the EVA concept [12–14] has also triggered research and interest in some other related biomarkers and in haemodynamic ageing [43]. Telomeres represent the end segment of the DNA helix with a shortening taking place with every cell division and therefore regarded as a marker of the biological clock of ageing [44, 45]. Even if discrepant results have sometimes been published, most studies support the notion that telomere length, or rather the telomere attrition rate over time, could represent an interesting aspect of vascular ageing [44, 45]. Previous studies have shown an association between telomere length and arterial stiffness, as measured by pulse pressure [46].

Other biomarkers of growing interest are, for example, aldosterone and vitamin D, both with implication for cardiovascular ageing. Studies have shown that elevated aldosterone levels are associated with cardiovascular changes including sclerosis and increase stiffness [47]. This is possible to counteract by use of aldosterone antagonist, for example, spironolactone or eplerenone. Large-scale intervention studies are needed before conclusions can be drawn regarding the reversibility of these changes.

Growing evidence has documented that vitamin D deficiency could play a role in the development of pathological changes within the arterial system. Observational studies have shown an increased risk associated with vitamin D deficiency, but it has been hard to show benefits by vitamin D supplementation [48]. Therefore, the role of vitamin D is still somewhat enigmatic in arterial disease.

In the future, more studies should elucidate on the role of arterial stiffness in relation to cognitive decline and risk of dementia, as an association exists between impaired arterial compliance, arterial stiffness, mild cognitive impairment and the occurrence of so-called white matter lesions (WML) in the cerebral white matter [49]. Probably the pulse wave propagation from the general circulation, with stiff arteries, cannot be accommodated in a normal way in the cerebral microcirculation. This leads to micro-bleeds and the development of tissue scaring and WML, a common finding in subjects with uncontrolled hypertension. Hypertension was observed in a Swedish study of 70-year-old people to predict dementia, both of the vascular type and Alzheimer-like dementia [50]. In a recent statement from the American Heart Association/American Stroke Association, risk factors for cognitive impairment have been discussed, including the role of hypertension [51].

Finally, intervention studies are needed to show the benefits of reducing arterial stiffness, over and above blood pressure control per se. In this respect new drugs will also be tested, for example, the vascular protection believed to be an effect of compound 21, a specific angiotensin-2 (AT2) receptor agonist [52], soon to be tested also in humans. Animal studies have been promising in showing a reduction of arterial stiffness, without significant effects on blood pressure in a mouse model [53]. Other new experimental drugs are being developed for vascular protection and blood pressure control [54] and could be combined with more traditional drugs for control of hypertension and hyperlipidaemia. A novel approach is also to retard ageing via influencing mammalian Sir2 (SIRT-1, a NAD+-dependent deacetylase), previously shown to extend the lifespan of lower organisms. This is a promising target molecule to influence some aspects of vascular ageing, and drug development is underway [55]. In summary, arterial ageing is a fruitful concept to be explored for new understanding of vascular biology and new mechanisms for potential intervention.

Acknowledgements This review was supported by a grant from the Research Council of Sweden.

References

1. Najjar SS, Scuteri A, Lakatta EG (2005) Arterial aging: is it an immutable cardiovascular risk factor? Hypertension 46:454–462
2. Vanhoutte PM (2009) Endothelial dysfunction: the first step toward coronary arteriosclerosis. Circ J 73:595–601
3. Gage MC, Yuldasheva NY, Viswambharan H et al (2013) Endothelium-specific insulin resistance leads to accelerated atherosclerosis in areas with disturbed flow patterns: a role for reactive oxygen species. Atherosclerosis 230:131–139
4. Reaven GM, Lithell H, Landsberg L (1996) Hypertension and associated metabolic abnormalities – the role of insulin resistance and the sympathoadrenal system. N Engl J Med 334:374–381
5. Hansson GK (2005) Inflammation, atherosclerosis, and coronary artery disease. N Engl J Med 352:1685–1695
6. Dodson RB, Rozance PJ, Fleenor BS et al (2013) Increased arterial stiffness and extracellular matrix reorganization in intrauterine growth-restricted fetal sheep. Pediatr Res 73:147–154
7. Vlachopoulos C, Aznaouridis K, Stefanadis C (2010) Prediction of cardiovascular events and all-cause mortality with arterial stiffness: a systematic review and meta-analysis. J Am Coll Cardiol 55:1318–1327
8. Ben-Shlomo Y, Spears M, Boustred C et al (2013) Aortic pulse wave velocity improves cardiovascular event prediction: an individual participant meta-analysis of prospective observational data from 17,635 subjects. J Am Coll Cardiol 63:636–646
9. Laurent S, Cockcroft J, Van Bortel L, European Network for Non-invasive Investigation of Large Arteries et al (2006) Expert consensus document on arterial stiffness: methodological issues and clinical applications. Eur Heart J 27:2588–2605
10. The Reference Values for Arterial Stiffness' Collaboration (2010) Determinants of pulse wave velocity in healthy people and in the presence of cardiovascular risk factors: 'establishing normal and reference values'. Eur Heart J 31:2338–2350
11. Van Bortel LM, Laurent S, Boutouyrie P, Artery Society; European Society of Hypertension Working Group on Vascular Structure and Function; European Network for Non-invasive Investigation of Large Arteries et al (2012) Expert consensus document on the measurement of aortic stiffness in daily practice using carotid-femoral pulse wave velocity. J Hypertens 30: 445–448
12. Nilsson PM, Lurbe E, Laurent S (2008) The early life origins of vascular ageing and cardiovascular risk: the EVA syndrome (review). J Hypertens 26:1049–1057
13. Nilsson PM, Boutouyrie P, Laurent S (2009) Vascular aging: a tale of EVA and ADAM in cardiovascular risk assessment and prevention. Hypertension 54:3–10
14. Nilsson PM, Boutouyrie P, Cunha P et al (2013) Early vascular ageing in translation: from laboratory investigations to clinical applications in cardiovascular prevention. J Hypertens 8: 1517–1526
15. Gottsäter M, Östling G, Persson M et al (2015) Non-hemodynamic predictors of arterial stiffness after 17 years of follow-up: the Malmö diet and cancer study. J Hypertens (in press)
16. Nilsson PM (2012) Genetic and environmental determinants of early vascular ageing (EVA). Curr Vasc Pharmacol 10:700–701
17. Ehret GB, Munroe PB, Rice KM, International Consortium for Blood Pressure Genome-Wide Association Studies et al (2011) Genetic variants in novel pathways influence blood pressure and cardiovascular disease risk. Nature 478:103–109
18. Tarasov KV, Sanna S, Scuteri A et al (2009) COL4A1 is associated with arterial stiffness by genome-wide association scan. Circ Cardiovasc Genet 2:151–158
19. Ong KT, Delerme S, Pannier B et al; on behalf of the investigators (2011) Aortic stiffness is reduced beyond blood pressure lowering by short-term and long-term antihypertensive treatment: a meta-analysis of individual data in 294 patients. J Hypertens 29:1034–1042

20. Laurent S, Mousseaux E, Boutouyrie P (2013) Arterial stiffness as an imaging biomarker: are all pathways equal? Hypertension 62:10–12
21. Franklin SS, Lopez VA, Wong ND et al (2009) Single versus combined blood pressure components and risk for cardiovascular disease: the Framingham Heart Study. Circulation 119: 243–250
22. Nilsson PM, Khalili P, Franklin SS (2014) Blood pressure and pulse wave velocity as metrics for evaluating pathologic ageing of the cardiovascular system. Blood Press 23:17–30
23. Rothwell PM, Howard SC, Dolan E et al (2010) Prognostic significance of visit-to-visit variability, maximum systolic blood pressure, and episodic hypertension. Lancet 375:895–905
24. Parati G, Ochoa JE, Salvi P et al (2013) Prognostic value of blood pressure variability and average blood pressure levels in patients with hypertension and diabetes. Diabetes Care 36(Suppl 2):S312–S324
25. Theilade S, Lajer M, Persson F et al (2013) Arterial stiffness is associated with cardiovascular, renal, retinal, and autonomic disease in type 1 diabetes. Diabetes Care 36:715–721
26. Mattace-Raso FU, van den Meiracker AH, Bos WJ et al (2007) Arterial stiffness, cardiovagal baroreflex sensitivity and postural blood pressure changes in older adults: the Rotterdam Study. J Hypertens 25:1421–1426
27. Swierblewska E, Hering D, Kara T et al (2010) An independent relationship between muscle sympathetic nerve activity and pulse wave velocity in normal humans. J Hypertens 28:979–984
28. Barrett-O'Keefe Z, Witman MA, McDaniel J et al (2013) Angiotensin II potentiates α-adrenergic vasoconstriction in the elderly. Clin Sci (Lond) 124:413–422
29. Chirinos JA, Rietzschel ER, De Buyzere ML, Asklepios Investigators et al (2009) Arterial load and ventricular-arterial coupling: physiologic relations with body size and effect of obesity. Hypertension 54:558–566
30. O'Rourke MF, Safar ME, Dzau V (2010) The Cardiovascular continuum extended: aging effects on the aorta and microvasculature. Vasc Med 5:461–468
31. Cecelja M, Chowienczyk P (2009) Dissociation of aortic pulse wave velocity with risk factors for cardiovascular disease other than hypertension: a systematic review. Hypertension 54: 1328–1336
32. Stehouwer CD, Henry RM, Ferreira I (2008) Arterial stiffness in diabetes and the metabolic syndrome: a pathway to cardiovascular disease. Diabetologia 51:527–539
33. Scuteri A, Cunha PG, Rosei EA, MARE Consortium et al (2014) Arterial stiffness and influences of the metabolic syndrome: a cross-countries study. Atherosclerosis 233:654–660
34. London GM, Pannier B, Marchais SJ (2013) Vascular calcifications, arterial aging and arterial remodeling in ESRD. Blood Purif 35(1–3):16–21
35. Shanahan CM (2013) Mechanisms of vascular calcification in CKD-evidence for premature ageing? Nat Rev Nephrol 9:661–670
36. Wang M, Jiang L, Monticone RE, Lakatta EG (2014) Proinflammation: the key to arterial aging. Trends Endocrinol Metab 25:72–79
37. Zhang Y, Agnoletti D, Xu Y et al (2014) Carotid-femoral pulse wave velocity in the elderly. J Hypertens 32:1572–1576
38. Safar ME, Nilsson PM (2013) Pulsatile hemodynamics and cardiovascular risk factors in very old patients: background, sex aspects and implications. J Hypertens 31:848–857
39. Beckett NS, Peters R, Fletcher AE, HYVET Study Group et al (2008) Treatment of hypertension in patients 80 years of age or older. N Engl J Med 358:1887–1898
40. Puca AA, Carrizzo A, Villa F et al (2013) Vascular ageing: the role of oxidative stress. Int J Biochem Cell Biol 45:556–559
41. Zanoli L, Rastelli S, Inserra G et al (2014) Increased arterial stiffness in inflammatory bowel diseases is dependent upon inflammation and reduced by immunomodulatory drugs. Atherosclerosis 234:346–351
42. Brunner EJ, Shipley MJ, Witte DR et al (2011) Arterial stiffness, physical function, and functional limitation: the Whitehall II Study. Hypertension 57:1003–1009

43. Nilsson PM (2014) Hemodynamic aging as the consequence of structural changes associated with Early Vascular Aging (EVA). Aging Dis 5:109–113
44. Fyhrquist F, Saijonmaa O, Strandberg T (2013) The roles of senescence and telomere shortening in cardiovascular disease. Nat Rev Cardiol 10:274–283
45. Nilsson PM, Tufvesson H, Leosdottir M, Melander O (2013) Telomeres and cardiovascular disease risk: an update 2013. Transl Res 162:371–380
46. Benetos A, Okuda K, Lajemi M et al (2001) Telomere length as an indicator of biological aging: the gender effect and relation with pulse pressure and pulse wave velocity. Hypertension 37(2 Pt 2):381–385
47. Brown JM, Underwood PC, Ferri C et al (2014) Aldosterone dysregulation with aging predicts renal vascular function and cardiovascular risk. Hypertension 63:1205–1211
48. Chowdhury R, Kunutsor S, Vitezova A et al (2014) Vitamin D and risk of cause specific death: systematic review and meta-analysis of observational cohort and randomized intervention studies. BMJ 348:g1903
49. Mitchell GF, van Buchem MA, Sigurdsson S et al (2011) Arterial stiffness, pressure and flow pulsatility and brain structure and function: the age, gene/environment susceptibility–Reykjavik study. Brain 134(Pt 11):3398–3407
50. Skoog I, Lernfelt B, Landahl S et al (1996) 15-year longitudinal study of blood pressure and dementia. Lancet 347:1141–1145
51. Gorelick PB, Scuteri A, Black SE, American Heart Association Stroke Council, Council on Epidemiology and Prevention, Council on Cardiovascular Nursing, Council on Cardiovascular Radiology and Intervention, and Council on Cardiovascular Surgery and Anesthesia et al (2011) Vascular contributions to cognitive impairment and dementia: a statement for healthcare professionals from the American Heart Association/American Stroke Association. Stroke 42:2672–2713
52. Steckelings UM, Paulis L, Namsolleck P, Unger T (2012) AT2 receptor agonists: hypertension and beyond. Curr Opin Nephrol Hypertens 21:142–146
53. Paulis L, Becker ST, Lucht K et al (2012) Direct angiotensin II type 2 receptor stimulation in Nω-nitro-L-arginine-methyl ester-induced hypertension: the effect on pulse wave velocity and aortic remodeling. Hypertension 59:485–492
54. Laurent S, Schlaich M, Esler M (2012) New drugs, procedures, and devices for hypertension. Lancet 380:591–600
55. Wang F, Chen HZ, Lv X, Liu DP (2013) SIRT1 as a novel potential treatment target for vascular aging and age-related vascular diseases. Curr Mol Med 13:155–164

Renal Arterial Aging

15

Adel E. Berbari, Najla A. Daouk, and Samir G. Mallat

15.1 Introduction

Over the past century, life expectancy at birth has increased significantly from less than 50 years to over 75 years in both developed and developing countries, with the elderly constituting a growing proportion of the population. Among diseases responsible for increased morbidity and mortality in this segment of the population, renal disorders play an important role [1, 2]. Estimated prevalence of chronic kidney disease (CKD) nears 40 % after the age of 70 years [3]. Furthermore, according to the United States Renal Data System (USRDS) data, the elderly population has the fastest growth of end-stage renal disease at 11 % for ages 65–74 years and 14 % for age 75 years and above [4].

Like other organs in the body, the kidneys undergo involutionary changes with age. In both humans and experimental animals, aging is associated with progressive impairment of the morphology and function of the kidneys [5–9].

In subjects without hypertension or diabetes mellitus, moderate to severe reduction in renal function (glomerular filtration rate – GFR – <60 ml/min/1.73 m^2) is common among those >70 years with an incidence of 16 % compared to 0.1 and 1.2 % in subjects of age group 20–39 and 40–59 years, respectively [10]. Furthermore, aside from hypertension and diabetes, age appears to be a key predictor of CKD: 11 % of subjects >65 years without hypertension or diabetes have stage 3 or more CKD [10].

In the elderly, several disorders are associated with CKD (Table 15.1) [10]. Cross-sectional and prospective studies have identified many factors that may accelerate

A.E. Berbari (✉) • N.A. Daouk • S.G. Mallat
Department of Internal Medicine, American University of Beirut Medical Center,
Beirut, Lebanon
e-mail: ab01@aub.edu.lb; nd00@aub.edu.lb; sm104@aub.edu.lb

© Springer International Publishing Switzerland 2015   203
A. Berbari, G. Mancia (eds.), *Arterial Disorders:*
Definition, Clinical Manifestations, Mechanisms and Therapeutic Approaches,
DOI 10.1007/978-3-319-14556-3_15

Table 15.1 Primary renal disease in the elderly

1. Primary renal parenchymal disorders
2. Diabetic kidney disease
3. Hypertension
4. Infections
5. Tumors of the kidney and renal pelvis
6. Renal arterial aging

age-related decline in renal function such as hypertension, diabetes mellitus, atherosclerosis, urinary tract obstruction, increased consumption of nephrotoxic drugs, increased use of radiological procedures using iodinated contrast media, and increased necessity of major surgery [11]. Among these contributing conditions, renal arterial aging is emerging as a powerful determinant of renal impairment in this age group [12, 13].

The present chapter is a summary of the state of knowledge about the morphological and functional features of the renal vasculature during the aging process. For this purpose, the focus will be mainly on studies in humans. Information obtained in animals is taken into consideration only if it contributes to the understanding of the problem in the human.

15.2   Renal Arterial Aging

15.2.1 Definition

Renal arterial aging can be defined as a measure of the cumulative impact of age, cardiovascular risk factors, and genetic background on the structure and function of the renal vascular system over the course of an individual's lifetime. Although these changes are not specific, they become more frequent as senescence is evolving [5, 6, 13].

15.2.2 Morphologic Alterations with Aging

15.2.2.1 Anatomy of the Aging Kidney

The aging process is associated with marked morphologic and functional alterations in several organ systems [7]. With the possible exception of the lungs, the changes in renal structure and function associated with normal aging are the most dramatic in any human organ system [7].

Normal aging results in relentless loss of renal mass. Renal mass increases from birth to adulthood and then progressively declines during aging. The average kidney weight increases from 50 g at birth, peaks at about 300–400 g at about 40–50 years, and then declines by about 20–30 % to 180–200 g between 70 and

90 years [5, 7, 13]. The loss of renal mass is primarily cortical with sparing of the medulla, leading to thinning of the renal cortical parenchyma [5, 7, 13].

15.2.2.2 Renal Vasculature in Aging

Renal Microvascular Disease

Several studies have documented age-related changes in the histopathology of the renal vessels [5, 6, 8]. Although they are not specific and pathognomonic for the aging process, they become more evident after the age of 40 years increasing in evidence and severity with the evolution of senescence [5]. These changes become distinctly more pronounced at the levels of the small arteries and arterioles [5, 6].

In a microangiographic and histologic study performed on 31 kidneys obtained from surgical specimen or autopsy on 28 subjects aged 20–79 years with no evidence of cardiovascular or renal disease, Ljungquist and Lagergren demonstrated that age-related changes in the renal arterial tree occur mainly at the level of small arteries [14]. The walls of the wider branches of the renal vasculature contain only dispersed subintimal plaques and slight subintimal fibrosis with local hyalinization [14].

The vessels most susceptible to histopathologic changes are the small arteries and arterioles [5, 6]. The aging kidney frequently displays two types of microvasculopathic lesions: (a) arterial sclerosis and (b) arteriolar hyalinization [5, 6, 8, 15, 16].

Arterial Sclerosis

This term is used to denote thickening of the wall of the artery associated with narrowing of the vascular lumen leading to increased wall/radius ratio [5].

Thickening of the arterial wall can be produced by different morphologic processes which include hyperplasia and/or hypertrophy of the medial vascular smooth muscles, fibrosis of the media, and/or fibrosis of the intima [6]. These lesions have been reported in hypertension, diabetes mellitus, and aging and increase in frequency with advancing age [5, 6].

Intimal fibrosis, also known as intimal fibroplasia, is the more specific lesion of the aging renal microvasculature [5, 6]. It involves small and larger interlobular arteries with a diameter of 80–300 μm. It is characterized by progressive thickening of the intima by reduplication of the elastic tissue and atrophy of the underlying media associated with loss of vascular smooth muscle cells [5, 6]. The media may even disappear almost completely when intimal thickening becomes maximal [17]. In contrast, in the very small interlobular arteries which give rise to the afferent arterioles, the intima becomes thicker by subendothelial deposition of hyaline and collagen [12].

Intimal fibroplasia which renders the vessel wall rigid is a universal finding in kidneys of elderly subjects [5, 6, 8]. Although it starts early in life, it becomes much more prominent after the age of 50 years [5, 6, 8].

Intimal fibroplasia is not limited to the renal vasculature but involves other organs such as the liver, the spleen, and the adrenal gland [8].

The etiology of intimal fibroplasia remains elusive. It may be enhanced or even precipitated by blood pressure elevation and hypertension [5, 6, 8]. It appears to be associated with global glomerulosclerosis rather than by hyaline arteriosclerosis and subsequent subcapsular injury [5, 6].

Arteriolar Hyalinization

Arteriolar hyalinization, also known as hyaline arteriolosclerosis, is another feature of the aging renal microvasculature [5, 6]. The frequent occurrence of hyaline arteriolosclerosis/arteriolar hyalinization with increasing age was first described by Moritz and Oldt. This lesion which involves mainly the 10–30 µm diameter afferent arterioles is characterized by deposition of hyaline, a term derived from the Greek word "hyalos," which is a glassy eosinophilic homogeneous material [18, 19]. Ultrastructurally, hyaline deposition is associated with (1) the presence of a homogeneous material which, by immunofluorescence, contains plasma proteins, (2) thinning of the media and atrophy of vascular smooth muscle cells, and (3) irregular thickening of the basement membrane and collagen [19]. Hyaline change occurs patchily along the length of the afferent arteriole and is predominant in its proximal portion and rarely extends into the glomerular capillaries [18, 19]. Further, hyaline deposition is rare in the interlobular arteries and when present occurs in the orifice of the afferent arteriole [18].

Hill and Bariety examined the relationship between hyaline arteriolosclerosis and glomerular structure in aging humans. They identified three types of changes in the afferent arterioles, namely, no hyaline deposition, non-obstructing hyaline, and obstructing hyaline. These investigators reported that, compared to those without hyaline lesions, afferent arterioles with nonoccluding hyaline deposits had a much larger lumen, twice as great (480 ± 240 µm^2 vs 204 ± 160 µm^2), with corresponding increases in diameter and outer circumference and a markedly reduced wall/lumen ratio (3.2 ± 1.8 vs 6.4 ± 6.1 %). In the areas involved by hyaline deposition, the wall thickness was thinner (7.4 ± 3.9 µm vs 15.9 ± 5.8 µm), and vascular smooth muscle cells were atrophic, which might impair the constricting capacity of the vessel [17].

The incidence and severity of hyaline afferent arteriolosclerosis is dependent on age and BP levels. In kidneys of normotensive subjects, Smith reported that minor degrees of sclerosis occur in the third to fourth decades, increasing gradually with age and becoming significant in the fifth to sixth decades [19] although these vascular changes remain minor [19]. However arteriolosclerosis increases as the blood pressure rises even with BP differences in the normal range. Arteriolosclerosis was found in 13.5 % of patients with systolic BP of 90–129 mmHg, in 22.1 % of those with BP of 130–139 mmHg, and in 34.1 % of those with BP above 140 mmHg [19]. Smith concluded that arteriolosclerosis of the afferent arteriole appears to be an age change that is enhanced by hypertension [19].

Arteriolar hyalinization involves also the efferent arterioles. However, in contrast to the afferent arterioles, subendothelial hyaline deposits on the efferent arterioles are scarce, occurring in only 7–9 % of kidneys of nondiabetic normotensive or hypertensive subjects [15, 16, 18]. They appear to be also age related, as they are not seen before the age of 40 years but increase in incidence with age [18]. They are independent of BP levels or presence of hypertension but are greatly enhanced by diabetes mellitus [18]. The hyaline deposits in the efferent arterioles occur patchily along the vascular wall and frequently surround and constrict the vascular lumen [18]. Although hyalinization of both afferent and efferent arterioles appears to be age related, they are greatly enhanced by diabetes mellitus [5, 6, 18].

An increased prevalence of other abnormalities in the renal vasculature has been reported. In postmortem angiographic studies in subjects beyond the seventh decade, tapering of interlobular arteries and increased tortuosity of intralobular arteries have been observed [20].

Vascular Disease of the Large Renal Arterial System

Primary diseases of the renal arteries often involve the large renal arteries and are associated with two most frequent clinical entities, fibromuscular dysplasia and atherosclerotic renal artery stenosis (RAS) [21].

Atherosclerosis accounts for about 90 % of cases of RAS and usually involves the ostium and proximal one third (1/3) of the renal artery and perirenal aorta [21]. In advanced cases, segmental and diffuse intrarenal atherosclerosis also occurs particularly in patients with ischemic nephropathy [21].

Atherosclerotic RAS is a common finding in subjects older than 50 years of age [21]. Its prevalence increases with age, particularly in patients with diabetes mellitus, hypertension, and/or aorto-occlusive disease [21]. An epidemiologic study involving one million subjects aged 67 years disclosed an estimated prevalence and incidence of renovascular disease (RVD) of 0.5 % and 3.7 per 1,000 subjects per year, respectively [11, 22]. Furthermore, occult RVD has been reported in about 24 % of patients with unexplained chronic or progressive renal failure [21].

Atherosclerotic RVD is a progressive disorder and a major cause of progressive renal failure in the elderly [23]. It has been estimated that 10–15 % of patients with atherosclerotic RAS develop end-stage renal disease [23].

Atherosclerotic RVD may occur alone (isolated anatomical RAS) or in association with hypertension and other comorbidities (ischemic nephropathy) [21]. Concurrent atherosclerotic coronary artery, renovascular, and peripheral vascular diseases are frequently present [11, 21].

Ischemic nephropathy represents a syndrome characterized by obstruction to renal blood flow leading to renal ischemia and renal excretory dysfunction associated with renal insufficiency, hypertension in 50 % of patients, recurrent attacks of flash pulmonary edema due to salt/water retention, and evidence of systemic atherosclerosis [21].

Atherosclerotic RVD comprises two clinical entities: (a) renal ischemia due to ostial or truncular atheromatous lesions and (b) distal systemic cholesterol embolism. It may be associated with renal microvascular lesions and glomerular hyalinization, raising the concept of a link between atherosclerosis and glomerular nephrosclerosis/ obsolescence [21]. Kasiske demonstrated that the severity of systemic atherosclerosis has a major impact on the degree of age-related glomerulosclerosis [24]. In the light of these findings, many authors have postulated that glomerulosclerosis may indicate the presence of subclinical RVD [25].

Cholesterol embolism is a direct consequence of disruption of atheromatous plaques and shedding of cholesterol crystals into the renal circulation resulting in microinfarcts and renal parenchymal scarring [21].

The pathogenesis of atherosclerotic RVD has not been completely elucidated. Combination of high BP activation of humoral factors and inflammation may contribute to acceleration of systemic and renovascular atherosclerosis [21, 26].

15.2.2.3 Aging Renal Glomerulus

Structural Changes
Several morphologic changes have been described in the glomerulus of aging subjects [5, 6, 8]. These alterations are characterized by glomerulopenia, glomerulosclerosis, and increase in size of the remnant intact glomeruli and impaired intrinsic glomerular properties.

Glomerulopenia
The number of glomeruli varies with age and gender [5, 6, 11, 27]. Several studies have documented a reduction in the number of glomeruli with aging in both human and experimental animals [5, 6, 8, 9]. Using an accurate and unbiased stereologic method, Nyengaard and Bendsten demonstrated that the number of glomeruli in kidneys in subjects coming to autopsy declines with age [27]. Subjects younger than 55 years had a greater number of glomeruli per kidney than those older than those of 55 years, 695×10^3 versus 560×10^3, respectively [27]. The reduction in the number of nephrons is thought to result from both glomerulosclerosis and resorption of obsolescent glomeruli [27].

In the senescent kidney, glomerular lobulations tend to disappear, and the length of the glomerular tuft perimeter decreases [28, 29]. Accordingly, these morphologic changes, associated with loss of nephrons, contribute to the observed age-related reduction in surface area available for filtration and reduction in glomerular filtration rate [28, 29].

Glomerulosclerosis
Sclerosis of the glomerulus is defined as acellular obliteration of the glomerular tufts leading to complete solidification of the glomerulus [5, 6]. This process is referred to as global glomerulosclerosis.

The incidence of sclerotic glomeruli rises with advancing age from less than 5 % at ages 40–45 years to 10–30 % of the total glomerular population by the eighth decade [5, 6, 8, 30].

The pattern of glomerular and vascular changes differs according to the renal zones. In the juxtamedullary glomeruli, the sclerosing damage in aging subjects results in a vascular connection between the afferent and efferent arterioles which, by shunting blood past the obsolescent glomeruli, maintains an adequate rate of medullary blood flow [30–34]. In contrast, in the cortex, global glomerulosclerosis is associated with obliteration of the arteriolar blood supply, eventually leading to resorption of the obsolescent sclerosed glomeruli [30–34].

There is some controversy as to the pathogenesis of glomerulosclerosis. In some studies, glomerulosclerosis and the associated tubulointerstitial changes are attributed to both intimal fibroplasia and hyaline arteriolosclerosis, while in others, the renal parenchymal changes appear to correlate better with intimal fibroplasia [15, 30].

The number of sclerosed glomeruli is linked to age and microvascular renal pathology [30]. However, age-related glomerular involution may occur independently of events in the renal microvasculature [30].

Totally sclerosed glomeruli are more frequent in aged men than in aged women [30–35].

Structure of the Remnant Intact Glomeruli

With the evolution of senescence, the number of remnant intact (nonsclerotic) glomeruli decreases with age while their size enlarges [30]. The enlarged (intact) glomeruli display specific morphologic features. They have increased tuft size, dilated hilar capillaries, increased mean area of individual capillaries, and increased total capillary area [17, 36]. They are served by markedly dilated afferent arterioles with non-obstructing luminal hyaline deposits [17, 36]. These morphologic features predispose glomeruli to hemodynamic and physical injury leading to global glomerulosclerosis [17, 30, 36].

There is, however, no unanimity as to the zonal distribution of enlarged glomeruli. Newbold et al. measured single cross-sectional areas of outer cortical and juxtamedullary glomeruli in 41 adults aged 22–92 years with a mean age of 61 year and reported that glomerulosclerosis was more severe in the outer cortex, while the juxtamedullary glomeruli had a significant greater glomerular area, and the enlargement of the juxtamedullary glomeruli was positively correlated with cortical glomerulosclerosis [33]. The authors postulated that the increased number of sclerotic glomeruli (glomerulosclerosis) in the superficial cortex shifts glomerular blood flow to the remnant nonsclerotic juxtamedullary nephrons leading to glomerular hypertension, hyperfiltration, and increased risk of glomerulosclerosis [33]. In contrast Samuel et al. using the dissector (Cavalieri method) to estimate the distribution and volumes of glomeruli in the superficial, middle, and juxtamedullary cortex in autopsy kidneys in 12 young male adults aged 20–30 years and 12 older males aged 51–69 years found that glomerular mean volume was 20 % larger in the superficial cortex than in juxtamedullary zone [34]. Global glomerulosclerosis was also more severe in the superficial cortex. In kidneys of young adults, there were no significant differences between superficial and juxtamedullary glomeruli [34].

Intrinsic Glomerular Ultrafiltration Properties

In a recent study, Hoang et al. evaluated the extent and mechanisms of age-related reduction in glomerular filtration rate (GFR) in healthy aging volunteers and in healthy transplant kidney donors [37]. The study included 159 healthy volunteers aged 18–88 years and 33 healthy transplant kidney donors aged 23–69 years. Glomerular dynamics were evaluated in the 159 healthy volunteers, while renal biopsy from 33 healthy kidney transplant donors was subjected to a morphometric analysis to determine glomerular hydraulic permeability and filtration surface area [37].

In their study, Hoang et al. reported that, compared to the healthy younger subjects, healthy elderly volunteers had a 22 % lower GFR (81 ± 17 vs 104 ± 15 ml/min/1.73 m^2) and a 28 % lower renal plasma flow (RPF) (413 ± 106 vs 576 ± 127 ml/min/1.73 m^2). Further, the computed Kf (two-kidney ultrafiltration coefficient) was significantly reduced below youthful levels by 21–53 % [37]. Morphometric studies in renal biopsy specimens from healthy kidney transplant donors revealed reduced filtration surface density (0.1 ± 0.01 vs 0.13 ± 0.04 μm^3/μm^3) and epithelial filtration slits ($1,110 \pm 17$ vs $1,272 \pm 182$ slits/mm) and increased glomerular basement membrane thickness (461 ± 81 vs 417 ± 61 mm). According to these investigators, this study indicates that the intrinsic hydraulic permeability is reduced in aging individual glomeruli, which contributes to the age-related renal functional impairment [37]. Thus, an overall reduction in the number of functioning glomeruli, increased glomerular base membrane thickness, and accumulation of mesangial matrix limit both glomerular filtration area and glomerular permeability [37].

Aglomerular Arterioles

An increased frequency of direct continuity between afferent and efferent arterioles is a prominent feature of aged kidneys [5, 6, 30]. In the juxtamedullary glomeruli, glomerular sclerosis is associated with formation of a direct channel between afferent and efferent arterioles, referred to as arteriolae rectae verae or aglomerular arterioles which maintain blood flow in juxtamedullary nephrons. In the cortex, a different pattern of change predominates. Degeneration of glomeruli results in atrophy of the afferent and efferent arterioles. This leads to a gradual reduction in blood flow in cortical nephrons and eventual global sclerosis [30].

15.2.2.4 Renal Tubulointerstitium in Aging

Tubulointerstitial changes are a common feature of the aging kidney. The decrease in renal size with senescence has been attributed to tubulointerstitial scarring, infarction, and fibrosis [5, 6, 11, 38]. The number, volume, and length of the tubules decrease with age [5, 6]. Tubular atrophy with thickening of the basement membrane and tubular "thyroidization" with dilatation of lumen and hyaline casts are a common feature. Simple renal cysts and tubular diverticula are more frequent in senescent kidneys [6].

The degree of renal functional impairment correlates not only with loss of glomeruli but also with severity of tubulointerstitial alterations [6].

Nephrosclerosis

Nephrosclerosis, defined as a primary vascular lesion associated with glomerular obsolescence, tubulointerstitial changes, and fibrosis, is a morphological entity with no specific clinical features [21, 39]. The etiology of this lesion remains elusive but appears to be multifactorial. It has been reported in aged normotensive subjects but is enhanced by hypertension, diabetes mellitus, and systemic atherosclerosis [21, 39].

In the elderly, nephrosclerosis is the most frequent diagnosis in patients with end-stage renal disease (ESRD) starting maintenance dialysis [11, 40, 41]. However, the high incidence of nephrosclerosis as a cause of ESRD in the elderly is due mainly to ischemic damage induced by atherosclerotic RVD [11, 21].

15.3   Pathogenesis of Age-Mediated Glomerulosclerosis

The mechanisms responsible for glomerulosclerosis and progressive nephrons loss in aged kidneys have not been completely elucidated but appear to be multifactorial. Impaired autoregulation of renal blood flow (RBF) has been shown to play an important role in this process [5, 6].

The renal circulation is characterized by a high resting renal blood flow, low afferent arteriole resistance, and minimal wave reflection in the renal artery [42]. Consequently, high flow and wave oscillations are transmitted through the low afferent arteriole resistance to the glomerular capillaries exposing these vessels to biotrauma [42].

These features of the renal circulation render the kidney more vulnerable to the harmful effects of aging and its associated disturbed large artery dynamics, namely, arterial stiffness and hypertension [43, 44].

15.3.1 Autoregulation of Renal Blood Flow

15.3.1.1 Definition
Autoregulation of RBF is defined as the mechanism that maintains intrarenal functional hemodynamic parameters, i.e., renal glomerular flow, glomerular filtration rate, and mean glomerular capillary hydraulic pressure relatively constant in the face of episodic or sustained increases in BP [45].

15.3.1.2 Physiology and Determinants
Renal autoregulation is mediated by two systems intrinsic to the kidney, a rapid myogenic response and a slow tubuloglomerular feedback (TGF) [45]. Although the myogenic and TGF systems act in concert to regulate BP and body fluid volumes, the myogenic response appears to be primarily involved in protecting morphologic integrity of the kidney from hypertensive injury [45, 46].

The myogenic mechanism describes the capacity of the preglomerular resistance vessels, primarily the afferent arterioles, to constrict or dilate in response to changes in intraluminal pressure [45]. Normally, increases in systemic arterial BP, either transient or sustained, result in proportionate increases in intrarenal vascular resistance to guard against excessive elevation in intraglomerular capillary pressure which remains normal [44, 45]. Thus, glomerular capillaries are protected from biotrauma as long as the renal autoregulatory mechanisms are intact [44, 45].

The myogenic mechanism responds rapidly, within seconds, and is elicited by changes in BP oscillations, mainly by variation in systolic and pulse pressures more than by changes in sustained mean arterial pressure [45].

15.3.1.3 Dysautoregulation of Renal Blood Flow

Dysautoregulation or impaired autoregulation of RBF is characterized by enhanced transmission of "inappropriate" BP levels through a poorly autoregulated preglomerular microcirculation leading to glomerular hypertension and ultimate glomerular injury [42–44, 47, 48]. This process may be associated with dilatation of the afferent and efferent arterioles and glomerular hypertrophy [17, 36].

Longitudinal and cross-sectional studies have documented an age-related loss of renal autoregulation which may promote acceleration of loss of renal function. In a recent study, morphologic changes consistent with impaired renal autoregulation have been reported in human kidneys taken from normotensive elderly subjects [17, 36]. Afferent arterioles exhibited nonocclusive or occlusive subendothelial hyaline deposits, although few were normal [17]. Afferent arterioles with nonocclusive subendothelial hyaline lesions were markedly dilated and were connected with hypertrophied glomeruli containing larger than normal capillary lumen particularly in the hilar region [17]. The medial vascular smooth muscle cells were atrophic or even completely absent. As a result, myogenic contraction induced by vessel distention would be impaired. The net effect is altered distal transmission of systemic blood pressure [17, 36].

Several factors have been postulated to disrupt renal autoregulation with advancing age (Table 15.2).

Hypertension: Blood Pressure Liability

Hypertension enhances the deterioration of renal function with aging. Linderman et al. reported that age reduction in GFR was more pronounced in elderly hypertensive subjects [49].

Although in mild to moderate hypertension, renal autoregulation is well preserved, exposure of the renal microcirculation to long-standing BP elevation levels leads to a preglomerular arteriopathy, impairment of renal autoregulation, and progressive glomerulosclerosis [44]. At necropsy, 68–97 % of elderly patients with well-established hypertension had histologically proven arteriolosclerosis [40].

Table 15.2 Determinants of impaired RBF in aging

1. Hypertension/BP lability
2. Large arterial stiffness
3. Preglomerular microvascular arteriolopathy
4. Atheroembolic renal disease
5. Reduced renal mass
6. Endothelial dysfunction
7. Salt sensitivity
8. Genetic susceptibility
9. Comorbid conditions
Diabetes mellitus
Hypertension
Atherosclerosis
10. Cardiovascular risk factors

Furthermore, a close negative relation between RBF and the severity of arteriolar nephrosclerosis was reported in a series of 100 renal biopsies [41].

Recent data suggest that hypertensive renal damage correlates most strongly with systolic and pulse pressures. In 4,736 subjects with isolated systolic hypertension (ISH) older than 65 years included in Systolic Hypertension in the Elderly Program (SHEP), systolic BP and to a lesser extent pulse pressure (PP) and mean arterial pressure (MAP) were significant predictors of a decrease in GFR within 5 years of follow-up [50]. In contrast, in a cross-sectional study of 212 patients with untreated ISH, high PP rather than MAP was associated with lower effective renal plasma flow (ERPF) and GFR in subjects 60 years of age or older [51]. These observations favor the assertion that PP, a parameter of BP pulsatility and a sign of arterial stiffness in the aged, modulates the tone of the afferent arteriole and autoregulation of RBF [45]. Thus, PP in the elderly is a determinant of pressure transmission to the glomerulus and may predispose to glomerulosclerosis and deterioration in renal function [51].

Arterial Stiffness/Cross Talk Between the Macrocirculation and the Microcirculation

Increased stiffness of the central (large) arteries which frequently occurs with advancing age is characterized by increased systolic BP and PP and high pulse wave velocity (PWV) [43]. Several studies indicate that arterial stiffness plays a major role in the pathogenesis of renal functional impairment and incident CKD in the elderly. In the Multi-Ethnic Study of Atherosclerosis which included 4,850 subjects, large artery stiffness and PP were associated with faster decline in GFR among participants with baseline GFR >60 ml/min/1.73 m^2 [52]. Likewise, in a cohort of 2,050 Japanese patients with GFR >60 ml/min/1.73 m^2 followed up for 5–6 years, higher baseline brachial ankle PWV was associated with lower GFR and a higher annual rate of decrease in GFR [53]. In the Health, Aging and Body Composition (Health ABC) study of 2,129 initially well-functioning elderly subjects aged 72–79 years followed up for about 9 years, higher baseline PWV was related to incident CKD and more rapid decrease in GFR as assessed by cystine C [54].

Several observational and clinical studies support the suggestion of an interaction between the large arterial system and the microcirculation in the pathogenesis of CKD and target organ involvement in the elderly, a phenomenon often referred to as cross talk between the macrocirculation and the microcirculation [43, 55, 56]. Stiffening of the aorta, a major determinant of an age-related alteration of the large arterial system, leads to an increase in PWV and premature reflected waves. These disturbed arterial functional parameters are associated with an increase in SBP and pulsatile hemodynamic load which favor damage to the peripheral and renal microcirculation. Further, the transmission of an elevated systemic BP to the glomerular capillaries due to impaired RBF autoregulation favors glomerular hypertension and damage and progression to CKD (Table 15.3) [43, 55, 56].

Studies have demonstrated that, in the elderly, aortic stiffness is also associated with endothelial dysfunction and abnormalities in systemic microvasculature [26, 56].

Table 15.3 Links between large artery stiffness and chronic kidney disease	1. Glomerular hypertension/glomerular injury/ glomerulosclerosis
	2. Preglomerular microvascular arteriopathy/thrombosis/ microinfarctions
	3. Systemic atherosclerosis

Miscellaneous

Advancing age is associated with decreased renal mass, salt sensitivity, genetic susceptibility, and presence of comorbid states and cardiovascular risk factors (Table 15.2) [47, 57]. These factors may impair pressure-induced myogenic vasoconstriction of the afferent arterioles and RBF autoregulation, favoring transmission of systemic BP to the glomerular capillaries, and lead to glomerular hypertension, glomerular injury, CKD, and preglomerular microvascular disease [47, 57, 58].

15.4 Renal Hemodynamics in Aging Kidneys

The morphologic changes that are associated with aging result in profound alterations in renal hemodynamics. They are characterized by: (a) reduction in RBF, GFR, and renal functional reserve and (b) increase in intrarenal vascular resistance [11, 31].

15.4.1 Renal Blood Flow

Several investigators using different techniques in healthy subjects free of comorbid conditions and renal disease have demonstrated that advancing age is associated with a reduction in RBF [5, 8, 11, 31]. Significant increase in filtration fraction and renal vascular resistance has also been reported in some of these studies [11, 31].

In a review of 38 renal hemodynamic studies which included 634 healthy subjects with varying age range, Wesson reported that total RBF was well maintained until the fourth decade [59]. Thereafter, there was a 10 % reduction per decade with the effective renal plasma flow falling from 600 ml/min/1.73 m² in young adults to about 300 ml/min/1.73 m² by the age of 80 years [58]. However, the reduction in RBF does not involve the renal regions to the same extent. In a study of 207 healthy kidney donors, Hollenberg et al. reported a significant decrease in the rapid (cortical) blood flow, while medullary blood flow was well preserved in aged subjects [11, 31]. This redistribution in blood flow from cortex to medulla may account, at least partly, for the increased filtration fraction reported with advancing age [31].

Structural and functional factors have been postulated to account for age-related reduction in RBF: (1) redistribution of RBF from the well-perfused cortex to lesser-perfused medulla [31]; (2) structural changes in the preglomerular microcirculation including tapering and increased irregularity and tortuosity of the arcuate, interlobular, and intralobular arteries [20]; (3) endothelial dysfunction [47, 56]; (4) defective angiogenesis resulting from impaired growth factors in the kidney (vascular endo-thelial growth factor (VEGF) and angiopoietin-1 factors) [47]; and (5) persistent renal vasoconstriction and increased renal vascular resistance [11, 31].

15.4.2 Intrarenal Renal Vascular Resistance

Resting intrarenal vascular resistance is increased in aging kidneys, even in normo-tensive subjects, but is enhanced by the presence of established hypertension and/or cardiovascular comorbidities [5, 6, 31, 47].

The enhanced age-related renal vascular resistance has been attributed both to functional and structural factors.

An imbalance between vasodilating and vasoconstricting responses has been reported in aged kidneys [26, 47]. In aging, there is an attenuated responsiveness to dilators such as nitric oxide (NO), endothelial-derived hyperpolarizing factor (EDHF), and prostacyclin [47]. In addition, renal vasodilatation after administration of acetylcholine and L-arginine is markedly impaired [60]. Since response to these vasoactive agents is dependent on NO, these findings suggest impaired NO genera-tion [61]. Kielstein et al. reported accumulation of endogenous NO inhibitor, asym-metric dimethylarginine, in senescent kidneys [61]. On the other hand, enhanced renal vasoconstriction to pressor substances, such as angiotensin II, has also been reported [47]. This imbalance may result in resting vasoconstriction of the renal circulation and high resting renal vascular resistance in aging [11, 31].

Structural changes in the renal microvasculature such as narrowing or obsoles-cence of pre- and postglomerular vessels, frequently observed in aging kidneys, may contribute to the high resting vascular resistance [20].

15.4.3 Glomerular Filtration Rate

A fall in glomerular filtration rate (GFR) with advancing age has been documented by both population-based and longitudinal studies [5, 6, 49, 59, 62].

GFR remains stable until the ages of 30–40 years and thereafter decreases at an average of about 8 ml/min/1.73 m^2/decade and is enhanced by increasing mean arte-rial pressure [5–8, 31]. The clinical significance of this age-related fall in GFR is minimal until an acute or chronic illness further impairs the already decreased renal reserve seen in aging [5–8]. However, with aging, the decline in renal function is not uniform but varies with each subject. In the Baltimore Longitudinal Study of Aging, Lindeman et al. evaluated renal function by repeated creatinine clearances in 446 subjects aged 22–96 years over 12–18-month intervals. They reported that 30–35 % of elderly subjects had no change in renal function [49].

GFR has been assessed by the clearance of creatinine and by the infused exoge-nous markers, such as inulin and iothalamate, and estimation formulae. The inulin clearance (C_{In}), the gold standard method, is cumbersome and requires special pro-cedures. The creatinine clearance (C_{cr}) in a timed urinary collection is commonly used to estimate GFR [11, 62, 63]. However, this method is fraught with significant inaccuracies in the elderly. With aging, as the muscle mass decreases, creatinine production, serum creatinine, and urinary creatinine excretion are reduced [30, 62, 63]. Therefore, in the aged, serum creatinine concentration is unreliable as a predictor of GFR and underestimates the degree of renal functional impairment in this group [30, 62, 63]. Despite these inaccuracies, studies revealed that true C_{cr} falls by 8 ml/min/1.73 m^2/decade beyond middle age [30].

To obviate the need for cumbersome and inaccurate 24-h urine sampling, prediction formulae are increasingly used to estimate GFR. In adults, C_{cr} is estimated by this Cockcroft-Gault (CG) equation and GFR by modification of diet in renal disease (MDRD) [62]. Estimation of C_{cr} from body weight and height and gender according to the CG equation has been shown to be unreliable especially in very old subjects [11, 30, 62]. In addition, there are no studies that evaluated the accuracy and precision of GFR evaluation by MDRD in the elderly. In a study involving 180 healthy elderly subjects aged 65–111 years, GFR values calculated by MDRD were much higher than those recorded by CG equation [64]. These observations suggest that, in the elderly, evaluation of GFR by estimation formulae may not reflect the exact status of renal function.

Several factors have been postulated to account for the progressive decrease in GFR with senescence: (1) increasing number of sclerotic glomeruli correlating with renal hemodynamic alterations [5–8]; (2) age-related atrophy involving the cortex more than the medulla, resulting in loss of great number of nephrons [5–8]; and (3) vascular lesions involving the small arteries rather than the arterioles favoring simultaneous reduction of filtration pressure in a large number of glomeruli [20].

15.4.4 Renal Functional Reserve

Renal functional reserve, defined as the capacity of the renal vasculature to dilate maximally in response to a vasodilating stimulus, is impaired with aging [65].

15.5 Acceleration of Renal Arterial Aging

Renal arterial aging is enhanced by risk factors of atherosclerosis such as hypertension, diabetes mellitus, smoking/nicotine, hyperlipidemia, and environmental toxic processes [47].

15.6 Premature Renal Arterial Aging

Renal arterial aging is not limited to senescence. Changes in the renal microvascular circulation, similar and indistinguishable from those in aging kidneys, have been reported in diabetes mellitus and in CKD in younger adults [47].

15.7 Therapeutic Strategies

There are no specific therapeutic measures to reverse age-related pathophysiologic macro- and microvascular changes [5, 6, 43]. However, lifestyle measures and normalization of systemic and glomerular hypertension may delay progression of renal functional impairment [5, 6]. Blockade of renin-angiotensin-aldosterone system (RAAS) affords better renoprotection [28]. Lipid-lowering and antiplatelet administration are also indicated [66, 67].

The management of atherosclerotic renal artery stenosis and ischemic nephropathy is by conservative measures. There is no evidence that revascularization of stenotic renal artery is associated with improvement in renal function and cardiovascular outcome [68].

Conclusion

Renal arterial aging represents a complex pathophysiologic state characterized by morphologic and functional changes in the renal macro-/microcirculation which lead to a wide spectrum of target organ involvement. Therapeutic measures are limited to normalization of systemic and glomerular hypertension; lipid-lowering, antiplatelet therapy; and lifestyle measures.

References

1. Bash LD, Astor BC, Coresh J (2010) Risk of incident ESRD: a comprehensive look at cardiovascular risk factors and 17 years of follow-up in the Arteriosclerosis Risk in Communities (ARIC) study. Am J Kidney Dis 55:31–41
2. Drey N, Roderick P, Mullee M, Rogerson M (2003) A population-based study of the incidence and outcomes of diagnosed chronic kidney disease. Am J Kidney Dis 42:677–684
3. Coresh J, Selvin E, Stevens LA et al (2007) Prevalence of chronic kidney disease in the United States. JAMA 298:2038–2047
4. United States Renal data System (2007) Annual data report, Bethesda
5. Silva FG (2005) The aging kidney: a review – part I. Int Urol Nephrol 37:185–205
6. Zhou XJ, Saxenia R, Liu Z, Vaziri ND, Silva FG (2008) Renal senescence in 2008: progress and challenges. Int Urol Nephrol 40:823–839
7. Epstein M (1996) Aging and the kidney. J Am Soc Nephrol 7:1106–1122
8. Martin JE, Sheaf MJ (2007) Renal ageing. J Pathol 211:198–205
9. Lopez Novoa JM, Montanes M (1987) Changes in renal function and morphology in aging laboratory animals. In: Macias Nuzez JF, Cameron JS (eds) Renal function and disease in the elderly. Buttersworths, London, pp 162–183
10. Coresh J, Astor BC, Green T et al (2003) Prevalence of chronic kidney disease and decreased kidney function in the adult US population: Third National Health and Nutrition Examination Survey. Am J Kidney Dis 41:1–12
11. Presta P, Lucisano G, Fuiano L, Fuisano G (2012) The kidney and the elderly: why does the risk increase. Int Urol Nephrol 44:625–632
12. Zhou XJ, Laszik ZG, Silva FG (2008) Anatomical changes in the aging kidney. In: Macias Nunez JF, Cameron JS, Oreopoulos DG (eds) The aging kidney in health and disease. Springer, New York, pp 39–54

13. Fliser D (2005) Ren sanus in corpore sano: the myth of the inexorable decline of renal function with senescence. Nephrol Dial Transplant 20:482–485
14. Ljungquist A, Lagergren C (1962) Normal intrarenal arterial pattern in adult and ageing human kidney: a micro-angiographical and histological study. J Anat 96(2):285–300
15. Tracy RE, Parra D, Eisaguirre W, Torresbalawza RA (2002) Influence of arteriolar hyalinization on arterial intima fibroplasia in the United States, Peru, and Bolivia, applicable also to other population. Am J Hypertens 15:1064–1073
16. Tracy RE, Ishii T (2000) Hypertensive renovasculopathies and the rise of blood pressure with age in Tokyo, Japan. Int Urol Nephrol 32:109–117
17. Hill GS, Heudes D, Bariety J (2003) Morphometric study of arterioles and glomeruli in the aging kidney suggests focal loss of autoregulation. Kidney Int 63:1027–1036
18. Tracy RE (2007) Age trends of renal arteriolar hyalinization explored with the aid of serial sections. Nephron Clin Pract 105:C171–C177
19. Smith JP (1955) Hyaline arteriolosclerosis in the kidney. J Pathol Bacteriol 69:147–168
20. Davidson AT, Talner LB, Downs WM (1969) A study of the angiographic appearance of the kidney in an ageing normotensive population. Radiology 92:975–983
21. Meyrier A (1996) Renal vascular lesions in the elderly: nephrosclerosis or atheromatous renal disease. Nephrol Dial Transplant 11(Suppl 9):45–52
22. Kalra PA, Guo H, Kausz AT et al (2005) Atherosclerotic renovascular disease in United States patients aged 67 years or older: risk factors, revascularization and prognosis. Kidney Int 68:293–301
23. Valderrabano F, Berthoux FC, Jones EH, Mehls O (1996) Report on management of renal failure in Europe, XXV, 1994 end stage renal disease and dialysis report. The EDTA ERA Registry. European Dialysis and Transplant Association-European Renal Association. Nephrol Dial Transplant 11(Suppl 1):2–21
24. Kasiske BL (1987) Relationship between vascular disease and age-associated changes in the human kidney. Kidney Int 31:1153–1159
25. Wright JR, Duggal A, Thomas R et al (2001) Clinicopathologic correlation in biopsy-proven atherosclerotic renovascular disease: implications for renal functional outcome in atherosclerotic renovascular disease. Nephrol Dial Transplant 16:765–770
26. Barton M (2005) Ageing as a determinant of renal and vascular disease: role endothelial factors. Nephrol Dial Transplant 20:485–490
27. Nyengaard JR, Bendtsen TF (1992) Glomerular number and size in relation to age, kidney weight, and body surface in normal man. Anat Rec 232:194–201
28. Heudes D, Michel O, Chevalier J et al (1994) Effect of chronic ANG I-converting enzyme inhibitor on aging processes-1 kidney structure and function. Am J Physiol 266:R1038–R1051
29. Anderson S, Brenner BM (1987) The aging kidney: structure, function, mechanisms and therapeutic implications. J Am Geriatr Soc 35:590–593
30. Fliser D, Ritz E (1996) Renal hemodynamics in the elderly. Nephrol Dial Transplant 11(Suppl 9):2–8
31. Hollenberg NK, Adams DF, Solomon HS et al (1974) Senescence and the renal vasculature in normal man. Circ Res 34:309–316
32. Kappel B, Olsen S (1980) Cortical interstitial tissue and sclerosed glomeruli in the normal human kidney, related to age and sex. A quantitative study. Virchows Arch A Pathol Anat Histol 387:271–277
33. Newbold KM, Sandison A, Howie AJ (1992) Comparison of size of juxtamedullary and outer cortical glomeruli in normal adult kidney. Virchows Arch A Pathol Anat Histopathol 420:127–129
34. Samuel T, Hoy WE, Douglas-Denton R et al (2005) Determinants of glomerular volume in different cortical zones of the human kidney. J Am Soc Nephrol 16:3102–3109
35. Hollenberg NK, Epstein M, Basch RI, Merrill JP (1969) "No Man's Land" of the renal vasculature an arteriographic and hemodynamic assessment of the interlobar and arcuate arteries in essential and accelerated hypertension. Am J Med 47:845–854

36. Hill GS, Heudes D, Jacquot C et al (2006) Morphometric evidence for impairment of renal autoregulation in advanced essential hypertension. Kidney Int 69:823–831
37. Hoang K, Jan JC, Derby G et al (2003) Determinants of glomerular hypofiltration in aging kidneys. Kidney Int 64:1417–1424
38. Dontas AS, Marketos SG, Papanayiotou P (1972) Mechanisms of renal tubular defects in old age. Postgrad Med J 48:295–303
39. Tracy RE, Ishii J (2000) What is nephrosclerosis? Lessons from the US, Japan, and Mexico. Nephrol Dial Transplant 15:1357–1366
40. Luke RG (1999) Hypertensive nephrosclerosis: pathogenesis and prevalence – essential hypertension is an important cause of end-stage renal disease. Nephrol Dial Transplant 14:2271–2278
41. Freedman BI, Iskandar SS, Appel RG (1995) The link between hypertension and nephrosclerosis. Am J Kidney Dis 25:207–221
42. Nichols WW, O'Rourke MF, Vlachopoulos C (2011) Special circulations. In: Nichols WW, O'Rourke MF, Vlachopoulos C (eds) McDonald's blood flow in arteries: theoretical, experimental and clinical principles, 6th edn. Taylor and Francis Ltd, London, pp 397–409
43. O'Rourke M, Safar M (2005) Relationship between aortic stiffening and microvascular disease in brain and kidney: cause and logic of therapy. Hypertension 46:200–204
44. Bidani AK, Polichnowski AJ, Loutzenhiser R, Griffin KA (2013) Renal microvascular dysfunction, hypertension and CKD progression. Curr Opin Nephrol Hypertens 22:1–9
45. Loutzenhiser R, Bidani A, Chilton L (2002) Renal myogenic response: kinetic attributes and psychological role. Circ Res 90:1316–1324
46. Bidani AK, Griffin KA, Williamson G et al (2009) Protective importance of the myogenic response in the renal circulation. Hypertension 54:393–398
47. Palmer BF (2004) Disturbances in renal autoregulation and the susceptibility to hypertension induced chronic kidney disease. Am J Med Sci 328:330–343
48. O'Rourke ME, Hashimoto J (2007) Mechanical factors in arterial ageing: a clinical perspective. J Am Coll Cardiol 5:1–13
49. Lindeman RD, Tobin J, Schock NW (1985) Longitudinal studies on the rate of decline in renal function with age. J Am Geriatr Soc 33:278–285
50. Young JH, Klag MJ, Muntner P et al (2002) Blood pressure and decline in kidney function: findings from the Systolic Hypertension in the Elderly program (SHEP). J Am Soc Nephrol 13:2776–2782
51. Verhave JC, Fesler P, du Cailar G et al (2005) Elevated pulse pressure is associated with low renal function in elderly patients with isolated systolic hypertension. Hypertension 45: 586–591
52. Peralta CA, Jacobs DR Jr, Katz R et al (2012) Association of pulse pressure, arterial elasticity, and endothelial function with kidney function decline among adults with estimated GFR>60 ml/min/1.73m^2: the Multi-Ethnic Study of Atherosclerosis (MESA). Am J Kidney Dis 59:41–49
53. Tomiyama H, Tanaka H, Hashimoto H et al (2010) Arterial stiffness and declines in individuals with normal renal function/early chronic kidney disease. Atherosclerosis 212:345–350
54. Madero M, Peralta C, Katz R et al (2013) Association of arterial rigidity with incidence kidney disease and kidney function decline: the Health ABC study. Clin J Am Soc Nephrol 8:424–433
55. Feihl F, Liaudet L, Waeber B (2009) The macrocirculation and microcirculation of hypertension. Curr Hypertens Rep 11:182–189
56. Yannoutsos A, Levy BI, Safar ME et al (2014) Pathophysiology of hypertension: interactions between macro and microvascular alterations through endothelial dysfunction. J Hypertens 32:216–224
57. Palmer BF (2001) Impaired autoregulation: implications for the genesis of hypertension and hypertension-induced renal injury. Am J Med Sci 321:388–400
58. James MA, Watt PA, Potter JF et al (1995) Pulse pressure and resistance artery structural in the elderly. Hypertension 26:301–306

59. Wesson LG Jr (1969) Renal hemodynamics in physiological states. In: Physiology of the human kidney. Grune and Stratton, New York, pp 96–108

60. Fuiano G, Sund S, Mazza G et al (2001) Renal hemodynamic response to maximal vasodilating stimulus in healthy older subjects. Kidney Int 59:1052–1058

61. Kielstein JJ, Bode-Böger SM, Frölich JC et al (2003) Asymmetric dimethylarginine, blood pressure, and renal perfusion in elderly subjects. Circulation 107:1891–1895

62. Muhlberg W, Platt D (1999) Age-dependent changes of the kidneys: pharmacological implications. Gerontology 45:243–253

63. Rowe JW, Andres R, Tobin JD (1976) The effect of age on creatinine clearance in men: a cross-sectional and longitudinal study. J Gerontol 31:155–163

64. Gill J, Malyuk R, Djurdjev O, Levin A (2007) Use of GFR equation to adjust drug doses in an elderly multi-ethnic group – a cautionary tale. Nephrol Dial Transplant 22:2894–2899

65. Fliser D, Zeler M, Nowick R, Ritz E (1993) Renal functional reserve in healthy elderly subjects. J Am Soc Nephrol 3:1371–1377

66. Ichihara A, Hayashi M, Koura Y et al (2005) Long-term effects of statins on arterial pressure and stiffness of hypertensives. J Hum Hypertens 19:103–109

67. Maki-Petaja KM, Wilkinson IB (2009) Antiinflammatory drugs and statins for arterial stiffness reduction. Curr Pharm Des 15:290–303

68. Cooper CJ, Murphy TP, Cutlip DE et al (2014) Stenting and medical therapy for atherosclerotic renal-artery stenosis. N Engl J Med 370:13–22

Diabetes Mellitus: Alterations in Vessel Wall Properties

16

Claudia R.L. Cardoso and Gil F. Salles

16.1 Introduction

Diabetes is considered as a major and growing health problem in most countries. According to the International Diabetes Federation Atlas, the estimated worldwide prevalence of diabetes in 2013 has risen to 382 million people, representing 8.3 % of the world adult population [1].

Type 2 diabetes is diagnosed and, mainly, defined by hyperglycemia. Nonetheless, the definition of diabetes and the pathologic characteristics of this disease often involve the vasculature, with hyperglycemia promoting microvascular and macrovascular complications. The clinical manifestations of microvascular disease are so characteristics of the disease that diabetes is defined by the glycated hemoglobin (HbA_{1c}) level that causes microvascular disease. However, while hyperglycemia is a key factor for microvascular complication development, it is only one of the multiple factors capable of increasing the risk of atherosclerotic macrovascular disease in diabetes. Indeed, diabetes-induced vascular complications are the major cause of morbidity and mortality in these subjects and provoke considerable amount of disability, premature mortality, loss of productivity, and increased demands on healthcare facilities [2–4]. There are two different types of vascular disease in diabetes, one affecting small resistance arteries, arterioles, and capillaries (microvascular disease) and the other affecting large conductance vessels (macrovascular disease).

Cardiovascular disease, including coronary, cerebral, and peripheral arterial disease, accounts for most of morbidity and mortality in type 2 diabetes. Coronary artery disease is the leading cause of mortality in type 2 diabetes [5]. Lower-limb amputations are at least ten times more frequent in diabetic than in nondiabetic

C.R.L. Cardoso • G.F. Salles (✉)
Department of Internal Medicine, School of Medicine, Universidade Federal do Rio de Janeiro, Rua Rodolpho Rocco, 255, Cidade Universitária, Rio de Janeiro 21941-913, Brazil
e-mail: claudiacardoso@hucff.ufrj.br; gilsalles@hucff.ufrj.br

© Springer International Publishing Switzerland 2015
A. Berbari, G. Mancia (eds.), *Arterial Disorders:*
Definition, Clinical Manifestations, Mechanisms and Therapeutic Approaches,
DOI 10.1007/978-3-319-14556-3_16

individuals worldwide [6, 7], and more than half of nontraumatic lower-limb amputations are due to diabetes. People with diabetes are two to four times more likely to develop cardiovascular disease in comparison to nondiabetic subjects [8, 9]. Otherwise, diabetes microvascular disease is a major contributing factor to morbidity, mortality, and costs in both type 1 and type 2 diabetes [10]. Diabetic nephropathy is the main cause of end-stage renal failure, both in low- and high-income populations [11]. Structural alterations of small vessels that supply peripheral nerves contribute to diabetic neuropathy, and damage of microvasculature of the eye is the leading cause of impairment and loss of vision in working age adults [10]. Given the impact of diabetic vascular disease, great effort has been directed towards reducing vascular outcomes in diabetes. While a better glucose control has a doubtless beneficial effect in reducing microvascular disease, its role in improving macrovascular outcomes is yet controversial.

This chapter will mainly discuss aspects of pathophysiology and pathogenesis involved in the development of vascular disease in diabetes, as well as the diagnosis of vascular disease and current therapy.

16.2   Pathophysiology of Diabetic Vascular Disease

Endothelial dysfunction, smooth muscle cell dysfunction, platelet hyperreactivity, impaired fibrinolysis with a trend for thrombosis and coagulation, and increased inflammation are among the physiological impairments that plausibly link diabetes with atherosclerotic vascular disease [12] (Fig. 16.1).

16.2.1 Endothelial Dysfunction

The endothelium has a central role in vascular homeostasis; it permits the vasculature to adapt to several stimuli and is fundamental for regulation of vascular tone and structure. Endothelial cells produce a broad spectrum of substances, of which the most characterized is nitric oxide (NO) that is generated from the metabolism of L-arginine by the endothelial NO synthase (eNOS) constitutively expressed by endothelial cells [13]. Under normal conditions, endothelial stimulation induces the production and release of NO, which diffuses to circumjacent tissue and cells and promotes its cardiovascular protective effects by relaxing media layer smooth muscle cells and by preventing adhesion molecule expression, leukocyte adhesion, and migration into the arterial wall, muscle cell proliferation, and platelet adhesion and aggregation [13]. The regulation of endothelial function is largely vascular area specific, hence promoting different responses in various organs and tissues. Within the same vascular area, it depends mainly on the vessel size, that is, large arteries (macrocirculation) and arterioles (microcirculation) [14]. In disease conditions, such as in diabetes, hypertension, and dyslipidemia, the endothelium undergoes functional and

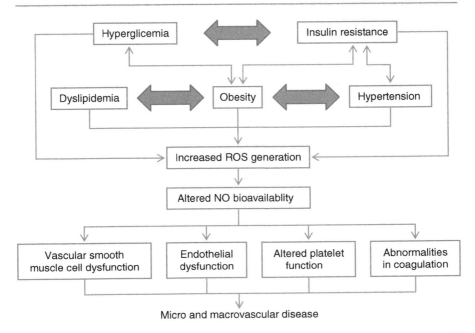

Fig. 16.1 Risks factors and mechanisms that plausibly link diabetes with vascular disease. *ROS* reactive oxygen species, *NO* nitric oxide

structural alterations and loses its protective vascular role, becoming a pro-atherothrombotic structure [12–14]. In the initial stages, the main endothelial alteration is functional and is referred as endothelial dysfunction. Impaired NO bioavailability is characteristic of this condition. It can be due to a reduced production of NO or, more frequently, to an increased breakdown by reactive oxygen species (ROS) [13]. The endothelium activates several pathways, trying to compensate NO deficiency. The production and release of other endothelium-derived vasodilators such as prostanoids and other endothelium-derived hyperpolarizing factors guarantee some, although impaired, endothelium-dependent vasodilatation. In association with NO deficiency, the endothelium produces substances and mediators that injure the arterial wall, including endothelin, thromboxane A_2, prostaglandin H_2, and ROS [13]. Diabetes-related endothelial dysfunction is present early at disease beginning or at prediabetic conditions and antecedes morphologic and structural vascular changes [13, 15], which includes accelerated disappearance of capillary endothelium [16], weakening of intercellular junctions [17], altered proteins synthesis, and altered expression/production of adhesion glycoproteins on endothelial cells [16–19], which promote attachment of monocytes and leukocytes and their transendothelial migration [17]. Endothelial dysfunction is the initial focus of atherosclerotic lesions that appears later during the course of diabetes [20, 21] and has itself been associated with adverse cardiovascular prognosis [22].

16.2.2 Biochemical Mechanisms Associated with Vascular Damage in Diabetes

In cells where glucose transport is not completely dependent on insulin (e.g., in vascular endothelial, renal, and retinal cells, as well as in peripheral nerves [23]), hyperglycemia increases glucose intracellular concentration and several other glycolytic intermediates [24] that are critical substrates for various important biochemical pathways [25]. In the presence of chronic hyperglycemia, there is an inappropriate down-regulation of insulin-dependent transporters, which exposes cells to the continuous influx of high amount of glucose from the extracellular space into cytosol. This promotes production of excess intracellular ROS [26–28]. ROS are the final inducers and also the initiating elements of, at minimum, four interrelated hyperglycemia-activated paths: (1) the polyol pathway, with its associated alterations in the redox state of nicotinamide-adenine dinucleotide phosphate (NADP) and its reduced form NADPH [28, 29]; (2) the covalent change of intracellular components by reactive advanced glycation end products (AGEs) [30, 31]; (3) the de novo synthesis of diacylglycerol, which makes active several protein kinase C isoforms [32, 33]; and (4) the augmented flux by the hexosamine path [27, 28]. The activation of these biochemical ways, at minimum partially mediated by glucose-related increased osmolarity [34], can explain why persistent elevation of glucose affects the biochemical homeostasis of cardiovascular cells, finally leading to the evolvement of diabetic vascular (mainly micro) complications [35]. Each of the pathways mentioned above is activated by hyperglycemia-induced ROS formation, in the form of an overproduction of superoxide anion through the mitochondrial electron transport chain [36], in conjunction with an overproduction of NO [37], which jointly lead to production of a toxic reaction product, the peroxynitrite anion [38, 39].

Hyperglycemia is related to increased oxidation stress [26], augmented leukocyte-endothelial interaction [40], and glycation of constitutional body proteins, including lipoproteins, apolipoproteins, and clotting factors, which progressively increase vasomotor tone, vascular permeability, growth, and remodeling [15–18]. Furthermore, hyperglycemia retards endothelial cell replication [15, 18] and increases extracellular matrix production [41], which may thicken the basal membrane. It also augments endothelial cell death [15, 18] and enzymes involved in collagen synthesis [41]. Long-term hyperglycemia, but not only this, leads to the formation of modified molecular species, by nonenzymatic reactions between the aldehydic group of reducing sugars with proteins, lipids, or nucleic acids [42]. The formation of these advanced glycation end products (AGEs) occurs mainly by glycation, by the polyol pathway, and by glycoxidation and oxidative stress [43]. All the conditions that promote AGEs formation are present in diabetes and are aggravated by the occurrence of renal failure [44]. AGEs promote proinflammatory cellular reactions that can damage tissues, frequently directed to specific organs. AGEs are involved in atherosclerosis development by at least two mechanisms: by direct tissue deposition and by interaction with the receptor of AGEs (RAGE) [43]. Due to tissue accumulation, AGEs directly cross-link with proteins of extracellular matrix (ECM), increasing arterial stiffness and entrapping other macromolecules [45]. The

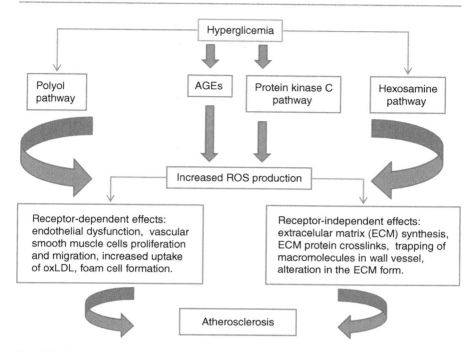

Fig. 16.2 Schematic model of vascular lesion associated with chronic hyperglycemia. *ROS* reactive oxygen species, *AGEs*, advanced glycation end products

other mechanism by which AGEs promote their harmful effects is by receptor mediated paths, and RAGE is the most investigated receptor [46]. The RAGE-AGE interaction alters cellular signaling, promotes gene expression, and increases the discharge of proinflammatory substances [47]. The RAGE interacts with AGEs and also with various different proinflammatory ligands that, like AGEs, augment the atherosclerotic process [48]. In atherogenesis, this multiligand receptor is highly expressed in activated endothelial cells, vascular smooth muscle cells, and inflammatory cells and, through interaction with its ligands, begins and maintains the pathologic process leading to atherosclerotic lesion in the arterial intima [48]. These mechanisms are summarized on Fig. 16.2.

16.2.3 Insulin Resistance

Insulin resistance, present in most of type 2 diabetic patients, is associated with impaired vascular insulin signaling and blunted vascular effects of insulin [49]. The mechanisms of insulin resistance are yet incompletely understood. Insulin resistance may reflect the combined influence of obesity, dietary patterns, and lifestyle and can also result in elevated blood pressure, impaired glucose, fat and lipid metabolism, inflammation, and a prothrombotic environment [50]. The most sensitive tissues for the insulin-glucose uptake reaction are the skeletal muscle and adipose tissue. However, insulin receptor signaling exerts important biological effects on vascular cells and regulates vessel dilation and contraction [51, 52]. Indeed, insulin resistance decreases blood flow to skeletal muscle [16, 53]. Moreover, insulin receptor signaling regulates monocyte differentiation into macrophages [54]. Hyperglycemia is not only a consequence but also a worsening factor for insulin resistance. Impaired insulin signaling in tissues impacts on vascular dysfunction, hypertension, hyperglycemia, dyslipidemia, and other metabolic disorders. These risk factors jointly contribute to endothelial dysfunction, an early event in atherosclerosis development [12, 13, 55].

16.3 The Link Between Micro- and Macrovascular Disease in Diabetes

Both types of vascular complications share common pathogenetic mechanisms [56–58]. The walls of the large arteries receive their nutrient and oxygen supply from the lumen and also from small vessels located in the adventitia. This plexus of microvessels in the arterial wall of the arteries is called the vasa vasorum [59]. Several studies suggested that microvascular disease may contribute to atherosclerotic progression in type 2 diabetes [56–58, 60–63]. By focusing on the role of neovascularization of vasa vasorum in promoting atherosclerosis progression and plaque rupture, these investigations support the link between micro- and macrovascular disease. Large-artery microvessels may also be targets to diabetic damage, in the same way it occurs in the microvessels of the retina, of the kidney glomerulus, and of the peripheral nerves [64]. A study including young patients with type 1 diabetes showed that the vasa vasorum of the aorta presented pathological characteristics of diabetic microvascular disease and that the lesion of vasa vasorum was an important determinant of aortic atherosclerosis development [65]. Another investigation also demonstrated increased microvessels in the aorta of diabetic patients in relation to nondiabetic individuals [66]. It is plausible that its physiopathological mechanisms involve a response of the microcirculation of the artery wall to ischemia and hypoxia [59], similar to which also leads to microvascular alterations in other territories, like the retina in diabetes [67]. Taking into account these previous investigations suggesting the participation of the vessel-wall microcirculation in the pathogenesis of diabetic atherosclerosis [56–58, 63, 64], Arcidiacono and colleagues proposed that the microangiopathy of the wall of large arteries could provide, at least in part, the explanation for the more severe and rapidly evolving form of atherosclerotic process observed in diabetes [64].

16.4 Screening for Vascular Disease in Diabetes

The presence of subclinical vascular disease confers an increased cardiovascular morbidity and mortality in patients with diabetes [68]. However, screening tests did not decrease the occurrence of cardiovascular events in patients with diabetes [69]. Nonetheless, several ways of evaluating noninvasively the presence of vascular disease may improve cardiovascular stratification risk, particularly, in patients at

Table 16.1 Summary of routine examinations that should be performed in patients with diabetes to identify the presence of macro- and microvascular complications

Physical examination
Palpation of dorsalis pedis and posterior tibial pulses
Ankle-brachial index measurement
Neurologic examination of lower limbs, including:
Patellar and Achilles tendinous reflexes
Evaluation of proprioception, vibration and monofilament sensation
Retinal fundoscopy
Laboratory exams
Urinary albumin excretion with spot urine albumin-to-creatinine ratio
Serum creatinine and estimated glomerular filtration rate
Resting electrocardiogram

intermediate risk [68]. These methods are better predictor than biomarkers, such as ultrasensitive reactive C protein and lipoprotein-associated phospholipase A2. The identification of patients at increased cardiovascular risk may permit interventions to reduce the burden of vascular disease, hence of vascular outcomes, and may improve compliance and adherence to treatment [68]. The measurement of common carotid intima-media thickness and plaques by ultrasonography and of central aortic arterial stiffness by carotid-femoral pulse wave velocity are among the simple, easily available and safe methods that can be employed for investigation of subclinical vascular disease [68]. Coronary calcium score, although can also improve cardiovascular risk stratification, has higher costs and a lower availability; so, its use is not easily implemented in clinical practice [70, 71]. The increase in the wall-to-lumen ratio of small arteries in adipose tissue of gluteal biopsies can refine evaluation of risk in diabetic patients [72]; nevertheless, because of its invasiveness, it is also not appropriate for general practice. Similarly, endothelial dysfunction has been associated with an increased risk of vascular outcomes [21], but it still lacks simpler and noninvasive techniques for investigating endothelial responsiveness to various stimuli. Additionally, the added value of using imaging methods to improving patient outcomes has not been demonstrated yet in randomized controlled studies [68].

Physical examination, fundoscopic exam performed by an ophthalmologist, electrocardiogram, and laboratory examination can identify the presence of asymptomatic micro- and macrovascular diabetic disease. Table 16.1 summarizes the routine exams that should be performed in diabetic patients to investigate the presence of micro- and macrovascular disease.

16.5   Treatment of Vascular Disease

There are various evidences from clinical trials that treatment of hyperglycemia, hypertension, dyslipidemia, and antiplatelet therapy are able to reduce morbidity and mortality related to vascular disease [73–76]. Indeed, multifactorial risk factors treatment seems to have greatest benefit on reducing cardiovascular morbidity and

Table 16.2 Schematic recommendations for glycemic, blood pressure, lipid, and antiplatelet treatment in diabetes

Parameter	Treatment target	Medication
Glycemic control – HbA$_{1c}$	<7 %[a]	Metformin plus other oral drugs or insulin in type 2 diabetes
Blood pressure control	<140/85–80 mmHg[b]	ACE inhibitors or ARBs as drugs of choice plus CCBs or diuretics
Lipid control – LDL-cholesterol	<100 mg/dl (individuals without CVD)	High-intensity statins
	<70 mg/dl (individuals with CVD)	
Antiplatelet treatment	Primary prevention[c]	Aspirin (75–162 mg)
	Secondary prevention	Aspirin (75–162 mg) clopidogrel (75 mg) for patients with aspirin contraindication
	Acute coronary syndromes	Consider double antiplatelet therapy for at least 1 year

Abbreviations: *HbA1c* glycated hemoglobin, *ACE* angiotensin-converting enzyme, *ARB* angiotensin II receptor blocker, *CCB* calcium channel blocker, *CVD* cardiovascular diseases
[a]Consider more or less stringent glycemic goals according to individual patients
[b]Lower blood pressure levels may be appropriate according to patients' characteristics
[c]Men >50 years or women >60 years or who have at least one major risk factor (family history of cardiovascular disease, hypertension, dyslipidemia, smoking, and albuminuria)

mortality in type 2 diabetes [77]. Table 16.2 summarizes the current treatment recommendations for diabetes aiming to reduce cardiovascular disease burden.

16.5.1 Hyperglycemia

The relation between glycemic control and development of microvascular complications is clearer than for macrovascular disease [5]. A meta-analysis, including 33,040 diabetic patients from five randomized clinical trials comparing conventional vs. tight glycemic control, demonstrated a 17 % reduction in myocardial infarction risk without effect on stroke or on all-cause mortality [74]. Based on three recent randomized studies [78–80] in high-risk patients with type 2 diabetes that could not demonstrate a reduction in cardiovascular risk with HbA$_{1c}$ values lower than 6.5 % in relation to standard values (7–7.9 %), current recommendation is a target HbA$_{1c}$ lower than 7 % [5].

16.5.2 Hypertension

Hypertension affects most of patients with type 2 diabetes and patients with type 1 diabetes with underlying nephropathy. It is a major risk factor for both micro- and macrovascular disease development and progression. In a meta-analysis, clinic blood pressure values >115/75 mmHg have been associated with increased cardiovascular events and mortality risks in general populations [81]. However, randomized clinical trials demonstrated beneficial effect of reduction of systolic blood pressure to lower than 140 mmHg and of diastolic pressure to lower than 80–85 mmHg [82–84]. Currently, there is not enough evidence of benefits of lower blood pressure thresholds in diabetes, and the present recommendation is a clinic blood pressure target of <140/80 mmHg [5]. Ambulatory blood pressure monitoring seems to provide better cardiovascular risk stratification than clinic blood pressures in type 2 diabetes, with lower blood pressure targets, and should be performed whenever available [85].

The renin-angiotensin system inhibitors may be particularly beneficial in initial hypertension treatment in patients with diabetes. They may have effects in atherogenesis prevention and renal protection beyond blood pressure lowering [86]. Although some studies have shown superiority of renin-angiotensin system antagonists in reducing cardiovascular risk over other antihypertensive drug classes in patients with diabetes [87–89], a meta-analysis demonstrated no significant differences among antihypertensive drugs in improving patient prognosis, suggesting that the blood pressure reduction is the most important effect of these medications [90]. Indeed, most diabetic patients with hypertension will need multiple drug therapies to achieve blood pressure targets and commonly will present resistant hypertension, but renin-angiotensin system antagonists remain the cornerstone of antihypertensive drug treatment in patients with diabetes [5].

16.5.3 Dyslipidemia

Diabetic patients have an increased prevalence of lipid abnormalities that augments their already high cardiovascular risk. Several interventions may help to achieve lipid level targets, such as physical activity, diet changes, and weight loss. Many clinical trials demonstrated a reduction in cardiovascular risk, both in primary and secondary prevention, with statins use in patients with diabetes [91–97]. A meta-analysis in diabetes, including 14 randomized trials of statins, confirmed a reduction of global and vascular mortality [98]. LDL-cholesterol shall be <100 mg/dl (2.6 mmol/L) in patients without manifest cardiovascular disease and <70 mg/dl (1.8 mmol/L) in those patients with clinical cardiovascular disease [5, 99]. As in nondiabetic individuals, the beneficial effects of statins are greater in diabetic patients with higher baseline risk [5].

The combination of low HDL-cholesterol and high triglycerides is the most common dyslipidemia in type 2 diabetes. There are few studies investigating if treating these lipid abnormalities reduces cardiovascular outcomes. A study using gemfibrozil, demonstrated a reduction in cardiovascular risk, in a subgroup analysis of diabetic patients [100]. However, a study performed in diabetic patients using fenofibrate did not demonstrate reduction in cardiovascular risk [101]. Therefore, unless there are severe hypertriglyceridemia (>1,000 mg/dl) and consequently an increased risk pancreatitis, the target should be reducing LDL-cholesterol with high-intensity statin treatment, because there is not sufficient evidence for benefits of HDL-cholesterol or triglycerides treatment as there is for statins [5]. Also, there is no current evidence that supports the association of statins with fibrates to reduce cardiovascular risk in diabetes [102, 103]. The association of statins with fibrates increases the risk of augment of aminotransferases, myositis, and rhabdomyolysis, particularly in patients with renal failure. This risk seems to be higher with gemfibrozil [104].

16.5.4 Antiplatelet Treatment

Aspirin was demonstrated to reduce cardiovascular mortality in patients with previous myocardial infarction and stroke (secondary prevention) [105]. Its beneficial effect is less clear in primary prevention [106, 107]. Aspirin is currently recommended (75–162 mg) in diabetic patients with a history of cardiovascular disease for secondary prevention. For primary prevention, they are recommended for type 1 or type 2 diabetes at increased cardiovascular risk (10-year risk of event greater than 10 %). This includes men >50 years or women >60 years and patients who have at least one major risk factor (family history of cardiovascular disease, hypertension, dyslipidemia, smoking, or albuminuria) [108]. In diabetic patients with cardiovascular disease with contraindication to aspirin use, clopidogrel 75 mg should be used. In patients with acute coronary syndromes, double antiplatelet therapy is recommended for at least 1 year [105].

16.5.5 Smoking Cessation

Studies support a causal relation between cigarette smoking and increased health risks [109]. Diabetic patients who are smokers should be counseled and helped to stop smoking together with the other therapeutic measures [5].

Conclusions

Currently, treatment is based on the control of the risk factors that begin the vasculopathy, by keeping strict glycemic, lipid, and blood pressures control, in conjunction with regular physical activity, changes in diet habits, weight control, and pharmacological interventions. In a near future, we hope basic research on the mechanisms of vascular disease may provide data to discover new therapeutic interventions that can further reduce the diabetic vascular disease burden and improve its prognosis.

References

1. International Diabetes Federation (2013) IDF diabetes atlas, 6th edn. International Diabetes Federation, Brussels, http://www.idf.org/diabetesatlas
2. Barceló A, Aedo C, Rajpathak S, Robles S (2003) The cost of diabetes in Latin America and the Caribbean. Bull World Health Organ 81:19–27

3. American Diabetes Association (2013) Economic costs of diabetes in the U.S. in 2012. Diabetes Care 36:1033–1046

4. Breton MC, Guénette L, Amiche MA et al (2013) Burden of diabetes on the ability to work: a systematic review. Diabetes Care 36:740–749

5. American Diabetes Association (2014) Standards of medical care in diabetes 2014. Diabetes Care 37(Suppl 1):S14–S77

6. Vamos EP, Bottle A, Edmonds ME et al (2010) Changes in the incidence of lower extremity amputations in individuals with and without diabetes in England between 2004 and 2008. Diabetes Care 33:2592–2597

7. Moxey PW, Gogalniceanu P, Hinchliffe RJ et al (2011) Lower extremity amputations– a review of global variability in incidence. Diabet Med 28:1144–1153

8. De Marco R, Locatelli F, Zoppini G et al (1999) Cause-specific mortality in type 2 diabetes: the Verona Diabetes Study. Diabetes Care 22:756–761

9. Wei M, Gaskill SP, Haffner SM, Stern MP (1998) Effects of diabetes and level of glycemia on all-cause and cardiovascular mortality: the San Antonio Heart Study. Diabetes Care 21:1167–1172

10. Blonde L (2007) State of diabetes care in the United States. Am J Manag Care 13(Suppl 2): S36–S40

11. Ritz E (2013) Clinical manifestations and natural history of diabetic kidney disease. Med Clin N Am 97:19–29

12. Rahman S, Rahman T, Ismail AA, Rashid AR (2007) Diabetes-associated macrovasculopathy: pathophysiology and pathogenesis. Diabetes Obes Metab 9:767–780

13. Taddei S, Ghiadoni L, Virdis A et al (2003) Mechanisms of endothelial dysfunction: clinical significance and preventive non-pharmacological therapeutic strategies. Curr Pharm Des 9:2385–2402

14. Versari D, Daghini E, Virdis A et al (2009) Endothelial dysfunction as a target for prevention of cardiovascular disease. Diabetes Care 32(Suppl 2):S314–S321

15. Brunner H, Cockcroft JR, Deanfield J et al., Working Group on Endothelins and Endothelial Factors of the European Society of Hypertension (2005) Endothelial function and dysfunction. Part II: association with cardiovascular risk factors and diseases. A statement by the Working Group on Endothelins and Endothelial Factors of the European Society of Hypertension. J Hypertens 23:233–246

16. Tooke JE (1995) Microvascular function in human diabetes. A physiological perspective. Diabetes 44:721–726

17. Rattan V, Sultana C, Shen Y, Kalra VK (1997) Oxidant stress-induced transendothelial migration of monocytes is linked to phosphorylation of PECAM-1. Am J Physiol 273 (3 Pt 1):E453–E461

18. Tesfamariam B, Brown ML, Cohen RA (1991) Elevated glucose impairs endothelium-dependent relaxation by activating protein kinase C. Clin Invest 87:1643–1648

19. Poston L, Taylor PD (1995) Endothelium-mediated vascular function in insulin-dependent diabetes mellitus. Clin Sci (Lond) 88:245–255

20. Creager MA, Lüscher TF, Cosentino F, Beckman JA (2003) Diabetes and vascular disease: pathophysiology, clinical consequences, and medical therapy: part I. Circulation 108: 1527–1532

21. Lüscher TF, Creager MA, Beckman JA, Cosentino F (2003) Diabetes and vascular disease: pathophysiology, clinical consequences, and medical therapy: part II. Circulation 108: 1655–1661

22. Lerman A, Zeiher AM (2005) Endothelial function: cardiac events. Circulation 111:363–368

23. Kaiser N, Sasson S, Feener EP et al (1993) Differential regulation of glucose transport and transporters by glucose in vascular endothelial and smooth muscle cells. Diabetes 42:80–89

24. Stevens VJ, Vlassara H, Abati A, Cerami A (1977) Nonenzymatic glycosylation of hemoglobin. J Biol Chem 252:2998–3002

25. Wolf BA, Williamson JR, Easom RA et al (1991) Diacylglycerol accumulation and microvascular abnormalities induced by elevated glucose levels. J Clin Invest 87:31–38

26. Baynes JW (1991) Role of oxidative stress in development of complications in diabetes. Diabetes 40:405–412
27. Brownlee M (2001) Biochemistry and molecular cell biology of diabetic complications. Nature 414(6865):813–820
28. Giacco F, Brownlee M (2010) Oxidative stress and diabetic complications. Circ Res 107:1058–1070
29. Tilton RG, Chang K, Pugliese G et al (1989) Prevention of hemodynamic and vascular albumin filtration changes in diabetic rats by aldose reductase inhibitors. Diabetes 38: 1258–1270
30. Farmer DG, Kennedy S (2009) RAGE, vascular tone and vascular disease. Pharmacol Ther 124:185–194
31. Yao D, Brownlee M (2010) Hyperglycemia-induced reactive oxygen species increase expression of the receptor for advanced glycation end products (RAGE) and RAGE ligands. Diabetes 59:249–255
32. Ishii H, Koya D, King GL (1998) Protein kinase C activation and its role in the development of vascular complications in diabetes mellitus. J Mol Med (Berl) 76:21–31
33. Thallas-Bonke V, Thorpe SR, Coughlan MT et al (2008) Inhibition of NADPH oxidase prevents advanced glycation end product-mediated damage in diabetic nephropathy through a protein kinase C-alpha-dependent pathway. Diabetes 57:460–469
34. Madonna R, Renna FV, Cellini C et al (2011) Age-dependent impairment of number and angiogenic potential of adipose tissue-derived progenitor cells. Eur J Clin Invest 41: 126–133
35. Setter SM, Campbell RK, Cahoon CJ (2003) Biochemical pathways for microvascular complications of diabetes mellitus. Ann Pharmacother 37:1858–1866
36. Nishikawa T, Edelstein D, Brownlee M (2000) The missing link: a single unifying mechanism for diabetic complications. Kidney Int Suppl 77:S26–S30
37. Cosentino F, Hishikawa K, Katusic ZS, Lüscher TF (1997) High glucose increases nitric oxide synthase expression and superoxide anion generation in human aortic endothelial cells. Circulation 96:25–28
38. Pacher P, Obrosova IG, Mabley JG, Szabó C (2005) Role of nitrosative stress and peroxynitrite in the pathogenesis of diabetic complications. Emerging new therapeutical strategies. Curr Med Chem 12:267–275
39. Madonna R, De Caterina R (2011) Cellular and molecular mechanisms of vascular injury in diabetes–part I: pathways of vascular disease in diabetes. Vascul Pharmacol 54:68–74
40. Morigi M, Angioletti S, Imberti B et al (1998) Leukocyte-endothelial interaction is augmented by high glucose concentrations and hyperglycemia in a NF-kB-dependent fashion. J Clin Invest 101:1905–1915
41. Cagliero E, Roth T, Roy S, Lorenzi M (1991) Characteristics and mechanisms of high-glucose-induced overexpression of basement membrane components in cultured human endothelial cells. Diabetes 40:102–110
42. Balletshofer BM, Rittig K, Enderle MD et al (2000) Endothelial dysfunction is detectable in young normotensive first-degree relatives of subjects with type 2 diabetes in association with insulin resistance. Circulation 101:1780–1784
43. Del Turco S, Basta G (2012) An update on advanced glycation endproducts and atherosclerosis. Biofactors 38:266–274
44. Daroux M, Prévost G, Maillard-Lefebvre H et al (2010) Advanced glycation end-products: implications for diabetic and non-diabetic nephropathies. Diabetes Metab 36:1–10
45. Yudkin JS, Eringa E, Stehouwer CD (2005) "Vasocrine" signalling from perivascular fat: a mechanism linking insulin resistance to vascular disease. Lancet 365(9473):1817–1820
46. Wendt T, Harja E, Bucciarelli L et al (2006) RAGE modulates vascular inflammation and atherosclerosis in a murine model of type 2 diabetes. Atherosclerosis 185:70–77
47. Basta G, Lazzerini G, Del Turco S et al (2005) At least 2 distinct pathways generating reactive oxygen species mediate vascular cell adhesion molecule-1 induction by advanced glycation end products. Arterioscler Thromb Vasc Biol 25:1401–1407

48. Basta G (2008) Receptor for advanced glycation endproducts and atherosclerosis: from basic mechanisms to clinical implications. Atherosclerosis 196:9–21
49. Jiang ZY, Lin YW, Clemont A et al (1999) Characterization of selective resistance to insulin signaling in the vasculature of obese Zucker(fa/fa) rats. J Clin Invest 104:447–457
50. Reaven GM, Chen YD (1988) Role of insulin in regulation of lipoprotein metabolism in diabetes. Diabetes Metab Rev 4:639–652
51. Feener EP, King GL (1997) Vascular dysfunction in diabetes mellitus. Lancet 350 (Suppl 1):SI9–SI13
52. Hsueh WA, Lyon CJ, Quinones MJ (2004) Insulin resistance and the endothelium. Am J Med 117:109–117
53. Steinberg HO, Brechtel G, Johnson A et al (1994) Insulin-mediated skeletal muscle vasodilation is nitric oxide dependent. A novel action of insulin to increase nitric oxide release. J Clin Invest 94:1172–1179
54. Malide D, Davies-Hill TM, Levine M, Simpson IA (1998) Distinct localization of GLUT-1, -3, and -5 in human monocyte-derived macrophages: effects of cell activation. Am J Physiol 274:E516–E526
55. Pansuria M, Xi H, Li L et al (2012) Insulin resistance, metabolic stress, and atherosclerosis. Front Biosci (Schol Ed) 4:916–931
56. Hayden MR, Tyagi SC (2004) Vasa vasorum in plaque angiogenesis, metabolic syndrome, type 2 diabetes mellitus, and atheroscleropathy: a malignant transformation. Cardiovasc Diabetol 3:1
57. Orasanu G, Plutzky J (2009) The pathologic continuum of diabetic vascular disease. J Am Coll Cardiol 53(5 suppl):S35–S42
58. Jax TW (2010) Metabolic memory: a vascular perspective. Cardiovasc Diabetol 9:51
59. Langheinrich AC, Kampschulte M, Buch T, Bohle RM (2007) Vasa vasorum and atherosclerosis – Quid novi? Thromb Haemost 97:873–879
60. Barger AC, Beeuwkes R 3rd, Lainey LI, Silverman KJ (1984) Hypothesis: vasa vasorum and neovascularization of human coronary arteries. A possible role in the pathophysiology of atherosclerosis. N Engl J Med 310:175–177
61. Barger AC, Beeuwkes R 3rd (1990) Rupture of coronary vasa vasorum as a trigger of acute myocardial infarction. Am J Cardiol 66:41G–43G
62. Kumamoto M, Nakashima Y, Sueishi K (1995) Intimal neovascularization in human coronary atherosclerosis: its origin and pathophysiological significance. Hum Pathol 26:450–456
63. Moreno PR, Fuster V (2004) New aspects in the pathogenesis of diabetic atherothrombosis. J Am Coll Cardiol 44:2293–2300
64. Arcidiacono MA, Traveset A, Rubinat E et al (2013) Microangiopathy of large artery wall: a neglected complication of diabetes mellitus. Atherosclerosis 228:142–147
65. Angervall L, Dahl I, Säve-Söderbergh J (1966) The aortic vasa vasorum in juvenile diabetes. Pathol Microbiol 29:431–437
66. Purushothaman KR, Purushothaman M, Muntner P et al (2011) Inflammation, neovascularization and intra-plaque hemorrhage are associated with increased reparative collagen content: implication for plaque progression in diabetic atherosclerosis. Vasc Med 16: 103–108
67. Cheung N, Mitchell P, Wong TY (2010) Diabetic retinopathy. Lancet 376:124–136
68. Shah PK (2010) Screening asymptomatic subjects for subclinical atherosclerosis: can we, does it matter, and should we? J Am Coll Cardiol 56:98–105
69. Young LH, Wackers FJ, Chyun DA et al (2009) Cardiac outcomes after screening for asymptomatic coronary artery disease in patients with type 2 diabetes: the DIAD study: a randomized controlled trial. JAMA 301:1547–1555
70. Budoff MJ, Shaw LJ, Liu ST et al (2007) Long-term prognosis associated with coronary calcification: observations with coronary calcification: observations from a registry of 25,253 patients. J Am Coll Cardiol 49:1860–1870
71. Detrano R, Guerci AD, Carr JJ et al (2008) Coronary calcium as a predictor of coronary events in four racial or ethnic groups. N Engl J Med 358:1336–1345

72. Schofield I, Malik R, Izzard A et al (2002) Vascular structural and functional changes in type 2 diabetes mellitus: evidence for the roles of abnormal myogenic responsiveness and dyslipidemia. Circulation 106:3037–3043
73. Holman RR, Paul SK, Bethel MA et al (2008) 10-year follow-up of intensive glucose control in type 2 diabetes. N Engl J Med 359:1577–1589
74. Ray KK, Seshasai SR, Wijesuriya S et al (2009) Effect of intensive control of glucose on cardiovascular outcomes and death in patients with diabetes mellitus: a meta-analysis of randomised controlled trials. Lancet 373(9677):1765–1772
75. ALLHAT Officers and Coordinators for the ALLHAT Collaborative Research Group (2002) Major outcomes in high-risk hypertensive patients randomized to angiotensin-converting enzyme inhibitor or calcium channel blocker vs. diuretic: the Antihypertensive and Lipid-Lowering Treatment to Prevent Heart Attack Trial (ALLHAT). JAMA 288:2981–2997
76. Colhoun HM, Betteridge DJ, Durrington PN et al (2004) CARDS investigators primary prevention of cardiovascular disease with atorvastatin in type 2 diabetes in the Collaborative Atorvastatin Diabetes Study (CARDS): multicentre randomised placebo-controlled trial. Lancet 364(9435):685–696
77. Gaede P, Lund-Andersen H, Parving HH, Pedersen O (2008) Effect of a multifactorial intervention on mortality in type 2 diabetes. N Engl J Med 358:580–591
78. Action to Control Cardiovascular Risk in Diabetes Study Group, Gerstein HC, Miller ME, Byington RP et al (2008) Effects of intensive glucose lowering in type 2 diabetes. N Engl J Med 358:2545–2559
79. ADVANCE Collaborative Group, Patel A, MacMahon S, Chalmers J et al (2008) Intensive blood glucose control and vascular outcomes in patients with type 2 diabetes. N Engl J Med 358:2560–2572
80. Duckworth W, Abraira C, Moritz T et al., VADT Investigators (2009) Glucose control and vascular complications in veterans with type 2 diabetes. N Engl J Med 360:129–139
81. Lewington S, Clarke R, Qizilbash N et al., Prospective Studies Collaboration (2002) Age-specific relevance of usual blood pressure to vascular mortality: a meta-analysis of individual data for one million adults in 61 prospective studies. Lancet 360:1903–1913
82. UK Prospective Diabetes Study Group (1998) Tight blood pressure control and risk of macrovascular and microvascular complications in type 2 diabetes: UKPDS38. BMJ 317:703–713
83. Hansson L, Zanchetti A, Carruthers SG et al., HOT Study Group (1998) Effects of intensive blood-pressure lowering and low-dose aspirin in patients with hypertension: principal results of the Hypertension Optimal Treatment (HOT) randomised trial. Lancet 351:1755–1762
84. Adler AI, Stratton IM, Neil HA et al (2000) Association of systolic blood pressure with macrovascular and microvascular complications of type 2 diabetes (UKPDS 36): prospective observational study. BMJ 321:412–419
85. Salles GF, Leite NC, Pereira BB et al (2013) Prognostic impact of clinic and ambulatory blood pressure components in high-risk type 2 diabetic patients: the Rio de Janeiro Type 2 Diabetes Cohort Study. J Hypertens 31:2176–2186
86. Beckman JA, Paneni F, Cosentino F, Creager MA (2013) Diabetes and vascular disease: pathophysiology, clinical consequences, and medical therapy: part II. Eur Heart J 34:2444–2456
87. Heart Outcomes Prevention Evaluation Study Investigators (2000) Effects of ramipril on cardiovascular and microvascular outcomes in people with diabetes mellitus: results of the HOPE study and MICRO-HOPE substudy. Lancet 355:253–259
88. Lindholm LH, Ibsen H, Dahlöf B et al., LIFE Study Group (2002) Cardiovascular morbidity and mortality in patients with diabetes in the Losartan Intervention For End point reduction in hypertension study (LIFE): a randomised trial against atenolol. Lancet 359:1004–1010
89. Berl T, Hunsicker LG, Lewis JB et al., Irbesartan Diabetic Nephropathy Trial, Collaborative Study Group (2003) Cardiovascular outcomes in the Irbesartan Diabetic Nephropathy Trial of patients with type 2 diabetes and overt nephropathy. Ann Intern Med 138:542–549
90. Turnbull F (2003) Effects of different blood-pressure-lowering regimens on major cardiovascular events: results of prospectively-designed overviews of randomised trials. Lancet 362:1527–1535

91. Pyorala K, Pedersen TR, Kjekshus J et al (1997) Cholesterol lowering with simvastatin improves prognosis of diabetic patients with coronary heart disease. A subgroup analysis of the Scandinavian Simvastatin Survival Study (4S). Diabetes Care 20:614–620
92. Peto R, Heart Protection Study Collaborative Group (2003) MRC/BHF Heart Protection Study of cholesterol-lowering with simvastatin in 5963 people with diabetes: a randomised placebo controlled trial. Lancet 361:2005–2016
93. Goldberg RB, Mellies MJ, Sacks FM et al., The Care Investigators (1998) Cardiovascular events and their reduction with pravastatin in diabetic and glucose intolerant myocardial infarction survivor with average cholesterol levels: subgroup analyses in the Cholesterol And Recurrent Events (CARE) trial. Circulation 98:2513–2519
94. Shepherd J, Barter P, Carmena R et al (2006) Effect of lowering LDL cholesterol substantially below currently recommended levels in patients with coronary heart disease and diabetes: the Treating to New Targets (TNT) study. Diabetes Care 29:1220–1226
95. Sever PS, Poulter NR, Dahlöf B et al (2005) Reduction in cardiovascular events with atorvastatin in 2,532 patients with type 2 diabetes: Anglo-Scandinavian Cardiac Outcomes Trial Lipid-Lowering Arm (ASCOT-LLA). Diabetes Care 28:1151–1157
96. Knopp RH, d'Emden M, Smilde JG, Pocock SJ (2006) Efficacy and safety of atorvastatin in the prevention of cardiovascular endpoints in subjects with type 2 diabetes: the Atorvastatin Study for Prevention of Coronary Heart Disease Endpoints in noninsulin- dependent diabetes mellitus (ASPEN). Diabetes Care 29:1478–1485
97. Colhoun HM, Betteridge DJ, Durrington PN et al., CARDS Investigators (2004) Primary prevention of cardiovascular disease with atorvastatin in type 2 diabetes in the Collaborative Atorvastatin Diabetes Study (CARDS): multicentre randomized placebo-controlled trial. Lancet 364:685–696
98. Kearney PM, Blackwell L, Collins R et al., Cholesterol Treatment Trialists' (CTT) Collaborators (2008) Efficacy of cholesterol lowering therapy in 18,686 people with diabetes in 14 randomised trials of statins: a meta-analysis. Lancet 371:117–125
99. Grundy SM, Cleeman JI, Merz CN et al., National Heart Lung, and Blood Institute, American College of Cardiology Foundation, American Heart Association (2004) Implications of recent clinical trials for the National Cholesterol Education Program Adult Treatment Panel III guidelines. Circulation 110:227–239
100. Rubins HB, Robins SJ, Collins D et al., Veterans Affairs High-Density Lipoprotein Cholesterol Intervention Trial Study Group (1999) Gemfibrozil for the secondary prevention of coronary heart disease in men with low levels of high-density lipoprotein cholesterol. N Engl J Med 341:410–418
101. Keech A, Simes RJ, Barter P et al., FIELD study investigators (2005) Effects of long-term fenofibrate therapy on cardiovascular events in 9795 people with type 2 diabetes mellitus (the FIELD study): randomised controlled trial. Lancet 366:1849–1861
102. Ginsberg HN, Elam MB, Lovato LC et al., ACCORD Study Group (2010) Effects of combination lipid therapy in type 2 diabetes mellitus. N Engl J Med 362:1563–1574
103. Boden WE, Probstfield JL, Anderson T, et al., AIM-HIGH Investigators (2011) Niacin in patients with low HDL-cholesterol levels receiving intensive statin therapy. N Engl J Med 365:2255–2267
104. Jones PH, Davidson MH (2005) Reporting rate of rhabdomyolysis with fenofibrate + statin versus gemfibrozil + any statin. Am J Cardiol 95:120–122
105. Vandvik PO, Lincoff AM, Gore JM et al (2012) Primary and secondary prevention of cardiovascular disease: antithrombotic therapy and prevention of thrombosis, 9th ed: American College of Chest Physicians Evidence-Based Clinical Practice Guidelines. Chest 141:e637S–e668S
106. Belch J, MacCuish A, Campbell I et al., Prevention of Progression of Arterial Disease and Diabetes Study Group, Diabetes Registry Group, Royal College of Physicians Edinburgh (2008) The Prevention of Progression of Arterial Disease and Diabetes (POPADAD) trial: factorial randomised placebo controlled trial of aspirin and antioxidants in patients with diabetes and asymptomatic peripheral arterial disease. BMJ 337:a1840

107. Kataja-Tuomola MK, Ogawa H, Nakayama M et al., Japanese Primary Prevention of Atherosclerosis with Aspirin for Diabetes (JPAD) Trial Investigators (2008) Low-dose aspirin for primary prevention of atherosclerotic events in patients with type 2 diabetes: a randomized controlled trial. JAMA 300:2134–2141
108. Pignone M, Alberts MJ, Colwell JA et al., American Diabetes Association, American Heart Association, American College of Cardiology Foundation (2010) Aspirin for primary prevention of cardiovascular events in people with diabetes: a position statement of the American Diabetes Association, a scientific statement of the American Heart Association, and an expert consensus document of the American College of Cardiology Foundation. Diabetes Care 33:1395–1402
109. Katsiki N, Papadopoulou SK, Fachantidou AI, Mikhailidis DP (2013) Smoking and vascular risk: are all forms of smoking harmful to all types of vascular disease? Pub Health 127: 435–441

Obesity and Metabolic Syndrome

17

Isabel Ferreira

Obesity, in particular central obesity, is a major risk factor for cardiovascular disease (CVD) [1]. A great portion of the adverse impact of (central) obesity on cardiovascular health may be explained through related haemodynamic and metabolic mediators such as blood pressure (BP), cholesterol and glucose [2]. These risk factors tend to cluster within individuals forming the metabolic syndrome (MetS) [3]. Obesity and/or MetS-related adverse changes in the arterial wall provide a structural and functional background for clinical events such as myocardial infarction, stroke and peripheral artery disease, all known to occur at higher rates in these conditions [4–7]. This chapter revises the current epidemiological evidence around the adverse effects that (central) obesity and the MetS may exert on large artery properties, particularly, arterial stiffening. Focus is put on evidence derived, whenever available, from representative prospective observational and intervention studies conducted over the last decade.

17.1 Body Fatness/Fat Distribution and Arterial Stiffness: An Early Phenomenon

Many studies have shown that higher levels of body fatness, in particular, a central pattern of fat distribution, are associated with arterial stiffness (reviewed in [6, 8]). These primarily cross-sectional studies may be fairly summarised into two key observations: firstly, deleterious adaptations related to increased adiposity seem to occur across all age categories [9–11]; secondly, such adaptations are observed with

I. Ferreira, PhD
Department of Clinical Epidemiology and Medical Technology Assessment,
CARIM School for Cardiovascular Diseases, Maastricht University Medical Centre,
P.Debyelaan 25, Maastricht 6202 AZ, The Netherlands
e-mail: i.ferreira@maastrichtuniversity.nl

© Springer International Publishing Switzerland 2015
A. Berbari, G. Mancia (eds.), *Arterial Disorders:*
Definition, Clinical Manifestations, Mechanisms and Therapeutic Approaches,
DOI 10.1007/978-3-319-14556-3_17

higher levels of adiposity even when within the ranges of normal weight and are thus not confined to obesity. Indeed, the increased levels of arterial stiffness observed already among children/adolescents [12–17] and young adults [9, 18, 19] suggest that higher levels of (central) adiposity do not need to be long lasting to have deleterious effects on the arterial system. In addition, the fact that higher levels of (central) adiposity at young(er) ages are associated with higher arterial stiffness later in life [18, 20–22] and that a favourable change in obesity status from childhood to adulthood is associated with less arterial stiffness in adulthood [23] emphasise the importance of healthy lifestyle promotion early in life. The strong tracking of (central) obesity throughout the life course [20] further corroborates this need because early and cumulative exposures to adverse levels of (central) body fatness may hamper considerable and sustainable improvements in arterial properties resulting from interventions targeting obese adults, given that such interventions will invariably be much shorter than a person's lifetime.

17.2   Do Changes in Body Fatness Affect Arterial Stiffness?

The extent to which changes in body fatness affect changes in arterial stiffness remains unclear because most of the longitudinal (observational or intervention) studies available thus far have been restricted to the appreciation of the impact of changes in body weight, which does not discern fat from lean body mass. Indeed, some observational studies have shown that increases in weight were associated with increases in arterial stiffness among young and healthy [24] and overweight middle-aged adults [25]. Several small intervention studies, all confined to individuals with obesity or diabetes, have shown that weight loss led to arterial de-stiffening [26–30]. More recent and larger randomised controlled trials (RCTs) confirmed the beneficial effects of weight loss attained by means of behavioural interventions (diet and/or exercise) among nondiabetic overweight/obese individuals with (e.g. the ENCORE study [31]) or without hypertension (e.g. the SAVE trial [32, 33]). Assuming that the weight loss attained indeed reflected reductions in body fatness, these findings support the view that body fatness may impact on arterial stiffness independently, at least in part, of related changes in BP. Still, it remains that arterial adaptations related to weight changes do not clarify the extent to which any of the favourable effects observed could be attributed to reductions in specific types of fat depots (e.g. *visceral* vs. *subcutaneous*) and/or its distribution (e.g. *central* vs. *peripheral*) or even be attenuated by concomitant loss of muscle mass.

17.2.1 Visceral Fat as Main Determinant of Arterial Stiffness

Abdominal visceral fat is thought to be more strongly associated with arterial stiffness than abdominal subcutaneous fat [34–37]. In an important proof of concept study, and despite its small sample and highly experimental setting, Orr et al. indeed showed that abdominal visceral (VAT), not subcutaneous adipose tissue (SAT), was associated with the increases in arterial stiffness resulting from 5 kg weight gain induced by overfeeding nonobese young adults for 6–8 weeks [38]. In addition, in a recent study in which the biopsies from visceral (greater omentum) and subcutaneous (abdominal) white adipose tissue samples were obtained from obese subjects scheduled for bariatric surgery, the visceral fat cell size (i.e. volume), but not number, was strongly associated with arterial stiffness, whereas no such association was found with SAT (volume or number) [39]. It must be mentioned that recent studies suggest that the adverse effect of VAT on arterial stiffness (as on metabolic disturbances relating central obesity to poorer cardiovascular outcome) may not only be due to the effects of omental hypertrophy of adipose tissue but also due to adipose tissue accumulating specifically around the epicardium [40–42] and/or in the liver (a typical feature of non-alcoholic fatty liver disease) [43–45]. Because this evidence derives from cross-sectional studies, the interrelations, relative contributions and specific pathobiological mechanisms through which these fat depots may impact on general and local arterial stiffening, and haemodynamic factors still need to be further investigated in prospective studies.

17.2.2 The Beneficial Role of Peripheral Fat on Arterial Stiffness

Studies examining the role of the whole-body fat distribution on arterial stiffness rather than of central fatness only have unveiled a complex scenario: in contrast to central fat (i.e. that accumulated in the trunk/abdominal areas), higher levels of peripheral fat mass (i.e. that accumulated in the limbs and thus stored mainly subcutaneously) may have an independent *favourable* impact on arterial stiffness [19, 46, 47]. Indeed, the different lipolytic activity of the two fat regions/tissues provides biological support for their opposite effects on arterial stiffness. These 'dysfunctional' [1] vs. 'functional' [48] effects of fat could explain why, in general, central fat estimates correlate more strongly with health outcomes than estimates of total body fatness. As such, adverse changes in *body fat distribution* may occur with ageing (i.e. increases in central accompanied by decreases in peripheral fat mass) without being detected by appreciable changes in total body weight or body mass index (BMI), though both contributing, additively, to accelerated arterial stiffening. This hypothesis was tested in the *Amsterdam Growth and Health Longitudinal Study*, in a first study to have examined in detail, how naturally occurring changes in body fat and its distribution (assessed by dual x-ray absorptiometry) correlated with changes in arterial stiffness indexed by a large set of valid estimates throughout the arterial tree [49]. The study had three key findings: first, throughout the 6-year longitudinal study (between the ages of 36 and 42), greater levels of central fat were *adversely* associated with carotid, femoral and aortic stiffness, whereas greater levels of peripheral fat were *favourably* associated with these stiffness estimates; these associations reflected the more 'chronic' (deleterious) effects of persistent adverse fat distribution over time. Second, increases in trunk fat were *adversely* associated with 6-year changes in carotid and aortic, though not femoral, stiffness, whereas increases in peripheral fat were *favourably* associated with changes in these stiffness estimates; these observations suggested a more 'acute' component to the deleterious effects of changes in body fat distribution on arterial stiffness of predominantly elastic arterial segments. Finally, the detrimental effects of *increases* in central fat and *decreases* in peripheral fat on arterial stiffness were independent of one another and concomitant changes in lean mass and other risk factors (including mean BP) and were accompanied by only minor increases in body weight [49]. Noteworthy, increases in trunk but decreases in peripheral fat mass formed a relatively prevalent phenotype (one third of the study population) that displayed the steepest rates of progression in carotid and aortic stiffness (Fig. 16.1a, b, *respectively*) despite changes in BMI that ranged within the limits assigned to normal weight (Fig. 16.1c). This phenotype is consistent with the existence of a relative prevalent subgroup of individuals at the population level designated as 'metabolically obese but normal weight', who are often characterised by elevated visceral adiposity (despite a BMI <25) and a more atherogenic lipid and/or glucose metabolism profile and who thus may be at a particular high risk for metabolic and arterial disease and in need of appropriate screening and preventive measures [50, 51].

17.2.3 The Role of Muscle Mass: The Need for Comprehensive Whole-Body Composition Studies

Adopting a whole-body composition (i.e. examining also the independent contribution of muscle mass in addition to body fat) rather than a body fat/fat distribution-only model has revealed that also appendicular muscle mass may be an independent beneficial determinant of arterial stiffness, particularly though not confined to the elderly [19, 46, 49, 52–55]. Currently, there is a great concern about the cardiometabolic consequences of the increasing prevalence of (central) obesity and sarcopenia (i.e. the degenerative loss of skeletal muscle mass and strength) associated with ageing, especially when occurring in combination – i.e. *sarcopenic obesity* [56]. How decreases in lean mass may affect arterial stiffness is not clear as the evidence so far has been mainly derived from cross-sectional studies [19, 46, 52–55]. It is possible that the relationship is not causal in the sense that higher muscle mass may simply reflect higher (lifelong) physical activity and/or less sedentary habits, better nutrient intake status and/or better glucose uptake/insulin sensitivity, all of which protect against arterial stiffness [57–61]. Alternatively, arterial stiffness may promote sarcopenia by reducing limb blood flow and inducing rarefaction and

Fig. 17.1 Comparisons of (**a**) changes in carotid Young's elastic modulus (cYEM), (**b**) changes in carotid-femoral pulse wave velocity (cfPWV) and (**c**) baseline and follow-up body mass index (BMI), between different phenotypes of change in body fat distribution as observed in a 6-year follow-up from the *Amsterdam Growth and Health Longitudinal Study*. BMI data were adjusted for sex; arterial data were adjusted for sex, body height and changes in mean arterial pressure, lean mass and other biological risk factors. Error bars indicate the standard errors of the means (Reproduced from Schouten et al. [49] with permission from the American Society of Nutrition)

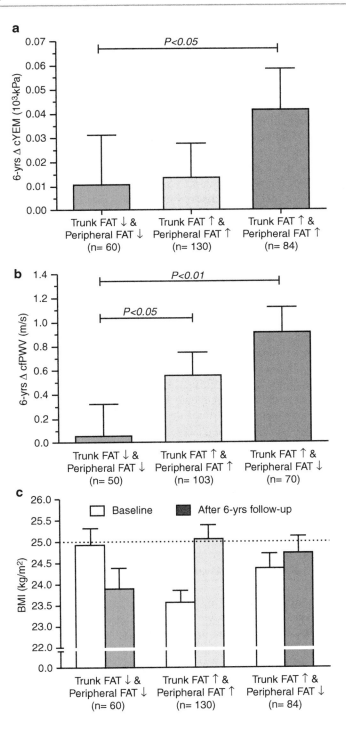

dysfunction in the microcirculation, thereby affecting muscle contraction and ultimately leading to muscle mass rarefaction. This hypothesis was supported by a recent prospective study from the *Health, Aging and Body Composition Study*, showing that older individuals with higher cfPWV at baseline had poorer levels of leg lean mass and sarcopenic index at baseline and over a 6-year follow-up period, independently of age, BMI, BP, diabetes, physical activity, smoking, total fat mass, low-grade inflammation, peripheral artery disease and CHD status [62]. Further longitudinal and intervention studies are needed to clarify the role of muscle mass on arterial stiffening (or vice versa), if any. Nevertheless, the existence of a link between muscle mass and arterial stiffness retains relevant clinical implications because it stresses the need to carefully monitor and secure that weight-loss interventions do not occur at the expense of muscle mass, particularly among the elderly.

17.3 Metabolic Syndrome and Arterial Stiffness: An Early Phenomenon

Increased arterial stiffness has been consistently reported in individuals with the MetS or with increasing clustered load or number of traits of the MetS (reviewed in [7]). Like for (central) fatness, a major force underlying the MetS risk factor clustering, such adverse arterial changes have been shown across all ages [63, 64], including young children and adolescents, with [65] or without overt obesity [12, 66], and young [67–71] and older adults [72], including those treated [73] or untreated for hypertension [74, 75]. The increased arterial stiffness in the MetS thus seems to be caused by subtle metabolic abnormalities that characterise prediabetic states but not necessarily fully developed diabetes. In addition, the recent findings from *the Cardiovascular Risk in Young Finns Study* showing higher levels of arterial stiffness among young adults who had the MetS during youth but also of arterial stiffness reduced to levels similar to those who had never had the MetS throughout the life course among those who, by adulthood, recovered from the MetS [76], support the potential reversibility of the adverse effects of the MetS if prevented/targeted early in life.

17.4 Do Changes in Metabolic Syndrome Status Affect Arterial Stiffness?

Confirming the suggestions derived from cross-sectional observations showing that the increases in arterial stiffness with advancing age were accentuated in the presence of the MetS [68, 64], recent prospective cohort studies have shown that individuals with the MetS not only have higher arterial stiffness at baseline but also display *steeper* increases in arterial stiffness with ageing as compared with those without the MetS [70, 77–80]. In addition, analyses of the impact of changes in MetS status among young [80, 81] and middle-aged [82] adults showed that those with incident and persistent MetS over the course of time displayed the steepest increases in arterial stiffness as compared with their peers who remained MetS-free throughout. Importantly, increases in arterial stiffness with ageing among those who recovered from the MetS tended to be somewhat less steep than those with persistent MetS [80] or even comparable to those who remained MetS-free throughout [82, 81]. An important observation in one of these longitudinal studies was that the MetS-related increase in carotid stiffness seemed to have preceded structural and local haemodynamic changes consistent with maladaptive (outward) carotid remodelling, an important process that may explain the increase risk of stroke in individuals with the MetS [80]. Taken together, the longitudinal data reviewed above [70, 76–82] demonstrate *accelerated arterial stiffening and maladaptive remodelling*, which may explain, at least in part, the increased CVD risk in individuals with the MetS [7]. These findings also emphasise the importance of primary prevention given the observed reversibility of the adverse impact of MetS on arterial structural and functional properties among those individuals who recovered from the MetS.

17.4.1 Specific Clusters of the Metabolic Syndrome's Traits and Arterial Stiffness

It is important to stress that the association between the MetS and arterial stiffness seems not only to be attributable to elevated BP, one of its most common traits and a main determinant of arterial stiffness. Indeed, in addition to (and independently of) elevated BP, (central) obesity and increased glucose levels are traits often associated with arterial stiffness [70, 72, 80, 83], whereas dyslipidaemia (as ascertained by elevated triglycerides and/or decreased HDL cholesterol) has been less or not consistently so. The clustering of central obesity, increased glucose levels and BP appears to be the most prevalent across several populations in the western world [64, 84, 83], and this phenotype is not only associated with the highest arterial stiffness levels [64, 83] but also with the greatest mortality risk [84].

17.5 Pathobiological Mechanisms Linking (Central) Obesity and the Metabolic Syndrome to Arterial Stiffening

The adverse association of the critical axis (central) obesity - MetS with arterial stiffness raises important questions about the potential underlying molecular processes. These may include some of the effects central obesity and related insulin resistance are known to exert at the vascular wall level, for instance, through inflammatory reactions, endothelial dysfunction and sympathetic activation [34, 32, 85]. These abnormalities are interrelated and affect vascular tone and stimulate vascular smooth muscle cell proliferation. In addition, changes in the type or structure of elastin and/or collagen in the arterial wall due to hyperglycaemia, particularly the formation of crosslinks through nonenzymatic glycosylation of proteins that generate advanced glycation end products, could constitute another mechanism [7]. Several of these putative mediators are thus likely to account for the obesity- or MetS-related increases in arterial stiffness, but currently we have only fragments of insight among a likely large set of players involved [5]. Teasing apart their individual contribution and/or identification of predominant operative pathways may provide key information for tailored interventions aiming at the treatment of arterial stiffening and related cardiovascular *sequelae* [6]. A comprehensive analysis of these issues in the context of representative prospective cohort studies or RCTs is still lacking and thus most warranted.

17.6 Summary

In this chapter, recent epidemiological evidence pertaining to the role of (central) obesity and the MetS on arterial stiffness was reviewed. Reinforced by recent prospective data, there is convincing evidence that these interrelated risk factors increase arterial stiffness, a mechanism that may explain the associated higher CVD risk. However, there is still relatively few data on (1) the molecular basis of greater arterial stiffness associated with these risk factors, (2) the prognostic significance of arterial stiffness indices in individuals with these risk factors and (3) the extent to which intervention on these risk factors improves cardiovascular outcome through beneficial impact on arterial stiffness. Given the high and increasing prevalence of obesity and the MetS, these questions constitute an important research agenda.

Acknowledgement Dr. Ferreira is supported by a senior postdoctoral fellowship from the Netherlands Heart Foundation (grant no. 2006T050).

References

1. Hajer GR, van Haeften TW, Visseren FL (2008) Adipose tissue dysfunction in obesity, diabetes, and vascular diseases. Eur Heart J 29(24):2959–2971
2. Global Burden of Metabolic Risk Factors for Chronic Diseases Collaboration, Lu Y, Hajifathalian K, Ezzati M et al (2014) Metabolic mediators of the effects of body-mass index, overweight, and obesity on coronary heart disease and stroke: a pooled analysis of 97 prospective cohorts with 1.8 million participants. Lancet 383(9921):970–983
3. Grundy SM (2000) Metabolic complications of obesity. Endocrine 13(2):155–165
4. Safar ME, Czernichow S, Blacher J (2006) Obesity, arterial stiffness, and cardiovascular risk. J Am Soc Nephrol 17(4 Suppl 2):S109–S111
5. Seals DR, Gates PE (2005) Stiffening our resolve against adult weight gain. Hypertension 45(2):175–177
6. Ferreira I, van de Laar RJ, Stehouwer CD (2014) Obesity, metabolic syndrome, diabetes and smoking. In: Safar ME, O'Rourke MF, Frohlich ED (eds) Blood pressure and arterial wall mechanics in cardiovascular diseases. Springer, London, pp 409–422
7. Stehouwer CD, Henry RM, Ferreira I (2008) Arterial stiffness in diabetes and the metabolic syndrome: a pathway to cardiovascular disease. Diabetologia 51(4):527–539
8. Stehouwer CD, Ferreira I (2006) Diabetes, lipids and other cardiovascular risk factors. In: Safar ME, O'Rourke MF (eds) Arterial stiffness in hypertension, vol 23, Handbook of hypertension. Elsevier, Amsterdam, pp 427–456
9. Wildman RP, Mackey RH, Bostom A et al (2003) Measures of obesity are associated with vascular stiffness in young and older adults. Hypertension 42(4):468–473

10. Zebekakis PE, Nawrot T, Thijs L et al (2005) Obesity is associated with increased arterial stiffness from adolescence until old age. J Hypertens 23(10):1839–1846
11. Scuteri A, Orru M, Morrell CH et al (2012) Associations of large artery structure and function with adiposity: effects of age, gender, and hypertension. The SardiNIA Study. Atherosclerosis 221(1):189–197
12. Whincup PH, Gilg JA, Donald AE et al (2005) Arterial distensibility in adolescents: the influence of adiposity, the metabolic syndrome, and classic risk factors. Circulation 112(12):1789–1797
13. Geerts CC, Evelein AM, Bots ML et al (2012) Body fat distribution and early arterial changes in healthy 5-year-old children. Ann Med 44(4):350–359
14. Urbina EM, Gao Z, Khoury PR et al (2012) Insulin resistance and arterial stiffness in healthy adolescents and young adults. Diabetologia 55(3):625–631
15. Sakuragi S, Abhayaratna K, Gravenmaker KJ et al (2009) Influence of adiposity and physical activity on arterial stiffness in healthy children: the lifestyle of our kids study. Hypertension 53(4):611–616
16. Urbina EM, Kimball TR, Khoury PR et al (2010) Increased arterial stiffness is found in adolescents with obesity or obesity-related type 2 diabetes mellitus. J Hypertens 28(8):1692–1698
17. Aggoun Y, Farpour-Lambert NJ, Marchand LM et al (2008) Impaired endothelial and smooth muscle functions and arterial stiffness appear before puberty in obese children and are associated with elevated ambulatory blood pressure. Eur Heart J 29(6):792–799
18. Ferreira I, Twisk JW, van Mechelen W et al (2004) Current and adolescent body fatness and fat distribution: relationships with carotid intima-media thickness and large artery stiffness at the age of 36 years. J Hypertens 22(1):145–155
19. Ferreira I, Snijder MB, Twisk JW et al (2004) Central fat mass versus peripheral fat and lean mass: opposite (adverse versus favorable) associations with arterial stiffness? The Amsterdam Growth and Health Longitudinal Study. J Clin Endocrinol Metab 89(6):2632–2639
20. Ferreira I, van de Laar RJ, Prins MH et al (2012) Carotid stiffness in young adults: a life-course analysis of its early determinants: the Amsterdam Growth and Health Longitudinal Study. Hypertension 59(1):54–61
21. McEniery CM, Spratt M, Munnery M et al (2010) An analysis of prospective risk factors for aortic stiffness in men: 20-year follow-up from the Caerphilly prospective study. Hypertension 56(1):36–43
22. Johansen NB, Vistisen D, Brunner EJ et al (2012) Determinants of aortic stiffness: 16-year follow-up of the Whitehall II study. PLoS One 7(5):e37165
23. Aatola H, Hutri-Kahonen N, Juonala M et al (2010) Lifetime risk factors and arterial pulse wave velocity in adulthood: the cardiovascular risk in Young Finns Study. Hypertension 55(3):806–811
24. Wildman RP, Farhat GN, Patel AS et al (2005) Weight change is associated with change in arterial stiffness among healthy young adults. Hypertension 45(2):187–192
25. Yamada J, Tomiyama H, Matsumoto C et al (2008) Overweight body mass index classification modifies arterial stiffening associated with weight gain in healthy middle-aged Japanese men. Hypertens Res 31(6):1087–1092
26. Goldberg Y, Boaz M, Matas Z et al (2009) Weight loss induced by nutritional and exercise intervention decreases arterial stiffness in obese subjects. Clin Nutr 28:21–25
27. Rider OJ, Tayal U, Francis JM et al (2010) The effect of obesity and weight loss on aortic pulse wave velocity as assessed by magnetic resonance imaging. Obesity (Silver Spring) 18(12):2311–2316
28. Barinas-Mitchell E, Kuller LH, Sutton-Tyrrell K et al (2006) Effect of weight loss and nutritional intervention on arterial stiffness in type 2 diabetes. Diabetes Care 29(10):2218–2222
29. Dengo AL, Dennis EA, Orr JS et al (2010) Arterial destiffening with weight loss in overweight and obese middle-aged and older adults. Hypertension 55(4):855–861
30. Ikonomidis I, Mazarakis A, Papadopoulos C et al (2007) Weight loss after bariatric surgery improves aortic elastic properties and left ventricular function in individuals with morbid obesity: a 3-year follow-up study. J Hypertens 25(2):439–447

31. Blumenthal JA, Babyak MA, Hinderliter A et al (2010) Effects of the DASH diet alone and in combination with exercise and weight loss on blood pressure and cardiovascular biomarkers in men and women with high blood pressure: the ENCORE study. Arch Intern Med 170(2): 126–135

32. Cooper JN, Buchanich JM, Youk A et al (2012) Reductions in arterial stiffness with weight loss in overweight and obese young adults: potential mechanisms. Atherosclerosis 223(2): 485–490

33. Hughes TM, Althouse AD, Niemczyk NA et al (2012) Effects of weight loss and insulin reduction on arterial stiffness in the SAVE trial. Cardiovasc Diabetol 11:114

34. Diamant M, Lamb HJ, van de Ree MA et al (2005) The association between abdominal visceral fat and carotid stiffness is mediated by circulating inflammatory markers in uncomplicated type 2 diabetes. J Clin Endocrinol Metab 90(3):1495–1501

35. Sutton-Tyrrell K, Newman A, Simonsick EM et al (2001) Aortic stiffness is associated with visceral adiposity in older adults enrolled in the study of health, aging, and body composition. Hypertension 38(3):429–433

36. Lee JW, Lee HR, Shim JY et al (2007) Viscerally obese women with normal body weight have greater brachial-ankle pulse wave velocity than nonviscerally obese women with excessive body weight. Clin Endocrinol (Oxf) 66(4):572–578

37. Ohashi N, Ito C, Fujikawa R et al (2009) The impact of visceral adipose tissue and high-molecular weight adiponectin on cardio-ankle vascular index in asymptomatic Japanese subjects. Metabolism 58(7):1023–1029

38. Orr JS, Gentile CL, Davy BM, Davy KP (2008) Large artery stiffening with weight gain in humans: role of visceral fat accumulation. Hypertension 51(6):1519–1524

39. Arner P, Backdahl J, Hemmingsson P et al (2014) Regional variations in the relationship between arterial stiffness and adipocyte volume or number in obese subjects. Int J Obes (Lond). doi:10.1038/ijo.2014.118

40. Kim BJ, Kim BS, Kang JH (2013) Echocardiographic epicardial fat thickness is associated with arterial stiffness. Int J Cardiol 167(5):2234–2238

41. Natale F, Tedesco MA, Mocerino R et al (2009) Visceral adiposity and arterial stiffness: echocardiographic epicardial fat thickness reflects, better than waist circumference, carotid arterial stiffness in a large population of hypertensives. Eur J Echocardiogr 10(4):549–555

42. Choi TY, Ahmadi N, Sourayanezhad S et al (2013) Relation of vascular stiffness with epicardial and pericardial adipose tissues, and coronary atherosclerosis. Atherosclerosis 229(1): 118–123

43. Huang Y, Bi Y, Xu M et al (2012) Nonalcoholic fatty liver disease is associated with atherosclerosis in middle-aged and elderly Chinese. Arterioscler Thromb Vasc Biol 32(9): 2321–2326

44. Vlachopoulos C, Manesis E, Baou K et al (2010) Increased arterial stiffness and impaired endothelial function in nonalcoholic fatty liver disease: a pilot study. Am J Hypertens 23(11): 1183–1189

45. Salvi P, Ruffini R, Agnoletti D et al (2010) Increased arterial stiffness in nonalcoholic fatty liver disease: the Cardio-GOOSE study. J Hypertens 28(8):1699–1707

46. Snijder MB, Henry RM, Visser M et al (2004) Regional body composition as a determinant of arterial stiffness in the elderly: the Hoorn study. J Hypertens 22(12):2339–2347

47. Lee M, Choh AC, Demerath EW et al (2012) Associations between trunk, leg and total body adiposity with arterial stiffness. Am J Hypertens 25(10):1131–1137

48. Frayn KN (2002) Adipose tissue as a buffer for daily lipid flux. Diabetologia 45(9): 1201–1210

49. Schouten F, Twisk JW, de Boer MR et al (2011) Increases in central fat mass and decreases in peripheral fat mass are associated with accelerated arterial stiffening in healthy adults: the Amsterdam Growth and Health Longitudinal Study. Am J Clin Nutr 94(1):40–48

50. Conus F, Rabasa-Lhoret R, Peronnet F (2007) Characteristics of metabolically obese normal-weight (MONW) subjects. Appl Physiol Nutr Metab 32(1):4–12

51. Ruderman N, Chisholm D, Pi-Sunyer X, Schneider S (1998) The metabolically obese, normal-weight individual revisited. Diabetes 47(5):699–713
52. Ochi M, Kohara K, Tabara Y et al (2010) Arterial stiffness is associated with low thigh muscle mass in middle-aged to elderly men. Atherosclerosis 212(1):327–332
53. Kim TN, Park MS, Lim KI et al (2011) Skeletal muscle mass to visceral fat area ratio is associated with metabolic syndrome and arterial stiffness: The Korean Sarcopenic Obesity Study (KSOS). Diabetes Res Clin Pract 93(2):285–291
54. Sanada K, Miyachi M, Tanimoto M et al (2010) A cross-sectional study of sarcopenia in Japanese men and women: reference values and association with cardiovascular risk factors. Eur J Appl Physiol 110(1):57–65
55. Kohara K, Ochi M, Tabara Y et al (2012) Arterial stiffness in sarcopenic visceral obesity in the elderly: J-SHIPP study. Int J Cardiol 158(1):146–148
56. Prado CM, Wells JC, Smith SR et al (2012) Sarcopenic obesity: a critical appraisal of the current evidence. Clin Nutr 31(5):583–601
57. Henry RM, Kostense PJ, Spijkerman AM et al (2003) Arterial stiffness increases with deteriorating glucose tolerance status: the Hoorn study. Circulation 107(16):2089–2095
58. van de Laar RJ, Ferreira I, van Mechelen W et al (2010) Lifetime vigorous but not light-to-moderate habitual physical activity impacts favorably on carotid stiffness in young adults: the Amsterdam Growth and Health Longitudinal Study. Hypertension 55(1):33–39
59. van de Laar RJ, Stehouwer CD, van Bussel BC et al (2013) Adherence to a Mediterranean dietary pattern in early life is associated with lower arterial stiffness in adulthood: the Amsterdam Growth and Health Longitudinal Study. J Intern Med 273(1):79–93
60. van de Laar RJ, Stehouwer CD, van Bussel BC et al (2012) Lower lifetime dietary fiber intake is associated with carotid artery stiffness: the Amsterdam Growth and Health Longitudinal Study. Am J Clin Nutr 96(1):14–23
61. van de Laar RJ, Stehouwer CD, Prins MH et al (2014) Self-reported time spent watching television is associated with arterial stiffness in young adults: the Amsterdam Growth and Health Longitudinal Study. Br J Sports Med 48(3):256–264
62. Abbatecola AM, Chiodini P, Gallo C et al (2012) Pulse wave velocity is associated with muscle mass decline: Health ABC study. Age (Dordr) 34(2):469–478
63. Scuteri A, Najjar SS, Muller DC et al (2004) Metabolic syndrome amplifies the age-associated increases in vascular thickness and stiffness. J Am Coll Cardiol 43(8):1388–1395
64. Scuteri A, Najjar SS, Orru M et al (2010) The central arterial burden of the metabolic syndrome is similar in men and women: the SardiNIA Study. Eur Heart J 31(5):602–613
65. Iannuzzi A, Licenziati MR, Acampora C et al (2006) Carotid artery stiffness in obese children with the metabolic syndrome. Am J Cardiol 97(4):528–531
66. Pandit D, Chiplonkar S, Khadilkar A et al (2011) Efficacy of a continuous metabolic syndrome score in Indian children for detecting subclinical atherosclerotic risk. Int J Obes (Lond) 35(10):1318–1324
67. Ferreira I, Henry RM, Twisk JW et al (2005) The metabolic syndrome, cardiopulmonary fitness, and subcutaneous trunk fat as independent determinants of arterial stiffness: the Amsterdam Growth and Health Longitudinal Study. Arch Intern Med 165(8):875–882
68. Li S, Chen W, Srinivasan SR, Berenson GS (2005) Influence of metabolic syndrome on arterial stiffness and its age-related change in young adults: the Bogalusa Heart Study. Atherosclerosis 180(2):349–354
69. Ferreira I, Boreham CA, Twisk JW et al (2007) Clustering of metabolic syndrome risk factors and arterial stiffness in young adults: the Northern Ireland Young Hearts Project. J Hypertens 25:1009–1020
70. Koskinen J, Magnussen CG, Viikari JS et al (2012) Effect of age, gender and cardiovascular risk factors on carotid distensibility during 6-year follow-up. The cardiovascular risk in Young Finns study. Atherosclerosis 224(2):474–479
71. Urbina EM, Srinivasan SR, Kieltyka RL et al (2004) Correlates of carotid artery stiffness in young adults: the Bogalusa Heart Study. Atherosclerosis 176(1):157–164

72. Della-Morte D, Gardener H, Denaro F et al (2010) Metabolic syndrome increases carotid artery stiffness: the Northern Manhattan Study. Int J Stroke 5(3):138–144
73. Protogerou AD, Blacher J, Aslangul E et al (2007) Gender influence on metabolic syndrome's effects on arterial stiffness and pressure wave reflections in treated hypertensive subjects. Atherosclerosis 193(1):151–158
74. Schillaci G, Pirro M, Vaudo G et al (2005) Metabolic syndrome is associated with aortic stiffness in untreated essential hypertension. Hypertension 45(6):1078–1082
75. Vyssoulis GP, Pietri PG, Karpanou EA et al (2010) Differential impact of metabolic syndrome on arterial stiffness and wave reflections: focus on distinct definitions. Int J Cardiol 138(2):119–125
76. Koivistoinen T, Hutri-Kahonen N, Juonala M et al (2011) Metabolic syndrome in childhood and increased arterial stiffness in adulthood: the cardiovascular risk in Young Finns Study. Ann Med 43(4):312–319
77. Nakanishi N, Suzuki K, Tatara K (2003) Clustered features of the metabolic syndrome and the risk for increased aortic pulse wave velocity in middle-aged Japanese men. Angiology 54(5):551–559
78. Safar ME, Thomas F, Blacher J et al (2006) Metabolic syndrome and age-related progression of aortic stiffness. J Am Coll Cardiol 47(1):72–75
79. Li CI, Kardia SL, Liu CS et al (2011) Metabolic syndrome is associated with change in subclinical arterial stiffness: a community-based Taichung Community Health Study. BMC Public Health 11:808
80. Ferreira I, Beijers HJ, Schouten F et al (2012) Clustering of metabolic syndrome traits is associated with maladaptive carotid remodeling and stiffening: a 6-year longitudinal study. Hypertension 60(2):542–549
81. Koskinen J, Magnussen CG, Taittonen L et al (2010) Arterial structure and function after recovery from the metabolic syndrome: the cardiovascular risk in Young Finns Study. Circulation 121(3):392–400
82. Tomiyama H, Hirayama Y, Hashimoto H et al (2006) The effects of changes in the metabolic syndrome detection status on arterial stiffening: a prospective study. Hypertens Res 29(9):673–678
83. Scuteri A, Cunha PG, Rosei EA et al (2014) Arterial stiffness and influences of the metabolic syndrome: a cross-countries study. Atherosclerosis 233(2):654–660
84. Guize L, Thomas F, Pannier B et al (2007) All-cause mortality associated with specific combinations of the metabolic syndrome according to recent definitions. Diabetes Care 30(9):2381–2387
85. Beijers HJ, Ferreira I, Bravenboer B et al (2014) Higher central fat mass and lower peripheral lean mass are independent determinants of endothelial dysfunction in the elderly: the Hoorn study. Atherosclerosis 233(1):310–318

Systemic Vasculitides

18

Dylan V. Miller and C. Taylor Duncan

18.1 Introduction/Overview

In this chapter, we will give a brief overview of the systemic vasculitides, excluding those directly caused by an infective agent. Systemic vasculitis is defined as widespread vascular inflammation, which may be a primary condition or consequent to another pathologic process. The vasculitides are a heterogenous group of diseases with poorly understood pathophysiology, making their classification a somewhat artificial and arbitrary attempt to segment entities along what is likely a continuous spectrum. In this chapter, we will examine systemic vasculitis syndromes according to the predominant size of the vessels it affects using the recently revised Chapel Hill Consensus Conference Nomenclature of Vasculitides standards [1].

Classifying vasculitides according to the type of affected vessel is clinically convenient, but also reflects differences in pathogenic mechanisms, since each division of the vascular tree has unique tissue architecture, cellular constituents, and dynamic physiology. The large vessels, namely, the aorta and its primary branches, are elastic arteries. These vessels function to accommodate the stroke volume from each ventricular contraction and then, by elastic recoil, maintain perfusion during diastole. Their structure reflects their highly elastic nature, being comprised almost entirely

D.V. Miller, MD (✉)
Pathology, Intermountain Medical Center/University of Utah,
Electron Microscopy Lab, Intermountain Central Lab,
5252 S Intermountain Dr., Murray, UT 84157, USA
e-mail: Dylan.Miller@imail.org

C.T. Duncan, MD
Internal Medicine, Intermountain Medical Center,
5121 S Cottonwood Street, Murray, UT 84157, USA
e-mail: ctaylorduncan@gmail.com

© Springer International Publishing Switzerland 2015
A. Berbari, G. Mancia (eds.), *Arterial Disorders:*
Definition, Clinical Manifestations, Mechanisms and Therapeutic Approaches,
DOI 10.1007/978-3-319-14556-3_18

by redundant layers of elastic tissue with intervening smooth muscle. Their thick walls require the presence of a rich network of vasa vasorum. The medium vessels are muscular arteries, most of which are named anatomically. These vessels experience pulsatile flow and have some elasticity, but also can dilate and constrict to modulate flow to downstream vascular beds. Their structure reflects these functions, being comprised of a thick muscular medial layer bounded by two distinct elastic lamellae. The small vessels include the remainder of the vessels – the arterioles, capillaries, venules, and veins (paradoxically including the larger named veins as well). This is a diverse group of vascular structures, but all lack a substantial medial smooth muscle and elastic component in comparison to the large- and medium-sized vessels. Tissue-level differences in the various divisions of the vascular tree likely account for differences in their observed pathology.

18.2 Large-Vessel Vasculitis

18.2.1 Giant Cell Arteritis

Giant cell arteritis (GCA), or temporal arteritis, largely affects the ascending aorta and extracranial branches of the carotid artery. This systemic vasculitis syndrome is characterized by segmental involvement of these vessels by granulomatous inflammation where histiocytes and T lymphocytes predominate. In the aorta, the inflammation leads to a loss of elastic tissue and progressive aneurysmal dilatation with risk of rupture. In smaller artery branches, the inflammation leads to progressive luminal occlusion and downstream ischemia.

18.2.1.1 Epidemiology
GCA is the most common of the systemic vasculitides with an incidence ranging from 1 in 100,000 individuals to 17.0 in 100,000 [2]. Affected patients are generally white (Scandinavian or other northern European ancestry) and 60 years or older. Women are affected two to three times more than men [3]. Approximately 50–75 % of patients are also affected by polymyalgia rheumatica, lending credence to an autoimmune hypothesis for this disease.

18.2.1.2 Pathology/Pathophysiology
GCA primarily affects the extracranial branches of the carotid arteries and less frequently the aorta and its proximal branches, particularly the subclavian artery. As noted previously, the pathologic findings in GCA include focal segments of granulomatous inflammation, often with skip areas of uninvolved artery. The term "granulomatous" reflects the predominance of histiocytes in the inflammatory milieu, including the occasional presence of the namesake multinucleated giant cell (Fig. 18.1). Despite the name, these giant cells are not always observed in GCA. While the term "granulomatous" is apt, true well-formed granulomas are not typically seen. Inflammation is associated with damage and destruction of elastic tissue. In the aorta, this leads to a pattern of vertical wrinkling that has been referred

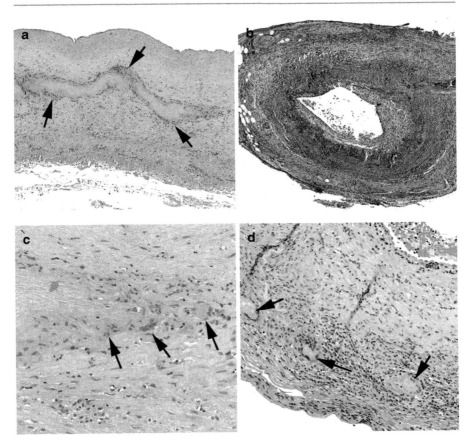

Fig. 18.1 Giant cell arteritis. (**a**) Low-power photomicrograph of aortitis due to giant cell arteritis with large-vessel involvement. In the middle of the aortic media (*arrows*) is a band of acellular collapsed elastic tissue surrounded by an inflammatory infiltrate. (**b**) Low-power photomicrograph of a temporal artery biopsy involved by giant cell arteritis. There is transmural inflammation, resulting in luminal narrowing. (**c**) Higher-power photomicrograph of the aortic wall seen in (**a**). The inflammation is rich in histiocytes and lymphocytes and includes multinucleated giant cells (*arrows*). (**d**) Higher-power photomicrograph of the temporal artery wall seen in (**b**). The inflammation is mixed but rich in histiocytes and lymphocytes and includes multinucleated giant cells (*arrows*)

to as having a "tree bark" appearance (Fig. 18.2). The pathophysiology is still being elucidated, but likely involves a loss of self-tolerance to antigens in the elastic artery walls and/or vasa vasorum due to senescence of the aging immune system. The apparent conundrum of discrete involvement of the largest artery as well as very peripheral branches has led to speculation that the aortic disease may be secondary to adventitial vasa vasorum involvement since these vessels are closer in caliber to the temporal artery.

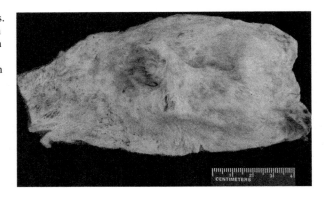

Fig. 18.2 Giant cell arteritis. An opened surgical resection specimen from a patient with ascending aortic aneurysm due to giant cell arteritis with large-vessel involvement. Note the linear wrinkles that have been described as having a "tree bark" appearance. These result from scar replacement of elastic tissue in the aortic wall

18.2.1.3 Presentation/Diagnosis

GCA is a clinical diagnosis, incorporating both symptoms and laboratory markers of inflammation. The gold standard for diagnosis remains temporal artery biopsy. Patients typically present with symptoms such as unilateral headache, fatigue, fever, jaw pain, myalgias, and diaphoresis [4]. High morbidity may occur from permanent vision loss due to inflammation of the ophthalmic artery. Additionally, there is a markedly increased risk of ascending aortic aneurysms and aortic rupture in patients diagnosed with GCA [5].

18.2.1.4 Treatment

Treatment consists of a long course of high-dose corticosteroids. Treatment is often started empirically, before biopsy results, as vision may be at risk (retinal artery occlusion) if treatment is delayed [6].

18.2.2 Takayasu Arteritis

Takayasu arteritis is a chronic granulomatous inflammatory disease of unknown etiology that affects the aorta and its primary branches, but not the small carotid artery branches. It is also distinguished from GCA in that it almost exclusively affects younger women, often of Asian ancestry [7].

18.2.2.1 Epidemiology

Takayasu arteritis has an estimated incidence of 1.2/1,000,000–2.6/1,000,000 individuals annually. It is a disease of adolescents and young adults. While the diagnostic age criterion is <50 years of age [2], the great majority have signs or symptoms decades before age 50.

18.2.2.2 Pathology/Pathophysiology

Like GCA, Takayasu arteritis is characterized by focal granulomatous inflammation of the large vessels. Unlike GCA, the adventitial inflammation is typically more impressive than medial inflammation (Fig. 18.3). Neutrophils and areas of necrosis may be seen as well. The etiology and pathogenesis are not well understood,

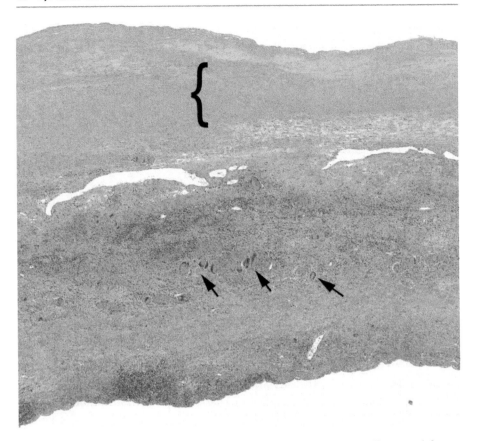

Fig. 18.3 Takayasu arteritis. Low-power photomicrograph of an aortic wall removed from a patient with Takayasu arteritis showing inflammation throughout the wall. The media is demarcated by a ({) symbol. Most of the wall thickness is a result of adventitial inflammation and fibrosis. Multinucleated giant cells (*arrows*) can be seen even at low magnification

although the apparent aggressiveness of this disease suggests a more active T-cell-mediated process with acute inflammation, followed by necrosis, neovascularization, intimal proliferation with smooth muscle integration, and finally giant cell formation in the remodeled vessel walls [7].

18.2.2.3 Presentation/Diagnosis

Aortitis with ascending aortic aneurysm is the most common presentation. The affected aortic branches (subclavian, carotid, renal, mesenteric) are prone to obstructive stenosis, so Takayasu arteritis is also known as "pulseless disease." Patients initially present with systemic symptoms such as fevers, chills, malaise, diaphoresis, myalgias, anorexia, and weight loss. Patients often progress to vascular complications such as stenosis, occlusions, and cerebrovascular events. Diagnostic criteria have been delineated by both the American College of Rheumatology and the Ishikawa Criteria.

18.2.2.4 Treatment

Treatment for Takayasu arteritis generally consists of a long course of immunosuppression with corticosteroids and additional immunomodulatory agents depending on disease severity and acuity [8].

18.3   Medium-Vessel Vasculitis

18.3.1 Polyarteritis Nodosa

Polyarteritis nodosa (PAN) is the prototypic medium-vessel vasculitis, showing transmural necrotizing arteritis of medium-sized arteries. It is not associated with antineutrophilic cytoplasmic antibodies (ANCAs). Arterioles, capillaries, venules, and glomeruli are spared. Additionally, the current definition of PAN excludes hepatitis B-associated vasculitis, a specific disease once considered a variant of PAN [1, 9].

18.3.1.1 Epidemiology

PAN is a relatively uncommon disease, occurring in an estimated 4–9/1,000,000 individuals [10]. Previous estimates were much higher prior to reclassification of the disease to exclude hepatitis B-associated vasculitis.

18.3.1.2 Pathology/Pathophysiology

PAN is a systemic, transmural necrotizing vasculitis of the medium-sized vessels. The transmural vessel wall damage leads to pseudoaneurysm (contained rupture) formation in the affected vessels. The size of the pseudoaneurysms is many times greater than the adjacent vessel diameter and they often thrombose, leading to the appearance of nodules, hence "nodosa" (Fig. 18.4). The majority of cases affect the kidneys, gastrointestinal tract, and skin [11]. CNS involvement is rare. Temporal variability (both recent and old lesions present at the time of diagnosis) is a hallmark of PAN. The etiology of PAN is unknown. Innate and humoral immunity likely participate given the rapid and destructive nature of the immune response. A large portion of previous PAN diagnoses were likely hepatitis B-associated vasculitis, confounding much of the previous research on PAN [12].

18.3.1.3 Presentation/Diagnosis

Patients often present with specific signs and symptoms due to ischemic or inflammatory damage to specific organs [9]. Additionally, constitutional symptoms are common with fevers, myalgias, skin lesions, and abdominal pain [13].

18.3.1.4 Treatment

Treatment of PAN involves high-dose corticosteroids with the addition of cyclophosphamide and other cytotoxic agents for more severe cases [14].

Fig. 18.4 Polyarteritis nodosa. (**a**) Mesenteric artery angiogram in a patient with polyarteritis nodosa showing multiple nodular pseudoaneurysms (*arrows*). (**b**) Low-power photomicrograph of a pseudoaneurysm in polyarteritis nodosa. The collapsed elastic laminae represent the former true lumen; the *arrow* indicates the aneurysm formed by contained rupture of the native artery

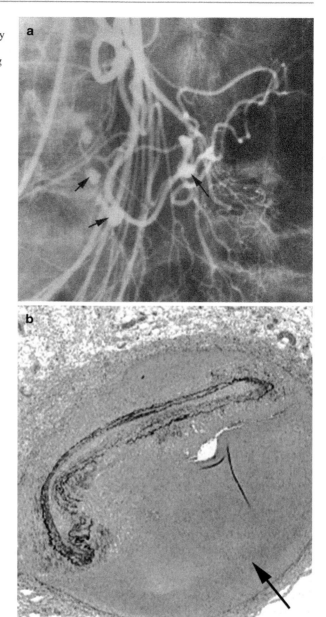

18.3.2 Kawasaki Disease

Kawasaki disease (KD) is an arteritis predominantly involving medium and small arteries. It is associated with mucocutaneous lymph node syndrome.

Fig. 18.5 Kawasaki disease.
Right coronary artery
angiogram showing a
pseudoaneurysm in an adult
patient who had Kawasaki
disease as a child

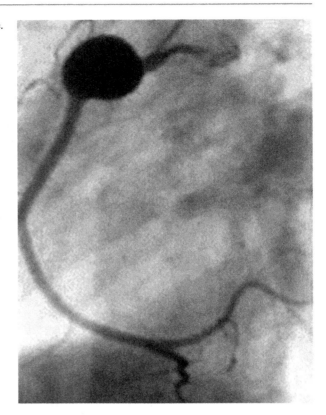

18.3.2.1 Epidemiology

KD is most common in infants and young children although its sequelae are life-long. KD incidence in the United States is approximately 17–20/100,000 individuals; however, it is significantly more common in East Asians with an incidence of approximately 220/100,000 [15]. In the developed world, as rheumatic heart disease has declined in recent decades, KD has become the leading cause of acquired cardiovascular disease in children [16].

18.3.2.2 Pathology/Pathophysiology

The etiology of KD is still unknown. A growing body of evidence indicates autoimmune reactivity to viral proteins (mimicry) influenced by a genetic predisposition [17]. The most important consequence of KD is acquired cardiovascular disease due to coronary artery vasculitis with pseudoaneurysm formation (Fig. 18.5). The vascular lesions consist of a transmural inflammation with eventual accumulation macrophages and IgA plasma cells [18]. Severe damage to all layers of the arterial wall occurs, weakening the wall and leading to pseudoaneurysm formation in a fashion similar to PAN [19].

18.3.2.3 Presentation/Diagnosis

KD is a clinical diagnosis based on these criteria: (1) fever for 5 or more days, (2) bilateral conjunctival congestion, (3) changes in the lips and oral cavity, (4) polymorphous exanthema, (5) changes in peripheral extremities including erythema or desquamation, and (6) acute non-purulent cervical lymphadenopathy [20]. Coronary pseudoaneurysms may not be present in the early phases of illness and coronary arteritis may not be apparent until later on.

18.3.2.4 Treatment

Treatment consists of high-dose intravenous immunoglobulin [21]. Prompt treatment decreases the likelihood of progression to coronary artery abnormalities. A variety of other immunomodulatory treatments have been attempted with varied success. High-dose intravenous immunoglobulin remains the first-line treatment [22].

18.4   Small-Vessel Vasculitis

18.4.1 ANCA Associated

18.4.1.1 Granulomatosis with Polyangiitis (Wegener's)

Granulomatosis with polyangiitis (GPA) also termed "Wegener's granulomatosis" is a necrotizing vasculitis of the respiratory tract and small- to medium-sized vessels. Renal involvement is common.

Epidemiology

GPA is a relatively uncommon systemic vasculitis with an estimated prevalence of 3/100,000 [23]. Mean age of diagnosis is approximately 50 years old with no clear sex predilection [24].

Pathology/Pathophysiology

Like PAN and KD, the inflammation in GPA and the other small-vessel vasculitis syndromes is acute and necrotizing. Small-vessel vasculitis typically manifests in capillary-sized vessels, particularly in the renal glomerulus and alveolar capillaries of the lung. GPA has three major pathologic features: necrotizing granulomas of the respiratory tract, granulomatous necrotizing vasculitis of small (and medium) vessels, and necrotizing crescentic glomerulonephritis [25] (Fig. 18.6).

Presentation/Diagnosis

Patients often present with respiratory complaints, both lower and upper respiratory tract. This includes nasal septum ulceration, subglottic stenosis, hemoptysis, pneumonias, and eye irritation. The so-called pulmonary-renal syndrome is the combination of these signs and symptoms with glomerulonephritis [24]. GPA is a clinical diagnosis with two or more of the following criteria to be met: nasal or oral inflammation, abnormal chest imaging, hematuria, and granulomatous inflammation on a biopsy specimen [26]. Antibodies against the neutrophil cytoplasmic protein

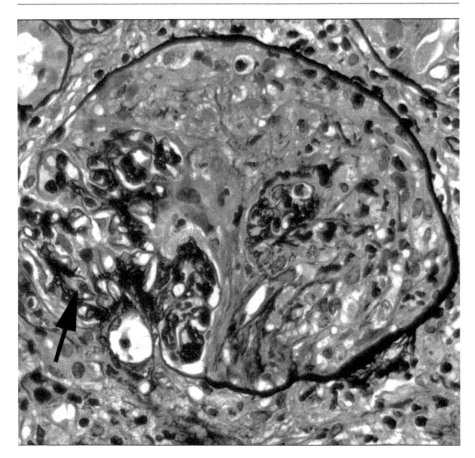

Fig. 18.6 Granulomatosis with polyangiitis. High-power photomicrograph of a glomerulus affected by necrotizing crescentic glomerulonephritis in a patient with positive PR3/c-ANCA. Residual intact glomerular capillaries are seen in the lower left (*arrow*). The rest of Bowman's space is occupied by proliferating parietal epithelial cells, leukocytes, and organizing fibrin

protease 3 (PR3) can be detected in the serum. In mouse neutrophil staining assays, this autoantibody yields a cytoplasmic staining pattern (c-ANCA) (Fig. 18.7).

Treatment
Treatment for GPA generally consists of a long course of cyclophosphamide and prednisone [27]. GPA portended an extremely high mortality prior to development of effective treatment strategies (mean survival of less than 5 months and a 2-year mortality of 93 % [27, 28]). This is no longer the case, although GPA can have relapsing-remitting nature with up to 50 % recurrence despite aggressive treatment. There is still significant disease morbidity as well [28, 29].

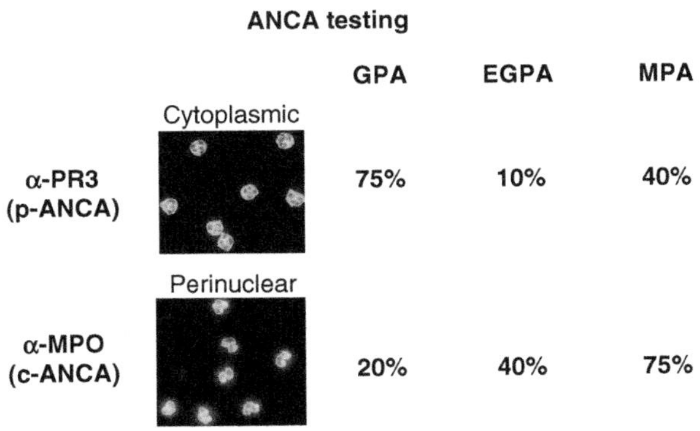

Fig. 18.7 Antineutrophil
cytoplasmic antibody testing.
(*Abbreviations*: *ANCA*
antineutrophil cytoplasmic
antibody, *PR3* proteinase 3,
MPO myeloperoxidase, *GPA*
granulomatosis with
polyangiitis, *EGPA*
eosinophilic granulomatosis
with polyangiitis, *MPA*
microscopic polyangiitis)

ANCA testing

	GPA	EGPA	MPA
α-PR3 (p-ANCA) Cytoplasmic	75%	10%	40%
α-MPO (c-ANCA) Perinuclear	20%	40%	75%

18.4.1.2 Eosinophilic Granulomatosis with Polyangiitis (Churg-Strauss Syndrome)

Eosinophilic granulomatosis with polyangiitis (EGPA), formerly Churg-Strauss syndrome, is a necrotizing granulomatous small-vessel vasculitis with extensive eosinophilia that is associated with asthma [1].

Epidemiology

EGPA typically develops in asthmatic patients in their fifth decade of life, and recent data indicate 5-year survival at greater than 90 % with appropriate therapy [30]. Epidemiologic data varies widely regarding EGPA with incidence reports ranging between 0.5 per million and 70 per million individuals [31], depending on the population.

Pathology/Pathophysiology

EGPA is a systemic vasculitis affecting small to medium vessels and is associated with asthma and eosinophilia. Necrotizing vasculitis with eosinophilia and a variable granulomatous component is found on histologic examination of affected tissues (e.g., lung and kidney) [32]. Lesions are often found in the upper airways, heart, skin, and neurovascular bundles as well. Antibodies directed against the neutrophil cytoplasmic protein myeloperoxidase (MPO) can be detected in the serum. In mouse neutrophil staining assays, this autoantibody yields a perinuclear staining pattern (p-ANCA). MPO-ANCA is detected in ~40 % of cases and indicates a worse prognosis [33] when present. The etiology is not well understood, but the association with asthma suggests a common underlying immune mechanism.

Presentation/Diagnosis

Patients almost always have preexisting asthma or develop adult-onset asthma. Patients then begin to experience systemic symptoms such as fevers, malaise, anorexia, and weight loss. Additional symptoms affecting the sinuses and upper respiratory system are frequent [34]. Diagnosis is made when a patient presents with a history of asthma, eosinophilia, and systemic vasculitis [35].

Treatment

Treatment for EGPA consists of a long course of corticosteroids with or without the addition of cyclophosphamide depending upon disease severity [36].

18.4.1.3 Microscopic Polyangiitis

Microscopic polyangiitis (MPA) is an uncommon necrotizing vasculitis affecting small vessels. Like GPA and EGPA, MPA is pauci-immune process. While ANCA may be detectable in serum, no bound antibody or immune complexes are demonstrated by tissue pathology techniques [1]. This is because antibody-mediated neutrophil damage occurs in the peripheral circulation, and the dying neutrophils lodge in the capillary beds (especially renal and pulmonary capillaries) and release their toxic contents. Antibody and immune complexes are absent in the tissue by immunofluorescence techniques at this stage of the disease.

Epidemiology

MPA is a relatively uncommon vasculitis, with prevalence estimates ranging from 2.7 to 94 cases per million individuals in Europe [37, 38]. Typical age of onset is in the fifth decade of life with no sex predilection [39].

Pathology/Pathophysiology

MPA is an ANCA-associated vasculitis with approximately 75 % of patients displaying p/MPO-ANCA in the serum [38]. One of the hallmarks of MPA is rapidly progressive glomerulonephritis, with corresponding crescentic glomerulonephritis on histologic examination [39]. Renal findings are indistinguishable from the other ANCA-associated vasculitides (GPA and EGPA). Pulmonary capillaritis may also be seen and often progresses to mild to moderate alveolar hemorrhage. Palpable purpura may develop, due to leukocytoclastic vasculitis on histologic examination of skin biopsies [40]. No more is known about the etiology of this syndrome than for the other ANCA-associated diseases.

Presentation/Diagnosis

Patients typically initially present with systemic symptoms, such as fever or weight loss, and a multitude of vague complaints that often delay diagnosis [41]. As the disease progresses, glomerulonephritis and pulmonary symptoms, such as shortness of breath and hemoptysis, develop [38]. Abdominal pain, peripheral neuropathy, and skin lesions are common [39].

Treatment

Treatment for MPA consists of a long course of corticosteroids with or without the addition of cyclophosphamide or other similar agents depending upon disease severity [38]. The 5-year survival rate is approximately 75 % with appropriate treatment [39, 41].

18.4.2 Autoantibody or Immune Complex Associated

18.4.2.1 Anti-GBM (Goodpasture's)

Anti-glomerular basement membrane (GBM) disease, or Goodpasture's syndrome, is a small-vessel vasculitis caused by direct binding of anti-GBM autoantibodies, primarily affecting the kidneys and/or lungs [1].

Epidemiology

Anti-GBM disease is very rare with an estimated prevalence of one case per one million individuals [42]. Men are affected slightly more than women and individuals with toxic pulmonary exposures such as smoking, cocaine, or inhaled solvents may have an increased risk of developing the disease [42, 43].

Pathology/Pathophysiology

The pathophysiology is better understood than for most of the small-vessel vasculitides. Autoantibodies are developed against type IV collagenous epitopes in basement membranes. These autoantibodies bind the basement membrane of the glomerular and pulmonary alveolar capillaries. Complement is activating by bound antibody and resulting cascade of cytotoxic and chemotactic events leads to significant vascular inflammation and destruction [44]. Crescentic glomerulonephritis is the hallmark lesion in the kidney and neutrophilic alveolitis is seen in the lung. Unlike the ANCA-mediated diseases, these patterns are accompanied by bright linear staining of basement membranes using immunofluorescence methods to detect bound immunoglobulin [45].

Presentation/Diagnosis

Patients typically present with shortness of breath, fatigue, hemoptysis, and hematuria with rapidly progressive nephritis [43]. Detecting anti-GBM autoantibodies in the serum is confirmatory [44].

Treatment

Treatment consists of plasmapheresis to remove the anti-GBM antibody and a long course of corticosteroids with or without the addition of cytotoxic agents depending upon disease severity [43, 46].

18.4.2.2 IgA Vasculitis (Henoch-Schönlein)

IgA vasculitis (IGAV) (including Henoch-Schönlein purpura) is an IgA-mediated small-vessel vasculitis [1]. Henoch-Schönlein purpura is a sub-variant of IGAV with a specific prototypical presentation that includes systemic manifestations in the skin, kidneys, and intestinal tract.

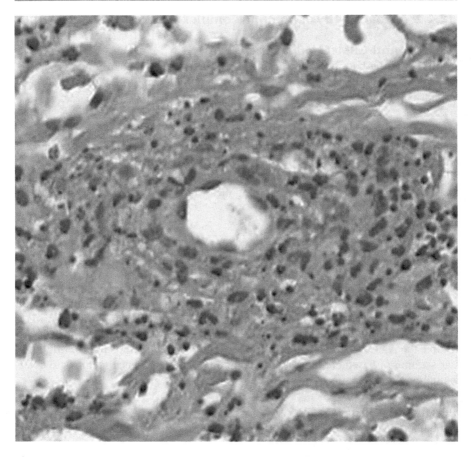

Fig. 18.8 Leukocytoclastic vasculitis. High-power photomicrograph of a small cutaneous vessel showing neutrophil-rich inflammation with fibrinoid necrosis and extravasation of red and white blood cells

Epidemiology

IGAV is the most common childhood vasculitis and one of the most common vasculitides in general. Its incidence is approximately 20 per 100,000 individuals. Ninety percent of patients are under the age of 10 with a male predominance of 2:1 [47].

Pathology/Pathophysiology

On histologic and immunopathologic examination, IgA immune deposits in vessel walls are seen with associated inflammation [48, 49]. Biopsy specimens of the typical palpable purpuric skin lesions show a leukocytoclastic vasculitis with prominent neutrophils, fibrinoid necrosis, and extravasation of capillary contents [48, 49] (Fig. 18.8). Patients are noted to have increased plasma levels of IgA and IgA immune complexes [50].

Presentation/Diagnosis

Patients typically present with palpable purpura on the lower extremities, arthralgias, abdominal pain, and occasional gastrointestinal bleeding [50]. Palpable purpura is present in almost all adult cases of IGAV/Henoch-Schönlein purpura [51].

Treatment

Treatment for IGAV is generally supportive [52, 53]. While short-term benefit may be seen in active disease and more severe Henoch-Schönlein purpura, studies of long-term corticosteroids have consistently shown little benefit [50, 54, 55]. In children, there is significant morbidity from permanent renal disease in a small subset of patients, but IGAV is typically a self-limiting disease with very low mortality [50, 54]. IGAV in adults, while much less common, has a worse prognosis with approximately 80 % of patients developing chronic kidney disease and 25 % mortality in some studies [51].

18.5 Variable-Vessel Vasculitis

18.5.1 Behcet's Disease

Intro/Etiology: Behcet's disease is a variable-vessel vasculitis (involving any size vessel, though small vessels are the most frequently involved) causing a variety of vascular pathologies in addition to recurrent oral and genital ulcers and diffuse inflammatory lesions [1].

Epidemiology: A wide range of prevalence figures have been reported for Behcet's, ranging from 1 to over 400 per 1,000,000. This disease is most common among patients with Mediterranean or Asian ancestry.

Pathology/Pathophysiology: Histology of the cutaneous/mucosal lesions in Behcet's shows leukocytoclastic vasculitis, fibrinoid necrosis of small vessels with abundant neutrophils. The etiology is largely unknown.

Presentation/Diagnosis: Although patients may have diffuse systemic symptoms including fatigue, weight loss, and fevers, inflammatory ophthalmic processes are often the initial diagnostic symptom in BD [56]. BD is a clinical diagnosis that requires oral ulcerations plus any two of eye lesions, skin lesions, positive pathergy test, or genital ulcerations [57, 58].

Treatment: The most appropriate therapy for Behcet's disease varies according to severity. For cutaneous/mucosal ulcers, topical steroids may be sufficient. For more systemic involvement, more aggressive immunosuppression may be warranted.

18.6 Other Vasculitis Syndromes

This chapter does not exhaustively cover of all described vasculitis syndromes. The small-vessel vasculitis syndromes in particular comprise a long and growing list including systemic lupus erythematosus, rheumatoid arthritis-associated vasculitis, sarcoid vasculitis, cryoglobulinemic vasculitis, hypocomplementemic urticarial vasculitis, and vasculitides associated with hepatitis B, hepatitis C, and certain drugs and as a paraneoplastic syndrome associated with a number of malignancies. Additional medium- and large-vessel vasculitis syndromes include Cogan syndrome, ankylosing spondylitis-associated vasculitis, and IgG4-related fibrosing disease. There are also a number of organ-confined (nonsystemic) forms of vasculitis, including cutaneous leukocytoclastic angiitis, primary CNS vasculitis, and isolated aortitis.

Conclusions

Systemic vasculitis syndromes represent a wide and varied array of entities, the great majority of which are poorly understood in terms of their underlying pathogenic mechanisms and most appropriate and effective therapies. Further investigation at the bench and bedside is needed to illuminate these and improve the care of patients living with and dying from these diseases.

References

1. Jennette JC, Falk RJ, Bacon PA et al (2013) 2012 revised International Chapel Hill Consensus Conference nomenclature of vasculitides. Arthritis Rheum 65:1–11
2. Richards BL, March L, Gabriel SE (2010) Epidemiology of large-vessel vasculidities. Best Pract Res Clin Rheumatol 24:871–883
3. Kisza K, Murchison AP, Dai Y et al (2013) Giant cell arteritis incidence: analysis by season and year in mid-Atlantic United States. Clin Experiment Ophthalmol 41:577–581
4. Borchers AT, Gershwin ME (2012) Giant cell arteritis: a review of classification, pathophysiology, geoepidemiology and treatment. Autoimmun Rev 11:A544–A554
5. Robson JC, Kiran A, Maskell J et al (2015) The relative risk of aortic aneurysm in patients with giant cell arteritis compared with the general population of the UK. Ann Rheum Dis. 74:129–135
6. Salvarani C, Cantini F, Hunder GG (2008) Polymyalgia rheumatica and giant-cell arteritis. Lancet 372:234–245
7. Vaideeswar P, Deshpande JR (2013) Pathology of Takayasu arteritis: a brief review. Ann Pediatr Cardiol 6:52–58
8. Keser G, Direskeneli H, Aksu K (2014) Management of Takayasu arteritis: a systematic review. Rheumatology (Oxford) 53:793–801
9. Colmegna I, Maldonado-Cocco JA (2005) Polyarteritis nodosa revisited. Curr Rheumatol Rep 7:288–296
10. Conn DL (1990) Polyarteritis. Rheum Dis Clin North Am 16:341–362
11. Stanson AW, Friese JL, Johnson CM et al (2001) Polyarteritis nodosa: spectrum of angiographic findings. Radiographics 21:151–159
12. Guillevin L, Mahr A, Callard P et al (2005) Hepatitis B virus-associated polyarteritis nodosa: clinical characteristics, outcome, and impact of treatment in 115 patients. Medicine (Baltimore) 84:313–322
13. Eleftheriou D, Dillon MJ, Tullus K et al (2013) Systemic polyarteritis nodosa in the young: a single-center experience over thirty-two years. Arthritis Rheum 65:2476–2485
14. De Menthon M, Mahr A (2011) Treating polyarteritis nodosa: current state of the art. Clin Exp Rheumatol 29:S110–S116
15. Uehara R, Belay ED (2012) Epidemiology of Kawasaki disease in Asia, Europe, and the United States. J Epidemiol 22:79–85

16. Newburger JW, Takahashi M, Gerber MA et al (2004) Diagnosis, treatment, and long-term management of Kawasaki disease: a statement for health professionals from the Committee on Rheumatic Fever, Endocarditis, and Kawasaki Disease, Council on Cardiovascular Disease in the Young, American Heart Association. Pediatrics 114:1708–1733
17. Rowley AH (2011) Kawasaki disease: novel insights into etiology and genetic susceptibility. Annu Rev Med 62:69–77
18. Takahashi K, Oharaseki T, Yokouchi Y et al (2010) Kawasaki disease as a systemic vasculitis in childhood. Ann Vasc Dis 3:173–181
19. Takahashi K, Oharaseki T, Yokouchi Y (2011) Pathogenesis of Kawasaki disease. Clin Exp Immunol 164(Suppl):20–22
20. Ayusawa M, Sonobe T, Uemura S et al (2005) Revision of diagnostic guidelines for Kawasaki disease (the 5th revised edition). Pediatr Int 47:232–234
21. Furusho K, Kamiya T, Nakano H et al (1984) High-dose intravenous gammaglobulin for Kawasaki disease. Lancet 2:1055–1058
22. Luca NJC, Yeung RSM (2012) Epidemiology and management of Kawasaki disease. Drugs 72:1029–1038
23. Cotch MF et al (1996) The epidemiology of Wegener's granulomatosis. Estimates of the five-year period prevalence, annual mortality, and geographic disease distribution from population-based data sources. Arthritis Rheum 39:87–92
24. Wung PK, Stone JH (2006) Therapeutics of Wegener's granulomatosis. Nat Clin Pract Rheumatol 2:192–200
25. Cabral DA, Uribe AG, Benseler S et al (2009) Classification, presentation, and initial treatment of Wegener's granulomatosis in childhood. Arthritis Rheum 60:3413–3424
26. Jennette JC, Falk RJ, Andrassy K et al (1994) Nomenclature of systemic vasculitides. Arthritis Rheum 37:187–192
27. Riccieri V, Valesini G (2004) Treatment of Wegener's granulomatosis. Reumatismo 56:69–76
28. Mahr A (2001) Analysis of factors predictive of survival based on 49 patients with systemic Wegener's granulomatosis and prospective follow-up. Rheumatology 40:492–498
29. Hoffman GS (1993) Wegener's granulomatosis. Curr Opin Rheumatol 5:11–17
30. Dunogué B, Pagnoux C, Guillevin L (2011) Churg-Strauss syndrome: clinical symptoms, complementary investigations, prognosis and outcome, and treatment. Semin Respir Crit Care Med 32:298–309
31. Noth I, Strek ME, Leff AR (2003) Churg-Strauss syndrome. Lancet 361:587–594
32. Vaglio A, Buzio C, Zwerina J (2013) Eosinophilic granulomatosis with polyangiitis (Churg-Strauss): state of the art. Allergy 68:261–273
33. Mahr A, Moosig F, Neumann T et al (2014) Eosinophilic granulomatosis with polyangiitis (Churg-Strauss): evolutions in classification, etiopathogenesis, assessment and management. Curr Opin Rheumatol 26:16–23
34. Comarmond C, Pagnoux C, Khellaf M et al (2013) Eosinophilic granulomatosis with polyangiitis (Churg-Strauss): clinical characteristics and long-term follow up of the 383 patients enrolled in the French Vasculitis Study Group cohort. Arthritis Rheum 65:270–281
35. Lanham JG, Elkon KB, Pusey CD, Hughes GR (1984) Systemic vasculitis with asthma and eosinophilia: a clinical approach to the Churg-Strauss syndrome. Med (Baltimore) 63:65–81
36. Samson M, Puechal X, Devilliers H et al (2013) Long-term outcomes of 118 patients with eosinophilic granulomatosis with polyangiitis (Churg-Strauss syndrome) enrolled in two prospective trials. J Autoimmun 43:60–69
37. Mohammad AJ, Jacobsson LTH, Mahr AD et al (2007) Prevalence of Wegener's granulomatosis, microscopic polyangiitis, polyarteritis nodosa and Churg-Strauss syndrome within a defined population in southern Sweden. Rheumatology (Oxford) 46:1329–1337
38. Chung SA, Seo P (2010) Microscopic polyangiitis. Rheum Dis Clin North Am 36:545–558
39. Guillevin L, Durand-Gasselin B, Cevallos R et al (1999) Microscopic polyangiitis: clinical and laboratory findings in eighty-five patients. Arthritis Rheum 42:421–430
40. Kawakami T, Soma Y, Saito C et al (2006) Cutaneous manifestations in patients with microscopic polyangiitis: two case reports and a minireview. Acta Derm Venereol 86:144–147

41. Agard C, Mouthon L, Mahr A, Guillevin L (2003) Microscopic polyangiitis and polyarteritis nodosa: how and when do they start? Arthritis Rheum 49:709–715
42. Salama AD, Levy JB, Lightstone L, Pusey CD (2001) Goodpasture's disease. Lancet 358: 917–920
43. Chan AL, Louie S, Leslie KO et al (2011) Cutting edge issues in Goodpasture's disease. Clin Rev Allergy Immunol 41:151–162
44. Hellmark T, Segelmark M (2014) Diagnosis and classification of Goodpasture's disease (anti-GBM). J Autoimmun 48–49:108–112
45. Syeda UA, Singer NG, Magrey M (2013) Anti-glomerular basement membrane antibody disease treated with rituximab: a case-based review. Semin Arthritis Rheum 42:567–572
46. Levin M, Rigden SP, Pincott JR et al (1983) Goodpasture's syndrome: treatment with plasma-pheresis, immunosuppression, and anticoagulation. Arch Dis Child 58:697–702
47. Gardner-Medwin JMM, Dolezalova P, Cummins C, Southwood TR (2002) Incidence of Henoch-Schönlein purpura, Kawasaki disease, and rare vasculitides in children of different ethnic origins. Lancet 360:1197–1202
48. Yang Y-H, Yu H-H, Chiang B-L (2014) The diagnosis and classification of Henoch-Schönlein purpura: an updated review. Autoimmun Rev. doi:10.1016/j.autrev.2014.01.031
49. Linskey KR, Kroshinsky D, Mihm MC, Hoang MP (2012) Immunoglobulin-A–associated small-vessel vasculitis: a 10-year experience at the Massachusetts General Hospital. J Am Acad Dermatol 66:813–822
50. Saulsbury FT (1999) Henoch-Schönlein purpura in children. Report of 100 patients and review of the literature. Med (Baltimore) 78:395–409
51. Pillebout E, Thervet E, Hill G et al (2002) Henoch-Schönlein Purpura in adults: outcome and prognostic factors. J Am Soc Nephrol 13:1271–1278
52. Chartapisak W, Opastirakul S, Hodson EM et al (2009) Interventions for preventing and treating kidney disease in Henoch-Schönlein Purpura (HSP). Cochrane database Syst Rev (3):CD005128. doi:10.1002/14651858.CD005128.pub2
53. Trnka P (2013) Henoch-Schönlein purpura in children. J Paediatr Child Health 49:995–1003
54. Trapani S, Micheli A, Grisolia F et al (2005) Henoch Schonlein purpura in childhood: epidemiological and clinical analysis of 150 cases over a 5-year period and review of literature. Semin Arthritis Rheum 35:143–153
55. Bayrakci US, Topaloglu R, Soylemezoglu O et al (2007) Effect of early corticosteroid therapy on development of Henoch-Schönlein nephritis. J Nephrol 20:406–409
56. Tugal-Tutkun I, Onal S, Altan-Yaycioglu R et al (2004) Uveitis in Behçet disease: an analysis of 880 patients. Am J Ophthalmol 138:373–380
57. International Study Group for Behçet's Disease (1990) Criteria for diagnosis of Behçet's disease. Lancet 335:1078–1080
58. O'Neill TW, Rigby AS, Silman AJ, Barnes C (1994) Validation of the International Study Group criteria for Behçet's disease. Br J Rheumatol 33:115–117

Marfan Syndrome and Related Heritable Thoracic Aortic Aneurysms and Dissections

19

Julie De Backer and Marjolijn Renard

In this chapter, we wish to provide an overview and address a number of recent developments regarding aetiology, clinical aspects and treatment of heritable thoracic aortic disease. We want to focus on monogenetic disorders related to aortic aneurysms which are admittedly rare but provide a unique basis for the study of underlying pathogenetic pathways in the complex disease process of aneurysm formation. Understanding these pathomechanisms may lead to the identification of new treatment targets and improved management.

Within this group of disease entities, Marfan syndrome is considered as a paradigm entity, and many insights are derived from the study of clinical, genetic and animal models for Marfan syndrome. We will therefore provide a detailed overview of the various aspects of Marfan syndrome and end with an overview of related syndromes.

19.1 Marfan Syndrome

19.1.1 Definitions and Diagnosis

Marfan syndrome (MFS) is an inherited connective tissue disorder, caused by mutations in the fibrillin-1 gene (*FBN1*) [1], affecting approximately 1 in 5,000 individuals with no gender, ethnic or racial predilection.

J. De Backer, MD, PhD (✉)
Department of Cardiology and Medical Genetics, University Hospital Ghent,
Belgium, De Pintelaan 185, Ghent 9000, Belgium
e-mail: Julie.debacker@ugent.be

M. Renard, PhD
Center for Medical Genetics, University Hospital Ghent,
Belgium, De Pintelaan 185, Ghent 9000, Belgium
e-mail: Marjolijn.renard@ugent.be

© Springer International Publishing Switzerland 2015
A. Berbari, G. Mancia (eds.), *Arterial Disorders:*
Definition, Clinical Manifestations, Mechanisms and Therapeutic Approaches,
DOI 10.1007/978-3-319-14556-3_19

267

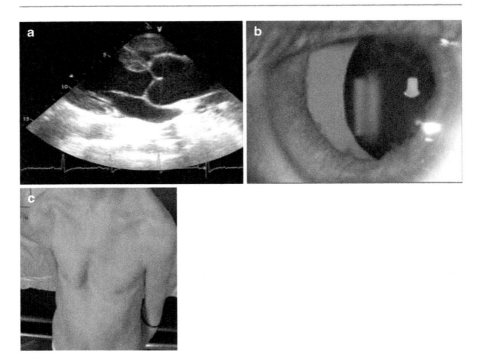

Fig. 19.1 Main clinical features of Marfan syndrome. (**a**) Aortic root dilatation; (**b**) ectopia lentis; (**c**) skeletal abnormalities

Marfan syndrome is diagnosed on the basis of distinct clinical criteria defined in the revised Ghent nosology [2] in which aortic root dilatation and ectopia lentis are the cardinal clinical features (Fig. 19.1). Genetic testing of the *FBN1* gene, although not mandatory, has greater weight in the diagnostic assessment when compared to the previous nosology.

In the absence of a family history of MFS, the diagnosis is confirmed when:

1. Ao ($Z \geq 2$) + EL = MFS
2. Ao ($Z \geq 2$) + FBN1 = MFS
3. Ao ($Z \geq 2$) + Syst (≥ 7 pts) = MFS
4. EL + FBN1 with known Ao = MFS

with Ao ($Z \geq 2$) as aortic root dilatation, defined as a diameter of the aorta at the level of the sinuses of Valsalva exceeding two standard deviations ($Z \geq 2$) above the mean; EL as ectopia lentis; Syst as systemic score, consisting of a list of features in different organ systems (see reference); and FBN1 as documented mutation in the *FBN1* gene.

In the presence of a family history (FH), criteria are slightly less strict:

5. EL + FH of MFS (as defined above) = MFS
6. Syst (≥ 7 pts) + FH of MFS (as defined above) = MFS
7. Ao ($Z \geq 2$ in adults, $Z \geq 3$ in children) + FH of MFS (as defined above) = MFS

MFS shows virtually complete penetrance but the clinical spectrum is highly variable, even within families. Modifiers of the clinical severity are largely unknown. Up to 30 % of cases are due to new dominant mutations.

To date, there are no reproducible genotype-phenotype correlations in MFS with the exception of the neonatal form being caused by mutations in the middle region of the gene (exons 24–32) [3]. Neonatal Marfan syndrome is the most severe form of the disorder, with death occurring early in life, often during the first year.

19.1.2 Clinical Cardiovascular Manifestations

19.1.2.1 Aortic Disease

Most of the morbidity and mortality associated with MFS is related to the cardio-vascular manifestations. The most common lesion is aortic root dilatation leading to aneurysm formation, which can be complicated by aortic dissection or rupture. It is estimated that aortic root dilatation is present in >80 % of adult MFS patients [1]. In surgical series, up to one-third of MFS patients present with aortic dissection, mainly Stanford type A dissection, indicating the persisting deficiency of timely diagnosis and adequate risk estimation [4].

The predilection for the ascending aorta to dilate is a result of both structural and local haemodynamic factors. Both the aortic root and the proximal part of the pulmonary artery are derived from the neural crest, whereas the more distal arterial structures stem from the mesodermis. It has been demonstrated that the elastic fibre content is higher in the ascending aorta than in any other region of the arterial tree [5]. Diseases such as MFS affecting elastic fibre integrity will therefore manifest more easily in this region. Furthermore, it is primarily the ascending portion of the aorta which is subjected to the repetitive stress of left ventricular ejection, eventually resulting in progressive dilatation [6, 7]. Since pressures in the aorta are significantly higher than in the pulmonary artery, dilatation will be more pronounced at the aortic root. Pulmonary artery dilatation occurs commonly in MFS but does not carry the same risk of dissection [8–10].

Up to now, complications in the descending aorta are limited to a minority of MFS patients, but the incidence of descending thoracic aortic dissection may increase since medical and surgical treatments of ascending aortic complications have significantly improved, hence leaving the descending aorta at risk [11, 12]. Marfan syndrome patients having thoraco-abdominal aortic aneurysm/dissection as a presenting manifestation are reported in a few case reports [13, 14], and it is notable that dissection in the descending part of the aorta is independent of the diameter of the ascending aorta [15]. Other data on the descending aorta in MFS patients are found in surgical reports describing the occurrence of primary or secondary complications in the descending aorta necessitating surgical intervention. Eight to fifteen percent of Marfan patients require initial surgery in the descending aorta [4, 11]. Patients with initial type B aortic dissection are at a significant higher risk for re-intervention (86 % for previous type B dissection versus 42 % for previous type A dissection). The majority of re-interventions are required in patients with previous dissection (48 % versus 11 % re-intervention in the patients presenting with aortic aneurysm) [4].

Altered anatomical features in the aorta of MFS patients, such as dilatation and/or dissection, are accompanied by functional impairment of the vessel, as reflected in increased aortic stiffness in MFS patients. Abnormal elastic properties – pulse wave velocity and local aortic distensibility – are not confined to the ascending aorta but are also detected in the normal-sized, more distal parts of the vessel [16, 17], and this as well in patients having previously undergone aortic root surgery as in unoperated MFS patients [18]. Interestingly, aortic stiffness seems to be an early marker of aortic disease as patients without thoracic aortic dilatation already demonstrate significant decreased aortic distensibility at proximal as well as distal levels of the aorta [17]. Local distensibility of the descending thoracic aorta appeared to be an independent predictor of progressive descending aortic dilatation [19].

19.1.2.2 Mitral Valve Prolapse

Mitral valve prolapse is another common cardiovascular complication of the Marfan syndrome occurring in up to 80 % of patients [10, 20, 21]. It is unclear whether the prevalence of MVP is increasing with age. In a large paediatric cohort, MVP occurred more commonly in females, but this female preponderance was not confirmed in adult series. A recent study showed that MFS patients have an increased risk of 28 % for MV-related clinical events at a younger age (endocarditis, surgery and heart failure) versus 13 % in idiopathic MVP [22]. Five to twelve percent of MFS patients will require mitral valve surgery as a primary cardiovascular intervention [23].

19.1.2.3 Cardiomyopathy and Arrhythmias

Although not commonly acknowledged in MFS, dilated cardiomyopathy, beyond that explained by aortic or mitral valve regurgitation, seems to occur with a higher prevalence, suggesting a role for the extracellular matrix protein fibrillin-1 in the myocardium. Significant LV dilatation and dysfunction leading to heart failure and necessitating heart transplantation has been described in a few cases and seems to be a very rare complication. Subclinical myocardial dysfunction on the other hand has been reported in larger subsets of MFS patients of various ages by several independent research groups [24–29], and mildly increased LV dimensions have been demonstrated in a subset of patients with MFS [30]. A study assessing genotype-phenotype correlations indicated that LV dilatation was more frequently observed in patients with a non-missense FBN1 mutation [31].

A feature that is closely related to ventricular dysfunction in MFS is an increased risk for adverse arrhythmogenic events as evidenced by several groups [32–34]. Hoffmann and co-workers found an association with increased NT-proBNP levels [33].

19.1.3 Aetiology and Pathophysiology

The pleiotropic clinical manifestations observed in MFS strongly suggested that the causal factor for the disease had to be found in a widespread tissue component such as the connective tissue. Applying monoclonal antibody studies in mice, Hollister, Sakai and their co-workers discovered a putative candidate, localized to numerous tissues including the aortic media and ciliary zonule, with the fibrils visualized termed fibrillin [35]. Fibrillin fibrils are a part of the 10 nm elastin-associated microfibrils. Immunohistochemical studies were the first to suggest that fibrillin is implicated in MFS [36]. The ultimate proof had to await the discovery of the gene encoding fibrillin (the fibrillin-1 gene, *FBN1*) and subsequent genetic linkage and mutation studies [37, 38]. To date more than 1,000 different mutations have been identified throughout the gene. Most mutations are unique to that individual or family.

The histological hallmark in the aorta of Marfan syndrome is the so-called cystic medial degeneration, with degeneration of the elastic fibres, irregular hypertrophy and apoptosis of vascular smooth muscle cells and increased basophilic ground substance within cell-depleted areas.

Conventional knowledge held that aneurysm formation in MFS results from an inherent structural weakness of connective tissues. Studies in different mouse models for MFS have extended this knowledge by demonstrating that fibrillin-1 also plays an important functional role in regulating transforming growth factor-beta (TGFβ) bioavailability. TGFβ is a multifunctional peptide that controls proliferation, differentiation and other functions in many cell types. Sakai and co-workers demonstrated that fibrillin-1 is homologous to the family of latent TGFβ-binding proteins (LTBPs), which serve to hold TGFβ in an inactive complex in various tissues, including the extracellular matrix [39], and it was known that fibrillin-1 binds TGFβ and LTBPs [40–42]. Increased TGFβ signalling has been demonstrated in several tissues in MFS patients.

More recent studies by Charbonneau and colleagues demonstrated that an *Fbn1* mouse in which the LTBP binding site was deleted (*Fbn1H1Δ*) did not present features of MFS [43]. Hence, instead of reduced TGFβ sequestration, mutant microfibrils probably influence TGFβ activation in a different way. More recent reports now suggest that this increased signalling is the result of a final common pathway in the disease process and that the role of the TGFβ signalling pathway may vary during the dynamic transition from aortic aneurysm predisposition to end-stage disease, such as dissection [44]. A recent and very interesting hypothesis states that in case of loss of extracellular matrix integrity by mutated microfibrils, mesenchymal cells, such as fibroblasts or smooth muscle cells, detect the defective matrix and respond by repairing the failed matrix through the generation of active TGFβ and production of the required activators of latent TGFβ as part of the repair process [45]. Other mechanisms such as mitochondrial dysfunction and compromised VSMC differentiation may also play an important role. A schematic overview of the pathogenesis is provided in Fig. 19.2.

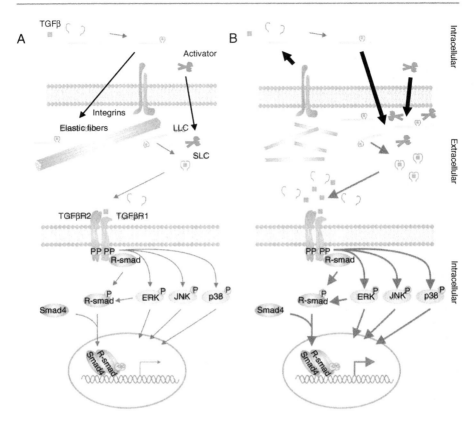

Fig. 19.2 Pathogenic mechanism of Marfan syndrome. (**a**) TGFβ signalling in healthy individuals. (**b**) Fragmented microfibres lead to a damaged ECM and initiate repair responses producing more (*enhanced arrows*) ECM constituents, SLCs and LLCs together with their activators; subsequently, enhanced (*bold arrows*) signalling through canonical (*purple*) and non-canonical (*green*) TGFβ signalling results in changes in target gene expression in MFS patients

The processes occurring in the aortic ECM due to mutated *FBN1* are further influenced by altered haemodynamic stress in the aorta. As such, mechano-transduction of haemodynamic stress further exacerbates the tissue-related activation of vascular smooth muscle cells, matrix metalloproteinases and TGFβ.

19.1.4 Management and Treatment of Marfan Syndrome

The pleiotropic nature of Marfan disease implies a multidisciplinary approach and appropriate treatment, involving among others ophthalmologists, physiotherapists, orthopaedic surgeons, cardiologists and cardiac surgeons. In this chapter, we will focus on the treatment of aortic disease, which mainly determines life expectancy in

MFS and has been a main clinical and research focus for many decades. Improved diagnosis and better medical and surgical treatment have already resulted in a spectacular increase in life expectancy of more than 30 years [46] – no other cardiovascular disease has seen a similar improvement. The cornerstone of adequate management in MFS is correct and timely diagnosis, necessitating adequate education of all involved healthcare workers and correct echocardiographic assessment of the aortic dimensions by (paediatric) cardiologists according to established guidelines [47]. CT or MRI can be used in case of insufficient visualization of the ascending aorta by echocardiography. Once the diagnosis is confirmed, a first reassessment of the aortic dimension is recommended after 6 months to assess evolutionary changes. Further follow-up is guided by the diameter, evolution, underlying diagnosis and family history. Stable diameters <45 mm in MFS patients without a family history of dissection require yearly follow-up. Biannual controls are recommended in all other cases. Despite rigorous follow-up and adherence to the guidelines, some MFS patients will still succumb to (fatal) aortic dissection, indicating the need for improved risk stratification. Ongoing studies are identifying potential circulating biomarkers, including fibrillin-1 fragments, which may be used in conjunction with imaging data to better identify patients at risk for aortic dissection [48].

The ultimate goal for the treatment of aortic complications in MFS is to obtain a reduction in the occurrence rate of (fatal) aortic dissection, and it is beyond any doubt that – up to now – prophylactic aortic root surgery is the most successful preventive intervention. Refinements of surgical techniques, mainly with the introduction of valve-sparing procedures, have led to excellent short- and middle-term results and have obviated the need for chronic use of anticoagulants [49]. Surgery is routinely recommended in MFS patients when the diameter of the aortic root attains 50 mm. A reduced threshold of 45 mm is warranted in cases of rapid growth (>0.2-0.5 cm/year), cases with a positive family history of aortic dissection and/or significant aortic valve regurgitation and in women with desire of pregnancy [50, 51].

Since aortic surgery is inherently associated with a (small) risk for complications and a prolonged rehabilitation period, attempts have been made to at least postpone the need for surgery. Ultimately, arresting aortic growth and, conceptually, interference with the underlying genetic defect are deemed to be the ideal solution, which is – alas – not (yet) feasible at the moment.

Slowing down aortic root growth may be achieved through reducing haemodynamic stress on the proximal aorta. The first report on the use of β-blockers in MFS dates from 1971 indicating that reduction in the rate of increase in aortic pressure over time (dP/dt) was more effective than could be explained by reduction of blood pressure alone [52]. Subsequent small studies with β-blockers in turkeys that are prone to aortic dissection and in uncontrolled human studies of MFS had varying results [53, 54].

Since then, no less than 1,583 Marfan patients have been included in at least 19 different trials since the late 1970s [6, 53, 55–71]. Only one trial, showing a reduction in aortic root growth with propranolol, had a placebo-controlled randomized design [57]. Many other trials have confirmed the effect of β-blockers on aortic growth, and in some trials, beneficial effects on the elastic properties of the aorta have been reported [58]. This notwithstanding, the beneficial effect of β-blockers has not been consistent in all studies. Differences in the populations studied, in the drug types and dosage and in the study design, render the interpretation and comparison of these trials particularly challenging.

Another aspect that remains elusive despite the numerous trials is the timing of initiation of treatment – some advocate treatment as soon as the diagnosis is made while others suggest to wait until some dilatation has occurred.

Alternatives for β-blockers have been suggested and studied in small series.

Calcium channel blockers have been investigated in a very small study [59], showing similar results as β-blockers. ACE inhibitors (ACEIs) were postulated to have therapeutic value in MFS because of their potential ability to block apoptotic pathways through inhibition of the AT2 receptor. An open-label, nonrandomized trial of ACEIs versus β-blockers in MFS showed apparent therapeutic value for ACEIs in terms of reduced aortic stiffness and smaller increases in aortic root diameter [61]. Another randomized trial of perindopril versus placebo in MFS revealed improved biomechanical properties of the aorta, slower aortic root growth and lower levels of circulating TGFβ [64].

A seemingly major breakthrough in the search for improved medical treatment in MFS patients was achieved with the documentation of the involvement of the TGFβ pathway in the process of aneurysm formation. This led to the insight that interference with TGFβ signalling may have a beneficial impact on aortic growth. Losartan, an ARB with known TGFβ-inhibiting potential, was tested in a mouse model for MFS showing normalization of aortic root growth and restoration of elastic fibre fragmentation [72]. Human trials published so far may suggest a beneficial effect of the combination of beta-blocker with losartan treatment [67, 70]. Very recently, the results of a large randomized trial in a young (1mo-25y) MFS cohort, conducted by the Pediatric Heart Network comparing Atenolol and Losartan were published showing no difference in aortic root growth rate between both groups [73].

19.2 Associated Thoracic Aortic Aneurysm Syndromes

Some patients and families do present with thoracic aortic disease but do not fulfil the diagnostic criteria for MFS and/or present with other clinical features that do not fit within the MFS spectrum. Moreover, since the more widespread availability of molecular genetic testing in MFS, it became clear that subgroups of patients and families exist that do not carry an *FBN1* mutation, suggesting the involvement of other genes.

Over the past decade, it has indeed been evidenced that heritable thoracic aortic disease (H-TAD) is genetically heterogeneous with a dozen genes being identified so far [74]. Most of these genetic conditions transmit as an autosomal dominant trait. Genes may be subdivided in three major categories: (1) genes involved in the extracellular matrix (*FBN1, COL3A1, FBNL4*), (2) genes involved in the TGFβ pathway (*TGFBR1* and *TGFBR2, SMAD3, TGFβ2, SKI*) and (3) genes involved in the vascular smooth muscle cell apparatus (*ACTA2, MYLK, MYH11, PRKG1*).

For most of these genes, both syndromic and non-syndromic disease entities have been described. Though some clinical features may be highly discriminative (e.g. lens luxation for MFS), there is substantial clinical overlap between these genetic entities. Molecular genetic testing is a helpful additional tool in many cases, not only for diagnostic purposes but also because medical management may vary according to the underlying condition.

The main clinical entities with their respective genes and clinical features are listed in Table 19.1. A brief description of the most notable clinical entities in the context of arterial disease is provided below.

The identification of new genes in H-TAD has offered important new opportunities for the diagnosis and gene-tailored management of patients and families. In addition, these new genes have offered us unique new insights into the pathogenesis of aneurysmal disease. Identification of mutations in the various components of the ECM, the TGFβ pathway and the contractile unit of vascular smooth muscle cells provide the ultimate proof for their involvement into the process of aneurysm formation as described above.

19.2.1 Loeys-Dietz Syndrome

Loeys-Dietz syndrome (LDS) is caused by mutations in either of the transforming growth factor-beta receptor genes (*TGFBR1* and *TGFBR2*). In its most typical form, LDS is characterized by aortic aneurysms and dissections, widespread arterial tortuosity/aneurysms, bifid uvula and hypertelorism (wide-spaced eyes) [76].

The cardiovascular lesions in LDS are more widespread, extending beyond the aorta, and may have a more aggressive course than in MFS with a higher annual increase in aortic root diameter in at least a subset of patients [77]. The expression of the disease is highly variable though, both between and within families. Milder presentations and even non-penetrance has been observed [90]. Larger-scale prospective registries are required to gain more insight into the course and presentation of the disease. Since aortic dissection has been reported in patients with aortic diameters well below conventional surgical thresholds, aortic root surgery in LDS is recommended at a diameter of 43–45 mm [50].

Williams et al. demonstrated that surgical outcome in LDS patients is good [91].

In view of the extent of cardiovascular lesions in LDS, more extended vascular studies such as MR angiography or CT scanning with 3D reconstruction from the head to the pelvis are required for the detection of distal aortic/arterial complications.

19.2.2 Aneurysm-Osteoarthritis Syndrome

Aneurysm-osteoarthritis syndrome (AOS) is caused by mutations in the *SMAD3* gene [78]. Since many patients with AOS present some degree of osteoarthritis, this feature is regarded as a discriminating feature. Aneurysms, dissections and

Table 19.1 Schematic overview of syndromic and non-syndromic TAAD (thoracic aortic aneurysm and dissections)

Disorder	Gene(s)	Main cardiovascular features	Additional clinical features
Syndromic H-TAD			
Marfan [1, 2, 37]	*FBN1*	**Aortic root aneurysm**, aortic dissection, mitral valve prolapse, main pulmonary artery dilatation, ventricular dysfunction	**Lens luxation**, skeletal features (arachnodactylia, pectus deformity, scoliosis, flat feet, increased arm span, dolichocephalia)
Vascular Ehlers-Danlos [75]	*COL3A1*	**Aortic and major branching vessel dissection/rupture, often without preceding dilatation**	**Thin, translucent skin, dystrophic scars, facial characteristics** (Madonna face, thin lips, deep-set eyes)
TGFβ-related vasculopathies	Loeys-Dietz [76, 77]	*TGFBR1/TGFBR2*	**Aortic root aneurysm**, aortic dissection, arterial aneurysms and dissections, **arterial tortuosity**, mitral valve prolapse, congenital cardiac malformations	**Bifid uvula/cleft palate, hypertelorism**, pectus abnormalities, scoliosis, club feet
	Aneurysm-osteoarthritis [78, 79]	*SMAD3*	**Aortic root aneurysm**, aortic dissection, arterial aneurysms and dissections, **arterial tortuosity**, mitral valve prolapse, congenital cardiac malformations	**Osteoarthritis**, soft skin, flat feet, scoliosis, recurrent hernias, hypertelorism, pectus abnormalities
	TGFβ2 [80, 81]	*TGFβ2*	**Aortic root aneurysm**, aortic dissection, arterial aneurysms and dissections, **arterial tortuosity, mitral valve prolapse**, congenital cardiac malformations	Club feet, soft translucent skin
	Shprintzen-Goldberg syndrome [82, 83]	*SKI*	**Mild aortic root dilatation**, mitral valve prolapse	Craniosynostosis, distinctive craniofacial features, skeletal changes, neurologic abnormalities, mild-to-moderate intellectual disability

Non-syndromic H-TAD

			Lack of syndromic features
Familial thoracic aortic aneurysm syndrome (FTAA) [84–88]	*TGFBR1/TGFBR2 (3–5%)*	Thoracic aortic aneurysm/dissection	Lack of syndromic features
	ACTA2 (10–14%)	Thoracic aortic aneurysm/dissection, BAV cerebrovascular disease, coronary artery disease	Lack of marfanoid skeletal features, **livedo reticularis, iris flocculi**
	MYLK	Thoracic aortic aneurysm/dissection	Gastrointestinal abnormalities
	SMAD3 (2%)	Intracranial and other arterial aneurysms	
	TGFβ2	**Mitral valve prolapse**	
	PRKG1	Thoracic aortic aneurysm/dissection, arterial aneurysms and dissections, arterial tortuosity	
FTAA with patent ductus arteriosus (PDA) [1, 89]	*MYH11*	**Patent ductus arteriosus**	

Distinctive features are indicated in bold

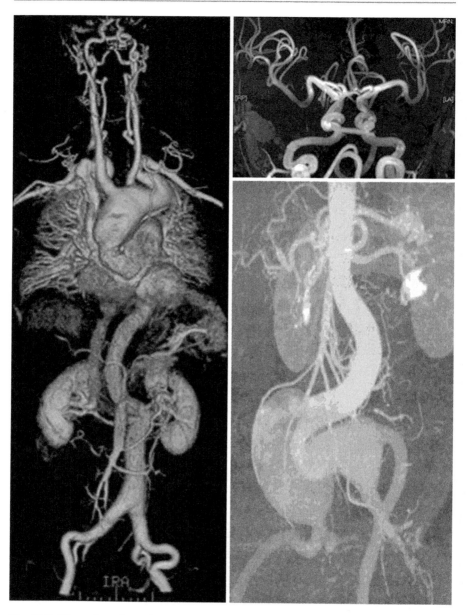

Fig. 19.3 Illustration of vascular anomalies in patients with LDS (*left and right-upper panel*) and with aneurysm-osteoarthritis syndrome (*right lower panel*)

tortuosity throughout the arterial tree are the main cardiovascular features. Arterial aneurysms may be very large with a predilection for visceral arteries and are often a presenting symptom [79, 92, 93]. An illustration is provided in Fig. 19.3.

19.2.3 Aortic Aneurysms Caused by TGFβ2 Mutations

Mutations in the TGFβ2 ligand were recently identified in patients presenting with a phenotype showing some overlap with the abovementioned syndromic TAA entities [80, 81]. Aortic dilatation may result in type A aortic dissection at diameters below classic surgical thresholds. We found significant mitral valve disease, possibly a signature feature that may direct molecular analyses [94].

19.2.4 Vascular Ehlers-Danlos Syndrome (EDS)

Vascular EDS, caused by mutations in the collagen type 3 gene (*COL3A1*), is a severe vascular connective tissue disorder clinically characterized by joint hypermobility, skin abnormalities (cigarette paper scars, easy bruising, soft velvety skin), fragility of intestinal and genito-urinary organs and vascular fragility leading to dissection or rupture of medium to large muscular arteries.

Typically in vascular EDS, dissections often occur without preceding dilatation/aneurysm formation. In a retrospective study, about half of the arterial complications in vascular EDS involved the thoracic or abdominal arteries, and the rest were divided equally between the head, the neck and the limbs [75].

Prophylactic treatment with celiprolol, a β1-adrenoceptor antagonist with β2 agonistic properties, is recommended based on the beneficial results in a randomized multicentre trial [95].

Surgical treatment of vascular lesions in vascular EDS is hazardous with a reported incidence of fatal complications during or immediately after vascular surgery at around 45 % [96].

Some authors advise not pursuing any additional investigation or surveillance, because a conservative approach will be adopted irrespectively and undue anxiety would be created [97]. Others recommend non-invasive cardiovascular imaging with echocardiography and vascular CT/MRI [96].

19.2.5 Non-syndromic Thoracic Aortic Aneurysms and Dissections (TAAD)

Non-syndromic TAAD is genetically heterogeneous with at least seven genes being identified so far. Genes include *TGFBR1*, *TGFBR2*, *ACTA2*, *MYH11*, *MYLK*, *SMAD3* and *PRKG1*. These genes account for disease in only 20 % of TAAD families, indicating that more genes are to be determined.

By definition, the entity of non-syndromic TAAD is restricted to those cases presenting with "isolated" TAAD – as opposed to the known syndromes such as MFS and LDS. In practice, many reported families also exhibit some mild additional clinical features as listed in Table 19.1.

References

1. Judge DP, Dietz HC (2005) Marfan's syndrome. Lancet 366:1965–1976
2. Loeys BL, Dietz HC, Braverman AC et al (2010) The revised Ghent nosology for the Marfan syndrome. J Med Genet 47:476–485
3. Faivre L, Masurel-Paulet A, Collod-Beroud G et al (2009) Clinical and molecular study of 320 children with Marfan syndrome and related type I fibrillinopathies in a series of 1009 probands with pathogenic FBN1 mutations. Pediatrics 123:391–398
4. Schoenhoff FS, Jungi S, Czerny M et al (2013) Acute aortic dissection determines the fate of initially untreated aortic segments in Marfan syndrome. Circulation 127:1569–1575
5. Apter JT (1967) Correlation of visco-elastic properties with microscopic structure of large arteries. IV. Thermal responses of collagen, elastin, smooth muscle, and intact arteries. Circ Res 21:901–918
6. Reed CM, Fox ME, Alpert BS (1993) Aortic biomechanical properties in pediatric patients with the Marfan syndrome, and the effects of atenolol. Am J Cardiol 71:606–608
7. Roman MJ, Rosen SE, Kramer-Fox R, Devereux RB (1993) Prognostic significance of the pattern of aortic root dilation in the Marfan syndrome. J Am Coll Cardiol 22:1470–1476
8. Keane MG, Pyeritz RE (2008) Medical management of Marfan syndrome. Circulation 117:2802–2813
9. Lundby R, Rand-Hendriksen S, Hald JK et al (2012) The pulmonary artery in patients with Marfan syndrome: a cross-sectional study. Genet Med 14:922–927
10. De Backer J, Loeys B, Devos D et al (2006) A critical analysis of minor cardiovascular criteria in the diagnostic evaluation of patients with Marfan syndrome. Genet Med 8:401–408
11. Finkbohner R, Johnston D, Crawford ES et al (1995) Marfan syndrome. Long-term survival and complications after aortic aneurysm repair. Circulation 91:728–733
12. Engelfriet PM (2006) Beyond the root: dilatation of the distal aorta in Marfan's syndrome. Heart 92:1238–1243
13. van Ooijen B (1988) Marfan's syndrome and isolated aneurysm of the abdominal aorta. Heart 59:81–84
14. Pruzinsky MS, Katz NM, Green CE, Satler LF (1988) Isolated descending thoracic aortic aneurysm in Marfan's syndrome. Am J Cardiol 61:1159–1160
15. Mimoun L (2011) Dissection in Marfan syndrome: the importance of the descending aorta. Eur Heart J 32:443–449
16. Groenink M, de Roos A, Mulder BJ et al (2001) Biophysical properties of the normal-sized aorta in patients with Marfan syndrome: evaluation with MR flow mapping. Radiology 219:535–540
17. Teixido-Tura G, Redheuil A, Rodríguez-Palomares J et al (2014) Aortic biomechanics by magnetic resonance: early markers of aortic disease in Marfan syndrome regardless of aortic dilatation? Int J Cardiol 171:56–61
18. Nollen GJ, Meijboom LJ, Groenink M et al (2003) Comparison of aortic elasticity in patients with the Marfan syndrome with and without aortic root replacement. Am J Cardiol 91:637–640
19. Nollen GJ, Groenink M, Tijssen JGP et al (2004) Aortic stiffness and diameter predict progressive aortic dilatation in patients with Marfan syndrome. Eur Heart J 25:1146–1152
20. Rybczynski M, Mir TS, Sheikhzadeh S et al (2010) Frequency and age-related course of mitral valve dysfunction in the Marfan syndrome. Am J Cardiol 106:1048–1053
21. Selamet Tierney ES, Levine JC, Chen S et al (2013) Echocardiographic methods, quality review, and measurement accuracy in a randomized multicenter clinical trial of Marfan syndrome. J Am Soc Echocardiogr 26:657–666
22. Rybczynski M, Treede H, Sheikhzadeh S et al (2011) Predictors of outcome of mitral valve prolapse in patients with the Marfan syndrome. Am J Cardiol 107:268–274
23. Pyeritz RE, Wappel MA (1983) Mitral valve dysfunction in the Marfan syndrome. Clinical and echocardiographic study of prevalence and natural history. Am J Med 74:797–807

24. Das BB, Taylor AL, Yetman AT (2006) Left ventricular diastolic dysfunction in children and young adults with Marfan syndrome. Pediatr Cardiol 27:256–258. doi:10.1007/s00246-005-1139-5
25. Savolainen A, Nisula L, Keto P et al (1994) Left ventricular function in children with the Marfan syndrome. Eur Heart J 15:625–630
26. Kiotsekoglou A, Moggridge JC, Bijnens BH et al (2009) Biventricular and atrial diastolic function assessment using conventional echocardiography and tissue-Doppler imaging in adults with Marfan syndrome. Eur J Echocardiogr 10:947–955
27. Alpendurada F, Wong J, Kiotsekoglou A et al (2010) Evidence for Marfan cardiomyopathy. Eur J Heart Fail 12:1085–1091
28. de Backer JF, Devos D, Segers P et al (2006) Primary impairment of left ventricular function in Marfan syndrome. Int J Cardiol 112:353–358
29. Rybczynski M, Koschyk DH, Aydin MA et al (2007) Tissue Doppler imaging identifies myocardial dysfunction in adults with Marfan syndrome. Clin Cardiol 30:19–24
30. Chatrath R (2003) Left ventricular function in the Marfan syndrome without significant valvular regurgitation. Am J Cardiol 91:914–916
31. Aalberts JJJ, van Tintelen JP, Meijboom LJ et al (2014) Relation between genotype and left-ventricular dilatation in patients with Marfan syndrome. Gene 534:40–43
32. Yetman AT, Bornemeier RA, McCrindle BW (2003) Long-term outcome in patients with Marfan syndrome: is aortic dissection the only cause of sudden death? J Am Coll Cardiol 41:329–332
33. Hoffmann BA, Rybczynski M, Rostock T et al (2013) Prospective risk stratification of sudden cardiac death in Marfan's syndrome. Int J Cardiol 167:2539–2545
34. Chen S, Fagan LF, Nouri S, Donahoe JL (1985) Ventricular dysrhythmias in children with Marfan's syndrome. Am J Dis Child 139:273–276
35. Sakai LY, Keene DR, Engvall E (1986) Fibrillin, a new 350-kD glycoprotein, is a component of extracellular microfibrils. J Cell Biol 103:2499–2509
36. Hollister DW, Godfrey M, Sakai LY, Pyeritz RE (1990) Immunohistologic abnormalities of the microfibrillar-fiber system in the Marfan syndrome. N Engl J Med 323:152–159
37. Dietz HC, Cutting GR, Pyeritz RE et al (1991) Marfan syndrome caused by a recurrent de novo missense mutation in the fibrillin gene. Nature 352:337–339
38. Lee B, Godfrey M, Vitale E et al (1991) Linkage of Marfan syndrome and a phenotypically related disorder to two different fibrillin genes. Nature 352:330–334
39. Isogai Z, Ono RN, Ushiro S et al (2003) Latent transforming growth factor beta-binding protein 1 interacts with fibrillin and is a microfibril-associated protein. J Biol Chem 278:2750–2757
40. Dallas SL, Miyazono K, Skerry TM et al (1995) Dual role for the latent transforming growth factor-beta binding protein in storage of latent TGF-beta in the extracellular matrix and as a structural matrix protein. J Cell Biol 131:539–549
41. Dallas SL, Keene DR, Bruder SP et al (2000) Role of the latent transforming growth factor beta binding protein 1 in fibrillin-containing microfibrils in bone cells in vitro and in vivo. J Bone Miner Res 15:68–81
42. Saharinen J, Hyytiäinen M, Taipale J, Keski-Oja J (1999) Latent transforming growth factor-beta binding proteins (LTBPs)–structural extracellular matrix proteins for targeting TGF-beta action. Cytokine Growth Factor Rev 10:99–117
43. Charbonneau NL, Carlson EJ, Tufa S et al (2010) In vivo studies of mutant fibrillin-1 microfibrils. J Biol Chem 285:24943–24955
44. Dietz HC (2010) TGF-beta in the pathogenesis and prevention of disease: a matter of aneurysmic proportions. J Clin Investig 120:403–406
45. Horiguchi M, Ota M, Rifkin DB (2012) Matrix control of transforming growth factor-β function. J Biochem 152:321–329
46. Silverman DI, Burton KJ, Gray J et al (1995) Life expectancy in the Marfan syndrome. Am J Clin Pathol 75:157–160
47. Evangelista A, Flachskampf FA, Erbel R et al (2010) Echocardiography in aortic diseases: EAE recommendations for clinical practice. Eur J Echocardiogr 11:645–658

48. Marshall LM, Carlson EJ, O'Malley J et al (2013) Thoracic aortic aneurysm frequency and dissection are associated with fibrillin-1 fragment concentrations in circulation. Circ Res 113: 1159–1168
49. Svensson LG, Blackstone EH, Alsalihi M et al (2013) Midterm results of David reimplantation in patients with connective tissue disorder. Ann Thorac Surg 95:555–562
50. Writing Group Members, Hiratzka LF, Bakris GL et al (2010) 2010 ACCF/AHA/AATS/ACR/ASA/SCA/SCAI/SIR/STS/SVM guidelines for the diagnosis and management of patients with thoracic aortic disease: a report of the American College of Cardiology Foundation/American Heart Association Task Force on Practice Guidelines, American Association for Thoracic Surgery, American College of Radiology, American Stroke Association, Society of Cardiovascular Anesthesiologists, Society for Cardiovascular Angiography and Interventions, Society of Interventional Radiology, Society of Thoracic Surgeons, and Society for Vascular Medicine. Circulation 121:e266–e369
51. Baumgartner H, Bonhoeffer P, De Groot NMS et al (2010) ESC guidelines for the management of grown-up congenital heart disease (new version 2010). Eur Heart J 31:2915–2957
52. Halpern BL, Char F, Murdoch JL et al (1971) A prospectus on the prevention of aortic rupture in the Marfan syndrome with data on survivorship without treatment. Johns Hopkins Med J 129:123–129
53. Ose L, McKusick VA (1977) Prophylactic use of propranolol in the Marfan syndrome to prevent aortic dissection. Birth Defects Orig Artic Ser 13:163–169
54. Simpson CF, Boucek RJ, Noble NL (1976) Influence of d-, l-, and dl-propranolol, and practolol on beta-amino-propionitrile-induced aortic ruptures of turkeys. Toxicol Appl Pharmacol 38:169–175
55. Salim MA, Alpert BS, Ward JC, Pyeritz RE (1994) Effect of beta-adrenergic blockade on aortic root rate of dilation in the Marfan syndrome. Am J Coll Cardiol 74:629–633
56. Tahernia AC (1993) Cardiovascular anomalies in Marfan's syndrome: the role of echocardiography and beta-blockers. South Med J 86:305–310
57. Shores J, Berger KR, Murphy EA, Pyeritz RE (1994) Progression of aortic dilatation and the benefit of long-term beta-adrenergic blockade in Marfan's syndrome. N Engl J Med 330: 1335–1341
58. Groenink M, de Roos A, Mulder BJ et al (1998) Changes in aortic distensibility and pulse wave velocity assessed with magnetic resonance imaging following beta-blocker therapy in the Marfan syndrome. Am J Cardiol 82:203–208
59. Rossi-Foulkes R, Roman MJ, Rosen SE et al (1999) Phenotypic features and impact of beta blocker or calcium antagonist therapy on aortic lumen size in the Marfan syndrome. Am J Cardiol 83:1364–1368
60. Rios AS, Silber EN, Bavishi N et al (1999) Effect of long-term beta-blockade on aortic root compliance in patients with Marfan syndrome. Am Heart J 137:1057–1061
61. Yetman AT, Bornemeier RA, McCrindle BW (2005) Usefulness of enalapril versus propranolol or atenolol for prevention of aortic dilation in patients with the Marfan syndrome. Am J Cardiol 95:1125–1127
62. Ladouceur M, Fermanian C, Lupoglazoff J-M et al (2007) Effect of beta-blockade on ascending aortic dilatation in children with the Marfan syndrome. Am J Cardiol 99:406–409
63. Selamet Tierney ES, Feingold B, Printz BF et al (2007) Beta-blocker therapy does not alter the rate of aortic root dilation in pediatric patients with Marfan syndrome. J Pediatr 150:77–82
64. Ahimastos AA, Aggarwal A, D'Orsa KM et al (2007) Effect of perindopril on large artery stiffness and aortic root diameter in patients with Marfan syndrome: a randomized controlled trial. JAMA 298:1539–1547
65. Brooke BS, Habashi JP, Judge DP et al (2008) Angiotensin II blockade and aortic-root dilation in Marfan's syndrome. N Engl J Med 358:2787–2795. doi:10.1056/NEJMoa0706585
66. Williams A, Kenny D, Wilson D et al (2012) Effects of atenolol, perindopril and verapamil on haemodynamic and vascular function in Marfan syndrome – a randomised, double-blind, crossover trial. Eur J Clin Invest 42:891–899

67. Chiu HH, Wu MH, Wang JK et al (2013) Losartan added to beta-blockade therapy for aortic root dilation in Marfan syndrome: a randomized, open-label pilot study. Mayo Clin Proc 88:271–276

68. Pees C, Laccone F, Hagl M et al (2013) Usefulness of Losartan on the size of the ascending aorta in an unselected cohort of children, adolescents, and young adults with Marfan syndrome. Am J Cardiol 112:1477–1483

69. Mueller GC, Stierle L, Stark V et al (2014) Retrospective analysis of the effect of angiotensin II receptor blocker versus β-blocker on aortic root growth in paediatric patients with Marfan syndrome. Heart 100:214–218

70. Groenink M, den Hartog AW, Franken R et al (2013) Losartan reduces aortic dilatation rate in adults with Marfan syndrome: a randomized controlled trial. Eur Heart J 34:3491–3500

71. Lacro RV, Dietz HC, Wruck LM et al (2007) Rationale and design of a randomized clinical trial of beta-blocker therapy (atenolol) versus angiotensin II receptor blocker therapy (losartan) in individuals with Marfan syndrome. Am Heart J 154:624–631

72. Habashi JP, Judge DP, Holm TM et al (2006) Losartan, an AT1 antagonist, prevents aortic aneurysm in a mouse model of Marfan syndrome. Science 312:117–121

73. Lacro RV, Dietz HC, Sleeper LA et al (2014) Atenolol versus Losartan in children and young adults with Marfan's Syndrome. N Engl J Med 371:2061–2071

74. Pyeritz RE (2014) Heritable thoracic aortic disorders. Curr Opin Cardiol 29:97–102

75. Pepin M, Schwarze U, Superti-Furga A, Byers PH (2000) Clinical and genetic features of Ehlers-Danlos syndrome type IV, the vascular type. N Engl J Med 342:673–680

76. Loeys BL, Chen J, Neptune ER et al (2005) A syndrome of altered cardiovascular, craniofacial, neurocognitive and skeletal development caused by mutations in TGFBR1 or TGFBR2. Nat Genet 37:275–281

77. Loeys BL, Schwarze U, Holm T et al (2006) Aneurysm syndromes caused by mutations in the TGF-beta receptor. N Engl J Med 355:788–798

78. van de Laar IMBH, Oldenburg RA, Pals G et al (2011) Mutations in SMAD3 cause a syndromic form of aortic aneurysms and dissections with early-onset osteoarthritis. Nat Genet 43:121–126

79. van der Linde D, van de Laar IMBH, Bertoli-Avella AM et al (2012) Aggressive cardiovascular phenotype of aneurysms-osteoarthritis syndrome caused by pathogenic SMAD3 variants. J Am Coll Cardiol 60:397–403

80. Lindsay ME, Schepers D, Bolar NA et al (2012) Loss-of-function mutations in TGFB2 cause a syndromic presentation of thoracic aortic aneurysm. Nat Genet 44:922–927

81. Boileau C, Guo DC, Hanna N et al (2012) TGFB2 mutations cause familial thoracic aortic aneurysms and dissections associated with mild systemic features of Marfan syndrome. Nat Genet 44:916–921

82. Carmignac V, Thevenon J, Adès L et al (2012) In-frame mutations in exon 1 of SKI cause dominant Shprintzen-Goldberg syndrome. Am J Hum Genet 91:950–957

83. Doyle AJ, Doyle JJ, Bessling SL et al (2012) Mutations in the TGF-β repressor SKI cause Shprintzen-Goldberg syndrome with aortic aneurysm. Nat Genet 44:1249–1254

84. Wang L, Guo D-C, Cao J et al (2010) Mutations in myosin light chain kinase cause familial aortic dissections. Am J Hum Genet 87:701–707

85. Guo D-C, Pannu H, Tran-Fadulu V et al (2007) Mutations in smooth muscle α-actin (ACTA2) lead to thoracic aortic aneurysms and dissections. Nat Genet 39:1488–1493

86. Akutsu K, Morisaki H, Okajima T et al (2010) Genetic analysis of young adult patients with aortic disease not fulfilling the diagnostic criteria for Marfan syndrome. Circ J 74: 990–997

87. Guo D-C, Regalado E, Casteel DE et al (2013) Recurrent gain-of-function mutation in PRKG1 causes thoracic aortic aneurysms and acute aortic dissections. Am J Hum Genet 93:398–404

88. Regalado ES, Guo D-C, Villamizar C et al (2011) Exome sequencing identifies SMAD3 mutations as a cause of familial thoracic aortic aneurysm and dissection with intracranial and other arterial aneurysms. Circ Res 109:680–686

89. Zhu L, Vranckx R, van Kien PK et al (2006) Mutations in myosin heavy chain 11 cause a syndrome associating thoracic aortic aneurysm/aortic dissection and patent ductus arteriosus. Nat Genet 38:343–349

90. Attias D, Stheneur C, Roy C et al (2009) Comparison of clinical presentations and outcomes between patients with TGFBR2 and FBN1 mutations in Marfan syndrome and related disorders. Circulation 120:2541–2549

91. Williams JA, Loeys BL, Nwakanma LU et al (2007) Early surgical experience with Loeys-Dietz: a new syndrome of aggressive thoracic aortic aneurysm disease. Ann Thorac Surg 83:S757–S763

92. van der Linde D, Verhagen HJM, Moelker A et al (2013) Aneurysm-osteoarthritis syndrome with visceral and iliac artery aneurysms. J Vasc Surg 57:96–102

93. Martens T, Van Herzeele I, De Ryck F et al (2013) Multiple aneurysms in a patient with aneurysms-osteoarthritis syndrome. Ann Thorac Surg 95:332–335

94. Renard M, Callewaert B, Malfait F et al (2012) Thoracic aortic-aneurysm and dissection in association with significant mitral valve disease caused by mutations in TGFB2. Int J Cardiol 165:584–587

95. Ong K-T, Perdu J, De Backer J et al (2010) Effect of celiprolol on prevention of cardiovascular events in vascular Ehlers-Danlos syndrome: a prospective randomised, open, blinded-endpoints trial. Lancet 376:1476–1484

96. Oderich GS, Panneton JM, Bower TC et al (2005) The spectrum, management and clinical outcome of Ehlers-Danlos syndrome type IV: a 30-year experience. J Vasc Surg 42:98–106

97. Bergqvist D, Björck M, Wanhainen A (2013) Treatment of vascular ehlers-danlos syndrome: a systematic review. Ann Surg 258:257–261

Arterial Alterations in Hypertension

20

Gino Seravalle, Guido Grassi, and Giuseppe Mancia

The hemodynamics of the circulation in humans display two important characteristics. First, the heart is beating, and therefore blood flow and blood pressure are characterized by pulsatile changes. Second, blood circulates via heterogeneous conduits progressively narrowing. Along this circuit the initial pulsatile pressure and flow become a continuous flow and pressure within the microcirculation.

The arterial tree consists of the aorta and large arteries (macrocirculation, elastic arteries), microcirculation (small arteries and arterioles; muscular arteries), and capillaries [1, 2]. The chapter will analyze the characteristics of the first two compartments and the changes associated with pathophysiological conditions.

G. Seravalle
Istituto Auxologico Italiano, IRCCS Ospedale San Luca,
Piazza Brescia 20, 20149 Milano, Italy
e-mail: g_seravalle@yahoo.com

G. Grassi
Department of Health Sciences, University of Milano-Bicocca,
Via Pergolesi, 33, 20900 Monza (MB), Italy
e-mail: guido.grassi@unimib.it

G. Mancia (✉)
Istituto Auxologico Italiano, IRCCS Ospedale San Luca, Piazza Brescia 20,
20149 Milano, Italy
e-mail: giuseppe.mancia@unimib.it

© Springer International Publishing Switzerland 2015
A. Berbari, G. Mancia (eds.), *Arterial Disorders:
Definition, Clinical Manifestations, Mechanisms and Therapeutic Approaches*,
DOI 10.1007/978-3-319-14556-3_20

20.1   Large Arteries: Structure and Physiology

Large arteries are close to the heart, and changes in flow, hydrostatic pressure, and diameter differ considerably [3]. The considerable variations in these parameters emphasize the importance of the tools developed to evaluate the physical properties of large arteries. The pressure wave that travels along conduit arteries increases from central to peripheral large arteries. In contrast the amplitude of the flow wave is more important in large than in peripheral arteries [4]. The relationship diameter/pressure is curvilinear because of the heterogeneous composition and properties of the arterial wall, which is different in central (elastic) and peripheral (muscular) arteries [5]. The profile of the pulse pressure wave varies from the thoracic aorta to peripheral vessels. In order to understand the profile of pulse pressure recordings, it is necessary to recognize the major physical components [6]. After ventricular contraction, an ejection wave travels from the heart to peripheral smaller vessels. Then, a reflection wave travels in the opposite directions after rebuttal at different potential sites of wave reflection. Determinants of the two critical components of the pressure curve are of physiological importance: the ejection wave is determined by the ventricular contractile force and by arterial stiffness, whereas the reflection component develops according to the bulk of distal reflection sites, in addition to arterial stiffness. Both ejection and reflection curves become superimposed under normal physiological conditions, but the breakdown of the two components may reveal several abnormalities of contour and suggest pathophysiological events originating from opposite directions [7] (Fig. 20.1). Both the shape and the amplitude of pulse pressure waves are influenced by the site within the arterial tree at which pressure measurements are

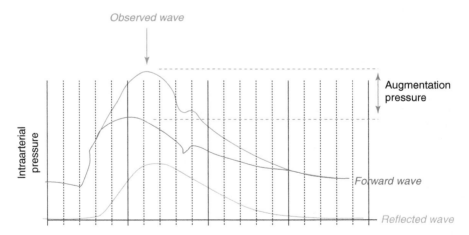

Fig. 20.1 Blood pressure curve in the ascending aorta with its forward and backward components. Augmentation pressure is the difference between systolic blood pressure and the peak of the forward wave and represents the additional systolic blood pressure increase in the ascending aorta due to wave reflections

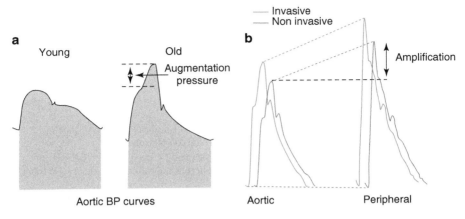

Fig. 20.2 (**a**) Physiological aspects of pulsatile blood pressure curves according to age: young (*left*) and old (*right*) subjects. (**b**) Difference between central and peripheral blood pressure curves: invasive (back waveform) or noninvasive (front waveform)

made. In peripheral arteries, close to the reflection sites, the incident and the reflected waves are in phase and produce an additive effect; conversely, in the ascending aorta and central arteries, the waves are not in phase. The return of the reflected wave is usually delayed to a degree that is dependent on the length of the arterial path and the pulse wave velocity (PWV) and is influenced by age. In mild and older individuals, the PWV increases, the reflecting sites appear to be closer to the ascending aorta, and the timing of the reflected waves is more closely in phase with the incident waves in the central region thus inducing an amplification of aortic and left ventricular pressures during systole and a reducing aortic pressure during diastole [3, 8–10] (Fig. 20.2).

20.1.1 Hemodynamic Patterns of Large Arteries: Methods of Measurement

The compliance, distensibility, or stiffness of an artery expresses the volume contained in the vasculature as a function of a given transmural pressure over a given physiological range [3, 11] (Table 20.1).

Measurement of large artery stiffness is of particular interest in the evaluation of the functions of large arteries. Many approaches have been applied to quantify stiffness. Frequently these approaches represent approximations due to the heterogeneity of the matrix composition, orientation, and smooth muscle types of the arterial wall and variability of arterial wall at different locations [5, 12]. As shown in Table 20.1 a consensus agreement has been established on the terminology used in the literature to describe large-artery stiffness and on the reproducible noninvasive methodology to use [13].

Table 20.1 Indices of arterial stiffness

Index	Definition
Elastic modulus	The pressure (P) step required for 100 % stretch from resting diameter (D) at fixed vessel length: $(\Delta P \cdot D)/\Delta D$ (mmHg)
Arterial distensibility	Relative diameter or area change for a pressure increment (inverse of elastic modulus): $\Delta D/(\Delta P \cdot D)$ (mmHg^{-1})
Arterial compliance	Absolute diameter or area change for a given pressure step at fixed vessel length: $\Delta D/\Delta P$ (cm/mmHg) or (cm^2/mmHg)
Volume elastic modulus	P step required for 100 % increase in volume (V) and no change in length: $\Delta P/(\Delta V/V)$ (mmHg) $\equiv \Delta P/(\Delta D/D)$ (mmHg)
Young's modulus	Elastic modulus per unit area, the pressure step per cm^2 required for 100 % stretch from resting length (h is the wall thickness): $\Delta P \cdot D/(\Delta D \cdot h)$ (mmHg/cm)
Pulse wave velocity	Speed of the pulse along an arterial segment: distance/Δt (cm/s)
Stiffness index	Ratio of logarithm (systolic/diastolic pressures) to (relative change in diameter): $\beta \equiv \ln\left(P_s / P_d\right) / \left(D_s - D_d\right) / D_d$

Three major noninvasive methodologies are available for (a) estimation of artery diameter and distending pressure, (b) analysis of the arterial pulse pressure, and (c) measurement of pulse transit time.

Estimation of artery diameter and distending pressures can be achieved noninvasively and expressing these parameters as distensibility and compliance (change in diameter caused by a given change in pressure), Peterson's elastic modulus (pressure change divided by the ratio of the change in diameter), and Young's modulus (longitudinal force per unit area divided by extension per unit area) [14].

The analysis of arterial pulse pressure involves computerized recording of arterial pressure, arterial diameter, and flow velocity using tonometry, echography, and Doppler techniques and application of three- or four-electrical Windkessel model [15].

The third noninvasive method of evaluating artery stiffness is based on the measurement of pulse transit time [16]. The pulse wave velocity (PWV) analysis involves measurement of arterial pulse transit time between two recording sites on the skin surface. The PWV can be related to the elastic modulus of the arterial wall by a mathematical relationship which involves blood density and arterial geometry.

20.2 Microcirculation

The microcirculatory network represents that part of vascular district in which the major part of energy dissipation in order to overcome resistance occurs, and it includes small arteries (diameter 100–300 μm) and arterioles (diameter <100 μm) [17]. Small arteries contribute for about 30–50 % of precapillary blood pressure drop, although an additional 30 % drop occurs at the arteriolar level with a distribution of resistance that varies among different vascular beds [18]. We can say that the principal function of the microcirculation is to optimize nutrient and oxygen supply

Angioadaptation

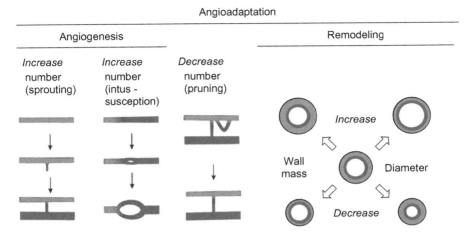

Fig. 20.3 Mechanisms of angioadaptation. The number of vessels is changed by the process of angiogenesis and pruning, while the vessel diameter and wall thickness are affected by remodeling

within the tissues in response to variations of demand and to minimize large fluctuations of hydrostatic pressure in the capillaries. Nevertheless it seems that the pulsatile behavior of blood pressure at the level of the small arteries has important functional consequences. First, pulsatility and myogenic tone are inversely related, implying that conduit arteries have no myogenic tone [19]. Second, the shear stress generated by each pulse wave excites release of endothelial nitric oxide, contributing to the degree of vasodilatation [20]. This allows forward progression of the pulse volume more distally and a change in reflection sites [21]. Thus the architectural design of the distal vascular tree has an influence on pulse pressure beyond the Windkessel (compliance/resistance) paradigm and implies a major role of wave reflections. The pulsatility of pressure exposes arteries in vivo to pulsed perfusion. The implication is that arteries are simultaneously exposed to phasic and static shear stress and stretch that activate different signal transduction pathways. Pressure oscillations elicit sustained afferent vasoconstriction, and the magnitude of the responses depends exclusively on the peak pressure [20, 22, 23]. It has been also shown that pulsed perfusion generates substantially different responses in endothelial nitric oxide synthesis, protein phosphorylation, and oxidative stress signaling [24].

Microvascular beds and their functional structure are maintained by processes named angioadaptation [25] (Fig. 20.3). New vessels are generated by two different modes: sprouting and splitting [26–28]. With the establishment of blood flow, control of vascular development is increasingly taken over by feedback signals derived from vascular function including blood flow (shear stress) and blood pressure (circumferential wall stress) in addition to those derived from the metabolic state of the tissue [29, 30]. This allows elimination of vessels which are functionally inadequate by the process of pruning and adjustment of vessel properties (diameter, wall thickness) by remodeling. For angioadaptations, responses of endothelial cells to shear stress by the activation of a number of signal transduction pathways are crucial [31–36]. As a result of angioadaptation, the properties of vascular beds are determined by the interplay between vascular and cellular reactions to hemodynamic and molecular signals and the functional implications of these reactions, constituting a complex feedback system. Pathophysiological changes of vascular response may lead to vascular maladaptation, e.g., inward remodeling and rarefaction in hypertension.

20.2.1 Evaluation of Structural and Functional Patterns of Microcirculation

The methods for the evaluation of microvascular structural and functional characteristics available in humans are relatively few: histology, plethysmography, wire and pressure myography, and scanning laser Doppler flowmetry.

Histological approaches are charged with substantial pitfalls, due to the artifacts introduced by fixation, staining, and dehydration [17].

Plethysmography has been one of the first methods used in the evaluation of forearm blood flow and vascular resistance. The plethysmographic technique needs the occlusion of the brachial artery of the dominant arm, through the inflation of a sphygmomanometric bladder up to 300 mmHg for 13 min and then a dynamic exercise (20–30 handgrips against resistance). The arterial occlusion is rapidly removed, while venous occlusion is maintained (around 60 mmHg of pressure in the sphygmomanometric bladder). Arterial flow is measured every 10 s for 3 min by a mercury strain gauge, which evaluates the increased volume of the forearm. In the absence of venous backward flow, the increased forearm volume is proportional to the arterial flow. The mean blood pressure divided by the maximum arterial flow allows the calculation of minimum vascular resistance [37].

The methodological approach that had the widest application is represented by the wire or pressure micromyography, as it allows a reliable evaluation of structural changes within the vascular wall and of functional aspects as well. Wire micromyography was developed by Mulvany and Halpern in the 1970s [38], and it was applied in several vascular districts (mesenteric, cerebral, coronary, renal, femoral) of different animal models. This technique was also used for the evaluation of morphology and function of small arteries obtained from biopsies of the subcutaneous tissue from the gluteal or anterior abdominal region, in normotensive as well as in hypertensive patients [39, 40]. Technically, small artery segments (diameter 100–300 µm), obtained by dissection and made free of periadventitial fat tissue, are cannulated with stainless steel wires and mounted on a micromyograph paying attention to preserve the endothelium. A mechanical stretch may be applied through a micrometric screw, while a force transducer records the passive tension developed. Adding various substances to the bath, such as norepinephrine, potassium, and serotonin, it is possible to measure the contractile responses of the vessels. Subsequently the vessel, in a relaxed condition, is transferred on the stage of an immersion lens microscope, and through a micrometric ocular the wall thickness and the internal diameter are evaluated and cross-sectional areas and volumes calculated. The most relevant and useful parameter obtained with this approach is the tunica media/internal lumen ratio that it appears independent from the vessel's dimensions [41].

An alternative to the wire micromyography is represented by perfusion-pressure micromyography. With this approach, isolated vessels are mounted in a pressurized myograph chamber and slipped into two glass microcannulae, connected to a perfusion system that allows a constant intraluminal pressure of 60 mmHg. Morphology of the vessels is evaluated by computer-assisted video analyzers. Vessels may be analyzed at a constant pressure or constant flow. Pressure micromyography allows a better evaluation of functional responses [42].

To avoid the invasiveness of these two methods, the interest of researchers was focused, in the last decade, on the retinal vascular district, as it represents the only microvascular bed that may be directly viewed with relatively simple approaches, such as an ophthalmoscope or a slit lamp [43]. One of the first attempts to precisely quantify structural alterations of retinal microcirculation was made by Wong et al. [44]. By means of an automated computerized method, they calculated the ratio between the arteriolar and venular external diameters (arterial-to-venular ratio, AVR) in circular segments of the retina. An additional approach was proposed by Hughes et al. [45] which demonstrated the possibility to quantify topological changes in retinal vascular architecture by means of a dedicated software. Harazny et al. [46, 47] proposed a method based on the association between confocal measurement of the external diameter of retinal arterioles and an evaluation of the internal diameter with a laser Doppler technique, with a comparison between the two images made by a dedicated software.

20.3 Arterial Changes in Pathophysiological Conditions

Hypertension is associated with important changes in the cross-sectional architecture (diameter and structure) of the arterial wall, influencing the quantitative (compliance and distensibility) or qualitative (stiffness) properties.

Hypertension enhances the arterial stiffening, and a chronic elevation of arterial pressure is accompanied by a reduction in overall arterial distensibility [48–50]. However, the effects of chronic blood pressure elevations on the mechanical properties of arteries of different structure and size are more complex. It has been shown that, compared to the values seen in normotensives, carotid and radial artery distensibilities were reduced in subjects with isolated systolic hypertension. This was not the case, however, in subjects with systo-diastolic hypertension in whom the reduction only involved carotid arterial distensibility [51]. Thus, alterations of arterial distensibility are not always uniform throughout the arterial tree. Several studies have also focused their attention on the functional factors modulating arterial distensibility in the absence of structural alterations. For example, it has been shown the radial artery distensibility can vary considerably in women throughout the menstrual cycle [52].

In the past, DBP was considered as the better guide to determine the severity of hypertension. Epidemiological studies have then directed attention to SBP as a more adequate for CV risk, and it has been shown that increased PP is an

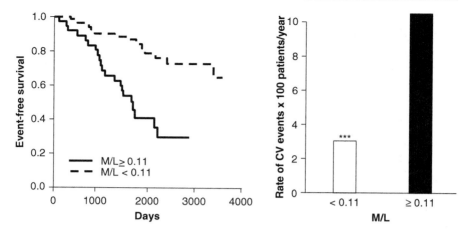

Fig. 20.4 Event-free survival (Kaplan-Meier curves) in a group of patients with essential hypertension and with a media lumen (*M/L*) ratio of subcutaneous small arteries ≥0.11 (*solid line*) or <0.11 (*dotted line*) (*left panel*). Incidence of cardiovascular (CV) events in the two groups (*right panel*) (modified from [64])

independent CV risk factor [53, 54]. Increased PP appears to be the most powerful measure available to identify those hypertensive patients at greatest risk for subsequent myocardial infarction [55, 56]. Because ventricular ejection and arterial stiffness are the main determinants of PP and because ventricular ejection tends to decrease with age, the question has arisen of whether pulse wave velocity, a classic marker of arterial stiffness, might be an independent predictor of CV mortality in subjects with hypertension. Calculation of CV risk using Framingham equations [57] indicates that in these subjects the 10-year CV mortality rate consistently increases with the increase in aortic PWV. After adjustment for age and other confounding variables, PWV is the best theoretical predictor of CV mortality.

The damaging effect of local pulse pressure has been well demonstrated on large and small arteries. Elevated pulse pressure can stimulate hypertrophy, remodeling (increase media: lumen ratio), or rarefaction in the microcirculation, leading to increased resistance to mean flow and a vascular reserve worsening which may have important clinical consequences. Several studies showed a close relationship between microvascular damage in the heart, brain, kidney, and retina and either PP or arterial stiffness. Significant relationships have been demonstrated between brachial PP, arterial stiffness and carotid stiffness, and several target organ damages. Several papers have shown a close relationship with glomerular filtration rate and microalbuminuria [58–60], with white matter lesions or cognitive function [61, 62], with myocardial ischemia [63–65] (Fig. 20.4), and with retinal arteriolar narrowing [46, 66, 67].

In the last decade, with the progress of retinal imaging techniques, a number of observational studies were conducted to characterize the different abnormalities encountered and to determine the factors contributing to their onset. The main findings were the association between retinal arteriolar narrowing and the presence of hypertension or risk of hypertension onset [68–72]. The increase in retinal venular diameter has not been proven to be linked with hypertension, while a correlation was found with the presence of diabetes, obesity, metabolic disorders, smoking, inflammatory markers, endothelial dysfunction, and atherosclerotic markers [73, 74]. The relationship between these abnormalities and cardiovascular risk was also studied in a number of longitudinal studies [75]. The main findings were the increased risk of cardiovascular morbidity and mortality predominantly in individuals <75 years old, correlation with cerebral white matter lesions detected by MRI, increased risk of stroke, and deterioration in cognitive function [76]. Concerning coronary artery disease, the MESA study [77] showed a correlation between the presence of reduced arteriolar caliber and coronary calcifications as observed by CT scan. The association between retinal microvascular abnormalities and the incidence of coronary artery disease, heart failure, and cardiovascular mortality has been observed in several prospective studies [44, 78, 79].

It needs to be mentioned the findings observed in two different pathophysiological conditions, such as obesity and diabetes, associated, with or without the hypertensive state, with an increased morbidity and mortality rate. Obesity is characterized by vascular alterations that involve not only large- and medium-sized arteries [80], but they extend also to the microcirculation as well [81]. The hypertrophic remodeling of the vessel wall is associated with a marked impairment in endothelium-dependent vasodilatation but with a preserved wall stiffness, presumably because the tunica media content of collagen/elastin is not markedly altered. In this condition neural (sympathetic activation) and metabolic (insulin, leptin, adipokines, tumor necrosis factor) factors seem to be the major candidates for the development and progression of vascular hypertrophy and endothelial dysfunction [81].

Similar observations can be reported in patients affected by diabetes mellitus. A marked alteration in small artery structure, an increase in media cross-sectional area (suggesting the presence of hypertrophic remodeling), a correlation between plasma insulin levels and media-to-lumen ratio of subcutaneous small arteries, and an impairment in myogenic response are present in diabetic patients [82, 83]. A functional and structural capillary rarefaction can also be observed in diabetic patients [84]. These alterations favor the target organ damage, particularly at the level of the eyes, kidneys, nerves, and heart. Several studies have clearly shown that these microvascular alterations in diabetic patients are associated with a significant increase in cardiovascular morbidity and mortality; diabetic retinopathy is associated with 1.7-fold increased risk and nephropathy with 2.0-fold increased risk [85].

References

1. Sjostrand T (1953) Volume and distribution of blood and their significance in regulating the circulation. Physiol Rev 33:202–257
2. Guyton AC, Coleman TG, Granger HJ (1972) Circulation: overall regulation. Annu Rev Physiol 34:13–46

3. Nichols WW, O'Rourke M, McDonald DA (1998) Blood flow in arteries: theoretical, experimental and clinical principles. Edward Arnold, London
4. Kelly R, Daley J, Avolio A, O'Rourke M (1989) Arterial dilatation and reduced wave reflection. Hypertension 14:14–21
5. Taylor MG (1964) Wave travel in arteries and the design of the cardiovascular system. In: Attinger EO (ed) Pulsatile blood flow. McGraw-Hill, New York, pp 343–347
6. London GM (1995) Large artery function and alterations in hypertension. J Hypertens 13:S35–S38
7. London GM, Guerin AP, Pannier B et al (1992) Arterial wave reflections and increased systolic and pulse pressure in chronic uremia. Study using non invasive carotid pulse wave-form registration. Hypertension 20:10–19
8. Safar ME, Levi BI, Struijker-Boudier H (2003) Current perspectives on arterial stiffness and pulse pressure in hypertension and cardiovascular diseases. Circulation 107:2864–2869
9. Cohn JN, Finkelstein S, McVeigh G (1995) Non invasive pulse wave analysis for the early detection of vascular disease. Hypertension 26:503–508
10. Herbert A, Cruickshank JK, Laurent S, Boutouyrie P, Reference Values for Arterial Measurements Collaboration (2014) Establishing reference values for central blood pressure and its amplification in a general healthy population and according to cardiovascular risk factors. Eur Heart J. doi:10.1093/eurheartj/ehu293
11. O'Rourke M (1995) Mechanical principles in arterial disease. Hypertension 26:2–9
12. Benetos A, Laurent S, Hoeks AP et al (1993) Arterial alterations with ageing and high blood pressure. A non invasive study of carotid and femoral arteries. Arterioscler Thromb 13:90–97
13. Pannier BM, Avolio AP, Hoeks APG, Mancia G, Tazakawa K (2002) Methods and devices for measuring arterial compliance in humans. Am J Hypertens 15:743–753
14. Lehmann ED (1999) Terminology for the definition of arterial elastic properties. Pathol Biol 47:656–664
15. Davies JI, Strueters AD (2003) Pulse wave analysis and pulse wave velocity: a critical review of their strengths and weaknesses. J Hypertens 21:463–472
16. Asmar R (1999) Arterial stiffness and pulse wave velocity: clinical applications. Elsevier, Amsterdam, pp 9–15
17. Mulvany MJ, Aalkjaer C (1990) Structure and function of small arteries. Physiol Rev 70:921–971
18. Christensen KL, Mulvany MJ (2001) Location of resistance arteries. J Vasc Res 38:1–12
19. Allen SP, Wade SS, Prewitt RL (1997) Myogenic tone attenuates pressure-induced gene expression in isolated small arteries. Hypertension 30:203–208
20. Peng X, Haldar S, Deshpande S et al (2003) Wall stiffness suppress Akt/eNOS and cytoprotection in pulse perfused endothelium. Hypertension 41:378–381
21. Paolocci N, Pagliaro P, Isoda T et al (2001) Role of calcium-sensitive K(+) channels and nitric oxide in in-vivo coronary vasodilation from enhanced perfusion pulsatility. Circulation 103: 119–124
22. Loutzenhiser R, Bidani AK, Wang X (2004) Systolic pressure and the myogenic response of the renal afferent arteriole. Acta Physiol Scand 181:407–413
23. Nakano T, Tominaga R, Nagano I et al (2000) Pulsatile flow enhances endothelium-derived nitric oxide release in the peripheral vasculature. Am J Physiol Heart Circ Physiol 278:H1098–H1104
24. Williams B (1998) Mechanical influences on vascular smooth muscle cell function. J Hypertens 16:1921–1929
25. Zakrzewicz A, Secomb TW, Pries AR (2002) Angioadaptation: keeping the vascular system in shape. News Physiol Sci 17:197–201
26. Carmeliet P (2005) Angiogenesis in life, disease and medicine. Nature 438:932–936
27. Burri PH, Hlushchuk R, Djonov V (2004) Intussusceptive angiogenesis: its emergence, its characteristics, and its significance. Dev Dyn 231:474–488
28. Gerhardt H, Golding M, Fruttiger M et al (2003) VEGF guides angiogenic sprouting utilizing endothelial tip cell filopodia. J Cell Biol 161:1163–1177

29. le Noble F, Klein C, Tintu A et al (2008) Neural guidance molecules, tip cells, and mechanical factors in vascular development. Cardiovasc Res 78:232–241
30. le Noble F, Fleury V, Pries A et al (2005) Control of arterial branching morphogenesis in embryogenesis: go with the flow. Cardiovasc Res 65:619–628
31. Lehoux S, Castier Y, Tedgui A (2006) Molecular mechanisms of the vascular responses to haemodynamic forces. J Intern Med 259:381–392
32. Kurz H, Burri PH, Djonov VG (2003) Angiogenesis and vascular remodeling by intussusception: from form to function. News Physiol Sci 18:65–70
33. Baum O, Da Silva-Azevedo L, Willerding G et al (2004) Endothelial NOS is main mediator for shear stress-dependent angiogenesis in skeletal muscle after prazosin administration. Am J Physiol Heart Circ Physiol 287:H2300–H2308
34. Hudlicka O, Brown MD, May S et al (2006) Changes in capillary shear stress in skeletal muscle exposed to long term activity: role of nitric oxide. Microcirculation 13:249–259
35. Hudlicka O (1998) Is physiological angiogenesis in skeletal muscle regulated by changes in microcirculation? Microcirculation 5:5–23
36. Ferrara N, Gerber HP, LeCouter J (2003) The biology of VGEF and its receptors. Nat Med 9:669–676
37. Greenfield ADM, Whitney RJ, Mowbray JF (1963) Methods for investigation of peripheral flow. Br Med Bull 19:101–109
38. Mulvany MJ, Halpern W (1977) Contractile properties of small resistance vessels in spontaneously hypertensive and normotensive rats. Circ Res 41:19–26
39. Aalkjaer C, Eiskjaer H, Mulvany MJ et al (1989) Abnormal structure and function of isolated subcutaneous resistance vessels from essential hypertensive patients despite antihypertensive treatment. J Hypertens 7:305–310
40. Agabiti-Rosei E, Rizzoni D, Castellano M et al (1995) Media: lumen ratio in human small resistance arteries is related to forearm minimal vascular resistance. J Hypertens 13:341–347
41. Schiffrin EL, Deng LY (1996) Structure and function of resistance arteries of hypertensive patients treated with a beta-blocker or a calcium channel antagonist. J Hypertens 14:1247–1255
42. Schiffrin EL, Hayoz D (1997) How to assess vascular remodeling in small and medium-sized muscular arteries in humans. J Hypertens 15:571–584
43. Mancia G, Fagard R, Narkiewicz K et al; Task Force Members (2013) 2013 ESH/ESC guidelines for the management of arterial hypertension: the Task Force for the management of arterial hypertension of the European Society of Hypertension (ESH) and of the European Society of Cardiology (ESC). J Hypertens 31:1281–1357
44. Wong TY, Klein R, Sharett AR et al (2002) Retinal arteriolar narrowing and risk of coronary heart disease in men and women. The Atherosclerosis Risk in Communities Study. JAMA 287:1153–1159
45. Hughes AD, Martinez-Perez E, Jabbar AS et al (2006) Quantification of topological changes in retinal vascular architecture in essential and malignant hypertension. J Hypertens 24:889–894
46. Harazny JM, Ritt M, Baleanu D et al (2007) Increased wall: lumen ratio of retinal arterioles in male patients with a history of a cerebrovascular events. Hypertension 50:623–629
47. Harazny JM, Raff U, Welzenbach J et al (2011) New software analyses increase the reliability of measurements of retinal arterioles morphology by scanning laser Doppler flowmetry in humans. J Hypertens 29:777–782
48. Beltran A, McVeigh G, Morgan D et al (2001) Arterial compliance abnormalities in isolated systolic hypertension. Am J Hypertens 14:1007–1011
49. Boutouyrie P, Tropeano AL, Asmar R et al (2002) Aortic stiffness is an independent predictor of primary coronary events in hypertensive patients: a longitudinal study. Hypertension 39:10–15
50. Blacher J, Asmar R, Djane S et al (1999) Aortic pulse velocity as a marker of cardiovascular risk in hypertensive patients. Hypertension 33:1111–1117
51. Stella ML, Failla M, Mangoni AA et al (1998) Effects of isolated systolic hypertension and essential hypertension on large and middle sized artery compliance. Blood Press 7:96–102

52. Giannattasio C, Failla M, Grappiolo A et al (1999) Fluctuations of radial artery distensibility throughout the menstrual cycle. Arterioscler Thromb Vasc Biol 19:1925–1929
53. Sagie A, Larson MG, Levy D (1993) The natural history of borderline isolated systolic hypertension. N Engl J Med 329:1912–1917
54. Darne B, Girerd X, Safar M et al (1989) Pulsatile versus steady component of blood pressure: a cross-sectional analysis and a prospective analysis on cardiovascular mortality. Hypertension 13:392–400
55. Franklin SS, Khan SA, Wong ND et al (1999) Is pulse pressure useful in predicting risk for coronary heart disease: the Framingham Heart Study. Circulation 100:354–360
56. Benetos A, Zureik M, Morcet J et al (2000) A decrease in diastolic blood pressure combined with an increase in systolic blood pressure is associated with high cardiovascular mortality. J Am Coll Cardiol 35:673–680
57. Anderson KM, Odell PM, Wilson PWF, Kannel WB (1991) Cardiovascular disease risk profiles. Am Heart J 121:293–298
58. Fesler P, Safar ME, du Cailar G et al (2007) Pulse pressure is an independent determinant of renal function decline during treatment of essential hypertension. J Hypertens 25:1915–1920
59. Briet M, Bozec E, Laurent S et al (2006) Arterial stiffness and enlargement in mild to moderate chronic kidney disease. Kidney Int 96:350–357
60. Hermans MM, Henry R, Dekker JM et al (2007) Estimated glomerular filtration rate and urinary albumin excretion are independently associated with greater arterial stiffness: the Hoorn Study. J Am Soc Nephrol 18:1942–1952
61. Henskens LH, Kroon AA, van Oostenbrugge RJ et al (2008) Increased aortic pulse wave velocity is associated with silent cerebral small vessel disease in hypertensive patients. Hypertension 52:1120–1126
62. Hanon O, Haulon S, Lenoir H et al (2005) Relationship between arterial stiffness and cognitive function in elderly subjects with complaints of memory loss. Stroke 36:2193–2197
63. Kaul S, Ito H (2004) Microvasculature in acute myocardial ischemia: part I: evolving concepts in pathophysiology, diagnosis and treatment. Circulation 109:146–149
64. Rizzoni D, Porteri E, Boari GEM et al (2003) Prognostic significance of small artery structure in hypertension. Circulation 108:2230–2235
65. Safar ME, Lacolley P (2007) Disturbance of macro- and microcirculation: relations with pulse pressure and cardiac organ damage. Am J Physiol Heart Circ Physiol 293:H1–H7
66. Cheung H, Sharrett AR, Klein R et al (2007) Aortic distensibility and retinal arteriolar narrowing: the multiethnic study of atherosclerosis. Hypertension 50:617–622
67. Masaidi M, Cuspidi C, Giudici V et al (2009) Is retinal arteriolar-venular ratio associated with cardiac and extracardiac organ damage in essential hypertension? J Hypertens 27:1277–1283
68. Grassi G, Buzzi S, Dell'Oro R et al (2013) Structural alterations of the retinal microcirculation in the "prehypertensive" high- normal blood pressure state. Curr Pharm Des 19(13):2375–2381
69. Wong TY, Klein R, Sharrett AR et al; Atherosclerosis Risk in Communities Study (2004) Retinal arteriolar diameter and risk for hypertension. Ann Intern Med 140:248–255
70. Wong TY, Shankar A, Klein R et al (2004) Prospective cohort study of retinal vessel diameters and risk of hypertension. BMJ 329:79
71. Smith W, Wang JJ, Wong TY et al (2004) Retinal arteriolar narrowing is associated with 5-year incident severe hypertension: the Blue Mountains Eye Study. Hypertension 44:442–447
72. Ikram MK, Witteman JC, Vingerling JR et al (2006) Retinal vessel diameters and risk of hypertension: the Rotterdam Study. Hypertension 47:189–194
73. Klein R, Sharrett AR, Klein BE et al (2000) Are retinal arteriolar abnormalities related to atherosclerosis? The Atherosclerosis Risk in Communities Study. Atherioscler Thromb Vasc Biol 20:1644–1650
74. Nguyen TT, Wong TY (2006) Retinal vascular manifestations of metabolic disorders. Trends Endocrinol Metab 17:262–268
75. Mimoun L, Massin P, Steg G (2009) Retinal microvascularisation abnormalities and cardiovascular risk. Arch Cardiovasc Dis 102:449–456

76. Wong TY, Klein R, Sharrett AR et al; ARIC Investigators (2002) Cerebral white matter lesions, retinopathy, and incident clinical stroke. JAMA 288:67–74
77. Wang L, Wong TY, Sharrett AR et al (2008) Relationship between retinal arteriolar narrowing and myocardial perfusion: multi-ethnic study of atherosclerosis. Hypertension 51:119–126
78. Wang JJ, Liew G, Wong TY et al (2006) Retinal vascular calibre and the risk of coronary heart disease-related death. Heart 92:1583–1587
79. Wong TY, Kamineni A, Klein R et al (2006) Quantitative retinal venular caliber and risk of cardiovascular disease in older persons: the cardiovascular health study. Arch Intern Med 166:2388–2394
80. Levy BI, Schiffrin EL, Mourad JJ et al (2008) Impaired tissue perfusion: a pathology common to hypertension, obesity, and diabetes mellitus. Circulation 118:968–976
81. Grassi G, Seravalle G, Scopelliti F et al (2009) Structural and functional alterations of subcutaneous small resistance arteries in severe human obesity. Obesity 18:92–98
82. Rizzoni D, Porteri E, Guelfi D et al (2001) Structural alterations in subcutaneous small arteries of normotensive and hypertensive patients with non insulin dependent diabetes mellitus. Circulation 103:1238–1244
83. Schofield I, Malik R, Izzard A et al (2002) Vascular structural and functional changes in type 2 diabetes mellitus. Evidence for the roles of abnormal myogenic responsiveness and dyslipidemia. Circulation 106:3037–3043
84. Clark MG, Barrett EJ, Wallis MG et al (2002) The microvasculature in insulin resistance and type 2 diabetes. Semin Vasc Med 2:21–31
85. Rosenson RS, Fioretto P, Dodson PM (2011) Does microvascular disease predict macrovascular events in type 2 diabetes? Atherosclerosis 218:13–18

Chronic Kidney Disease and Renovascular Interactions

21

Adel E. Berbari, Najla A. Daouk, and Majida M. Daouk

21.1 Introduction

Chronic kidney disease (CKD) is a significant public health concern [1]. CKD is associated with a markedly increased risk of cardiovascular disease (CVD) [2, 3]. Cardiovascular complications are the major cause of the enhanced morbidity and mortality in patients with CKD and in particular in end-stage renal disease (ESRD) [4–6].

Similar findings have been reported in the pediatric age group. Cardiovascular morbidity and even mortality seem to be enhanced among children and adolescents with CKD and ESRD, despite much lower exposure to classical risk factors for atherosclerosis such as hypertension, dyslipidemia, diabetes mellitus, and smoking [7, 8].

These observations suggest that different pathophysiologic mechanisms appear to be involved in the arteriopathy of CKD and ESRD in pediatric and adult age groups [7].

The aims of this chapter are to: (1) define the clinical characteristics and risk profile in CKD and (2) discuss the spectrum of cardiovascular disorders associated with renal functional impairment and the pathophysiologic mechanisms underlying renovascular associations.

21.2 Chronic Kidney Disease

21.2.1 Definition

CKD encompasses a large group of heterogeneous disorders which affect the structure and function of the kidney. Current definitions of CKD include the presence of markers of kidney damage (albuminuria, abnormalities of urinary sediment,

A.E. Berbari (✉) • N.A. Daouk • M.M. Daouk
Department of Internal Medicine, American University of Beirut Medical Center, Beirut, Lebanon
e-mail: ab01@aub.edu.lb; nd00@aub.edu.lb; md00@aub.edu.lb

© Springer International Publishing Switzerland 2015
A. Berbari, G. Mancia (eds.), *Arterial Disorders:*
Definition, Clinical Manifestations, Mechanisms and Therapeutic Approaches,
DOI 10.1007/978-3-319-14556-3_21

imaging tests, and/or biopsy) and impaired function [rising serum creatinine levels, decreased glomerular filtration rate (GFR $\leq$60 ml/min/1.73 m²), and low urine output] for over 3 months [9, 10]. Based on these criteria, it has been estimated that the population prevalence of CKD is 10–15 % worldwide [9, 10].

21.2.2 Classification and Staging

The aim of this section is not an extensive discussion of the classification and staging of CKD but to present an overview of the salient features which characterize each stage of CKD.

According to the National Kidney Foundation (NKF) guidelines, the stage of CKD is defined by the level of GFR, with higher stages representing lower GFR levels and/or by the presence of markers of CKD damage [9].

21.2.2.1   Levels of GFR (Table 21.1)
GFR $\geq$90 ml/min/1.73 m²
Individuals with GFR $\geq$90 ml/min/1.73 m² may or may not have CKD depending on the presence of evidence of kidney damage. Those with this level of renal function with or without hypertension and no markers of kidney damage are considered to have no CKD, although an elevation of BP may predispose to adverse renal and cardiovascular outcomes [9]. However, GFR $\geq$90 ml/min/1.73 m² with markers of kidney damage are considered to have CKD and are classified as stage 1.

GFR = 60–89 ml/min/1.73 m²
Individuals with GFR = 60–89 ml/min/1.73 m² are classified as stage 2 and may or may not have CKD. Such levels of GFR are frequently observed at extremes of age (infants and elderly). Whether such GFR levels without markers of kidney damage suggest CKD is unclear. However there is no definite evidence of increased risk of progression to CKD and or cardiovascular events in such individuals [9].

GFR <60 ml/min/1.73 m²
All individuals with a GFR <60 ml/min/1.73 m² for over 3 months are classified as having CKD independent of the presence of kidney damage [9]. These individuals, who have lost over 50 % of their renal function, appear to be at increased risk of cardiovascular complications [9].

Decreasing levels of GFR are classified as stages 3, 4, and 5 depending on the level of renal function (refer to Table 21.1). Such patients are at increased risk of progression to ESRD and cardiovascular events [9, 10].

21.2.2.2   Kidney Damage
Presence of markers of kidney damage which include albuminuria, abnormal urine sediment, or imaging tests and kidney biopsy findings is classified as CKD, independent of the level of GFR [9] (Table 21.1).

Table 21.1 Classification/staging of chronic kidney disease modified from National Kidney Foundation guidelines [10]

Stage	GFR (ml/min/1.73 m²)	HT	Kidney damage	CKD	CVD risk
	Glomerular filtration rates				
1	≥90	+	0	0	±
	≥90	±	+	+	+
2	60–89	0	0	±	±
	60–89	±	+	+	+
3	30–59	±	+	+	+
4	15–29	+	+	+	+
5	<15	+	+	+	+
	Presence of kidney damage classified as CKD irrespective of GFR level				

HT hypertension, *CKD* chronic kidney disease, *CVD* cardiovascular disease, *GFR* glomerular filtration rate

21.2.2.3 Renovascular Associations

The advent of adequate renal replacement therapy (dialysis and renal transplantation) over the past several decades has been associated with increased life span of patients with end-stage renal disease (ESRD). As those patients survive longer, they tend to develop and die of cardiovascular disease [11, 12].

Compared to the general population, the mortality rate from CVD is 500-fold higher in younger patients on dialysis and five times greater among older patients [11, 12].

The increased risk of poor cardiovascular outcome is not limited to patients with ESRD. Patients with early CKD are more likely to die from cardiovascular comorbidities than to progress to ESRD [13, 14]. Similarly, patients with reduced GFR tend to die from cardiovascular disease than to develop ESRD [13, 14].

21.3 Spectrum of Vascular Diseases in Adults

21.3.1 Renovascular Associations

The pathophysiologic mechanisms of the exclusively elevated cardiovascular morbidity and mortality in CKD/ESRD have not been completely elucidated. Patients with CKD have a high burden of cardiovascular risk factors [15, 16]. They share both traditional and uremia-related risk factors [15, 16]. As a result, CKD populations display a wide spectrum of vascular pathologies [12, 17]. The kidney appears to act as a perceiver and modulator of cardiovascular disease [18].

Among various system/organ disorders, renal functional impairment is unique in that it involves almost every segment of the cardiovascular system. Vascular changes involve both the macrocirculation and microcirculation [12, 17] (Fig. 21.1).

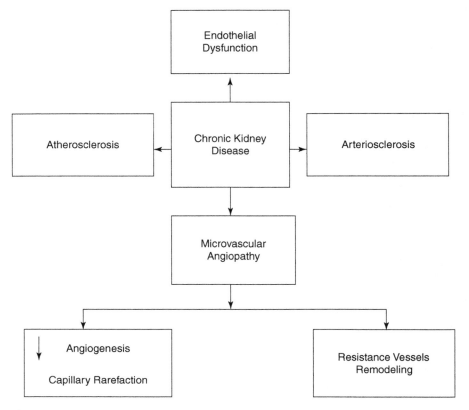

Fig. 21.1 Spectrum of vascular disease in chronic kidney disease

21.3.2 Macrovascular Diseases

21.3.2.1 Atherosclerosis

Atherosclerosis which refers to an intimal disease, more frequent in CKD/ESRD than in nonrenal populations, is characterized by the presence of plaques and occlusive vascular lesions [12, 18, 19]. Calcifications, when present, involve the intima [18, 19]. However, in CKD, the atherosclerotic lesions have a distinct morphology. They are frequently calcified with a relatively increased media thickness, whereas in the general population, they are fibroatheromatous with thickening of the intima [18, 19].

Intimal calcification is observed in older patients with a clinical history of atherosclerotic complications and even before the initiation of dialysis therapy [20]. In contrast, medial calcification occurs more frequently in young and middle-aged patients with CKD, and its severity increases with the degree of uremia-related cardiovascular risk profile [20, 21].

In CKD, as in the general population, traditional cardiovascular risk factors have been postulated to initiate the atherosclerotic process [5, 11]. Among these factors, dyslipidemia appears to be a major determinant [22–24]. However the atherogenic dyslipidemia pattern, which is characterized by increased triglycerides, low high-density lipoprotein cholesterol (HDL-C), and normal or near-normal total serum cholesterol levels, plays a critical role in the pathogenesis of the atherosclerotic process only in patients with mild renal functional impairment [25, 26]. In contrast, in patients with more severe renal functional impairment, the atherogenic dyslipidemia pattern becomes a weaker predictor of atherosclerosis and cardiovascular disease [25, 26]. In moderate to severe renal insufficiency, there appears to be no relationship between renal function and progression of the atherosclerotic process [27]. No difference in atheroma plaque volume and growth could be demonstrated in patients with GFR >60 ml/min/1.73 m^2 versus those with GFR <60 ml/min/1.73 m^2. These observations suggest that in more severe renal functional impairment, pathobiologic processes other than or in addition to the known traditional factors may be involved in the initiation and progression of cardiovascular disease [26–28].

Atherosclerotic lesions tend to be patchy in distribution along the length of the artery and more frequent in the CKD population and tend to be more occlusive [25–28]. Clinical presentations include ischemic heart disease (angina, myocardial infarction, and sudden cardiac death), cerebrovascular disorders, and heart failure [25, 26].

21.3.2.2 Arteriosclerosis

Arteriosclerosis is a frequent vascular lesion in CKD/ESRD. It is defined as hardening or stiffening of the arteries, particularly the elastic arteries (aorta/major branches and common carotid artery), and is characterized by increased luminal diameter, media thickness, and extracellular matrix, destruction of the elastic lamellae, and extensive medial calcification [20, 21, 29, 30]. These structural modifications, often referred to as remodeling, reduce elasticity and compliance and increase stiffness of the elastic arteries, impairing the cushion function and capacity to smooth out the pulsatile flow associated with intermittent ventricular ejection [29, 30].

Arterial aging impaired renal function and elevated BP levels are the major determinants of increased arterial stiffness [29].

Factors that link arterial stiffness to renal function have not been completely elucidated. Disturbed mineral metabolism associated with renal functional impairment has been postulated to account for remodeling process [20, 28]. In CKD/ESRD, the mineral metabolism, characterized by hyperphosphatemia, increased calcium phosphorous product, hyperparathyroidism, and reduced 1,25 vitamin D(OH) 25, appears to induce medial calcification and arterial stiffening [20, 28, 31–33]. However the relationship between increased arterial stiffness and renal function is not limited to patients with substantially impaired renal function and ESRD. An inverse relationship between arterial stiffness and renal function has been reported in a group of never-treated individuals with mild renal insufficiency (serum creatinine ≥1.47 mg/dl) and normal or mildly elevated BP levels [34]. It has been postulated that in such individuals changes in serum phosphate levels, although still within the normal reference range, may trigger arterial calcification and cause increased arterial stiffness [34].

Ejection of left ventricular stroke volume into stiff elastic arteries results in an increase in amplitude of the systolic and a decrease in diastolic blood pressures, enhanced pulse wave velocity and early return of the reflected pulse wave into late systole, and a wide pulse pressure [35, 36]. Clinically, these alterations in arterial function are associated with isolated systolic hypertension, left ventricular hypertrophy, coronary hypoperfusion, and damage to highly perfused target organs such as the brain and the kidneys. These patients are prone to develop coronary events, heart failure, impaired cognitive function and dementia, and renal dysfunction [35, 36].

21.3.2.3 Vascular Diseases in ESRD/Uremia

Patients on renal replacement therapy often exhibit both atherosclerosis and arteriosclerosis. Both lesions are more severe and more widespread. A significantly higher prevalence of calcified plaques has been reported in the common carotid artery [23, 24, 28, 29, 37].

The arteriosclerotic changes which involve the large central elastic arteries are characterized by luminal dilatation, increased intima-media thickness, and significant increase in arterial stiffness. In uremic patients, the altered arterial stiffness appears to be more apparent in younger than in older individuals, since aging may mask the uremia-related elevation in the wall properties of the vessel [7, 28, 29].

The high incidence of cardiovascular events in dialyzed and uremic patients has been attributed to the severe macrovascular disease in this population [37, 38].

21.3.2.4 Calcific Uremic Arteriolopathy/Calciphylaxis

Calcific uremic arteriolopathy (CUA), also known as calciphylaxis, is a rare life-threatening microvascular calcific disorder which affects predominantly adult patients with ESRD and uremia or with CKD [39, 40]. It is characterized both by specific histopathologic findings and clinical presentation. Histopathologic findings include media calcification of the small- and medium-sized vessels, extravascular calcification, intimal proliferation, microthrombus formation, epidermal ulceration, and subdermal and dermal necrosis [39]. The obliterative vasculopathy also involves both venules and capillaries [39]. The clinical manifestations are characterized by painful, violaceous, mottled skin lesions which may progress to tissue necrosis, nonhealing ulcers, and gangrene, possibly leading to amputation, sepsis, and/or death [39]. Multiple risk factors, such as female gender, diabetes, obesity, warfarin use, hyperphosphatemia, hyperparathyroidism, use of calcium-containing phosphate binders, and severe CKD, have been postulated to act as pathophysiologic factors [39–41]. The prognosis of CUA is poor, being determined by the underlying cardiovascular disease [39, 40].

21.3.2.5 Uremic Cardiomyopathy

Cardiovascular disease (CVD), the leading cause of mortality in patients with end-stage renal disease (ESRD), accounts for over 40 % of all deaths [42]. Of all of these various complications, heart failure, often referred to as uremic cardiomyopathy, appears to be the most frequent [43–46].

The pathophysiologic mechanism of uremic cardiomyopathy has not been completely elucidated. In contrast to the general population, the contribution of atherosclerotic coronary artery disease is less important in CKD [43–46]. In an autopsy study of 94 uremic patients dying from heart failure, presence of coronary heart disease was absent to minimal in 40 % [42].

Hemodynamic, structural, and uremia-related humoral and metabolic factors have been postulated to account for uremic cardiomyopathy. With worsening renal function and onset of heart failure, uremic patients often exhibit hypertension, anemia, and overactive circulation associated with the creation of an arteriovenous fistula in those on hemodialysis treatment, increased arterial stiffening, left ventricular hypertrophy, and dilatation resulting from pressure and volume overload [45, 46]. Structural changes in autopsied uremic hearts include intracardiac coronary artery thickening, decreased myocardial capillary density, increased myocardial fibrosis, and inhibition of apoptosis in hearts of experimental uremic animals [42–46]. Clinically these patients present heart failure resistant to therapy, evidence of myocardial ischemia and arrhythmias, and sudden cardiac death [45].

21.3.3 Microvascular Diseases

21.3.3.1 Impairment of Endothelial Function
Endothelial dysfunction, a major determinant of cardiovascular disease, is frequently reported in CKD/ESRD [47].

Endothelial function is assessed by dilatation of the brachial artery in response to hyperemia or administration of sublingual glyceryl trinitrate (nitroglycerine) [48]. Maximal brachial artery dilatation to hyperemia assesses endothelium-dependent vasodilatation while the response to nitroglycerine evaluates the endothelium-independent vascular function [48].

In CKD, the endothelium-dependent vasodilatation is defective, while the endothelium-independent vascular function remains intact [48].

In CKD, impairment of endothelial function has been reported even in mild decrease in renal function and becomes progressively severe with further deterioration in renal function [48].

Several factors have been implicated in the pathophysiology of endothelial function in CKD [47–50]: (1) impaired nitric oxide release or bioavailability due to accumulation and elevation of asymmetric dimethylarginine (ADMA) levels, (2) oxidative stress associated with accumulation of oxidative stress markers, (3) activation of renin-angiotensin system which induces oxidative stress, (4) chronic inflammation, (5) homocysteinemia, (6) hyperuricemia, (7) dyslipidemia, and (8) deficiency of endothelial progenitor cells.

21.3.3.2 Remodeling of the Resistance Arteries and Capillary Rarefaction
Changes in the structural properties of the microcirculation have been documented in CKD and ESRD. These structural modifications are characterized by remodeling of the resistance arteries and arterioles and capillary rarefaction.

Remodeling of the Small Arteries/Arterioles

Remodeling of the small arteries and arterioles is characterized by increased wall thickness, luminal narrowing, and increased wall/lumen ratio [51]. These structural features may be associated with a reduced wall cross-sectional area in eutrophic remodeling and increased wall cross-sectional area in hypertrophic remodeling [51].

Although both types of these structural alterations are often associated with hypertension, they have been reported also in CKD/ESRD [51]. In a model of uremic hypertension in rats, systemic resistance arteries (cremasteric and mesenteric) exhibited inward eutrophic remodeling while the cerebral arteries were spared [51]. Similar observations were made in normotensive rats with renal failure [52]. In these animals, intramyocardial arterioles were thickened although their BP was not elevated [52]. These observations suggest that renal functional impairment may provoke remodeling of resistance arteries even in the absence of hypertension [51–54].

Capillary Rarefaction

Capillary rarefaction defined as a reduction in the number or length of capillaries or both appears to be a histopathologic feature of advanced renal functional impairment [54–56]. In experimental animals, in addition to the intramyocardial arteriolar wall thickening, capillary rarefaction has been reported in experimental uremic animals [55]. These changes were independent of BP levels [55].

Similar histopathologic findings involving the microcirculation have been reported in patients with uremic cardiomyopathy [43].

The altered morphologic features of renal functional impairment and uremia have been attributed to uremia-related factors or to cross talk between the macrocirculation and microcirculation [37, 38].

21.4   Chronic Kidney Disease in Pediatric and Young Adults

21.4.1 Epidemiology

As in adults, the life expectancy of pediatric, adolescent, and young adult patients with CKD is significantly shortened [8, 58, 59]. Several studies have indicated that in the United States, children on dialysis live 40–60 years less than their nonrenal counterparts [8, 58, 59]. Similarly, the mortality of young adults (aged 25–34 years) on dialysis is 700-fold higher than in age-related subjects in the general population [8, 58–60]. Analysis of data from Australia and New Zealand Dialysis and Transplant Registry has also demonstrated that in all children and adolescents who were 20 years of age or younger at the initiation of renal replacement therapy, mortality rates were 30 times higher than in age-matched individuals in the general population [8, 58–60].

The United States Renal Data System (USRDS) Annual Data Report revealed a persistently elevated mortality rate from cardiovascular causes in children on chronic dialysis [55]. Cardiac death is the second most common cause of death among pediatric patients with ESRD, accounting for 25 % of those deaths [58]. Cardiac death rates varied in an inconsistent pattern in the various age groups although the youngest age groups (<5 years) had the highest rate, accounting for about 10 % [8, 59, 60]. In all age groups, cardiac arrest was the most common cause of death followed by arrhythmias, cardiomyopathy, other cardiac disorders, and myocardial infarction [8, 59, 60].

21.4.2 Spectrum of Cardiovascular Disease

Cardiovascular disease is an important determinant of premature death in the pediatric CKD population [8, 59, 60]. It is due to three separate, although interrelated, disease processes: (a) atherosclerosis, (b) arteriosclerosis, and (c) myocardial disease [8, 60]. However, myocardial consequences of atherosclerosis barely exist in children [61].

21.4.2.1 Arteriosclerosis and Atherosclerosis
Both atherosclerosis and arteriosclerosis characterize the arterial damage in CKD in pediatric and young adult populations [8, 60–63]. In both lesions, vascular wall calcification is a major feature involving the tunica intima in atherosclerosis and tunica media in arteriosclerosis [60, 65].

Calcific arteriopathy is an active process and is regulated by mineral, metabolic, mechanical, infectious, and inflammatory influences [39]. An altered mineral metabolism, characterized by high serum phosphorous levels, elevated calcium phosphate product, and an imbalance between promoters and inhibitors of serum calcium phosphate complex uptake and precipitation in the vascular wall, has been identified as a major determinant of vascular calcification [60, 63].

Healthy children have phosphorous and calcium above the reference values and have a calcium/phosphate product above the recommended value (>55 mg^2/dl^2) [60, 63]. However, crystallization is prevented by inhibitors [60]. Several studies have demonstrated that in CKD and ESRD, the concentration of circulatory inhibitors such as fetuin-A and osteoprotegerin is reduced [64]. The reduced concentration of fetuin-A, a highly potent inhibitor of calcium phosphate complex formation, may favor arterial calcification [64, 65].

Atherosclerosis and arteriosclerosis represent two arterial lesions exhibiting different histopathologic cardiovascular risk factors, clinical manifestation profile, and age of onset of CKD.

Atherosclerotic lesions are characteristically intimal and patchy, associated with formation of occlusive plaques, dependent on the presence of traditional risk factors [58, 60]. Patients often present signs of decreased perfusion of target organs [62]. On the other hand, arteriosclerosis is a diffuse process, involving both intima and media of the vessel wall, resulting from a disturbed mineral metabolism [60]. Clinical manifestations are related to stiffening of the wall of elastic arteries [62, 64]. In pediatric CKD, arteriosclerosis can occur in the absence of atherosclerosis [66].

In pediatric CKD patients, younger than 20 years of age, arteriosclerosis appears to be the initial arteriopathy which develops during the course of progressive decline in renal function [60]. Evidence of atherosclerosis lesions are often absent as these children have no traditional cardiovascular risk factors [60, 66].

However, with increasing age and appearance of traditional risk factors, young adult patients with childhood CKD exhibit evidence of atherosclerotic lesions in coronary and carotid arteries and occlusive cardiovascular events [66, 67].

These observations suggest that in pediatric CKD, cardiovascular pathology is bimodal. In patients younger than 20 years of age, both the uremia-related risk factors and absence of traditional risk factors promote the development of arteriosclerosis and stiffening of the central elastic arteries. With increasing age in young adult patients with childhood CKD, the traditional cardiovascular risk factors become prominent [60, 61, 63]. Presence of both types of risk factors favors the development of the two types of arterial lesions and their associated clinical manifestation [60, 61, 63, 66, 67].

21.4.2.2 Cardiomyopathy

With advancing renal failure and ESRD, the uremia-related factors become prominent, leading to dilated especially hypertrophic cardiomyopathy. Macroscopic and microscopic structural abnormalities include fibrosis and cellular hypertrophy which predispose to electrical instability and arrhythmia which is the leading cause of death in CKD pediatric patients [8, 63]. In addition, the severe left ventricular hypertrophy which frequently occurs in children on prolonged dialysis may predispose to coronary microvascular disease, favoring treatment-resistant congestive heart failure [68].

Cardiomyopathy is a terminal myocardial disorder in CKD pediatric patients and carries an ominous prognosis [68].

21.4.2.3 Endothelial Dysfunction

Endothelial dysfunction as determined by impaired flow-mediated dilatation is frequently present in children with advanced renal failure [63, 69]. As in adult CKD, several factors have been postulated to account for impaired endothelial function in pediatric and young adult CKD [70].

Although well established in severe CKD/ESRD, it is unclear whether impairment of endothelial function occurs in early stages of pediatric CKD.

21.5   Renovascular Continuum

Children, adolescents, and adults are prone to develop CKD with its adverse cardiovascular outcome [57, 58]. However the natural history of the vasculopathy is different in these various age groups. In pediatric CKD/ESRD, the pathophysiologic mechanisms of the vascular disease is related to both the presence of uremia-related and absence of traditional risk factors leading to the development of arteriosclerosis and cardiomyopathy [63] (Fig. 21.2). With increasing age and appearance of

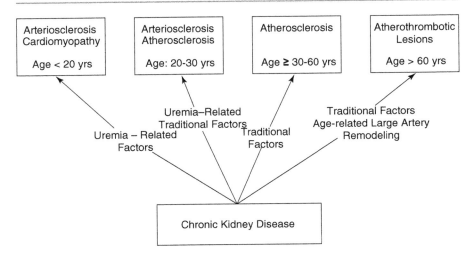

Fig. 21.2 Renovascular continuum

traditional risk factors in young adults, atherosclerosis becomes a prominent feature of the vasculopathy [61]. In the elderly CKD patients, age-related disease of the elastic arteries plays an increasing role in the development and progression of cardiovascular disease [11, 12] (Fig. 21.2).

Conclusion
Chronic kidney disease is characterized by the presence and interplay of traditional and uremia-related risk factors, a wide spectrum of vascular pathologies, and a markedly elevated cardiovascular morbidity and mortality. The initial vascular lesion appears to be age related, with children and adolescents exhibiting arteriosclerosis and cardiomyopathy, while in their older counterparts, both atherosclerosis and arteriosclerosis become more dominant.

References

1. Castro AF, Coresh J (2009) CKD surveillance rising laboratory data from the population-based National Health and Nutrition Examination Survey (NHANES). Am J Kidney Dis 53:S46–S55
2. Fried LF, Shlipak MG, Crump C et al (2003) Renal insufficiency as a predictor of cardiovascular outcomes and mortality in elderly individuals. J Am Coll Cardiol 41:1364–1372
3. Sarnak M, Levey A, Schoolworth A, Coresh J (2003) Kidney disease as a risk factor for development of cardiovascular disease: a statement from American Heart Association. Circulation 108:2154–2159
4. Astor BC, Hallan SI, Miller ER 3rd et al (2008) Glomerular filtration rate, albuminuria, and risk of cardiovascular and all cause mortality in the US population. Am J Epidemiol 167:1226–1234
5. Foley RN, Parfrey PS, Sarnak MJ (1998) Clinical epidemiology of cardiovascular disease in chronic renal disease. Am J Kidney Dis 32(Suppl B):S112–S119

6. Foley RN, Parfrey PS (1998) Cardiovascular disease and mortality in ESRD. J Nephrol 11:239–245
7. Querfeld U (2002) Is atherosclerosis accelerated in young patients with end-stage renal disease? The contribution of pediatric nephrology. Nephrol Dial Transplant 17:719–722
8. Chavers BM, Li S, Collins AJ, Herzog CA (2002) Cardiovascular disease in pediatric chronic dialysis patients. Kidney Int 62:648–653
9. Levey AS, Levin A, Kellum JA (2013) Editorial: definition and classification of kidney diseases. Am J Kidney Dis 61:686–688
10. National Kidney Foundation (2002) K/DOQI clinical practice guidelines for chronic kidney disease: evaluation, classification and stratification. Am J Kidney Dis 39(Suppl 1):S1–S266
11. Foley RN, Parfrey PS, Sarnak MJ (1998) Cardiovascular disease in chronic renal disease: clinical epidemiology of cardiovascular disease in chronic renal disease. Am J Kidney Dis 32:S112–S119
12. Sarnak MJ (2003) Cardiovascular complications in chronic kidney disease. Am J Kidney Dis 41(Suppl 5):S11–S17
13. Collins AJ, Li S, Gilbertson DT et al (2003) Chronic kidney disease and cardiovascular disease in the Medicare population. Kidney Int Suppl 87:S24–S31
14. Shulman NB, Ford CE, Hall WD et al; Hypertension Detection and Follow-Up Program Cooperative Group (1989) Prognostic value of serum creatinine and effect of treatment on renal function: results from the hypertension detection and follow-up program. Hypertension 13(Suppl 5):S180–S193
15. Yerram P, Karuparthi PR, Hesemann L et al (2007) Chronic kidney disease and cardiovascular risk. J Am Soc Hypertens 1:178–184
16. Sarnak MJ, Levey AS (2000) Cardiovascular disease and chronic renal disease: a new paradigm. Am J Kidney Dis 35(Suppl 1):S117–S131
17. Kooman JP, Leunissen KM (1993) Cardiovascular aspects in renal disease. Curr Opin Nephrol Hypertens 2:791–797
18. Schwarz U, Buzello M, Eberhard R et al (2000) Morphology of coronary atherosclerotic lesions in patients with end-stage renal failure. Nephrol Dial Transplant 15:218–223
19. Gross ML, Myer H-P, Ziebart H et al (2007) Calcification of coronary intima and media: immunohistochemistry, backscatter imaging, and x-ray analysis in renal and nonrenal patients. Clin J Am Soc Nephrol 2:121–134
20. Shroff R, Long DA, Shanahan C (2013) Mechanistic insights into vascular calcification in CKD. J Am Soc Nephrol 24:179–189
21. London GM (2003) Cardiovascular calcifications in uremic patients: clinical impact on cardiovascular function. J Am Soc Nephrol 14:S305–S309
22. Avram MM, Fein PA, Antignani A et al (1989) Cholesterol and lipid disturbances in renal disease: the natural history of uremic dyslipidemia and the impact of hemodialysis and continuous ambulatory peritoneal dialysis. Am J Med 87(5N):55N–60N
23. Jungers P, Khoa TN, Massy ZA et al (1999) Incidence of atherosclerotic arterial occlusive accidents in predialysis and dialysis patients: a multicentric study in the Ile de France district. Nephrol Dial Transplant 14:898–902
24. Drueke TB (1999) Genesis of atherosclerosis in uremic patients. Miner Electrolyte Metab 25:251–257
25. Menon V, Sarnak MJ (2005) The epidemiology of chronic kidney disease stages 1 to 4 and cardiovascular disease: a high risk combination. Am J Kidney Dis 45:223–232
26. Nogueira J, Weir M (2007) The unique character of cardiovascular disease in chronic kidney disease and its implications for treatment with lipid-lowering drugs. Clin J Am Soc Nephrol 2:766–785
27. Rigatto C, Levin A, House AA et al (2009) Atheroma progression in chronic kidney disease. Clin J Am Soc Nephrol 4:291–298
28. London G, Marchais SJ, Metivier F, Guerin AP (2000) Cardiovascular risk in end-stage renal disease: vascular aspects. Nephrol Dial Transplant 15(Suppl 5):97–105

29. London G, Marchais SJ, Guerin AP, Metivier F (2005) Arteriosclerosis, vascular calcification and cardiovascular disease in uremia. Curr Opin Nephrol Hypertens 14:525–531
30. London GM, Guérin AP, Marchais SJ et al (2003) Arterial media calcification in end-stage renal disease: impact on all-cause and cardiovascular mortality. Nephrol Dial Transplant 18:1731–1740
31. Burger D, Levin A (2013) 'Shedding' light on mechanisms of hyperphosphatemic vascular dysfunction. Kidney Int 83:187–189
32. Moe SM, Chen NX (2004) Pathophysiology of vascular calcification in chronic kidney disease. Circ Res 95:560–567
33. London GM, Pannier B, Marchais SJ (2010) Disturbed calcium- phosphorus metabolism/arterial calcifications: consequences on cardiovascular function and clinical outcome. In: Berbari A, Mancia G (eds) Cardiorenal syndrome: mechanisms, risk and treatment. Springer, Milan, pp 269–278
34. Mourad JJ, Pannier B, Blacher J et al (2001) Creatinine clearance, pulse wave velocity, carotid compliance and essential hypertension. Kidney Int 59:1834–1841
35. Zieman SJ, Melenovsky V, Kass DA (2005) Mechanism, pathophysiology and therapy of arterial stiffness. Arterioscler Thromb Vasc Biol 25:932–943
36. Briet M, Boutouyrie P, Laurent S, London GM (2012) Arterial stiffness and pulse pressure in CKD and ESRD. Kidney Int 82:388–400
37. Go AS, Chertow GM, Fan D et al (2004) Chronic kidney disease and the risks of death, cardiovascular events and hospitalization. N Engl J Med 351:1296–1305
38. Van Kuijk JP, Flu WJ, Chonchol M et al (2010) The prevalence and prognostic implications of polyvascular atherosclerotic disease in patients with chronic kidney disease. Nephrol Dial Transplant 25:1882–1888
39. Rogers NM, Coates PTH (2008) Calcific uraemic arteriolopathy: an update. Curr Opin Nephrol Hypertens 17:629–634
40. Angelis M, Wong LL, Myers SA et al (1997) Calciphylaxis in patients on hemodialysis: a prevalence study. Surgery 122:1083–1090
41. Brandenberg VM, Sinha S, Specht P, Ketteler M (2014) Calcific uraemic arteriolopathy: a rare disease with a potentially high impact on chronic kidney disease-mineral and bone disorder. Pediatr Nephrol. doi:10.1007/s00467-013-2746-7
42. Clyne N, Lins LE, Pehrsson SK (1986) Occurrence and significance of heart disease in uraemia. Scand J Urol Nephrol 20:307–311
43. De Santo NG, Cirillo M, Perna A et al (2001) The heart in uremia: role of hypertension, hypotension, and sleep apnea. Am J Kidney Dis 38(Suppl 1):S38–S46
44. Semple D, Smith K, Bhandari S et al (2011) Uremic cardiomyopathy and insulin resistance: a critical role for Akt? J Am Soc Nephrol 22:207–215
45. Foley RN, Parfrey PS, Kent GM et al (1998) Long-term evolution of cardiomyopathy in dialysis patients. Kidney Int 54:1720–1725
46. Wang AWM, Sanderson JE (2011) Current perspectives on diagnosis of heart failure in long-term dialysis patients. Am J Kidney Dis 57:308–319
47. Zoccali C (2010) Endothelial dysfunction, nitric oxide bioavailability, and asymmetric dimethyl arginine. In: Berbari A, Mancia G (eds) Cardiorenal syndrome: mechanisms, risk and treatment. Springer, Milan, pp 235–244
48. Yilmaz MI, Saglam M, Caglar K et al (2006) The determinants of endothelial dysfunction in CKD: oxidative stress and asymmetric dimethylarginine. Am J Kidney Dis 47:42–50
49. Landray MJ, Wheeler DC, Lip GYH et al (2004) Inflammation, endothelial dysfunction and platelet activation in patients with chronic kidney disease: the chronic renal impairment in Birmingham (CRIB) study. Am J Kidney Dis 43:244–253
50. Burger D, Touyz RM (2012) Cellular biomarkers of endothelial health: microparticles, endothelial progenitor cells and circulating endothelial cells. J Am Soc Hypertens 6:85–99
51. New DI, Chesser AM, Thuraisingha MC, Yaqoob MM (2004) Structural remodeling of resistance arteries in uremic hypertension. Kidney Int 65:1818–1825

52. Amann K, Neusub R, Ritz E et al (1995) Changes of vascular architecture independent of blood pressure in experimental uremia. Am J Hypertens 8:409–417
53. Amann K, Wiest G, Zimmer G et al (1992) Reduced capillary density in the myocardium of uremic rats-a stereological study. Kidney Int 42:1079–1085
54. Amann K, Tyralla K (2002) Cardiovascular changes in chronic renal failure- pathogenesis and therapy. Clin Nephrol 58(Suppl 1):S62–S72
55. Törnig J, Amann K, Ritz E et al (1996) Arteriolar wall thickening capillary rarefaction and interstitial fibrosis in the heart of rats with renal failure: the effects of Ramipril, nifedipine and moxonidine. J Am Soc Nephrol 7:667–675
56. Levy B, Schiffrin E, Mourad JJ et al (2008) Impaired tissue perfusion a pathology common to hypertension, obesity and diabetes mellitus. Circulation 118:968–976
57. Parekh RS, Carroll CE, Wolfe RA, Port FK (2002) Cardiovascular mortality in children and young adults with end-stage kidney disease. J Pediatr 141:191–197
58. Mitsnefes MM (2008) Cardiovascular complications of pediatric chronic kidney disease. Pediatr Nephrol 23:27–39
59. Schroff R (2009) Monitoring cardiovascular risk factors in children on dialysis. Perit Dial Int 29(S2):S173–S175
60. Schroff R, Quinlan C, Mitsenefes MM (2011) Uremic vasculopathy in children with chronic kidney disease: prevention or damage limitation. Pediatr Nephrol 26:853–865
61. Berenson G, Srinivasan SR, Bao W et al (1998) Association between multiple cardiovascular risk factors and atherosclerosis in children and young adults. N Engl J Med 338:1650–1656
62. Litwin M, Wuhl E, Jourdan C et al (2005) Altered morphologic properties of large arteries in children with chronic renal failure and after renal transplantation. J Am Soc Nephrol 16:1494–1500
63. Wilson AC, Mitsnefes MM (2009) Cardiovascular disease in CKD in children: update on risk factors, risk assessment, and management. Am J Kidney Dis 54:345–360
64. Mitsnefes MM, Kimball TR, Kartal J et al (2005) Cardiac and vascular adaptation in pediatric patients with chronic kidney disease: role of calcium-phosphorus metabolism. J Am Soc Nephrol 16:2796–2803
65. Shanahan CM (2006) Vascular calcification – a matter of damage limitation? Nephrol Dial Transplant 21:1166–1169
66. Oh J, Wunsch R, Turzer M et al (2002) Advanced coronary and carotid arteriopathy in young adults with childhood-onset chronic renal failure. Circulation 106:100–105
67. Mitsenefes MM (2005) Cardiovascular disease in children with chronic kidney disease. Adv Chronic Kidney Dis 12:397–405
68. Mitsnefes MM, Kimball TR, Witt SA et al (2004) Left ventricular mass and systolic performance in pediatric patients with chronic renal failure. Circulation 107:864–868
69. Wilson AC, Urbina E, Witt SA et al (2008) Flow-mediated vasodilatation of brachial artery in children with chronic kidney disease. Pediatr Nephrol 23:1297–1302
70. Kari J, Donald AE, Vallance DT (1997) Physiology and biochemistry of endothelial function in children with chronic renal failure. Kidney Int 52:468–472

Pulmonary Arterial Hypertension

22

Thenappan Thenappan and Daniel Duprez

22.1 Introduction

Pulmonary arterial hypertension (PAH) is a debilitating disease characterized by progressive adverse remodeling of the resistance pulmonary arteries, ultimately leading to right ventricular (RV) failure and death [1]. It is defined by increases in pulmonary arterial pressures (PAP), pulmonary vascular resistance (PVR), and ultimately, right ventricular failure. The field of PAH has made remarkable progress in the last two decades with understanding in the pathogenesis and improvements in therapeutic and prognostic tools. In this chapter, we will review the definition, pathogenesis, epidemiology, clinical presentation, management, and prognostication of PAH in the current era.

22.2 Definition and Classification

Pulmonary hypertension (PH) is defined as mean PAP $\geq$25 mmHg at rest. The most recent World Health Organization (WHO) classification has categorized PH into five different groups based on the underlying mechanism (Table 22.1). WHO group

T. Thenappan, MD • D. Duprez, MD, PhD (✉)
Division of Cardiovascular, University of Minnesota, Medical School,
420 Delaware street SE, MMC 508, Minneapolis, MN 55455, USA
e-mail: dupre007@umn.edu

© Springer International Publishing Switzerland 2015
A. Berbari, G. Mancia (eds.), *Arterial Disorders:
Definition, Clinical Manifestations, Mechanisms and Therapeutic Approaches*,
DOI 10.1007/978-3-319-14556-3_22

Table 22.1 Updated 2013 clinical classification of pulmonary hypertension

1. Pulmonary arterial hypertension (PAH)
1. Idiopathic PAH
2. Heritable PAH
1.2.1 BMPR2
1.2.2 ALK-1, ENG, SMAD9, CAV1, KCNK3
1.2.3 Unknown
1.3 Drug and toxin induced
1.4 Associated with
1.4.1 Connective tissue disease
1.4.2 HIV infection
1.4.3 Portal hypertension
1.4.4 Congenital heart diseases
1.4.5 Schistosomiasis
1′ Pulmonary venoocclusive disease and/or pulmonary capillary hemangiomatosis
1″ Persistent pulmonary hypertension of the newborn (PPHN)
2. Pulmonary hypertension due to left heart disease
1. Left ventricular systolic dysfunction
2. Left ventricular diastolic dysfunction
3. Valvular disease
4. Congenital/acquired left heart inflow/outflow tract obstruction and congenital cardiomyopathies
3. Pulmonary hypertension due to lung diseases and/or hypoxia
1. Chronic obstructive pulmonary disease
2. Interstitial lung disease
3. Other pulmonary diseases with mixed restrictive and obstructive pattern
4. Sleep-disordered breathing
5. Alveolar hypoventilation disorders
6. Chronic exposure to high altitude
7. Developmental lung diseases
4. Chronic thromboembolic pulmonary hypertension (CTEPH)
5. Pulmonary hypertension with unclear multifactorial mechanisms
1. Hematologic disorders: chronic hemolytic anemia, myeloproliferative disorders, splenectomy
2. Systemic disorders: sarcoidosis, pulmonary histiocytosis, lymphangioleiomyomatosis
3. Metabolic disorders: glycogen storage disease, Gaucher disease, thyroid disorders
4. Others: tumoral obstruction, fibrosing mediastinitis, chronic renal failure, segmental PH

Adapted with permission from Simonneau et al. [72]
BMPR bone morphogenetic protein receptor, *ALK* activin receptor-like kinase, *ENG* endoglin, *Smad* mothers against decapentaplegic, *CAV* caveolin, *KCNK3* potassium channel superfamily K member-3, *HIV* human immunodeficiency virus, and *CTEPH* chronic thromboembolic pulmonary hypertension

I PH or PAH is defined as mean PAP ≥25 mmHg, pulmonary capillary wedge pressure (PCWP) <15 mmHg, and PVR ≥3 Wood units. PAH includes a group of disorders that share similar pulmonary vascular pathophysiological mechanisms and clinical characteristics. PAH can be idiopathic, hereditable, or associated with other conditions such as connective tissue disease, congenital heart disease, portal hypertension, HIV infection, anorexigen exposure, or schistosomiasis.

22.3 Pathology

22.3.1 The Pulmonary Vasculature

PAH predominantly affects the small resistance pulmonary arteries, characterized by intimal hyperplasia, medial hypertrophy, adventitial proliferation, in situ thrombosis, and inflammation (Fig. 22.1) [2]. Plexiform arteriopathy, which refers to capillary-like, angioproliferative vascular channels within the lumina of small muscular arteries, is the pathognomonic histopathological lesion of

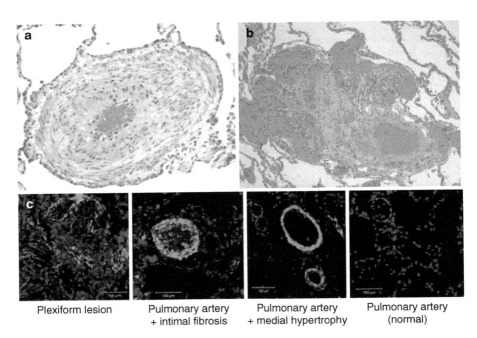

| Plexiform lesion | Pulmonary artery + intimal fibrosis | Pulmonary artery + medial hypertrophy | Pulmonary artery (normal) |

Fig. 22.1 Histopathological changes of the pulmonary vasculature in pulmonary arterial hypertension. (**a**) A small branch of pulmonary artery with severe medial hypertrophy and mild intimal fibrosis causing severe luminal obstruction (hematoxylin-eosin stain, original magnification ×20). (**b**) A characteristic plexiform lesion surrounded by dilated, thin-walled vessels (hematoxylin-eosin stain, original magnification ×4). (**c**) Immunofluorescent staining for proliferating cell nuclear antigen (*PNCA*) (*red*) indicative of ongoing vascular proliferation. The bright staining (*green*) is smooth muscle actin. The staining of the pulmonary vasculature from another patient who died without pulmonary vascular disease is shown for comparison as a normal control. Staining for PNCA is absent in the normal control. *PAH* pulmonary arterial hypertension (Reproduced with permission from the American College of Chest Physicians [2])

Adaptive RVH   Maladaptive RVH

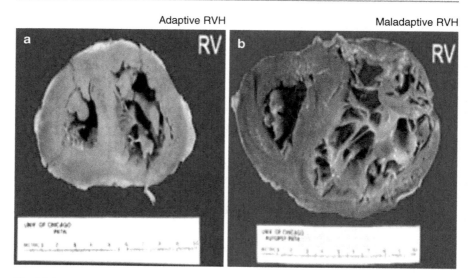

Fig. 22.2 Adaptive vs. maladaptive right ventricular hypertrophy in pulmonary arterial hypertension. (**a**) Adaptive right ventricular hypertrophy (*RVH*) characterized by concentric hypertrophy and minimal dilatation. (**b**) Maladaptive right ventricular hypertrophy characterized by eccentric dilatation. *RV* right ventricle, *RVH* right ventricular hypertrophy (Reproduced with permission from the American College of Chest Physicians [2])

PAH [2]. Plexiform lesions often appear at branch points, frequently have fibrin thrombi within the lumen, and have varying channel diameter, giving them a disordered appearance.

22.3.2 The Right Ventricle (RV)

The chronic elevation in RV afterload due to increased PVR induces right ventricular hypertrophy (RVH), which can be either adaptive or maladaptive (Fig. 22.2). Adaptive RVH, characterized by concentric hypertrophy with minimal eccentric dilatation and fibrosis, maintains normal ejection fraction, cardiac output, and filling pressures [2]. However, in contrast, maladaptive RVH illustrates eccentric dilatation, increased fibrosis, and capillary rarefaction with reduction in ejection fraction and cardiac output and elevation in filling pressures [2, 3]. At a metabolic level, maladaptive RVH is characterized by increased aerobic glycolysis and glutaminolysis [4]. In addition, maladaptive RVH is associated with increased sympathetic activation and downregulation of α, β, and dopaminergic receptors in the RV myocytes [5]. Some patients, especially those with congenital heart disease associated PAH, remain stable with adaptive RVH for a prolonged period. However, in contrast, certain PAH patients, specifically those with scleroderma-associated PAH, develop maladaptive RVH relatively early, leading to RV failure and death [6]. The mechanisms that switch the adaptive, compensatory hypertrophy of the RV to maladaptive

RV dilatation and ultimately RV failure are unclear and are under investigation [5, 7]. Long-term outcomes in PAH are largely determined by the response of the RV to the increased afterload [8].

22.4 Pathogenesis

The pathogenesis of PAH likely involves multiple pathways rather than a single mechanism [1]. First, there is endothelial dysfunction characterized by an imbalance of vasoactive and vasodilator substances in the small pulmonary arteries. There is increased production of thromboxane and decreased synthesis of prostacyclin. Thromboxane is a potent vasoconstrictor and activates proliferation of platelets, whereas prostacyclin is a potent vasodilator, inhibits smooth muscle proliferation, and has antiplatelet properties [1]. In addition, there is an increased level of endothelin, which is a strong vasoconstrictor and stimulates pulmonary artery smooth muscle proliferation [1]. Furthermore, there is a decreased level of nitric oxide, which is a potent vasodilator, inhibits smooth muscle proliferation, and inhibits platelet activation. Other vasoactive substances that have been implicated in the pathogenesis of PAH include serotonin and vasoactive intestinal polypeptide.

Second, there are several changes in the pulmonary artery smooth muscle cells that favor increased proliferation and decreased apoptosis including inappropriate activation of transcription factors hypoxia-inducible factor (HIF)-1 alpha and nuclear factor of activated T cells (NFAT), decreased expression of voltage-gated potassium channels (e.g., Kv1.5 and Kv2.1), de novo expression of the antiapoptotic protein survivin, and increased expression of transient receptor potential channels (TRPC) leading to calcium overload. Third, there increased activation of adventitial metalloproteinases, leading to adventitial remodeling. Finally, there are inflammatory infiltrates and activation of proinflammatory cytokines, suggesting that inflammation may play a role in the pathogenesis of PAH [9].

PAH can also be inherited. Approximately, 10 % of patients have hereditable PAH. Mutations in three genes involved in the transforming growth factor beta (TGF-ß) pathway, bone morphogenetic protein receptor (BMPR2), activin-like kinase, and endoglin have been identified in patients with hereditable PAH [10]. BMPR2 regulates vascular smooth muscle cell growth by activating the intracellular pathways of SMAD and LIM kinase. Loss of function mutation of the BMPR2 gene leads to decreased activation of SMAD, ultimately leading to increased proliferation of pulmonary artery smooth muscle cells. Recently, mutations in caveolin-1 and KCNK3 genes have also been identified in patients with hereditable PAH without mutations in genes encoding BMPR2 or other TGF-ß superfamily members [10]. Caveolin-1 is a membrane protein that forms caveolae, which are flask-shaped invaginations of the plasma membrane. Caveolae regulates membrane trafficking, cell signaling, cholesterol homeostasis, and mechanotransduction [10]. KCNK3 gene encodes a two-pore potassium channel expressed in pulmonary artery smooth muscle cells. This potassium channel modulates resting membrane potential, pulmonary vascular tone, and hypoxic pulmonary vasoconstriction [10].

22.5   Epidemiology

The landmark NIH registry initiated in 1981 collected data prospectively from 32 centers in the United States between 1981 and 1985 [11]. One hundred eighty seven patients with idiopathic PAH, heritable PAH, or anorexigen-associated PAH were included in this registry. The mean age at the time of presentation was 36 ± 15 years, and female to male ratio was 1.7:1. The predominant race was white (85.4 %) followed by African Americans (12.3 %) and Hispanics (2.3 %). The mean time interval between onset of symptoms and diagnosis was 2 years.

Since there has been a considerable change in the understanding of the pathogenesis and classification of PAH in the last three decades, several contemporary PAH registries were developed to advance our knowledge on PAH epidemiology. Data from these contemporary PAH registries suggest that the epidemiology of PAH has changed significantly in the current era [12]. PAH continues to remain as an orphan disease. The incidence and prevalence of PAH vary between 2–7.6 cases per million population and 10.6–26 cases per million population, respectively. In the contemporary PAH registries, nearly half of the patients had idiopathic or heritable PAH, and the rest had associated PAH. The most common etiology of associated PAH is connective tissue disease followed by congenital heart disease [13–15]. Scleroderma is the most common connective tissue disease associated with PAH. The mean age of the patients with idiopathic or heritable PAH enrolled in the contemporary registries is significantly higher when compared to the NIH registry (45–65 years vs. 36 years). The female to male ratio continues to remain high in the contemporary PAH registries, especially in the US-based registries [12, 16]. In the REVEAL registry, 72.8 % were Caucasians, 12.2 % were African Americans, 8.9 % were Hispanics, 3.3 % were Asians or Pacific Islanders, and 2.8 were others or unknown [15].

Unfortunately, despite increasing awareness of PAH, there is still a significant delay between the onset of symptoms and the diagnosis of PAH. The mean interval between onset of symptoms and diagnosis of PAH in the contemporary registries ranged from 18 to 32 months (vs. 2 years in the NIH registry) [17, 18]. In the REVEAL registry, 20 % of patients had symptoms >2 years before diagnosis [18]. Unlike the NIH registry, patients in the contemporary registries have several comorbidities that include systemic hypertension, diabetes, coronary artery disease, and the metabolic syndrome.

22.6   Clinical Manifestations

Dyspnea at rest or with exertion is the most common presenting symptom of PAH. Other symptoms include fatigue, chest pain or pressure with exertion, light-headedness, dizziness, syncope, and fluid retention. Typical physical exam findings of PAH include elevated jugular venous distension with a prominent "A" wave; a palpable right ventricular heave; a loud pulmonic component of the second heart sound; a right-sided S4; a holosystolic murmur secondary to tricuspid regurgitation and an early diastolic murmur, due to pulmonary regurgitation; and a right-sided S4. The presence of a prominent "V" wave in the jugular vein distension, a right-sided S3 gallop rhythm, hepatomegaly, ascites, and lower extremity edema may suggest underlying right heart failure.

22.7 Diagnostic Evaluation

The classic chest x-ray findings of PAH are prominent central pulmonary artery, decreased peripheral pulmonary vascular markings (vascular pruning), and reduced retrosternal space on a lateral projection suggestive of RVH [9]. The typical EKG findings of PAH include right atrial enlargement, RVH with strain pattern, right axis deviation of the QRS complex, and QT interval prolongation. Both chest x-ray and EKG findings are neither sensitive nor specific for the diagnosis of PAH [9].

Transthoracic echocardiogram is the initial screening test of choice in patients suspected of having PAH based on history, physical examination, chest x-ray, and electrocardiogram or in patients with substrates, which increase the chances of pulmonary vascular disease (connective tissue disease, portal hypertension, HIV infection, etc.) [9]. A Doppler-estimated systolic PAP >40 mmHg, the presence of right atrial enlargement, RV enlargement, and flattened interventricular septum (D-shaped) should prompt further evaluation for PAH. Echocardiogram also helps to exclude other common cardiovascular causes of unexplained dyspnea including left ventricular systolic and diastolic dysfunction and valvular heart disease, which are commonly associated with PAH (WHO group 2 PAH). In patients suspected to have underlying congenital heart disease, a bubble study should be performed to identify intracardiac shunt. Transthoracic echocardiogram is a useful screening test; however, Doppler estimates of PAP can be inaccurate and should not be relied upon solely to make a definitive diagnosis of PAH. Doppler-based methods have been shown to either overestimate or underestimate systolic PAP by 10 mmHg in nearly half of the patients [19, 20].

Echocardiographic findings suggestive of PAH should prompt further thorough systematic evaluation to exclude other WHO categories of PH and to identify the presence of associated causes of PAH including congenital heart disease, connective tissue disease, portal hypertension, HIV infection, and exposure to anorexigen use. Idiopathic PAH should be a diagnosis of exclusion.

Pulmonary function test should be performed to exclude obstructive and restrictive lung disease, which are commonly associated with PH (WHO group 3). Although not sensitive or specific, a very low diffusion capacity for carbon monoxide would suggest PAH [21]. Overnight, polysomnography is recommended to exclude sleep-disordered breathing, which can lead to PH [22]. V/Q scan is the diagnostic test of choice for excluding chronic pulmonary thromboembolic disease (WHO group 4) [23]. A low or intermediate probability scan excludes chronic thromboembolic disease, whereas a high probability scan should prompt invasive pulmonary angiogram or CT angiogram of the chest for confirmatory diagnosis. It is important to exclude chronic thromboembolic PH since it can be potentially cured by surgical pulmonary thromboendarterectomy in suitable candidates. Although chest CT angiogram is highly sensitive and specific for diagnosis proximal pulmonary embolism, it is less sensitive for excluding distal chronic thromboembolic disease compared to V/Q scan. Evaluation should also include testing to exclude common conditions associated with PAH. Patients should be tested for human immunodeficiency virus (HIV) infection, antinuclear antibody to exclude connective tissue disease, and liver function tests to rule out portal hypertension.

Right heart catheterization is the gold standard test for diagnosing PAH [9]. It helps to confirm the diagnosis, to assess the severity, and to test for acute vasodilator response. PAH is defined as mean PAP greater than 25 mmHg at rest with a PCWP ≤15 mmHg and a PVR >3 Wood units. Accurate measurement of PCWP is crucial for the distinction of PAH (WHO group 1) from PH due to left heart disease (WHO group 2). A PCWP ≤15 mmHg excludes left heart disease. Left ventricular end-diastolic pressure should be measured if the accuracy of wedge pressure measurement is questionable [24]. Cardiac output measured by thermodilution method correlates well with the Fick method even in the presence of severe tricuspid regurgitation and low cardiac output in patients with PAH [25]. Acute vasodilator challenge with inhaled nitric oxide, inhaled epoprostenol, or intravenous adenosine should be performed after confirming the diagnosis of PAH, especially in patients with idiopathic PAH. A positive vasodilator response is defined as a fall in the mean PAP by 10 mmHg with an absolute value less than 40 mmHg and no change or increase in cardiac output.

Cardiac magnetic resonance imaging (CMRI) is the gold standard imaging modality for accurate and reproducible measurement of RV volumes, mass, and other markers of RV function. Patients with PAH typically have late gadolinium enhancement in the interventricular septum at the RV free-wall insertion sites, which has been associated with PAH severity and has been shown to be a univariate predictor of mortality [26].

22.8 Treatment

Management of patients with PAH includes general supportive measures and PAH-specific vasodilator therapy. The goals of therapy are to decrease symptoms, improve hemodynamics, reduce hospitalizations, and ultimately prolong survival.

22.8.1 General Supportive Measures

The general supportive treatment measures for PAH include supplemental nasal oxygen, diuretics as needed for right heart failure, and long-term anticoagulation with warfarin. A systematic review and meta-analysis based on two prospective and seven retrospective studies regarding warfarin in PAH suggest a survival benefit [27]. Long-term anticoagulation is recommended mainly for patients with PAH, especially idiopathic PAH [9]. The target INR is 1.5–2.5. There is limited data to support the role of digoxin for right ventricular failure from PAH. It is used in the presence of atrial arrhythmias.

22.8.2 Calcium Channel Blockers

Calcium channel blockers are indicated in patients with idiopathic PAH who have a positive response during acute vasodilator testing at the time of diagnostic right heart catheterization. Compared to nonresponders, in prospective nonrandomized studies, patients with a positive vasodilator response had a sustained and significant reduction in mean PAP on long-term oral calcium channel blocker therapy and a better prognosis [28, 29]. Only 5–10 % of patients with idiopathic PAH have a positive vasodilator response [13]. Patients treated with calcium channel blockers should be closely monitored for adequate response. The prevalence of responders in patients with associated PAH is very uncommon.

22.8.3 PAH-Specific Vasodilator Therapies

Four classes of pulmonary vasodilator therapy have been approved for the treatment of PAH: phosphodiesterase-5A-inhibitors, endothelin receptor antagonists, soluble guanylyl cyclase stimulators, and prostanoids. These approved drugs act primarily on the three primary pathways implicated in the pathogenesis of PAH: the prostanoid pathway, the endothelin pathway, and the nitric oxide pathway.

22.8.3.1 Phosphodiesterase-5A-inhibitors (PDE5A-Inhibitors)

PDE5A-inhibitors increase cyclic guanine monophosphate (cGMP), by inhibiting its hydrolysis by the enzyme PDE-5, which has vasodilators, antiproliferative, and proapoptotic effects. Currently, there are two oral PDE5A inhibitors, sildenafil and tadalafil approved for the treatment of PAH in patients with WHO functional class II or III symptoms. Sildenafil was approved based on the SUPER-1 trial that randomized sildenafil 20, 40, and 80 mg three times daily vs. placebo for 12 weeks in 278 patients with PAH [30]. Sildenafil increased 6-min walk distance, improved functional class, reduced mean PAP, increased cardiac output, and decreased PVR. A long-term extension study reported sustained improvement in 6-min walk distance at 1 year in 229 PAH patients treated with sildenafil 80 mg three times daily [30]. Tadalafil was approved based on the PHIRST trial that randomized 409 patients with PAH to placebo vs. 2.5, 10, 20, and 40 mg once daily [31]. In this trial, tadalafil increased 6-min walk distance, improved time to clinical worsening, incidence of clinical worsening, and health-related quality of life. PHIRST 2, an uncontrolled 52-week extension study, showed sustained improvement in 6-min walk distance with tadalafil [32].

22.8.3.2 Endothelin Receptor Antagonists (ERA)

Bosentan, ambrisentan, and macitentan are the three ERAs that are currently approved as a first-line therapy for PAH. Bosentan is a dual endothelin receptor antagonist that blocks both the endothelin A and B receptors. BREATH 2 randomized 213 patients with PAH either to receive placebo or bosentan 62.5 mg twice daily for 4 weeks followed by 125 mg twice daily or 250 mg twice daily for a minimum of 12 weeks. Bosentan increased 6-min walk distance, improved functional class, and increased time to clinical worsening [33]. Ambrisentan is a specific endothelin A receptor antagonists approved for PAH patients with WHO functional class II or III symptoms based on the ARIES 1 and ARIES 2 clinical trials [34]. ARIES 1 randomized 202 patients with PAH to placebo vs. 5 or 10 mg once daily dose of ambrisentan. ARIES 2 randomized 102 patients with PAH to placebo vs. 2.5 or 5 mg once daily dose of ambrisentan. Six-minute walk distance improved across all doses of ambrisentan with sustained benefits in a 48-week long-term extension study. Macitentan is a dual endothelin receptor antagonist that was recently approved for use in PAH patients with WHO functional class II or III symptoms. Macitentan significantly reduced morbidity and mortality in an event-driven long-term, placebo-controlled clinical trial [35].

22.8.4 Soluble Guanylyl Cyclase Stimulators

Riociguat, a soluble guanylyl cyclase stimulator, increases cGMP by directly stimulating the enzyme soluble guanylyl cyclase independent of nitric oxide. Increased cGMP causes vasodilatation and reduced inflammation and thrombosis. In the PATENT trial, compared to placebo, riociguat improved 6-min walk distance, increased time to clinical worsening, and decreased both PVR and NT-proBNP levels [36]. Riociguat is approved as a first-line therapy in PAH patients with WHO functional II or III symptoms.

22.8.5 Parenteral Prostanoids

Parental prostacyclin therapy remains the first-line treatment for PAH patients with WHO functional classification IV symptoms due to right ventricular failure. Epoprostenol improved exercise capacity, hemodynamics, quality of life, and delayed lung transplantation in PAH patients with functional class III/IV symptoms A [37]. Long-term observational studies have reported improved survival with epoprostenol treatment compared to historical controls and risk model predicted survival [38, 39]. Epoprostenol has a half-life of only 3–5 min, as it is very unstable at room temperature. Hence, it requires continuous intravenous infusion through central venous catheter, portable pump, and ice packs to maintain the stability. In general, only designated PAH centers with experienced physicians administer epoprostenol because of the complexity involved. Treprostinil is a tricyclic benzene prostacyclin analog. Its pharmacological properties are similar to epoprostenol but it has a longer half-life, and it is stable in room temperature, allowing it to be administered either by subcutaneous or intravenous routes and alleviating the need for ice packs. Treprostinil improved exercise capacity, hemodynamics, and long-term survival compared to survival predicted by the NIH equation [40, 41].

22.8.6 Inhaled Prostanoids

Iloprost is an inhalational prostacyclin approved for treatment of patients with PAH and WHO functional class III symptoms. Iloprost improved exercise capacity either as monotherapy or add on therapy to patients on background [42]. It has a much shorter half-life requiring six to nine times daily dosing. Treprostinil can also be administered by inhalation. In the TRIUMP study, inhaled treprostinil added on to patients with persistent symptoms on background sildenafil or bosentan therapy improved exercise capacity and quality of life [43]. Unlike iloprost, inhaled treprostinil is administered four times daily, which increases patient compliance.

22.8.7 Oral Prostanoids

Treprostinil diolamine, a sustained release oral formulation of treprostinil, is approved in the United States as a first-line therapy in PAH patients with WHO functional II and III symptoms. In the Freedom C trial, oral treprostinil improved exercise capacity in patients not on background therapy [44]. In the subsequent Freedom C2 trial, oral treprostinil added to background ERA and PDE5A-inhibtior therapy did not result in a statistically significant improvement in exercise capacity [45]. Beraprost is an oral prostanoid approved for use only in Japan. It is currently under investigation in the United States.

22.8.8 Combination Therapy

There is limited data on the role of combination therapy in PAH. In the PACES trial, addition of oral sildenafil in patients who were having persistent or worsening symptoms on background intravenous epoprostenol therapy improved 6-min walk distance, hemodynamics, time to clinical worsening, and quality of life [46]. In the TRIUMP study, addition of inhaled treprostinil in symptomatic patients on background bosentan or sildenafil improved 6-min walk distance and quality of life [43]. There are several ongoing clinical trials evaluating the role of various combination therapies including add-on therapy and upfront combination therapy. At present, upfront combination therapy at the time of diagnosis is still investigational.

22.8.9 Lung Transplantation

Lung transplantation is a potential therapeutic option for patients with PAH who do not respond to pulmonary vasodilator therapy. There is no consensus on single lung transplant vs. double lung transplant. Donor lung reperfusion injury has been reported in patients with PAH patients who undergo single lung transplants. Patients with severe right ventricular failure may need combined heart-lung transplant [9].

22.8.10 Monitoring and Goal-Oriented Therapy

PAH patients should be followed every 3–6 months. During follow-up, patients are characterized into three categories based on the clinical symptoms and signs, non-invasive evaluation, and invasive evaluation: stable and satisfactory, stable but not satisfactory, and unstable and deteriorating [47].

Patients are considered stable and satisfactory when they have functional class I or II symptoms, no signs of right heart failure, normal or near normal NT-ProBNP, 6-min walk distance >440 m, normal or near normal RV function and no pericardial effusion, and cardiac index >2.5 l/min and right atrial pressure <8 mmHg. Such patients need regular follow-up but no alteration in their therapy. A patient is considered stable but not satisfactory when they meet some but not all the above-mentioned criteria for stable and satisfactory. Such patients need reevaluation in a short time period or escalation of their therapy. Patients are considered unstable and deteriorating, if they have functional IV symptoms, signs of right heart failure, 6-min walk distance <300 m, significantly elevated NT-ProBNP, moderate-severely reduced RV function or presence of pericardial effusion, cardiac index <2 l/min/m^2 or right atrial pressure >15 mmHg. These patients require escalation of PAH-specific therapy, usually institution of parental prostacyclin therapy.

22.9 Prognosis

22.9.1 Survival

In the original NIH registry from the 1980s, the estimated median survival was 2.8 years with a 1-year survival of 68 %, 3-year survival of 48 %, and a 5-year survival of 34 % [48]. Although survival has improved in the contemporary PAH registries, it still remains low. In the contemporary PAH registries, 1-year survival in the incident population was 85–89 %. The 1-, 3-, and 5-year survival rates in the total cohort including both prevalent and incident PAH patient cohorts were 85–87 %, 67–69 %, and 57–61 %, respectively [49–53]. The improvement in survival in PAH in the current era is attributed to increased awareness of PAH, greater use of long-term anticoagulation, and finally due to the availability of PAH-specific therapies. Two meta-analyses that evaluated the effect of PAH-specific therapy on short-term survival suggest a reduction in mortality when all treatment strategies are pooled together, but no individual class of drug produced a statistically significant reduction in mortality [54, 55].

22.9.2 Prognosticators in PAH

Prognostic factors play an important role in identifying high-risk PAH patients at baseline and at different time points in the disease course for making important clinical decision including initiation or escalation of PAH-specific vasodilator therapies and lung transplant evaluation. Observational PAH registries and clinical trials have identified several prognosticators in PAH including clinical, noninvasive imaging (echocardiography or cardiac MRI), and invasive hemodynamics parameters along with several other biomarkers. Although there is no clear consensus on which variable best predicts survival in PAH, measures of functional capacity and right ventricular function have been consistently shown to predict long-term survival in PAH.

22.9.3 Clinical Prognosticators

Age is an independent predictor of mortality in PAH [51]. Younger patients had a better survival when compared to older patients despite having more severe hemodynamic impairment [17]. Female gender was associated with a better survival compared to male [51, 56]. Scleroderma-associated PAH had a worse survival compared to idiopathic PAH likely due to maladaptive RV remodeling and intrinsic RV dysfunction [53]. Similarly, patients with portopulmonary hypertension, anorexigen-associated PAH, and hereditable PAH have a poor survival compared to those with idiopathic PAH [53]. In contrast, patients with PAH associated with congenital heart disease have a much better survival compared to idiopathic PAH probably due to chronic adaptive right ventricular hypertrophy [53].

22.9.4 Prognostic Value of Functional Capacity

Measures of functional capacity, both subjective New York Heart Association (NYHA)/WHO functional class and exercise testing, are important prognostic factors in the management of PAH. Patients with WHO functional class I/II symptoms have been shown to have a better survival compared to those with WHO functional class III/IV symptoms [38, 50]. There is also clear survival discrimination between WHO functional class III and IV PAH patients even as early as at the time of initial diagnostic right heart catheterization [38, 50]. In addition, patients who have worsening functional class overtime have poorer survival postworsening compared to those who have stable WHO functional class symptoms [57].

Six-minute walk distance (6MWD), the most commonly used method for objective assessment of exercise capacity in PAH, predicts long-term outcomes. In the REVEAL registry, 6MWD greater than 440 m was associated with longer survival, whereas less than 165 m was associated with increased mortality [53]. In the French national registry, 6MWD was an independent predictor of mortality, albeit, the hazards ratio was close to 1 (0.996; 95 % CI 0.993–0.995; P value 0.004) [51]. Six MWT is simple to perform and inexpensive, but it has several limitations. It is effort dependent and susceptible to motivational factors. It is less sensitive for detecting clinically meaningful change in less sick patients with WHO functional class I/II symptoms because of "ceiling effects." A meta-analysis of PAH clinical trials found no association between change in 6MWD overtime with treatment and survival [58].

Treadmill exercise testing and cardiopulmonary exercise testing have also been evaluated as prognostic tools in PAH. Reduced exercise capacity on a Naughton-Balke exercise treadmill testing was independently associated with abnormal hemodynamics and increased risk of death [59]. More importantly, exercise treadmill testing was able to risk stratify even less sick patients with WHO functional class I/II symptoms in whom the prognostic value of 6MWT is limited.

Cardiopulmonary exercise testing is used less commonly in patients with PAH. Reduced aerobic capacity (VO2), reduced ventilatory efficiency (VE/VCO2), hypoxemia, hypocapnia, and exercise-induced shunt predicts adverse outcomes in PAH patients [60].

22.9.5 Noninvasive Imaging Prognosticators

Several echocardiographic measures predict outcomes in PAH. Tricuspid annular plane systolic excursion (TAPSE), a measure of RV longitudinal motion, reflects RV systolic function. TAPSE <18 mm correlates with right heart remodeling and severe RV dysfunction and has been associated with poor 1- and 2-year survival [61]. PAH patients with TAPSE <18 mm had a 5.7-fold higher risk of death when compared to those with TAPSE >18 mmHg [61]. Tei index is a Doppler-derived measure of global RV function reflecting both systolic and diastolic functions. It is defined as the sum of isovolumetric contraction and relaxation times divided by ejection time. Every 0.1 unit increase in Tei index increases the odds of adverse outcome by 1.3 folds. Both the presence and the severity of pericardial effusion on 2D echocardiography have been shown to predict adverse outcomes in PAH [62–64]. Other echocardiographic predictors of adverse outcomes in PAH include right atrial enlargement and interventricular septal displacement [63].

CMRI measures of RV function have prognostic value in patients with PAH. RV stroke volume index ≤ 25 mL/m^2, RV end-diastolic volume index ≥ 84 mL/m^2, and LVEDV ≤ 40 mL/m^2 were associated with poor long-term survival in PAH [65]. In addition to the baseline measures, change in RVEF by cardiac MRI overtime has been shown to be a better predictor of long-term outcomes compared to invasively measured PVR [8]. Late gadolinium enhancement at the RV insertion point in the interventricular septum correlates with RV dilatation, reduced RVEF, severe hemodynamics, and predicts time to clinical worsening [26].

22.9.6 Invasive Hemodynamic Prognosticators

Invasive hemodynamic measures at the time of diagnosis and during follow-up assessment play a crucial role in risk-stratifying PAH patients. In the original NIH registry, mean right atrial pressure, cardiac index, and mean PAP were the independent predictors of mortality [48]. PAH patients with a positive acute vasodilator response had a significantly better long-term survival compared to those with no response [28, 39]. Invasive measures of right heart function, especially, mean right atrial pressure and cardiac index have been consistently shown to be an independent predictor of long-term adverse outcomes in PAH [49, 51, 53]. Unlike in the NIH registry, mean PAP was not found to be an independent predictor of survival in the recent PAH registries. Some studies have associated low mean PAP with increased mortality, conceivably due to severe RV dysfunction and a low-flow state [39]. PVR [53], mixed venous oxygen saturation [65], pulmonary arterial compliance [66], and stroke volume are the other hemodynamic parameters that have been demonstrated to predict long-term outcomes in patients with PAH.

22.9.7 Biomarkers with Prognostic Value in PAH

Elevated plasma levels of BNP, NT-proBNP, and cardiac troponin T reflect advanced disease and have been associated with increased mortality in PAH [67]. Other biomarkers that have been shown to have negative prognostic value in PAH include serum uric acid, serum creatinine, diffusing capacity of lung for carbon monoxide, C-reactive protein, von Willebrand factor, and circulating angiopoietins [67].

22.9.8 Survival Prediction Models in PAH

Survival prediction models help physicians to identify high-risk PAH patients to make evidence-based clinical decisions for optimization of treatment strategies. The NIH registry developed a regression equation to predict survival based on the baseline hemodynamics (mean right atrial pressure, cardiac index, and mean PAP) at the time of diagnosis [48]. This equation was used in many clinical trials to demonstrate long-term survival benefit with a drug therapy in patients with PAH by comparing observed survival rates on a study drug versus survival rates predicted by the NIH equation [38, 40, 68, 69]. However, the NIH equation underestimates survival in the current era, and it is no longer valid [49]. As a result, several novel survival prediction models have been developed to estimate survival in PAH in the current era [49, 51, 53] (Table 22.2).

22.9.9 The French Model

The French equation was developed from 190 patients with idiopathic PAH, heritable PAH, and anorexigen-associated PAH treated in France between 2002 and 2006 [51]. Of the 190 patients, 56 were incident cases and 134 were prevalent cases diagnosed <3 years before enrolling in the registry. On multivariate analysis, gender, cardiac output, and 6MWD were the independent predictors of mortality that were included in the model.

Table 22.2 Contemporary survival prediction equations in pulmonary arterial hypertension

Registry	Equation	
French equation	$P(t; x, y, z) = H(t) A(x, y, z)$	$H(t)$ = baseline survival = $e(a + b \cdot t)$, where a and b are parameters estimated from the multivariate Cox proportional hazards model, and t is the time from diagnosis measured in years.
		$A(x,y,z)$ = where x is the distance walked (m) at diagnosis, $y = 1$ if female, $y = 0$ if male, and z is the cardiac output (l/min) at diagnosis.
		$A(x,y,z) = e(-(c \cdot x + d \cdot y + e \cdot z)$, where c, d, and e were parameters obtained from the Cox proportional hazards model
PHC	$P(t) = e - A(x, y, z)t$	$P(t)$ is the probability of survival, t is the time interval in years.
		$A(x,y,z) = e(-1.270 - 0.0148x + 0.0402y - 0.361z)$, x = mean pulmonary artery pressure, y = mean right atrial pressure, z = cardiac index
REVEAL	$P(1 - \text{year}) = S0(1) \exp(Z'\beta)$	$S0(1)$ is the baseline survivor function (0.9698), $Z'\beta$ is the linear component, and β is the shrinkage coefficient (0.939)

PHC pulmonary hypertension connections, *REVEAL* Registry to Evaluate Early and Long-Term PAH Disease Management

22.9.10 The Pulmonary Hypertension Connection (PHC) Model

The PHC equation was derived using exponential regression in 249 patients with idiopathic PAH, hereditable PAH, and anorexigen-associated PAH (both incident and prevalent cases) referred to a single US center [49]. Although mean PAP was not a univariate predictor of mortality, it was included a priori in the multivariate model along with the other univariate predictors. The final model contained mean right atrial pressure, mean PAP, and cardiac index, similar to the NIH equation, however, with different coefficients.

The PHC and French equations have been validated in external cohorts [17, 70]. The French equation had a C-index of 0.57 for differentiating PAH patients who will die vs. those who will be alive. C-index was not calculated for the PHC model. Since there is a significant survival difference between patients with idiopathic PAH vs. associated PAH, the utility of these equations in other WHO category I PAH patient cohorts is unclear at present and needs further validation in the future. The ability of these equations to predict survival at an individual patient level is not well studied [70], and it needs further testing before it can be reliably used as a management tool in making clinical decision in an individual patient. However, the external validation of the PHC and the French equation justifies its use for clinical trial cohort comparisons [70].

22.9.11 The REVEAL Model

The REVEAL equation was created using data from 2,716 PAH patients consecutively enrolled in the REVEAL registry [53]. Unlike the PHC and French equation, patients with any WHO category I PAH were included in the REVEAL prediction model. The equation was generated using the 19 independent predictors of survival on the Cox proportional hazard multivariable model. REVEAL model predicts only 1-year survival. The strengths of the REVEAL model include the large sample size of the derivation cohort, its applicability in WHO group I PAH as a whole, and its flexibility to allow for individuals to be missing independent tests. The REVEAL model had a better discriminatory C-index of 0.77 compared to the French and the NIH model. It is also validated externally in other WHO category I PAH cohort with a good discriminatory power [52, 71].

Conclusion
Pulmonary arterial hypertension is becoming a serious health-economical major burden in our society. Diagnostic tools have facilitated the detection of PAH. The prognosis of this disease is often devastating. During the last decade, intensive research has contributed to the development of new medical therapy for PAH. Further research is needed in order to obtain more evidence-based medicine results, which can then be incorporated in the guidelines for diagnosis and treatment of PAH.

References

1. Farber HW, Loscalzo J (2004) Pulmonary arterial hypertension. N Engl J Med 351:1655–1665
2. Rich S, Pogoriler J, Husain AN et al (2010) Long-term effects of epoprostenol on the pulmonary vasculature in idiopathic pulmonary arterial hypertension. Chest 138:1234–1239
3. Ryan JJ, Archer SL (2014) The right ventricle in pulmonary arterial hypertension: disorders of metabolism, angiogenesis and adrenergic signaling in right ventricular failure. Circ Res 115:176–188
4. Archer SL, Fang YH, Ryan JJ, Piao L (2013) Metabolism and bioenergetics in the right ventricle and pulmonary vasculature in pulmonary hypertension. Pulm Circ 3:144–152
5. Piao L, Fang YH, Parikh KS et al (2012) GRK2-mediated inhibition of adrenergic and dopaminergic signaling in right ventricular hypertrophy: therapeutic implications in pulmonary hypertension. Circulation 126:2859–2869
6. Tedford RJ, Mudd JO, Girgis RE et al (2013) Right ventricular dysfunction in systemic sclerosis associated pulmonary arterial hypertension. Circ Heart Fail 6:953–963
7. Drake JI, Gomez-Arroyo J, Dumur CI et al (2013) Chronic carvedilol treatment partially reverses the right ventricular failure transcriptional profile in experimental pulmonary hypertension. Physiol Genomics 45:449–461
8. van de Veerdonk MC, Kind T, Marcus JT et al (2011) Progressive right ventricular dysfunction in patients with pulmonary arterial hypertension responding to therapy. J Am Coll Cardiol 58:2511–2519
9. McLaughlin VV, Archer SL, Badesch DB et al (2009) ACCF/AHA 2009 expert consensus document on pulmonary hypertension a report of the American College of Cardiology Foundation Task Force on Expert Consensus Documents and the American Heart Association

developed in collaboration with the American College of Chest Physicians; American Thoracic Society, Inc.; and the Pulmonary Hypertension Association. J Am Coll Cardiol 53: 1573–1619

10. Best DH, Austin ED, Chung WK, Elliott CG (2014) Genetics of pulmonary hypertension. Curr Opin Cardiol 29:520–527

11. Rich S, Dantzker R, Ayres S et al (1987) Primary pulmonary hypertension: a national prospective study. Ann Intern Med 107:216–223

12. Frost AE, Badesch DB, Barst RJ et al (2011) The changing picture of patients with pulmonary arterial hypertension in the United States: how REVEAL differs from historic and non-US Contemporary Registries. Chest 139:128–137

13. Thenappan T, Shah SJ, Rich S, Gomberg-Maitland M (2007) A USA-based registry for pulmonary arterial hypertension: 1982–2006. Eur Respir J 30:1103–1110

14. Humbert M, Sitbon O, Chaouat A et al (2006) Pulmonary arterial hypertension in France: results from a national registry. Am J Respir Crit Care Med 173:1023–1030

15. Badesch DB, Raskob GE, Elliott CG et al (2010) Pulmonary arterial hypertension: baseline characteristics from the REVEAL registry. Chest 137:376–387

16. McGoon MD, Benza RL, Escribano-Subias P et al (2013) Pulmonary arterial hypertension: epidemiology and registries. J Am Coll Cardiol 62:D51–D59

17. Ling Y, Johnson MK, Kiely DG et al (2012) Changing demographics, epidemiology, and survival of incident pulmonary arterial hypertension: results from the pulmonary hypertension registry of the United Kingdom and Ireland. Am J Respir Crit Care Med 186:790–796

18. Brown LM, Chen H, Halpern S et al (2011) Delay in recognition of pulmonary arterial hypertension: factors identified from the REVEAL Registry. Chest 140:19–26

19. Fisher MR, Forfia PR, Chamera E et al (2009) Accuracy of Doppler echocardiography in the hemodynamic assessment of pulmonary hypertension. Am J Respir Crit Care Med 179: 615–621

20. Rich JD, Shah SJ, Swamy RS et al (2011) Inaccuracy of Doppler echocardiographic estimates of pulmonary artery pressures in patients with pulmonary hypertension: implications for clinical practice. Chest 139:988–993

21. Chandra S, Shah SJ, Thenappan T et al (2010) Carbon monoxide diffusing capacity and mortality in pulmonary arterial hypertension. J Heart Lung Transplant 29:181–187

22. Atwood CW Jr, McCrory D, Garcia JG et al (2004) Pulmonary artery hypertension and sleep-disordered breathing: ACCP evidence-based clinical practice guidelines. Chest 126:72S–77S

23. Hoeper MM, Mayer E, Simonneau G, Rubin LJ (2006) Chronic thromboembolic pulmonary hypertension. Circulation 113:2011–2020

24. Halpern SD, Taichman DB (2009) Misclassification of pulmonary hypertension due to reliance on pulmonary capillary wedge pressure rather than left-ventricular end-diastolic pressure. Chest 136:37–43

25. Hoeper M, Maier R, Tongers J et al (1999) Determination of cardiac output by the Fick method, thermodilution, and acetylene rebreathing in pulmonary hypertension. Am J Respir Crit Care Med 160:535–541

26. Freed BH, Gomberg-Maitland M, Chandra S et al (2012) Late gadolinium enhancement cardiovascular magnetic resonance predicts clinical worsening in patients with pulmonary hypertension. J Cardiovasc Magn Reson 14:11

27. Caldeira D, Loureiro MJ, Costa J et al (2014) Oral anticoagulation for pulmonary arterial hypertension: systematic review and meta-analysis. Can J Cardiol 30:879–887

28. Rich S, Kaufman E, Levy P (1992) The effect of high doses of calcium-channel blockers on survival in primary pulmonary hypertension. N Engl J Med 327:76–81

29. Sitbon O, Humbert M, Jais X et al (2005) Long-term response to calcium channel blockers in idiopathic pulmonary arterial hypertension. Circulation 111:3105–3111

30. Galie N, Ghofrani HA, Torbicki A et al (2005) Sildenafil citrate therapy for pulmonary arterial hypertension. N Engl J Med 353:2148–2157

31. Galie N, Brundage BH, Ghofrani HA et al (2009) Tadalafil therapy for pulmonary arterial hypertension. Circulation 119:2894–2903

32. Oudiz RJ, Brundage BH, Galie N et al (2012) Tadalafil for the treatment of pulmonary arterial hypertension: a double-blind 52-week uncontrolled extension study. J Am Coll Cardiol 60: 768–774
33. Rubin L, Badesch D, Barst R et al (2002) Bosentan therapy for pulmonary arterial hypertension. N Engl J Med 346:896–903
34. Galie N, Olschewski H, Oudiz RJ et al (2008) Ambrisentan for the treatment of pulmonary arterial hypertension: results of the ambrisentan in pulmonary arterial hypertension, randomized, double-blind, placebo-controlled, multicenter, efficacy (ARIES) study 1 and 2. Circulation 117:3010–3019
35. Pulido T, Adzerikho I, Channick RN et al (2013) Macitentan and morbidity and mortality in pulmonary arterial hypertension. N Engl J Med 369:809–818
36. Ghofrani HA, Galie N, Grimminger F et al (2013) Riociguat for the treatment of pulmonary arterial hypertension. N Engl J Med 369:330–340
37. Barst R, Rubin L, Long W et al (1996) A comparison of continuous intravenous epoprostenol (prostacyclin) with conventional therapy for primary pulmonary hypertension. N Engl J Med 334:296–301
38. McLaughlin VV, Shillington A, Rich S (2002) Survival in primary pulmonary hypertension: the impact of epoprostenol therapy. Circulation 106:1477–1482
39. Sitbon O, Humbert M, Nunes H et al (2002) Long-term intravenous epoprostenol infusion in primary pulmonary hypertension: prognostic factors and survival. J Am Coll Cardiol 40:780–788
40. Barst RJ, Galie N, Naeije R et al (2006) Long-term outcome in pulmonary arterial hypertension patients treated with treprostinil. Eur Respir J 28:1195–1203
41. Lang I, Gomez-Sanchez M, Kneussl M et al (2006) Efficacy of long-term subcutaneous treprostinil sodium therapy in pulmonary hypertension. Chest 129:1636–1643
42. Olschewski H, Simonneau G, Galie N et al (2002) Inhaled iloprost for severe pulmonary hypertension. N Engl J Med 347:322–329
43. McLaughlin VV, Benza RL, Rubin LJ et al (2010) Addition of inhaled treprostinil to oral therapy for pulmonary arterial hypertension: a randomized controlled clinical trial. J Am Coll Cardiol 55:1915–1922
44. Jing ZC, Parikh K, Pulido T et al (2013) Efficacy and safety of oral treprostinil monotherapy for the treatment of pulmonary arterial hypertension: a randomized, controlled trial. Circulation 127:624–633
45. Tapson VF, Jing ZC, Xu KF et al (2013) Oral treprostinil for the treatment of pulmonary arterial hypertension in patients receiving background endothelin receptor antagonist and phosphodiesterase type 5 inhibitor therapy (the FREEDOM-C2 study): a randomized controlled trial. Chest 144:952–958
46. Simonneau G, Rubin LJ, Galie N et al (2008) Addition of sildenafil to long-term intravenous epoprostenol therapy in patients with pulmonary arterial hypertension: a randomized trial. Ann Intern Med 149:521–530
47. Galie N, Hoeper MM, Humbert M et al (2009) Guidelines for the diagnosis and treatment of pulmonary hypertension. Eur Respir J 34:1219–1263
48. D'Alonzo GE, Barst RJ, Ayres SM et al (1991) Survival in patients with primary pulmonary hypertension: results from a national prospective registry. Ann Intern Med 115:343–349
49. Thenappan T, Shah SJ, Rich S et al (2010) Survival in pulmonary arterial hypertension: a reappraisal of the NIH risk stratification equation. Eur Respir J 35:1079–1087
50. Humbert M, Sitbon O, Chaouat A et al (2010) Survival in patients with idiopathic, familial, and anorexigen-associated pulmonary arterial hypertension in the modern management era. Circulation 122:156–163
51. Humbert M, Sitbon O, Yaici A et al (2010) Survival in incident and prevalent cohorts of patients with pulmonary arterial hypertension. Eur Respir J 36:549–555
52. Benza RL, Gomberg-Maitland M, Miller DP et al (2012) The REVEAL Registry risk score calculator in patients newly diagnosed with pulmonary arterial hypertension. Chest 141:354–362
53. Benza RL, Miller DP, Gomberg-Maitland M et al (2010) Predicting survival in pulmonary arterial hypertension: insights from the Registry to Evaluate Early and Long-Term Pulmonary Arterial Hypertension Disease Management (REVEAL). Circulation 122:164–172

54. Macchia A, Marchioli R, Tognoni G et al (2010) Systematic review of trials using vasodilators in pulmonary arterial hypertension: why a new approach is needed. Am Heart J 159:245–257
55. Galie N, Manes A, Negro L et al (2009) A meta-analysis of randomized controlled trials in pulmonary arterial hypertension. Eur Heart J 30:394–403
56. Shapiro S, Traiger GL, Turner M et al (2012) Sex differences in the diagnosis, treatment, and outcome of patients with pulmonary arterial hypertension enrolled in the registry to evaluate early and long-term pulmonary arterial hypertension disease management. Chest 141:363–373
57. Frost AE, Badesch DB, Miller DP et al (2013) Evaluation of the predictive value of a clinical worsening definition using 2-year outcomes in patients with pulmonary arterial hypertension: a REVEAL Registry analysis. Chest 144:1521–1529
58. Macchia A, Marchioli R, Marfisi R et al (2007) A meta-analysis of trials of pulmonary hypertension: a clinical condition looking for drugs and research methodology. Am Heart J 153:1037–1047
59. Shah S, Thenappan T, Rich S et al (2009) Value of exercise treadmill testing in the risk stratification of patients with pulmonary hypertension. Circ Heart Fail 2:278–286
60. Wensel R, Opitz C, Anker S et al (2002) Assessment of survival in patients with primary pulmonary hypertension. Circulation 106:319–324
61. Forfia PR, Fisher MR, Mathai SC et al (2006) Tricuspid annular displacement predicts survival in pulmonary hypertension. Am J Respir Crit Care Med 174:1034–1041
62. Hinderliter A, Willis PW IV, Long W et al (1999) Frequency and prognostic significance of pericardial effusion in primary pulmonary hypertension. Am J Cardiol 84:481–484
63. Raymond R, Hinderliter A, Willis P et al (2002) Echocardiographic predictors of adverse outcomes in primary pulmonary hypertension. J Am Coll Cardiol 39:1214–1219
64. Fenstad ER, Le RJ, Sinak LJ et al (2013) Pericardial effusions in pulmonary arterial hypertension: characteristics, prognosis, and role of drainage. Chest 144:1530–1538
65. van Wolferen SA, Marcus JT, Boonstra A et al (2007) Prognostic value of right ventricular mass, volume, and function in idiopathic pulmonary arterial hypertension. Eur Heart J 28:1250–1257
66. Mahapatra S, Nishimura RA, Sorajja P et al (2006) Relationship of pulmonary arterial capacitance and mortality in idiopathic pulmonary arterial hypertension. J Am Coll Cardiol 47:799–803
67. Agarwal R, Gomberg-Maitland M (2012) Prognostication in pulmonary arterial hypertension. Heart Fail Clin 8:373–383
68. McLaughlin VV (2006) Survival in patients with pulmonary arterial hypertension treated with first-line bosentan. Eur J Clin Invest 36(Suppl 3):10–15
69. McLaughlin VV, Sitbon O, Badesch DB et al (2005) Survival with first-line bosentan in patients with primary pulmonary hypertension. Eur Respir J 25:244–249
70. Thenappan T, Glassner C, Gomberg-Maitland M (2012) Validation of the pulmonary hypertension connection equation for survival prediction in pulmonary arterial hypertension. Chest 141:642–650
71. Cogswell R, Kobashigawa E, McGlothlin D et al (2012) Validation of the Registry to Evaluate Early and Long-Term Pulmonary Arterial Hypertension Disease Management (REVEAL) pulmonary hypertension prediction model in a unique population and utility in the prediction of long-term survival. J Heart Lung Transplant 31:1165–1170
72. Simonneau G, Gatzoulis MA, Adatia I (2013) Updated clinical classification of pulmonary hypertension. J Am Coll Cardiol 62(25 Suppl):D34–D41

Cerebrovascular Interactions in Cerebral Disorders (Stroke, Transient Ischaemic Attacks, Microvascular Disease, Migraine)

23

Elio Clemente Agostoni and Marco Longoni

23.1 Macrovascular Disease

Transient Ischaemic Attack and Ischaemic Stroke

23.1.1 Definition

Strokes are a heterogeneous group of disorders involving cerebral circulation that causes a sudden neurologic deficit. Stroke can be ischaemic (80 %), typically resulting from thrombosis or embolism, or haemorrhagic (20 %), resulting from vascular rupture (e.g. subarachnoid or intracerebral haemorrhage) [1].

The World Health Organization defines stroke as the sudden onset of focal neurological signs, of presumed vascular origin, lasting longer than 24 h or causing death. After neuroradiological examinations (CT scan or MRI), stroke can be further classified as ischaemic or haemorrhagic. The term "brain attack" might also be used and seems appropriate to emphasise that stroke is a medical emergency.

Transient stroke symptoms (typically lasting <1 h) without evidence of acute cerebral infarction (based on diffusion-weighted MRI) are termed a transient ischaemic attack (TIA) [1].

23.1.2 Clinical Manifestation

Initial symptoms occur suddenly. Generally, they include numbness, weakness or paralysis of the contralateral limbs and the face, aphasia, confusion, visual disturbances in one or both eyes and dizziness or loss of balance and coordination.

E.C. Agostoni • M. Longoni (✉)
Neurology and Stroke Unit, A.O Niguarda Ca' Granda Milano,
Piazza dell'Ospedale Maggiore 3, Milan 20162, Italy
e-mail: Elioclemente.agostoni@ospedaleniguarda.it; marco.longoni@ospedaleniguarda.it

© Springer International Publishing Switzerland 2015
A. Berbari, G. Mancia (eds.), *Arterial Disorders:*
Definition, Clinical Manifestations, Mechanisms and Therapeutic Approaches,
DOI 10.1007/978-3-319-14556-3_23

Neurologic deficits reflect the area of brain involved. Anterior circulation stroke typically causes unilateral symptoms. Posterior circulation stroke can cause unilateral or bilateral deficits and is more likely to affect consciousness, especially when the basilar artery is involved.

Various clinical classification systems have been proposed for ischaemic stroke. The Oxford clinical classification is often used because it is simple to apply and is of prognostic use. It describes four subtypes of stroke [2]:

(i) Total anterior circulation stroke (TACS) which includes one of the following: contralateral motor or sensory deficit, homonymous hemianopia or higher cortical dysfunction (e.g. aphasia, visuospatial disturbances, etc.)
(ii) Partial anterior circulation stroke (PACS) which is characterised by two of following manifestations: contralateral motor or sensory deficit, homonymous hemianopia or higher cortical dysfunction (e.g. aphasia, visuospatial disturbances, etc.)
(iii) Posterior circulation stroke (POCS) characterised by one of the following: isolated homonymous hemianopia, brainstem signs, or cerebellar ataxia
(iv) Lacunar stroke (LACS) characterised by one of the following: pure motor deficit, pure sensory deficit or sensorimotor deficit

It is important to rapidly distinguish stroke or TIA from one of the numerous conditions that resemble it ("stroke mimics") to allow evidence-based treatment to be started early and to refer alternative conditions to the appropriate team.

Conditions that mimic stroke might be seizure, sepsis, toxic/metabolic accident (e.g. hypoglycaemia), space-occupying lesion, syncope, delirium, vestibular disease, mononeuropathy, migraine and functional symptoms [3].

23.1.3 Mechanism

The underlying cause in most cerebral ischaemic events is embolic due to a cardiac source or atheroembolic due to arterial disease (atherosclerosis or arterial dissection), which can cause either in situ thrombosis or distal embolism. Other causes are represented by small-vessel diseases (see further on), haemodynamic changes (stroke due to hypoperfusion), or rarer causes such as inflammation of cerebral vessels, hyperviscosity, etc.

Among cardiac sources of emboli atrial fibrillation, mural thrombus and valvular heart disease are the commonest, and they typically involve the territory of the large intracerebral arteries, particularly the middle cerebral artery [1]. Atherosclerotic disease typically affects the extracranial internal carotid artery but also the vertebral and basilar arteries. Lacunar infarction results from occlusion of deep perforating arteries, which arise from both the anterior and posterior circulation, and supplies the white matter of the cerebral hemispheres and brainstem.

Once a cerebral artery is occluded, the perfusion of that cerebral area is diminished.

Inadequate blood flow in a single brain artery can often be compensated by an efficient collateral system, particularly between the carotid and vertebral arteries via anastomoses at the circle of Willis and, to a lesser extent, between leptomeningeal anastomoses of arteries supplying the surrounding brain tissue. However, anatomical differences in the circle of Willis and in the calibre of various collateral vessels, atherosclerosis and other acquired arterial lesions can interfere with collateral flow, increasing the chance that a single arterial occlusion will cause brain ischaemia. The amount of perfusion deficit is linked to the extent of damage [1, 4]. If it is mild, damage proceeds slowly; thus, even if perfusion is 40 % of normal, 3–6 h may elapse before brain tissue is completely lost. However, if severe ischaemia (i.e. decrease in perfusion) persists >15–30 min, all the affected tissue is irreversibly damaged [5]. If tissues are ischaemic but not yet necrotic, promptly restoring blood flow may reduce or reverse injury. Intervention may be able to salvage the moderately ischaemic areas (penumbras) that often surround areas of severe ischaemia (these areas exist because of collateral flow). During ischaemic injury, several pathogenetic mechanisms play a role in neuronal loss. First of all, energy impairment produces cytotoxic oedema due to loss of ionic homeostasis (including intracellular Ca accumulation). Second, brain inflammation takes place with release of mediators (e.g. IL-1B, tumour necrosis factor alpha) that contribute to microvascular thrombosis and free radicals release causing cell membrane damage. Moreover, excitatory neurotoxins (e.g. glutamate) and programmed cell death (apoptosis) contribute to the extension of brain lesion [6].

23.1.4 Therapeutic Approach

Therapy for ischaemic stroke or TIA is based on multistep approach:

(i) Primary prevention. Indeed medical treatment of risk factors such as hypertension, diabetes, dyslipidemia, obesity, cigarette smoking, etc. plays a key role for the reduction of stroke incidence.
(ii) Secondary prevention considering that relapse is not rare.
(iii) Rehabilitation, is another cornerstone in stroke therapy.
(iv) Therapeutic approaches during the acute phase of ischaemic event [8]:
    (a) Reperfusion strategies (intravenous fibrinolytics and/or in selected cases mechanical removal of thrombus or ultrasound disruption of thrombus)
    (b) Admission to a stroke unit care
    (c) Antiplatelet agents (for patients not eligible to reperfusion strategies)

Figure 23.1 shows the flow chart for acute stroke management [7].

23.1.4.1 Thrombolysis

Intravenous Fibrinolytic Therapy
Intravenous fibrinolytic therapy for acute stroke is widely accepted. The US FDA approved the use of intravenous recombinant tissue plasminogen activator (rtPA) in 1996, in part on the basis of the results of the two-part NINDS rtPA Stroke Trial, in which 624 patients with ischaemic stroke were treated with placebo or intravenous rtPA (0.9 mg/kg IV, maximum 90 mg) within 3 h of symptom onset, with approximately one half treated within 90 min. From the trial it was clearly shown that the

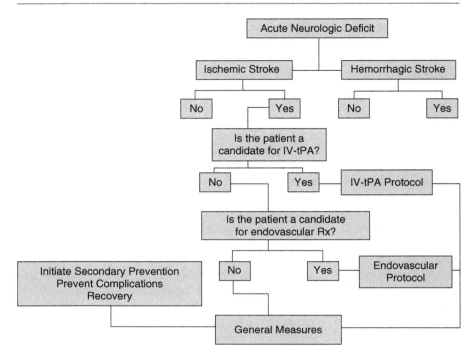

Fig. 23.1 Flow chart for acute stroke management (Reproduced with permission from Goldstein [7])

major risk of intravenous rtPA treatment was symptomatic haemorrhage (sICH) and also that the earlier the treatment is initiated, the better the result. Indeed treatment with intravenous rtPA initiated within 90 min of symptom onset was associated with an OR of 2.11 (95 % CI, 1.33–3.55) for favourable outcome instead of 1.69 (95 % CI, 1.09–2.62) for patients treated within 90–180 min [9]. From these results it appears that stroke is an emergency and time is one of the key points for the best therapeutic approach. Among complications after rtPA administration, angioedema merits attention. It is estimated to occur in 1.3–5.1 % of all patients who receive intravenous rtPA treatment. Risk of angioedema is associated with concomitant use of angiotensin-converting enzyme inhibitor [10] and with infarctions that involve the insular and frontal cortex.

The largest community experience, the SITS-ISTR (Safe Implementation of Thrombolysis in Stroke-International Stroke Thrombolysis Register), reported on 11,865 patients treated within 3 h of onset at 478 centres in 31 countries worldwide. The frequency of early neurological deterioration temporally associated with substantial parenchymal haematoma after intravenous rtPA was 1.6 % (95 % CI, 1.4–1.8 %). The frequency of favourable outcome (combined mRS scores of 0, 1 and 2) at 90 days was 56.3 % (CI, 55.3–57.2 %) [11]. These findings appear to confirm the safety of intravenous rtPA within the 3-h window at sites that have an institutional commitment to acute stroke care. Finally since ECASS 3 trial in 2008 has demonstrated that patients treated with rtPA within 3–4.5 h had a more favourable outcome than with placebo (52.4 % vs. 45.2 %; odds ratio, 1.34; 95 % confidence interval [CI], 1.02–1.76; $P=0.04$), rtPA use is now approved within 4.5 h from disease onset [12].

Endovascular Approach

The combination of pharmacological fibrinolysis and mechanical thrombectomy appears to have the highest rate of recanalisation without any difference in rate of intracranial haemorrhage. As the rate of recanalisation has increased, new challenges such as reocclusion, distal fragmentation and lack of clinical benefit despite complete recanalisation have been identified. Recently three different trials comparing endovascular approach instead of or after endovenous thrombolysis have failed to show a better outcome in the subgroup of patients treated with mechanical thrombectomy [13]. Since then the endovascular therapy might be considered in strictly selected patients in which rtPA is not effective or with contraindication to endovenous thrombolysis (e.g. therapy with anticoagulants).

23.1.4.2 Stroke Units

Numerous studies, performed mainly in Europe and Canada, demonstrate the utility of stroke units in lessening the rates of mortality and morbidity after stroke [14]. The positive effects persist for years. The benefits from treatment in a stroke unit are comparable to the effects achieved with intravenous administration of rtPA [15]. European stroke units usually do not include intensive care unit-level treatment, including ventilatory assistance. Regular communications and coordinated care are also key aspects of the stroke unit. Standardised stroke orders or integrated stroke pathways improve adherence to best practices for treatment of patients with stroke. Hospitals with a stroke unit compared with nondesignated hospitals led to lower overall 30-day mortality rates (10.1 % versus 12.5 %) and increased use of fibrinolytic therapy (4.8 % versus 1.7 %) [16]. Approximately 25 % of patients may have neurological worsening during the first 24–48 h after stroke, and it is difficult to predict which patients will deteriorate. In addition to the potential progression of the initial stroke, the need to prevent neurological or medical complications also means that patients with acute stroke should be admitted to the hospital in almost all circumstances. The goals of treatment after admission to the stroke unit are to (1) observe for changes in the patient's condition that might prompt initiation of medical or surgical interventions, (2) provide observation and treatment to reduce the likelihood of bleeding complications after the use of intravenous rtPA, (3) facilitate medical or surgical measures aimed at improving outcome after stroke, (4) begin measures to prevent subacute complications, (5) initiate long-term therapies to prevent recurrent stroke, and (6) start efforts to restore neurological function through rehabilitation and good supportive care [17].

23.1.4.3 Antiplatelets

During the acute phase of stroke for patient non-eligible to rtPa treatment, aspirin might be promptly administered. Currently available data demonstrate a small but statistically significant decline in mortality and unfavourable outcomes with the administration of aspirin within 48 h after stroke [18, 19]. It appears that the primary effects of aspirin are attributable to a reduction in early recurrent stroke. Data regarding the utility of other antiplatelet agents, including clopidogrel alone or in combination with aspirin, for the treatment of acute ischaemic stroke are limited. In addition, data on the safety of antiplatelet agents when given within 24 h of intravenous fibrinolysis are lacking.

23.2 Microvascular Disease

Cerebral Small-Vessel Disease

23.2.1 Definition

Cerebral small-vessel disease (SVD) is the term commonly used to describe a syndrome of clinical, cognitive, neuroimaging and neuropathological findings thought to arise from disease affecting the perforating cerebral arterioles, capillaries and venules and the resulting brain damage in the cerebral white and deep grey matter [20]. These perforating vessels are essential to maintain optimum functioning of the brain's most metabolically active nuclei and complex white matter networks [21]. However, misleadingly, the term small-vessel disease is used to describe only the ischaemic component of the pathological process (i.e. lacunar infarcts and white matter lesions). Instead, a broader view of small-vessel disease should be kept in mind, particularly for therapeutic aspects, because patients with small-vessel disease also have a risk of haemorrhage.

23.2.2 Clinical Features

The disease is very common and causes impairment in cognitive function [22] thus contributing up to 45 % of dementias. SVD is responsible for about a fifth of all strokes worldwide [23]; it more than doubles the future risk of stroke and produces physical disabilities. Overall, strokes caused by small-vessel disease are less severe than other types of stroke in terms of the clinical picture during the acute-phase and short-term prognosis. However, the long- term outcome of these patients cannot be thought of as benign in terms of mortality and functional impairment. The clinical manifestations are diverse and include sudden-onset stroke symptoms or syndromes; covert neurological symptoms that include mild, largely ignored, neurological symptoms and signs; self-reported cognitive difficulties; progressive cognitive decline; dementia; depression; and physical disabilities.

23.2.3 Mechanisms

The mechanisms that link small-vessel disease with parenchyma damage are heterogeneous and not completely known. Pathological changes in the small vessels can lead to both ischaemic and haemorrhagic consequences. The reason why some vessel ruptures and leads to major haemorrhage while others lead to microhaemorrhage is unknown. In cerebral amyloid angiopathy, differences in thickness of vessel walls are thought to explain the differences in haemorrhage, with thicker walls associated with more microhaemorrhages [24].

Although the mechanisms underlying haemorrhagic forms of small-vessel disease are more clear, in ischaemic lesions caused by small-vessel disease, vessel lumen tightening is thought to lead to a state of chronic hypoperfusion of the white matter [25], eventually resulting in degeneration of myelinated fibres as a consequence of repeated selective oligodendrocyte death. Alternatively, acute occlusion of a small vessel is hypothesised to occur, leading to focal and acute ischaemia and complete tissue necrosis (pannecrosis): this is the putative mechanism of lacunar infarcts. Although this theory was proposed many years ago in the seminal papers by Fisher [26], the so-called lacunar hypothesis remains unproven, and there is scarce pathological documentation for this hypothesis [27]. Other mechanisms such as blood–brain barrier damage, local subclinical inflammation and oligodendrocytes apoptosis could be involved in the so-called ischaemic forms of small-vessel disease and contribute to the final pathological picture.

A number of lines of evidence support a pathogenic role of endothelial activation and dysfunction of blood–brain barrier [28]. Genetic predisposition has also been implicated. Associations with genes involved in endothelial function, including those regulating the renin–angiotensin system, endothelial nitric oxide and homocysteine levels, have been reported.

23.2.4 Therapeutic Approaches

No specific treatment for strokes caused by small-vessel disease in the acute phase has yet been proposed, and there are no data to support the suggestion that any of the three approaches with recognised evidence-based efficacy in the acute setting (aspirin, thrombolysis, admission to a stroke unit) are effective in strokes caused by small-vessel disease. The presence of small-vessel disease is instead a marker of a poor outcome in some specific therapeutic settings, including acute-phase thrombolysis [29]. With regard to other pharmacological preventive measures, results from the Stroke Prevention by Aggressive Reduction of Cholesterol Levels (SPARCL) study have shown that patients with small-vessel disease and increased low-density lipoprotein cholesterol have a similar risk of stroke recurrence as do patients with large-vessel strokes and that treatment with atorvastatin 80 mg daily is equally effective in reducing this risk, implying that patients with small-vessel disease also benefit from statin therapy [30].

Finally data from SPS3 trial have shown that clopidogrel and aspirin, as compared with aspirin alone, in patients with a recent lacunar stroke identified on MRI, was not linked to a significant reduction in the risk of stroke recurrence; moreover, there was an unexpected increase in mortality [31].

23.3   Migraine

23.3.1 Definition and Clinical Manifestation

Migraine is a clinical condition characterised by recurrent headache disorder manifested by attacks lasting 4–72 h. Typical characteristics of the headache are unilateral in location, pulsating quality, moderate or severe in intensity, aggravated by routine physical activity and associated with nausea and/or photophobia and phonophobia.

If a transient neurological deficit precedes headache, it is called migraine with an aura; otherwise if cranial pain is the only symptom, the definition is migraine without aura.

Diagnostic criteria for migraine have been established in 1988, revised in 2004 and confirmed in 2013 by the International Headache Society (IHS) on the basis of expert consensus [32].

23.3.1.1 Diagnostic Criteria for Migraine Without Aura
At least five attacks fulfil these criteria:

  (i) Headache attacks lasting 4–72 h (untreated or unsuccessfully treated)
 (ii) Headache with at least two of the following characteristics:
   - Unilateral location
   - Pulsating quality
   - Moderate or severe pain intensity
   - Aggravation by or causing avoidance of routine physical activity (e.g. walking or climbing stairs)
(iii) The headache episode may be associated with at least one of the following:
   - Nausea and/or vomiting
   - Photophobia and phonophobia
 (iv) Not attributed to another disorder

23.3.1.2 Diagnostic Criteria for Migraine with Aura
At least two attacks fulfils the following criteria:

  (i) Aura consisting of at least one of the following, but no motor weakness:
   - Fully reversible visual symptoms including positive features (e.g. flickering lights, spots or lines) and/or negative features (i.e. loss of vision)
   - Fully reversible sensory symptoms including positive features (i.e. pins and needles) and/or negative features (i.e. numbness)
   - Fully reversible dysphasic speech disturbance
 (ii) At least two of the following:
   - Homonymous visual symptoms and/or unilateral sensory symptoms.
   - At least one aura symptom develops gradually over ≥5 min, and/or different aura symptoms occur in succession over ≥5 min.
   - Each symptom lasts ≥5 and ≤60 min.

(iii) Headache[1] begins during the aura or follows aura within 60 min.
(iv) Not attributed to another disorder

23.3.2 Mechanisms

Although a large number of recent studies have tried to establish the migraine pathophysiology [33, 34], the role of the neural and vascular mechanisms in this process has been largely discussed in the literature. As a matter of fact, there is still a debate whether the source of the pain is in the nerves around the cranial arteries, CNS or both [35, 36].

It has been generally accepted that calcitonin gene-related peptide (CGRP) plays an important role in the migraine pathophysiology [37]. CGRP is expressed throughout the CNS, particularly the striatum, amygdala, colliculi and cerebellum, as well as the peripheral nervous system. Recently, CGRP receptor antagonists have emerged as promising drugs to treat migraine. They could act by either blocking CGRP-induced vasodilation of meningeal blood vessels or inhibiting CGRP-mediated pain transmission in the CNS [37]. The fact that CGRP receptor antagonists, such as olcegepant and telcagepant, apparently require very high doses to produce significant clinical effects in migraine patients raises the possibility that those promising components have to cross the blood–brain barrier (BBB) in order to exert their effects [37]. Thus, according to some authors, it could support the concept that CNS mechanisms are predominantly involved in the migraine pathophysiology [38]. Conversely, the results of a functional neuroimaging study have indicated that changes in cortical blood flow, measured by blood oxygenated level (BOLD) signal variations, occur during episodes of migraine with aura. In addition, dilatation of both extracranial (middle meningeal) and intracranial (middle cerebral), as demonstrated by high-resolution direct MRA, has been shown after a migraine attack induced by infusion of CGRP. Remarkably, headache and vasodilatation occurred at the same side, and the administration of sumatriptan, a selective antimigraine drug, not only reduced the pain but also resulted in contraction of the middle meningeal artery. Collectively, those results suggest a key role of cranial blood vessels in the migraine pathophysiology. In fact, meningeal arteries lack BBB and represent much more permeable structures, compared with cortical vessels [39]. There have been considerable advances in the understanding of the sequence of events that lead to a migraine headache. Nevertheless, the specific structural and functional alterations that occur in the brains of patients affected by this disorder still need clarification, and BBB dysfunction has emerged as a possible mechanism.

---

[1] A headache occurring after aura may sometimes be of non-migrainous semiology or even absent (aura without headache). Aura may sometimes occur during the headache.

Table 23.1 Medications used as preventive strategies in migraine

Level A: medications with established efficacy (>2 class I trials)		
Divalproex sodium	Sodium valproate	Topiramate
Metoprolol	Propranolol	Timolol
Level B: medications are probably effective (1 class I or 2 class II studies)		
Amitriptyline	Venlafaxine	Atenolol
Nadolol		
Level C: medications are possibly effective (1 class II study)		
Lisinopril	Candesartan	Clonidine
Guanfacine	Carbamazepine	
Level U: inadequate or conflicting data to support or refute medication use		
Acetazolamide	Antithrombotics (e.g. Coumadin)	Fluvoxamine
Fluoxetine	Gabapentin	Verapamil
Other: medications that are established as possibly or probably ineffective		
Lamotrigine	Clomipramine	Acebutolol
Clonazepam	Nabumetone	Oxcarbazepine
Telmisartan	Montelukast	

Reproduced with permission from Loder et al. [41]
Adapted from American Headache Society/American Academy of Neurology 2012 guideline

23.3.3 Therapeutic Approach

Two pharmacological treatment options exist for migraine: preventive and symptomatic treatment.

23.3.3.1 Symptomatic Treatment

Symptomatic or acute treatment is necessary for all patients with migraine. The symptomatic treatment options include simple analgesics, nonsteroidal anti-inflammatory drugs (NSAIDs), ergotics and serotonin receptor (subunit 1B/1D) agonists (known as "triptans"). Except in children or in adults with mild attacks, the effectiveness of simple analgesics is very poor. On the other hand, because of efficacy and tolerability reasons, ergotics are not considered as the standard medication for migrainous patients. The symptomatic treatment of migraine lies, therefore, in the wise use of NSAIDs and triptans. In general, NSAIDs are indicated in mild-to-moderate attacks, whereas triptans are the medication of choice in the treatment of moderate-to-severe attacks and in those patients who do not respond to or do not tolerate NSAIDs.

Triptans

They have three main mechanisms of action: cranial vasoconstriction, peripheral trigeminal inhibition and inhibition of transmission through second-order neurons of the trigeminocervical complex. The relative importance of each of these mechanisms remains uncertain. By contrast with ergots, triptans have selective pharmacology, simple and consistent pharmacokinetics, evidence-based prescribing instructions, well-established efficacy, modest side effects and a well-established safety record [40]; they are, however, also contraindicated in the presence of cardiovascular disease.

23.3.3.2 Preventive Treatment

If the average of migraine attacks is high (6–8 days in a month with migraine), prevention of headache might be pursued considering the high risk of triptans and NSAIDs' abuse. Table 23.1 [41] shows the evidence-based medicine preventive therapies.

Anti-epileptic Drugs (AEDs)

Valproate and topiramate are both potent therapies that prevent migraine. Dosing can reach levels used in epilepsy, although typically the migraine doses are lower. Serious and significant side effects are possible with each, and nuisance side effects are common. There is some evidence that lamotrigine is effective in the prevention of migraine with aura [42].

Tricyclic Antidepressants (TCAs)

Of the TCAs, the best evidence overall is for amitriptyline. In addition, there is a strong clinical impression of their utility, especially in patients with coexistent sleep disruption, often characterised by fragmented sleep. Generally, low doses of 10–25 mg are used in migraine prevention, rather than higher antidepressant doses.

Beta-Blockers

Propranolol and timolol are generally considered safe and effective. Dosing may be similar to or lower than those used in the treatment of hypertension. Although often mentioned as first choices in a patient with migraine and hypertension, in practice, achieving the ideal dose of one medication for two separate conditions is often not possible.

Calcium Channel Antagonists

Of the various members of this heterogeneous group, verapamil is probably the most commonly used in migraine prevention and seems, based largely on clinical experience but with some research support, to have surpassed propranolol in the management of migraine with aura. Verapamil has been shown to be effective in vestibular migraine [41].

References

1. Mohr JP, Wolf PA, Grotta JC et al (2011) Stroke: pathophysiology, diagnosis, and management, 5th edn. Elsevier, Philadelphia
2. Bamford J, Sandercock P, Dennis M et al (1991) Classification and natural history of clinically identifiable subtypes of cerebral infarction. Lancet 337:1521–1526
3. Fernandes PM, Whiteley WN, Hart SR et al (2013) Strokes: mimics and chameleons. Pract Neurol 13(1):21–28. doi:10.1136/practneurol-2012-000465

4. Eilaghi A, d'Esterre CD, Lee TY et al (2014) Toward patient-tailored perfusion thresholds for prediction of stroke outcome. AJNR Am J Neuroradiol 35:472–477
5. Powers WJ, Grubb RL, Darriet D et al (1985) Cerebral blood flow and cerebral metabolic rate of oxygen requirements for cerebral function and viability in humans. J Cereb Blood Flow Metab 5:600–608
6. Brouns R, De Deyn PP (2009) The complexity of neurobiological processes in acute ischemic stroke. Clin Neurol Neurosurg 111(6):483–495
7. Goldstein LB (2007) Contemporary reviews in cardiovascular medicine acute ischemic stroke treatment in 2007. Circulation 116:1504–1514
8. Jauch EC, Saver JL, Adams HPJ et al (2013) Guidelines for the early management of patients with acute ischemic stroke: a guideline for healthcare professionals from the American Heart Association/American Stroke Association. Stroke 44:870–947
9. The National Institute of Neurological Disorders and Stroke rt-PA Stroke Study Group (1995) Tissue plasminogen activator for acute ischemic stroke. N Engl J Med 333:1581–1588
10. Hill MD, Lye T, Moss H et al (2003) Hemi-orolingual angioedema and ACE inhibition after alteplase treatment of stroke. Neurology 60:1525–1527
11. Külkens S, Hacke W (2007) Thrombolysis with alteplase for acute ischemic stroke: review of SITS-MOST and other phase IV studies. Expert Rev Neurother 7(7):783–788
12. Hacke W M.D., Kaste M M.D., Bluhmki E et al (2008) Thrombolysis with alteplase 3 to 4.5 hours after acute ischemic stroke. N Engl J Med 359:1317–1329
13. Chimowitz MI (2013) Endovascular treatment for acute ischemic stroke — still unproven. N Engl J Med 368:952–955
14. Rønning OM, Guldvog B (1998) Stroke unit versus general medical wards, II: neurological deficits and activities of daily living: a quasi-randomized controlled trial. Stroke 29:586–590
15. Gilligan AK, Thrift AG, Sturm JW et al (2005) Stroke units, tissue plasminogen activator, aspirin and neuroprotection: which stroke intervention could provide the greatest community benefit? Cerebrovasc Dis 20:239–244
16. Xian Y, Holloway RG, Chan PS et al (2011) Association between stroke center hospitalization for acute ischemic stroke and mortality. JAMA 305:373–380
17. Stroke Unit Trialists' Collaboration (2007) Organised inpatient (stroke unit) care for stroke. Cochrane Database Syst Rev (4):CD000197
18. CAST (Chinese Acute Stroke Trial) Collaborative Group (1997) CAST: randomised placebo-controlled trial of early aspirin use in 20,000 patients with acute ischaemic stroke. Lancet 349:1641–1649
19. International Stroke Trial Collaborative Group (1997) The International Stroke Trial (IST): a randomised trial of aspirin, subcutaneous heparin, both, or neither among 19435 patients with acute ischaemic stroke. Lancet 349:1569–1581
20. Pantoni L (2010) Cerebral small vessel disease: from pathogenesis and clinical characteristics to therapeutic challenges. Lancet Neurol 9(7):689–701
21. Bullmore E, Sporns O (2012) The economy of brain network organization. Nat Rev Neurosci 13(5):336–349
22. van der Flier WM, van Straaten EC, Barkhof F et al (2005) Small vessel disease and general cognitive function in nondisabled elderly: the LADIS study. Stroke 36:2116–2120
23. Sudlow CLM, Warlow CP (1997) Comparable studies of the incidence of stroke and its pathological types. Results from an international collaboration. Stroke 28:491–499
24. Greenberg SM, Nandigam RN, Delgado P et al (2009) Microbleeds versus macrobleeds: evidence for distinct entities. Stroke 40:2382–2386
25. Pantoni L, Garcia JH, Gutierrez JA (1996) Cerebral white matter is highly vulnerable to ischemia. Stroke 27:1641–1647
26. Fisher CM (1965) Lacunes: small, deep cerebral infarcts. Neurology 15:774–784
27. Boiten J, Lodder J (1991) Lacunar infarcts. Pathogenesis and validity of the clinical syndromes. Stroke 22:1374–1378
28. Hawkins BT, Davis TP (2005) The blood-brain barrier/neurovascular unit in health and disease. Pharmacol Rev 57(2):173–185

29. Cocho D, Belvís R, Martí-Fàbregas J et al (2006) Does thrombolysis benefit patients with lacunar syndrome? Eur Neurol 55:70–73
30. Amarenco P, Benavente O, Goldstein LB, SPARCL Investigators et al (2009) Results of the Stroke Prevention by Aggressive Reduction in Cholesterol Levels (SPARCL) trial by stroke subtypes. Stroke 40:1405–1409
31. The SPS3 Investigators (2012) Effects of clopidogrel added to aspirin in patients with recent lacunar stroke. N Engl J Med 367:817–825
32. Headache Classification Committee of the International Headache Society (2013) The International Classification of Headache Disorders, 3rd edition (beta version). Cephalalgia 33:629–808
33. Bhaskar S, Saeidi K, Borhani P et al (2013) Recent progress in migraine pathophysiology: role of cortical spreading depression and magnetic resonance imaging. Eur J Neurosci 38: 3540–3551
34. Noseda R, Burstein R (2013) Migraine pathophysiology: anatomy of the trigeminovascular pathway and associated neurological symptoms, CSD, sensitization and modulation of pain. Pain 154(Suppl 1):S44–S53
35. Goadsby PJ, Charbit AR, Andreou AP et al (2009) Neurobiology of migraine. Neuroscience 161:327–341
36. Olesen J, Burstein R, Ashina M et al (2009) Origin of pain in migraine: evidence for peripheral sensitisation. Lancet Neurol 8:679–690
37. Bell IM (2014) Calcitonin gene-related peptide receptor antagonists: new therapeutic agents for migraine. J Med Chem 57:7838–7858
38. Tfelt-Hansen P, Olesen J (2011) Possible site of action of CGRP antagonists in migraine. Cephalalgia 31:748–750
39. Edvinsson L, Tfelt-Hansen P (2008) The blood–brain barrier in migraine treatment. Cephalalgia 28:1245–1258
40. Ferrari M, Roon K, Lipton R, Goadsby P (2001) Oral triptans (serotonin 5-HT1B/1D agonists) in acute migraine treatment: a meta-analysis of 53 trials. Lancet 358:1668–1675
41. Loder E, Burch R, Rizzoli P (2012) The 2012 AHS/AAN Guidelines for prevention of episodic migraine: a summary and comparison with other recent clinical practice guidelines. Headache 52:930–945
42. Lampl C, Katsarava Z, Diener HC, Limmroth V (2005) Lamotrigine reduces migraine aura and migraine attacks in patients with migraine with aura. J Neurol Neurosurg Psychiatry 76: 1730–1732

Pre-eclampsia: A Multifaceted Disorder of Pregnancy

Catherine E.M. Aiken and Jeremy C. Brockelsby

24.1 Introduction

Pre-eclampsia is one of the most commonly occurring complications of pregnancy worldwide, affecting approximately 4.6 % (2.7–8.2 %) [1] of all pregnancies. Pre-eclampsia constitutes a complex syndrome of pregnancy-specific hypertensive disease, with multisystem involvement. Previous definitions of the syndrome have included strict criteria to measure proteinuria; however, recent guidance from the American College of Obstetricians and Gynecologists recognizes the multiplicity of different clinical presentations that may arise, including thrombocytopaenia, impaired renal or hepatic function, pulmonary oedema and cerebral or visual disturbance [2]. Overall 10–15 % of direct maternal deaths are attributable to pre-eclampsia and eclampsia [3]. The neonate is also at risk of significant short- and long-term morbidity from pre-eclampsia, particularly where iatrogenic early delivery is required [4]. The aetiology of pre-eclampsia however remains poorly understood.

The vasculature of both the mother and the fetoplacental unit is critical in the development of pre-eclampsia. The initiating event is thought to be impairment of the physiological conversion of the uterine spiral arteries in early pregnancy. This is then followed by a systemic inflammatory response-type reaction in the mother, which is likely driven by arterial endothelial dysfunction. How the two vascular events in the natural history of pre-eclampsia are linked, however, remains somewhat uncertain.

C.E.M. Aiken
Department of Obstetrics and Gynaecology, Cambridge University Hospitals NHS Foundation Trust, Hills Road, Cambridge, Cambridgeshire CB2 0QQ, UK
e-mail: Cema2@cam.ac.uk

J.C. Brockelsby (✉)
Department of Fetal Medicine, Cambridge University Hospitals NHS Foundation Trust, Hills Road, Cambridge, Cambridgeshire CB2 0QQ, UK
e-mail: jeremy.brockelsby@addenbrookes.nhs.uk

© Springer International Publishing Switzerland 2015
A. Berbari, G. Mancia (eds.), *Arterial Disorders:*
Definition, Clinical Manifestations, Mechanisms and Therapeutic Approaches,
DOI 10.1007/978-3-319-14556-3_24

24.2   Placental Development and Pre-eclampsia

The placenta has long been regarded as key to the aetiology of pre-eclampsia, particularly as the disorder does not resolve prior to its delivery. The idea that pathological maladaptation of the process of spiral artery transformation might underlie the development of pre-eclampsia was first suggested over 60 years ago. During the process of normal placentation, a vastly increased blood supply to the decidua basalis and underlying myometrium is required to support fetal and placental growth. The usual physiological adaptation to this increase in demand is conversion of the spiral arteries, which run through the myometrium to the developing placenta. This process involves a remarkable change in vessel morphology from small thick-muscled arteriolar walls to thin vessels, whose walls consist merely of a fibrous matrix containing invasive cytotrophoblast cells. These cytotrophoblast cells adopt a vascular morphology as they differentiate [5]. In uncomplicated pregnancies, virtually no structures resembling conventional arteries are detectable within the decidual or myometrial layers at term. The cytotrophoblasts in situ within these transformed maternal vessels alter their surface adhesion receptors to mimic maternal vascular endothelium, which allows them to adopt a vasculogenic role [6]. This change allows a constant, low-pressure flow of maternal blood to the placental bed. The intervillous space is thus perfused with a high-flow, low-pressure system, which ensures an adequate stream of nutrients and enables gas exchange with the fetal system.

The observation of reduced maternal blood flow in placentas of pregnancies affected by hypertensive disease [7] has stimulated close histological examinations of placentas from pre-eclamptic pregnancies. It was noted that structures with distinct arterial morphology remained present in the inner myometrium in pre-eclamptic pregnancies [8], giving rise to the hypothesis that incomplete conversion of the spiral arteries might be the driving factor behind development of the disorder. The careful and impressive studies of Pijnenborg et al., in the 1980s, on a unique collection of whole pregnant uteri demonstrated in detail how normal spiral artery invasion proceeds [9, 10]. More recently, better clinical correlation of the pre-eclampsia phenotype with a decreased disruption of the muscular arterial walls of the myometrial vessels and reduced intramural extravillous cytotrophoblast has been established [11]. As our understanding of the nature of placental vascular lesions improves, new subtypes of lesions can be identified particular to pregnancies complicated by pre-eclampsia [12]. In particular it has been suggested that acute atherosis, an accumulation of subendothelial lipid-filled foam cells usually in the decidual parts of the spiral arteries, may have a greater correlation with the phenotype of pre-eclampsia than previously described [13]. Whilst acute atherosis may occur in normotensive pregnancy, it may be that the disruption to normal placental blood flow caused by acute atherosis only becomes sufficient to cause a clinical syndrome in the additional presence of suboptimal spiral artery remodelling [14].

It is unclear precisely what drives invasion of the cytotrophoblast, much less why in pregnancies with pre-eclampsia the depth of invasion should be less. The process is known to depend on complex interactions between growth factors, adhesion proteins and proteases, among others [15]. A number of factors regulating cell signalling have recently been suggested as possibilities for impairing normal cytotrophoblast migration in pre-eclampsia [16]. Putative mechanisms influencing cytotrophoblast invasion include the Notch signalling pathway [17], which regulates cell-cell interactions and has a role in vasculogenesis elsewhere. The STOX1 signalling pathway, which may induce other cellular adhesion molecules including α-T-catenin [18], has also been suggested as a putative candidate for disruption in pre-eclampsia. The epidemiological evidence that links STOX1 polymorphisms with propensity to develop pre-eclampsia is, however, somewhat conflicting [19, 20]. Elsewhere, local angiotensin II from the maternal decidual tissue has been postulated to influence trophoblastic migration and invasion [21]. Recently, interest has been generated in the putative role of corin, a protease that activates atrial natriuretic peptide and which may promote trophoblast invasion [22].

There may also be important interactions between successful spiral artery conversion and an immunological component to the development of pre-eclampsia. The role of the immune system in the pathogenesis of pre-eclampsia is gradually emerging, as more is understood regarding the interaction between trophoblasts and uterine natural killer cells [23].

24.3   Maternal Vascular Adaptations to Pregnancy

Vascular tone during pregnancy is mediated at an endothelial level by a number of factors, which overlap in physiological function. The major driver of the maternal cardiovascular adaptations to pregnancy is the fall in the total peripheral resistance [24], hence the importance of availability of vasodilatory factors. The compensatory rise in plasma volume (30–40 % above the non-pregnant state) is essential for ensuring adequate organ perfusion, particularly of the low-pressure placental bed. In normal pregnancy, a careful balance is maintained between vasodilatory and vasoconstrictive factors, allowing for the cardiovascular changes of early pregnancy to be accommodated without significant blood pressure increase. In pre-eclamptic pregnancy, it is evident from the first trimester that maternal cardiovascular adaptation to pregnancy does not occur fully. Between 14 and 17 weeks, the plasma volume expansion in pre-eclamptic pregnancy is reduced [25], and the increase in cardiac output is less than in normal pregnancy [26]. In normotensive pregnancy, the renin-angiotensin-aldosterone system is upregulated, to allow an aldosterone-mediated increase in plasma volume. However, the normal pressor response to the upregulation of angiotensin II appears to be blunted, preventing a corresponding rise in blood pressure [24]. In pre-eclamptic pregnancy, all of these responses are reduced compared to the normotensive state, although the relationship between the renin-angiotensin-aldosterone system and the final rise in blood pressure seen later in pre-eclamptic pregnancy is very complex, particularly as different vascular beds may have different responses, and remains to be fully elucidated [24]. There is evidence that the apparent complexity of the relationship might be at least partly explained by the presence of angiotensin II receptor-stimulating antibodies in pre-eclamptic pregnancy [27]. It has been demonstrated that subtypes of agonistic angiotensin I receptor autoantibodies may be present in up to 95 % of cases of pre-eclampsia, giving potential for a role not only in disease pathogenesis but possible use as biomarkers and in diagnosis to reliably identify pre-eclamptic pregnancies [28].

24.4   Placental Perfusion and Ischaemia

Whilst the problems of fetoplacental circulation and the problems of the maternal vascular response are well described in pre-eclampsia, the mechanism linking the two aspects of pre-eclampsia remains to be elucidated. The answer may be oxidative stress-mediated endothelial damage and perturbations to angiogenic signalling, via a reperfusion-type injury from the relatively ischaemic placenta [29]. The failure of spiral artery conversion results in a placenta where flow is reduced, converting an already relatively hypoxic environment to one of chronic ischaemia.

The production of excess free radical species is a common finding where chronic ischaemia exists [30]. Free radical species without, and sometimes despite, appropriate upregulation of antioxidant defence mechanisms cause significant damage at both cellular and tissue levels. In the pre-eclamptic placenta, there is evidence of elevated levels of a number of tissue markers of oxidative stress [31]. The maternal arterial endothelium appears particularly sensitive to these changes [32], and this may be key to linking the initiating events of pre-eclampsia in the placenta with the clinical syndrome. There is further experimental evidence of reduced defences against oxidative stress associated with the pre-eclamptic placenta, including decreased levels of nitric oxide synthase and superoxide dismutase, both of which are prominent features of the normal cellular response to oxidative stress [33]. A contributory factor to the development of pre-eclampsia at the maternal-fetal interface may be increased stress-related expression of advanced glycation end products (AGEs) and their receptors (RAGEs) [34], which are known to initiate local inflammatory reactions at the placental bed and systemically [35]. RAGEs are abundantly expressed not only at the uterine-placental interface but also in the maternal serum and hence may contribute to both the local initiation of abnormal placentation and the systemic disease state in the mother.

Accompanying the increased reactive oxygen species production caused by relative placental ischaemia is a release of other vasoactive, angiogenic and inflammation-provoking substances into the maternal circulation [16]. Particularly implicated is the release of HIF-1α (hypoxia-inducible factor-1α) and TGF-β1 (transforming growth factor-β1). These in turn stimulate further production of indirectly vasoactive factors including a soluble splice variant of the VEGF receptor-1, sFlt-1 (soluble fms-like tyrosine kinase-1) [36]. This soluble receptor (sFlt-1) plays a crucial role in removing important angiogenic factors from the peripheral circulation by binding and inactivating them, particularly VEGF (vascular endothelial growth factor) and PIGF (placental growth factor) [37]. VEGF and PIGF have vital roles in maintaining vascular endothelial function and in vasculogenesis in both the pregnant and the non-pregnant state [38]. The inactivation of these factors is thought to have profound effects on the maternal vascular endothelium and its adaptations to pregnancy. The importance of the role of sFlt-1 in reducing plasma levels of VEGF and PlGF is demonstrated by the phenotype of hypertension and proteinuria that occurs when sFlt-1 levels are experimentally increased in animal models [36, 39], possibly via the upregulation of renal preproendothelin. Altered levels of sFlt-1 and PlGF are detectable in maternal plasma prior to the development of the clinical syndrome of pre-eclampsia, suggesting a possible future use for measuring these levels as a biomarker [40]. Further, removal of sFlt-1 from the peripheral circulation by plasmapheresis has been suggested as a novel new therapy for pre-eclampsia [41]. In addition to therapies targeted at reducing sFlt-1 levels, the possibility of countering its action by iatrogenically restoring VEGF has been explored. Studies in animal models of pre-eclampsia have demonstrated that VEGF infusion in rats with placental ischaemia-induced hypertension results in an improvement in both endothelial and glomerular function [42].

24.5   Maternal Endothelial Dysfunction

Widespread dysregulation of maternal endothelial function is well described in pre-eclampsia [38, 43, 44], likely due to oxidative stress from the hypoxic-ischaemic placenta [16]. The loss of normal regulatory function of the maternal endothelium in pre-eclampsia may be a form of the systemic inflammatory response syndrome, which occurs in a number of severe physiological insults [29]. Proinflammatory debris from the surface of the placenta, which can interact with the maternal endothelium, may be important in regulating and modulating the maternal response to pre-eclampsia. Many of these particles are microvesicles and nanoparticles, and it is an important area for future research to attempt classification of these and full investigation as to their role [45]. There are, however, a number of factors of more conventional vasoactive factors that have been implicated in the dysregulation of maternal endothelial function, including those which vasoconstrict, vasodilate, influence platelet function and regulate coagulation/fibrinolysis. The role of several of the better-understood vasoactive factors in pre-eclampsia is considered:

24.5.1 Nitric Oxide

One of the major vasodilatory factors is nitric oxide (NO), which causes a relaxation of vascular smooth muscle cells. Nitric oxide levels are elevated during normal pregnancy, as the vasculature relaxes to accommodate the increase in plasma volume. The relatively reduced bioavailability of NO in pre-eclampsia is thought to be key to the blood pressure rise in the third trimester [46]; however, direct assaying of NO in vivo is problematic. Lack of NO also has subsidiary effects on promoting platelet aggregation and activation [47] and inhibiting smooth muscle proliferation [48]. Recently, attention has focused on whether exogenous nitric oxide administration might prove a viable treatment strategy to address the clinical problem of pre-eclampsia at a molecular level [49]. An alternative strategy, which has been successful in some trials, is to supplement with L-arginine, a NO precursor [50].

24.5.2 Endothelin

In addition to the reduced vasodilator availability in pre-eclampsia, there is also a significant effect of increased responsiveness to vasoconstrictive agents [51]. Endothelin-1 (ET-1) is an extremely potent vasoconstrictive factor, the efficacy of which is dependent on the availability of its receptors, particularly the ET-A receptor in vascular smooth muscle. The circulating levels of ET-1 are elevated in pre-eclamptic pregnancy [52], although circulating levels of ET-1 do not appear to correlate well with the concentration of available factor at the tissue level. Work on animal models however has supported the idea that tissue concentrations of ET-1 are elevated in pre-eclamptic pregnancy [39]. The ET-A receptor is thus a potential target for pre-eclamptic therapy, but disruption of the ET-A receptor is detrimental in early pregnancy, and hence any therapy would have to be targeted only to the maternal circulation.

24.5.3 Haem Oxygenase

Haem oxygenase-1 (HO-1) is crucial for the in vivo breakdown of haem to a number of products including carbon monoxide (CO), biliverdin and free iron. Carbon monoxide, which is an inhibitor of sFlt-1 production and has vasodilatory effects [53], is primarily responsible for the angiogenic and antioxidant effects of HO-1 [54]. Furthermore, placental HO-1 expression is reduced in women experiencing severe pre-eclampsia [55]. Research in animal models suggests that in vivo induction of haem oxygenase-1 can enhance the availability of circulating VEGF and can reduce sFlt-1-mediated hypertension [56].

24.5.4 Prostacyclin

Prostacyclin (PGI$_2$) is a product of arachidonic acid metabolism and has a key role in vasodilatation in normotensive pregnancy. Derivation of PGI2 from arachidonic acid is mediated by cyclooxygenases 1 and 2, which may be downregulated in response to pre-eclampsia [57], hence reducing the vasodilatory response in pre-eclampsia. Experimental evidence however regarding PGI2 production is somewhat conflicting, with in vitro experiments demonstrating no difference in PGI2 production from placental trophoblasts between normotensive and pre-eclamptic pregnancies [58], whereas in vivo experiments have found reduced circulating levels in women with pre-eclampsia [59].

24.6   Pre-eclampsia and Macrovascular Disease

The diverse range of maternal macrovascular complications of pre-eclampsia, including malignant hypertension, stroke and eclampsia, is thought to be secondary to the generalized arterial endothelial dysfunction [60]. Thirty-nine percent of all pre-eclampsia deaths are due to cerebrovascular events [61]. Other rarer cerebrovascular syndromes are also increased during pregnancy complicated by pre-eclampsia, including posterior reversible encephalopathy syndrome and reversible cerebral vasoconstrictive syndrome [60]. It may be the case that normal pregnancy alters the permeability of the cerebral vasculature and that the elevated blood pressure in pre-eclamptic pregnancy inflicts secondary damage [62]. In particular, the decreased systemic vascular resistance of normal pregnancy may be synergistic with a decrease in myogenic tone in pre-eclamptic pregnancy [63] to produce increased cerebral blood flow and susceptibility to cerebral oedema.

Whilst it is known that women who develop pre-eclampsia in pregnancy are at greater risk of cardiovascular diseases and cardiovascular-related death later in life [64], it remains unclear whether this is attributable to an underlying propensity to arterial disease that predisposes to both pre-eclampsia and later cardiovascular disease or whether having had pre-eclampsia is itself a causative factor for later disease. Women who have an underlying condition that predisposes to a systemic inflammatory response (e.g. obesity, chronic kidney disease or essential hypertension) are significantly more susceptible to the development of pre-eclampsia, and even a normal or mildly abnormal placentation in these most susceptible women can be sufficient to develop clinical symptoms of pre-eclampsia [65]. The later risk of cardiovascular disease is related to the severity of the pre-eclampsia experienced [66], with women who had severe pre-eclampsia associated with intrauterine growth restriction experiencing a sevenfold increased risk of cardiovascular disease above the population baseline [67].

There is some evidence for the view that pre-eclamptic pregnancy has lasting effects on maternal arterial wall inflammation [68]. It is significant that altered endothelial function and altered angiogenic factors remain detectable in the circulation of women who have had pre-eclampsia for over 5 years following delivery [69]. Some changes in circulating markers of early endothelial dysfunction could be detected even at 10 years following the index pregnancy [70]. The risk of stroke following a pregnancy complicated by pre-eclampsia remains elevated in the year following delivery [71]. The persistence of the maternal arterial effects of pre-eclampsia has been demonstrated by an increase in common carotid artery intimal thickness compared to controls in women several years following pre-eclamptic pregnancy [72]. However, the mechanisms by which such changes persist remain unclear, and the ability to accurately predict the subset of women who will develop later cardiovascular disease as yet remains elusive.

Conclusions

We do not fully understand why the initiating event of pre-eclampsia, failure of extravillous cytotrophoblastic invasion of the spiral arteries, should occur in some pregnancies (up to 8 %) and not in others. There are known risk factors

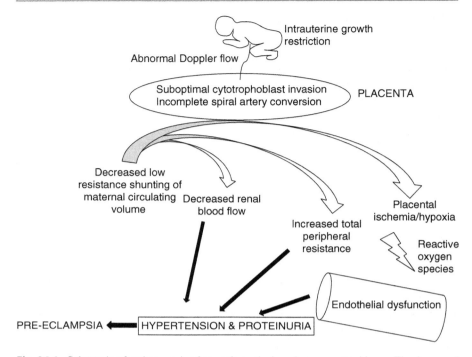

Fig. 24.1 Schematic of pathogenesis of pre-eclampsia, based on current evidence. The decreased low-resistance shunting of maternal blood, due to a disruption of the maternal-fetal interface, at the placenta has profound effects on maternal vascular adaptations to pregnancy. In a patient with susceptible endothelium, this leads to the development of the clinical syndrome of pre-eclampsia

including diabetes, obesity and genetic predisposition, but many pregnancies without these factors are also affected. Despite the advances in understanding of the vascular pathogenesis of pre-eclampsia outlined in this chapter and summarized in Fig. 24.1, the worldwide morbidity to both mothers and neonates remains high. Therapeutic options available presently are limited and are focused mainly on reducing seizure threshold and lowering blood pressure. Whilst these are useful therapies, they fail to address the underlying pathogenesis. The development of novel therapies including exogenous nitric oxide or glutathione donors may hold promise in this regard.

References

1. Abalos E, Cuesta C, Grosso AL et al (2013) Global and regional estimates of pre-eclampsia and eclampsia: a systematic review. Eur J Obstet Gynecol Reprod Biol 170(1):1–7
2. Task Force on Hypertension in Pregnancy (2013) Hypertension in pregnancy: American College of Obstetricians and Gynecologists. Hypertension in Pregnancy: Executive Summary Obstetrics & Gynecology 122(5):1122–1131. doi: 10.1097/01.AOG.0000437382.03963.88

3. Duley L (2009) The global impact of pre-eclampsia and eclampsia. Semin Perinatol 33(3): 130–137
4. Turner JA (2010) Diagnosis and management of pre-eclampsia: an update. Int J Wom Health 2:327–337
5. Zhou Y, Fisher SJ, Janatpour M et al (1997) Human cytotrophoblasts adopt a vascular phenotype as they differentiate. A strategy for successful endovascular invasion? J Clin Invest 99(9):2139–2151
6. Damsky CH, Fisher SJ (1998) Trophoblast pseudo-vasculogenesis: faking it with endothelial adhesion receptors. Curr Opin Cell Biol 10(5):660–666
7. Browne JC, Veall N (1953) The maternal placental blood flow in normotensive and hypertensive women. J Obstet Gynaecol Br Emp 60(2):141–147
8. Brosens IA, Robertson WB, Dixon HG (1972) The role of the spiral arteries in the pathogenesis of pre-eclampsia. Obstet Gynecol Ann 1:177–191
9. Pijnenborg R, Dixon G, Robertson WB, Brosens I (1980) Trophoblastic invasion of human decidua from 8 to 18 weeks of pregnancy. Placenta 1(1):3–19
10. Pijnenborg R, Bland JM, Robertson WB et al (1981) The pattern of interstitial trophoblastic invasion of the myometrium in early human pregnancy. Placenta 2(4):303–316
11. Lyall F, Robson SC, Bulmer JN (2013) Spiral artery remodeling and trophoblast invasion in pre-eclampsia and fetal growth restriction: relationship to clinical outcome. Hypertension 62(6):1046–1054
12. Kovo M, Schreiber L, Bar J (2013) Placental vascular pathology as a mechanism of disease in pregnancy complications. Thromb Res 131(Suppl 1):S18–S21
13. Stevens DU, Al-Nasiry S, Bulten J, Spaanderman ME (2012) Decidual vasculopathy and adverse perinatal outcome in pre-eclamptic pregnancy. Placenta 33(8):630–633
14. Staff AC, Dechend R, Redman CW (2013) Review: pre-eclampsia, acute atherosis of the spiral arteries and future cardiovascular disease: two new hypotheses. Placenta 34(Suppl):S73–S78
15. Norwitz ER, Schust DJ, Fisher SJ (2001) Implantation and the survival of early pregnancy. N Engl J Med 345(19):1400–1408
16. Palei AC, Spradley FT, Warrington JP et al (2013) Pathophysiology of hypertension in pre-eclampsia: a lesson in integrative physiology. Acta Physiol (Oxf) 208(3):224–233
17. Hunkapiller NM, Gasperowicz M, Kapidzic M et al (2011) A role for Notch signaling in trophoblast endovascular invasion and in the pathogenesis of pre-eclampsia. Development 138(14):2987–2998
18. Doridot L, Passet B, Mehats C et al (2013) Pre-eclampsia-like symptoms induced in mice by fetoplacental expression of STOX1 are reversed by aspirin treatment. Hypertension 61(3): 662–668
19. van Dijk M, Mulders J, Poutsma A et al (2005) Maternal segregation of the Dutch pre-eclampsia locus at 10q22 with a new member of the winged helix gene family. Nat Genet 37(5):514–519
20. Berends AL, Bertoli-Avella AM, de Groot CJ et al (2007) STOX1 gene in pre-eclampsia and intrauterine growth restriction. BJOG 114(9):1163–1167
21. Hering L, Herse F, Geusens N et al (2010) Effects of circulating and local uteroplacental angiotensin II in rat pregnancy. Hypertension 56(2):311–318
22. Cui Y, Wang W, Dong N et al (2012) Role of corin in trophoblast invasion and uterine spiral artery remodelling in pregnancy. Nature 484(7393):246–250
23. Colucci F, Boulenouar S, Kieckbusch J, Moffett A (2011) How does variability of immune system genes affect placentation? Placenta 32(8):539–545
24. Verdonk K, Visser W, Van Den Meiracker AH, Danser AH (2014) The renin-angiotensin-aldosterone system in pre-eclampsia: the delicate balance between good and bad. Clin Sci (Lond) 126(8):537–544
25. Salas SP, Marshall G, Gutierrez BL, Rosso P (2006) Time course of maternal plasma volume and hormonal changes in women with pre-eclampsia or fetal growth restriction. Hypertension 47(2):203–208

26. Visser W, Wallenburg HC (1991) Central hemodynamic observations in untreated preeclamptic patients. Hypertension 17(6 Pt 2):1072–1077
27. LaMarca B, Parrish MR, Wallace K (2012) Agonistic autoantibodies to the angiotensin II type I receptor cause pathophysiologic characteristics of pre-eclampsia. Gen Med 9(3):139–146
28. Siddiqui AH, Irani RA, Blackwell SC et al (2010) Angiotensin receptor agonistic autoantibody is highly prevalent in pre-eclampsia: correlation with disease severity. Hypertension 55(2):386–393
29. Redman CW, Sargent IL (2009) Placental stress and pre-eclampsia: a revised view. Placenta 30(Suppl A):S38–S42
30. Birben E, Sahiner UM, Sackesen C et al (2012) Oxidative stress and antioxidant defense. World Allergy Organ J 5(1):9–19
31. Staff AC, Ranheim T, Khoury J, Henriksen T (1999) Increased contents of phospholipids, cholesterol, and lipid peroxides in decidua basalis in women with pre-eclampsia. Am J Obstet Gynecol 180(3 Pt 1):587–592
32. Mitchell BM, Cook LG, Danchuk S, Puschett JB (2007) Uncoupled endothelial nitric oxide synthase and oxidative stress in a rat model of pregnancy-induced hypertension. Am J Hypertens 20(12):1297–1304
33. Hung TH, Burton GJ (2006) Hypoxia and reoxygenation: a possible mechanism for placental oxidative stress in pre-eclampsia. Taiwan J Obstet Gynecol 45(3):189–200
34. Daffu G, del Pozo CH, O'Shea KM et al (2013) Radical roles for RAGE in the pathogenesis of oxidative stress in cardiovascular diseases and beyond. Int J Mol Sci 14(10):19891–19910
35. Guedes-Martins L, Matos L, Soares A et al (2013) AGEs, contributors to placental bed vascular changes leading to pre-eclampsia. Free Radic Res 47(Suppl 1):70–80
36. Maynard SE, Min JY, Merchan J, Lim KH et al (2003) Excess placental soluble fms-like tyrosine kinase 1 (sFlt1) may contribute to endothelial dysfunction, hypertension, and proteinuria in pre-eclampsia. J Clin Invest 111(5):649–658
37. Wang A, Rana S, Karumanchi SA (2009) Pre-eclampsia: the role of angiogenic factors in its pathogenesis. Physiology (Bethesda) 24:147–158
38. Gilbert JS, Ryan MJ, LaMarca BB et al (2008) Pathophysiology of hypertension during pre-eclampsia: linking placental ischemia with endothelial dysfunction. Am J Physiol Heart Circ Physiol 294(2):H541–H550
39. Murphy SR, LaMarca BB, Cockrell K, Granger JP (2010) Role of endothelin in mediating soluble fms-like tyrosine kinase 1-induced hypertension in pregnant rats. Hypertension 55(2):394–398
40. Romero R, Nien JK, Espinoza J et al (2008) A longitudinal study of angiogenic (placental growth factor) and anti-angiogenic (soluble endoglin and soluble vascular endothelial growth factor receptor-1) factors in normal pregnancy and patients destined to develop pre-eclampsia and deliver a small for gestational age neonate. J Matern Fetal Neonatal Med 21(1):9–23
41. Thadhani R, Kisner T, Hagmann H et al (2011) Pilot study of extracorporeal removal of soluble fms-like tyrosine kinase 1 in pre-eclampsia. Circulation 124(8):940–950
42. Gilbert JS, Verzwyvelt J, Colson D et al (2010) Recombinant vascular endothelial growth factor 121 infusion lowers blood pressure and improves renal function in rats with placental ischemia-induced hypertension. Hypertension 55(2):380–385
43. Roberts JM, Taylor RN, Goldfien A (1991) Clinical and biochemical evidence of endothelial cell dysfunction in the pregnancy syndrome pre-eclampsia. Am J Hypertens 4(8):700–708
44. Krauss T, Kuhn W, Lakoma C, Augustin HG (1997) Circulating endothelial cell adhesion molecules as diagnostic markers for the early identification of pregnant women at risk for development of pre-eclampsia. Am J Obstet Gynecol 177(2):443–449
45. Redman CW, Tannetta DS, Dragovic RA et al (2012) Review: does size matter? Placental debris and the pathophysiology of pre-eclampsia. Placenta 33:S48–S54
46. Conrad KP, Kerchner LJ, Mosher MD (1999) Plasma and 24-h NO(x) and cGMP during normal pregnancy and pre-eclampsia in women on a reduced NO(x) diet. Am J Physiol 277(1 Pt 2): F48–F57

47. Konijnenberg A, Stokkers EW, van der Post JA et al (1997) Extensive platelet activation in pre-eclampsia compared with normal pregnancy: enhanced expression of cell adhesion molecules. Am J Obstet Gynecol 176(2):461–469
48. Jeremy JY, Rowe D, Emsley AM, Newby AC (1999) Nitric oxide and the proliferation of vascular smooth muscle cells. Cardiovasc Res 43(3):580–594
49. Johal T, Lees CC, Everett TR, Wilkinson IB (2013) The nitric oxide pathway and possible therapeutic options in pre-eclampsia. Br J Clin Pharmacol. doi:10.1111/bcp.12301
50. Alexander BT, Llinas MT, Kruckeberg WC, Granger JP (2004) L-arginine attenuates hypertension in pregnant rats with reduced uterine perfusion pressure. Hypertension 43(4): 832–836
51. Gant NF, Daley GL, Chand S, Whalley PJ, MacDonald PC (1973) A study of angiotensin II pressor response throughout primigravid pregnancy. J Clin Invest 52(11):2682–2689
52. George EM, Granger JP (2011) Endothelin: key mediator of hypertension in pre-eclampsia. Am J Hypertens 24(9):964–969
53. Cudmore M, Ahmad S, Al-Ani B et al (2007) Negative regulation of soluble Flt-1 and soluble endoglin release by heme oxygenase-1. Circulation 115(13):1789–1797
54. Levytska K, Kingdom J, Baczyk D, Drewlo S (2013) Heme oxygenase-1 in placental development and pathology. Placenta 34(4):291–298
55. Barber A, Robson SC, Myatt L et al (2001) Heme oxygenase expression in human placenta and placental bed: reduced expression of placenta endothelial HO-2 in pre-eclampsia and fetal growth restriction. FASEB J 15(7):1158–1168
56. George EM, Arany M, Cockrell K et al (2011) Induction of heme oxygenase-1 attenuates sFlt-1-induced hypertension in pregnant rats. Am J Physiol Regul Integr Comp Physiol 301(5): R1495–R1500
57. Beausejour A, Bibeau K, Lavoie JC et al (2007) Placental oxidative stress in a rat model of pre-eclampsia. Placenta 28(1):52–58
58. Zhao S, Gu Y, Lewis DF, Wang Y (2008) Predominant basal directional release of thromboxane, but not prostacyclin, by placental trophoblasts from normal and pre-eclamptic pregnancies. Placenta 29(1):81–88
59. Lewis DF, Canzoneri BJ, Gu Y (2010) Maternal levels of prostacyclin, thromboxane, ICAM, and VCAM in normal and pre-eclamptic pregnancies. Am J Reprod Immunol 64(6): 376–383
60. Block HS, Biller J (2014) Neurology of pregnancy. Handb Clin Neurol 121:1595–1622
61. MacKay AP, Berg CJ, Atrash HK (2001) Pregnancy-related mortality from pre-eclampsia and eclampsia. Obstet Gynecol 97(4):533–538
62. Warrington JP, George EM, Palei AC et al (2013) Recent advances in the understanding of the pathophysiology of pre-eclampsia. Hypertension 62(4):666–673
63. Ryan MJ, Gilbert EL, Glover PH et al (2011) Placental ischemia impairs middle cerebral artery myogenic responses in the pregnant rat. Hypertension 58(6):1126–1131
64. Irgens HU, Reisaeter L, Irgens LM, Lie RT (2001) Long term mortality of mothers and fathers after pre-eclampsia: population based cohort study. BMJ 323(7323):1213–1217
65. Myatt L, Miodovnik M (1999) Prediction of pre-eclampsia. Semin Perinatol 23(1):45–57
66. Newstead J, von Dadelszen P, Magee LA (2007) Pre-eclampsia and future cardiovascular risk. Expert Rev Cardiovasc Ther 5(2):283–294
67. Smith GC, Pell JP, Walsh D (2001) Pregnancy complications and maternal risk of ischaemic heart disease: a retrospective cohort study of 129,290 births. Lancet 357(9273):2002–2006
68. Martin U, Davies C, Hayavi S et al (1999) Is normal pregnancy atherogenic? Clin Sci (Lond) 96(4):421–425
69. Kvehaugen AS, Dechend R, Ramstad HB et al (2011) Endothelial function and circulating biomarkers are disturbed in women and children after pre-eclampsia. Hypertension 58(1): 63–69
70. Sandvik MK, Leirgul E, Nygard O et al (2013) Pre-eclampsia in healthy women and endothelial dysfunction 10 years later. Am J Obstet Gynecol 209(6):569 e1–569 e10

71. Tang CH, Wu CS, Lee TH et al (2009) Preeclampsia-eclampsia and the risk of stroke among peripartum in Taiwan. Stroke 40(4):1162–1168
72. Akhter T, Larsson M, Wikstrom AK, Naessen T (2013) Ultrasonographic individual artery wall layer dimensions indicate increased cardiovascular risk in previous severe pre-eclampsia. Ultrasound Obstet Gynecol. doi:10.1002/uog.13289

Kidney Transplantation: Indices of Large Arterial Function in Recipients and Donors

25

Sola Aoun Bahous, Yazan Daaboul, Serge Korjian, and Michel E. Safar

Renal transplantation confers a great advantage over other renal replacement modalities in the amelioration of patient cardiovascular profile. In the United States, more than 180,000 subjects are alive with a functioning transplanted kidney [1]. A meta-analysis of 16 studies showed that the general quality of life, physical functioning, and psychosocial functioning significantly improved following transplantation when compared to hemodialysis [2]. Nonetheless, only a minority of patients with end-stage renal disease (ESRD) are offered renal transplantation due to the scarcity of available donations. Approximately 17,000 kidney transplants are performed annually in the United States, with a relatively stable annual transplant rate since 2005, countered by a much more rapidly increasing waiting list of patients with ESRD [1].

Renal transplantation significantly reduces the cardiovascular disease burden observed in patients with ESRD. While cardiovascular death rates continuously increase over time in patients on dialysis, they are found to be persistently lower in the transplant patients with good graft function. Significant survival benefits of renal transplantation are evident in as early as 3 months post transplantation. In

S. Aoun Bahous, MD, PhD (✉)
Division of Nephrology, Department of Medicine, Lebanese American University Medical Center – Rizk Hospital, May Zahhar Street, Ashrafieh, Beirut 11-3288, Lebanon
e-mail: solabahous@hotmail.com; sola.bahous@lau.edu.lb

Y. Daaboul, MD • S. Korjian, MD
Gilbert and Rose Marie Chagoury School of Medicine, Lebanese American University, Lebanese American University Medical Center – Rizk Hospital, May Zahhar Str, Ashafieh, Beirut 11-3288, Lebanon
e-mail: yazan.daaboul@gmail.com; serge.korjian@gmail.com

M.E. Safar, MD
Publique des Hôpitaux de Paris, Hôtel-Dieu Hospital, Diagnosis and Therapeutics Center, Paris Descartes University, 1 Place du Parvis Notre-Dame, Paris 75004, France
e-mail: michel.safar@htd.aphp.fr

© Springer International Publishing Switzerland 2015
A. Berbari, G. Mancia (eds.), *Arterial Disorders:*
Definition, Clinical Manifestations, Mechanisms and Therapeutic Approaches,
DOI 10.1007/978-3-319-14556-3_25

3–6 months post transplantation, the age-adjusted cardiovascular and overall death rates, even in patients with hypertension and diabetes as primary diagnoses, were reduced to less than half. In contrast, cardiovascular death rates approximately doubled for patients with ESRD after only 1 year on dialysis [3].

Despite the substantial reduction in cardiovascular risk following transplantation, cardiovascular events remain the most common cause of death in renal transplant recipients. In fact, cardiovascular disease accounts for approximately one-third to one-half of all deaths after transplantation; and rates of cardiovascular events are still more than three times higher in renal transplant recipients compared to the age- and gender-matched general population [4–6].

25.1   Arterial Stiffness in Renal Transplant Patients

Stiffness of the large arterial system, estimated by the noninvasive measurement of pulse wave velocity (PWV) and central augmentation index (AI), is a reproducible predictor of early cardiovascular disease in the healthy population and in the renal transplant patients [7–9]. Unfortunately, the literature on arterial stiffness in renal transplant subjects is still insufficient because most data is derived from cohort and cross-sectional studies. In 2003, Covic and colleagues showed that the mean AI among renal transplant recipients at 3 months after live-related transplantation was significantly lower compared to those on hemodialysis. Mean AI levels were measured to be 15.9 and 25.1 %, respectively. Similarly, the mean PWV measurements were significantly higher in patients on hemodialysis (mean PWV = 7.19 m/s) compared to control patients with hypertension (mean PWV = 6.34 m/s) and to renal transplant recipients (mean PWV = 6.59 m/s) [10]. Ignace et al. found that improvement of carotid-femoral PWV (cfPWV) is probably age dependent, with a significant posttransplant benefit mostly seen in patients above the age of 50 years [11]. One study compared measurements of brachial-ankle PWV (baPWV) prior to transplantation and 6 months after transplantation among 58 renal transplant subjects with stable graft function [12]. The authors concluded that baPWV and systolic and diastolic blood pressures significantly decreased following transplantation.

The long-term arterial protective effect conferred by transplantation is highly suggested, but solid conclusions in that regard require more elaborate studies. It is believed that although transplantation improves arterial stiffness in comparison to ESRD, arterial stiffness in recipients of renal transplantation is still considered significantly higher than the age- and gender-matched general population. Bahous and colleagues demonstrated that carotid-femoral PWV (cfPWV) was increased in renal transplant patients independently of age and mean blood pressure compared to healthy controls. During a mean follow-up duration of 54 months, the authors concluded that higher PWV levels were also associated with higher rates of cardiovascular events [7]. Findings by Verbeke and colleagues confirmed that, even after adjustment for confounding factors, PWV was approximately 7.4 % higher in the renal transplant patients compared to healthy persons, corresponding to what they described as a difference in vascular age of approximately 10 years [13].

Finally, results by Strozecki et al. showed that in a mean follow-up period of 28 months starting at least 3 years after transplantation, cfPWV significantly increased from a mean of 9.1 m/s at baseline to a follow-up mean of 9.8 m/s [14]. The authors demonstrated that the calculated mean PWV increase of 0.7 m/s over 2 years in renal transplant recipients was markedly higher than the physiological increase of 0.1 m/s per year attributed to normal aging in the general population [14, 15]. The difference in cfPWV was further accentuated in patients above 50 years of age, increasing at a mean of 1 m/s in the follow-up period. Similarly, pulse pressure was significantly higher at follow-up, whereas systolic, diastolic, and mean blood pressures did not show any significant reduction [14].

Today, the concern is whether the beneficial effects of transplantation on arterial disorders are long lasting or simply a temporary improvement following the withdrawal of the uremic burden observed in ESRD that can be offset by the immune status of transplantation and donor factors. The overall effect of renal transplantation on arterial stiffness is probably beneficial but requires further investigation.

25.2 Factors Associated with Arterial Disorders in Renal Transplant Recipients

Arterial stiffness has been associated with specific transplant, recipient, and donor-related factors. In addition to the traditional risk factors observed in the normal aging population and in patients with ESRD, renal transplant recipients comprise a unique category of patients with unparalleled exposures and incomparable risk factors. To date, numerous studies have shown varying and sometimes contradictory findings and associations to arterial stiffness in these patients. Nonetheless, the true relationship between arterial stiffness and these associations is yet to be revealed with the help of ongoing basic and clinical research.

Although traditional recipient risk factors, such as age, male gender, smoking, diabetes, dyslipidemia, elevated mean arterial pressure, and hypertension, are also strong influences in the renal transplant population, the increased cardiovascular risk is unlikely to be fully explained by conventional risk factors alone [16–18]. In fact, the Framingham risk equation seems to underestimate the true cardiovascular risk among the transplant population due to the presence of unique risk factors that are not accounted for in the original equation [18].

Increased vascular calcification was linked to prolonged duration of dialysis in patients with ESRD [19]. Likewise, dialysis vintage was shown to be independently associated with aortic calcification at the time of transplantation and a predictor for future cardiovascular morbidity and mortality in the renal transplant population [20]. Using pulse wave analysis to measure aortic augmentation in 250 transplant patients with stable renal function, Ferro et al. showed that the total time on renal replacement therapy is positively correlated with the aortic AI [21]. The investigators revealed that a total time of more than 10 years was significantly associated with increased aortic AI. Cosio and colleagues studied the survival of patients over a mean duration of 84 months after transplantation. They showed that the length of time on dialysis is a significant factor in determining patient survival after transplant [22]. These findings have suggested that pre-transplant burden may persist even after transplantation and may have a substantial role in the development of arterial stiffness.

Immunosuppressive therapy seems to be an important factor of arterial function after renal transplantation. Generally, cyclosporine therapy in renal transplant patients is believed to be associated with endothelial dysfunction, reduced production of endothelial vasoactive substances, and loss of nocturnal blood pressure dipping, contributing to hypertension in these patients [23, 24]. AI in renal transplant patients was significantly higher in patients receiving cyclosporine immunosuppressive therapy compared to those receiving tacrolimus or non-calcineurin-inhibitor-based immunosuppressive regimen [21, 25]. These findings were later confirmed by Strozecki et al. who measured cfPWV in cadaveric renal transplant recipients [26]. Finally, two randomized controlled trials showed that indices of arterial stiffness, including cfPWV, were significantly higher post transplantation in patients who continued using cyclosporine versus those who switched to sirolimus and everolimus [27, 28]. The effect of newer immunosuppressive therapy on arterial disorders in the renal transplant population is under way, and results are yet to be released.

Cold ischemia time (CIT), defined as the time interval between graft icing after retrieval and its subsequent removal prior to transplantation, has been associated with arterial stiffening. Strozecki et al. showed that prolonged CIT ($\geq$24 h) was associated with increased PWV [29]. Although the mechanism is still poorly understood, the authors hypothesized that the increased association of acute graft rejection, chronic allograft nephropathy, or graft loss in patients with prolonged CIT may be attributable to the increased arterial stiffness seen in these patients [29, 30]. Although other studies have incorporated CIT in the evaluation of arterial stiffness, additional research to confirm the association between CIT and arterial stiffness has not been conducted. On the other hand, the association between arterial stiffness and warm ischemia time, defined as all remaining times of organ ischemia outside ice perfusion, has yet to be studied.

The relationship between arterial stiffness and allograft function has been poorly described in the literature. Although the association between renal function and arterial stiffness is well documented in ESRD, data is still conflicting for renal transplantation [31]. Although Delahousse et al. found no clear association between glomerular filtration rate (GFR) reduction and arterial stiffness, both Verbeke et al. and Kneifel et al. have reported an independent association between elevated PWV and lower GFR levels and emphasized on the importance of renal allograft function on vascular reactivity and arterial stiffness [13, 32, 33]. Also, Bahous et al. showed that increased PWV is independently associated with acute rejection, in addition to other classical parameters. The authors defined acute rejection as an increase of serum creatinine of greater or equal to 0.3 mg/dL either with biopsy-proven acute rejection or when other diagnoses seemed unlikely. Although not clinically proven, they postulated that renal insufficiency mediated by rejection episodes may be responsible for the associated arterial stiffness perceived in their study [34].

The roles of emerging risk factors, such as infections, AV fistulas, hyperhomocysteinemia, hypomagnesemia, hyperparathyroidism, erythropoietin therapy, low levels of folic acid and fibrinogen, hypovitaminosis, subclinical inflammation, and inflammatory and bone markers, have been variably described with insufficient evidence that needs further validation [21, 35–37].

Although still insufficiently explored, donor characteristics are an important aspect of arterial integrity in recipients. In this connection, traditional risk factors associated with arterial disorders rarely carry through from donors to recipients or are rather not classically observed in donors given the good health status of the selected donors. However, the increase in demand for kidney transplantation has led to the use of kidneys from expanded criteria donors (ECD) and from patients with death due to cardiac causes, termed donation after cardiac death (DCD). An ECD, defined by the Organ Procurement and Transplantation Network/United Network for Organ Sharing, is any donor older than 60 years or older than 50 years with at least two of the following: hypertension, serum creatinine greater than 1.5 mg/dL, or death due to a cerebrovascular event [38]. This expansion of the donor pool ushers in a new population of recipients that may be influenced by traditional risk factors in donors. Evidence such as decreased graft and recipient survival, as well as increased hospital admissions compared to recipients of kidneys from standard criteria donors, suggests a stronger influence of the donor profile [39, 40].

Two main donor characteristics have been associated with recipient arterial stiffness, namely, donor age at transplantation and donor large artery stiffness. Kneifel et al. first reported an association between donor age and recipient arterial stiffness measured by means of applanation tonometry. Recipients of kidneys from older donors had significantly stiffer large arteries 17 months after transplantation [33]. The results were validated by Delahousse et al. who measured central PWV in 74 recipients of kidneys from cadaveric donors. The authors showed that the adjusted PWV was 1 m/s higher at 1 year after transplantation in recipients of old-donor kidneys (greater than 53 years of age) compared to other patients [32].

Donor arterial stiffness has also been linked to recipient cardiovascular outcome. Bahous et al. studied 95 renal transplant recipients with a mean follow-up of 56 months and showed that higher PWV measurements in donors were associated with worse composite recipient outcome, corresponding to doubling of serum creatinine and development of ESRD, myocardial infarction, stroke, and cardiovascular death [41]. This underlines the relation between the kidney and the vascular system and a possible vascular profile carried by the transplanted kidney. Nevertheless, such associations are still poorly understood due to lacking data. With the advent of ECD, better-powered investigations and longer follow-up periods are needed to outline the exact link between donor parameters and recipient arterial dysfunction and outcome (Table 25.1).

Table 25.1 Factors associated with increased arterial stiffness in the transplant population

Factor	Study
Recipient-related factors	
Increased age	Barenbrock et al. (1998) [36]
	Ferro et al. (2002) [21]
	Bahous et al. (2004) [7]
	Bahous et al. (2006) [34]
	Delahousse et al. (2008) [32]
	Strozecki et al. (2010) [25]
	Strozecki et al. (2011) [14]
	Van Laecke et al. (2011) [35]
Higher fasting blood glucose	Opazo Saez et al. (2008) [42]
	Strozecki et al. (2010) [25]
	Van Laecke et al. (2010) [35]
Higher mean arterial pressure	Barenbrock et al. (1998) [36]
	Ferro et al. (2002) [21]
	Bahous et al. (2004) [7]
	Bahous et al. (2006) [34]
	Delahousse et al. (2008) [32]
	Opazo Saez et al. (2008) [42]
	Strozecki et al. (2010) [25]
	Van Laecke et al. (2011) [35]
Smoking	Bahous et al. (2004) [7]
	Bahous et al. (2006) [34]
Increased dialysis vintage	Ferro et al. (2002) [21]
Functioning AV fistula	Ferro et al. (2002) [21]
Hypomagnesemia	Van Laecke et al. (2011) [35]
Elevated CRP	Van Laecke et al. (2011) [43]
Elevated iPTH	Barenbrock et al. (1998) [36]
Transplantation-related factors	
Lower eGFR	Barenbrock et al. (1998) [36]
	Kneifel et al. (2006) [33]
	Verbeke et al. (2007) [13]
Cyclosporine therapy	Ferro et al. (2002) [21]
	Zoungas et al. (2004) [44]
	Strozecki et al. (2007) [26]
	Seckinger et al. (2008) [27]
	Strozecki et al. (2010) [25]
Acute rejection episodes	Bahous et al. (2004) [7]
	Bahous et al. (2006) [34]
Elevated cold ischemia time	Strozecki et al. (2009) [29]
Donor-related factors	
Older donor age	Kneifel et al. (2006) [33]
	Delahousse et al. (2008) [32]
Donor large artery stiffness	Bahous et al. (2012) [41]

25.3   Factors Associated with Arterial Disorders in Living Kidney Donors

Living donors have gradually become a vital source of transplanted kidneys in the past two decades. With the expansion of the living donor pool, a closer look at the short- and long-term effects of uninephrectomy was warranted. Several concerns regarding the outcome of uninephrectomized patients have been raised considering the risk of hyperfiltration injury reported in other debatably similar models. In rats, a significant reduction in nephron mass was associated with subsequent proteinuria and hypertension with a gradual decline in renal function [45, 46]. Physiologically, renal adaptation to nephron loss is through augmented filtration per single nephron. With hyperfiltration, glomerular hypertension and glomerulosclerosis ensue and eventually compromise renal function. Clinically, the observed effect of donor uninephrectomy does not seem to parallel that seen in other models of nephron loss. The exact underlying physiology is yet unknown, although it appears that the excision of half of the functional nephrons does not seem to bring about a maladaptive hyperfiltration, essentially due to the lack of a significant upsurge in glomerular capillary pressure. In other words, the required increase in single nephron glomerular filtration (SNGFR) brought on by uninephrectomy is fairly tolerated by the remaining nephrons due to an increase in glomerular plasma flow rather than an increase in pressure [47].

In kidney donors, initial cross-sectional studies made little to advance our understanding of the long-term outcomes following kidney donation particularly considering the variable methods and definitions used, conflicting results, significant losses to follow-up, and modest follow-up periods. Nevertheless, no significant risks were reported following kidney donation. In 2009, Ibrahim et al. presented a follow-up of 3,698 donors with time since donation ranging from 3 to 45 years. The authors found no significant long-term consequences compared to the general population. When donors were compared to their age-, sex-, and gender-matched controls, no significant increase in mortality was noted. Furthermore, the risk of developing hypertension, proteinuria, and ESRD was comparable to the general population [48].

Criticism concerning the choice of controls in prior studies led to newer investigations targeting healthy matched controls that would have been eligible for donation themselves. Two such studies conducted by Mjøen et al. in 2013 and Muzaale et al. in 2014 found a significant increase in long-term adverse outcomes in donors following donation [49, 50]. Mjøen et al. showed that comparing donors to matched non-donors eligible for donation yielded a higher hazard ratio for the development of ESRD (11.38) in donors over a median follow-up period of 15.1 years [49]. Overall, the study showed that ESRD, cardiovascular, and all-cause mortality is significantly increased in donors compared to non-donors who meet the criteria for donation. Similarly to previous studies, all-cause mortality was not increased in donors in the first 5–10 years, but it significantly increased thereafter [49, 51–53]. Unfortunately, Mjøen et al. did not evaluate for the presence of comorbidities and risk factors that may contribute to the increased cardiovascular risk in the donor population. Since ESRD in kidney donors was mostly due to a primary renal disease and most donors are first-degree relatives of patients with ESRD, the authors eventually raised the concern whether genetic familial factors, rather than uninephrectomy, may have guided their novel findings [49].

In another study, Muzaale et al. also reported a slightly elevated risk of ESRD with similarly profiled controls. The estimated lifetime risk of ESRD was 90 per 10,000 donors, compared to 14 per 10,000 in healthy matched controls. The investigators also pointed out the problematic comparisons previously made to the general population. When compared to unscreened controls (comparable to the general population), the risk of ESRD was threefold lower in donors given the increased prevalence of comorbidities in the unscreened cohort. At 15 years, donors who were 50 years of age and older, those of black ethnicity, and male donors had significantly higher cumulative incidence of ESRD than younger donors, donors of white ethnicity, and female donors [50]. Similarly to Mjøen et al., the authors did not incorporate other comorbidities in assessing the etiology of the increased risk of ESRD in the donor group [49, 50].

Beyond renal function in donors, alterations in arterial structure and function have recently become a major point of interest given the link between reduced kidney function and cardiovascular disease. Evaluating a proposed arterial dysfunction brought on by reduced renal mass has been attempted by several investigators primarily by assessing the risk for higher blood pressure and hypertension in the donor population. Following donor nephrectomy, studies have inconsistently shown an increased risk for the development of hypertension. Furthermore, despite a documented increase in systolic and/or diastolic blood pressure values in certain donors, most were still below a hypertensive-range blood pressure. Albeit, with findings of increased cardiovascular mortality with elevated blood pressure readings even below the hypertensive threshold, additional investigations in the kidney donor population are needed [54]. A meta-analysis by Boudville et al. pooling 48 studies on blood pressure following kidney donation showed a 5 mmHg increase beyond the expected for normal aging over a 5–10-year follow-up period. A higher risk for developing hypertension was documented in patients with male sex, older age at donation, higher pre-donation blood pressure, and lower pre-donation GFR [55]. Still, the tendency toward a higher blood pressure in donors has been contested by other investigators that documented a similar prevalence of hypertension compared to matched controls [48].

A similar trend was observed in studies reporting the estimated cardiovascular risk in donors. Variable results have been reported even with well-matched controls. Garg et al. showed a lower risk of death or a major cardiovascular event in a cohort of 2,028 donors and 20,280 healthy matched non-donors with a median follow-up of 6.5 years [53]. Conversely, Mjøen et al. reported results for a similar-sized cohort with a longer median follow-up of 15.1 years. The study showed an elevated hazard ratio for all-cause and cardiovascular mortality in donors compared to matched controls fitting classical donor selection criteria [49].

Although not yet clearly outlined, uninephrectomy may have some effect on the arterial dysfunction implicated in cardiovascular outcome in donors. The identification of surrogate measures to identify arterial integrity and to recognize early subclinical cardiovascular disease is thus essential in this unique population. The utility of arterial stiffness, a well-established predictor of cardiovascular outcome in patients with ESRD and renal transplant recipients, has been scarcely utilized among kidney donors. Bahous et al. were the first to report increased arterial stiffness in a cohort of kidney donors compared to healthy matched controls by means of cfPWV and pulse pressure (PP). The investigators showed that donors had a significantly higher mean cfPWV (9.5 ± 2.5 m/s) compared to healthy matched controls (8.5 ± 1.5). In addition to the association between elevated cfPWV and older donor age, higher mean arterial pressure, higher fasting plasma glucose, and smoking, unique renal factors such as longer time since kidney donation were also implicated in arterial stiffness post nephrectomy. Interestingly, the study postulated that the involvement of these renal factors in arterial stiffness might ultimately suggest a role for uninephrectomy in the worsening of arterial stiffness. In their study, the authors questioned whether the gradual development of the abovementioned factors could be in fact partly attributed to the "age" of unilateral nephrectomy, speculating a temporal relation between uninephrectomy and increased cfPWV. These results were the first to usher the association between uninephrectomy and elevated aortic PWV independently of other classically reported risk factors. Additionally, the investigators also described an independent positive relationship between PP and macroalbuminuria and/or microalbuminuria in donors, further strengthening a link between renal function and large artery stiffness [34]. Nonetheless, the real link between uninephrectomy and arterial stiffness remains poorly defined due to paucity of available data. Studies with a larger population of donors and a longer follow-up period are required to verify the association between donor uninephrectomy and increased arterial stiffness.

Conclusion

In conclusion, renal transplantation remains the renal replacement modality of choice for patients with ESRD. It confers great advantage in the amelioration of cardiovascular disease risk and arterial stiffness compared to other renal replacement therapies. Nonetheless, it was shown that arterial stiffness might still be greater in renal transplant recipients compared to age- and gender-matched subjects from the general population. This significant increase may be attributable to recipient, transplant, and donor characteristics that cumulatively predispose these patients to an increased cardiovascular disease burden.

While earlier studies focused on arterial stiffness in transplant recipients, emerging data is scrutinizing into arterial stiffness in the donor pool as well. However, the literature to date is still conflicting, and more long-term research is indeed warranted to better outline the true relation between arterial stiffness and cardiovascular risk in both renal transplant recipients and donors. Needless to say, kidney donation is undeniably an altruistic unrivaled act that confers better outcome to recipients and does not carry a significant risk for the living donor. Support of this act should remain unequivocal.

References

1. United States Renal Data System (2014) 2013 USRDS annual data report: atlas of chronic kidney disease and end-stage renal disease in the United States: transplantation. Am J Kidney Dis 63(1):e283–e294
2. Landreneau K, Lee K, Landreneau MD (2010) Quality of life in patients undergoing hemodialysis and renal transplantation–a meta-analytic review. Nephrol Nurs J 37(1):37–44
3. Meier-Kriesche HU, Schold JD, Srinivas TR et al (2004) Kidney transplantation halts cardiovascular disease progression in patients with end-stage renal disease. Am J Transplant 4(10):1662–1668
4. Sarnak MJ, Levey AS, Schoolwerth AC et al (2003) Kidney disease as a risk factor for development of cardiovascular disease: a statement from the American Heart Association Councils on Kidney in Cardiovascular Disease, High Blood Pressure Research, Clinical Cardiology, and Epidemiology and Prevention. Hypertension 42(5):1050–1065
5. Dimeny EM (2002) Cardiovascular disease after renal transplantation. Kidney Int Suppl 80:78–84
6. Ojo AO, Hanson JA, Wolfe RA et al (2000) Long-term survival in renal transplant recipients with graft function. Kidney Int 57(1):307–313
7. Bahous S, Stephan A, Barakat W et al (2004) Aortic pulse wave velocity in renal transplant patients. Kidney Int 66(4):1486–1492
8. Barenbrock M, Kosch M, Jöster E et al (2002) Reduced arterial distensibility is a predictor of cardiovascular disease in patients after renal transplantation. J Hypertens 20(1):79–84
9. Mitchell A, Opazo Saez A, Kos M et al (2010) Pulse wave velocity predicts mortality in renal transplant patients. Eur J Med Res 15(10):452–455
10. Covic A, Goldsmith DJ, Gusbeth-Tatomir P et al (2003) Successful renal transplantation decreases aortic stiffness and increases vascular reactivity in dialysis patients. Transplantation 76(11):1573–1577
11. Ignace S, Utescu MS, De Serres SA et al (2011) Age-related and blood pressure-independent reduction in aortic stiffness after kidney transplantation. J Hypertens 29(1):130–136
12. Hotta K, Harada H, Sasaki H et al (2012) Successful kidney transplantation ameliorates arterial stiffness in end-stage renal disease patients. Transplant Proc 44(3):684–686
13. Verbeke F, Van Biesen W, Peeters P et al (2007) Arterial stiffness and wave reflections in renal transplant recipients. Nephrol Dial Transplant 22(10):3021–3027
14. Strozecki P, Adamowicz A, Kozlowski M et al (2011) Progressive arterial stiffening in kidney transplant recipients. Ann Transplant 16(3):30–35
15. McEniery CM, Yasmin HIR et al (2005) Normal vascular aging: differential effects on wave reflection and aortic pulse wave velocity: the Anglo-Cardiff Collaborative Trial (ACCT). J Am Coll Cardiol 46(9):1753–1760
16. Bachelet-Rousseau C, Kearney-Schwartz A, Frimat L et al (2011) Evolution of arterial stiffness after kidney transplantation. Nephrol Dial Transplant 26(10):3386–3391
17. Culleton BF, Wilson PW (1998) Cardiovascular disease: risk factors, secular trends, and therapeutic guidelines. J Am Soc Nephrol 9(12 Suppl):S5–S15
18. Kasiske BL, Chakkera HA, Roel J (2000) Explained and unexplained ischemic heart disease risk after renal transplantation. J Am Soc Nephrol 11(9):1735–1743
19. Guerin AP, London GM, Marchais SJ, Metivier F (2000) Arterial stiffening and vascular calcifications in end-stage renal disease. Nephrol Dial Transplant 15(7):1014–1021
20. DeLoach SS, Joffe MM, Mai X et al (2009) Aortic calcification predicts cardiovascular events and all-cause mortality in renal transplantation. Nephrol Dial Transplant 24(4):1314–1319
21. Ferro CJ, Savage T, Pinder SJ, Tomson CR (2002) Central aortic pressure augmentation in stable renal transplant recipients. Kidney Int 62(1):166–171
22. Cosio FG, Alamir A, Yim S et al (1998) Patient survival after renal transplantation: I. The impact of dialysis pre-transplant. Kidney Int 53(3):767–772
23. van den Dorpel MA, van den Meiracker AH, Lameris TW et al (1996) Cyclosporin A impairs the nocturnal blood pressure fall in renal transplant recipients. Hypertension 28(2):304–307

24. Morris ST, McMurray JJ, Rodger RS et al (2000) Endothelial dysfunction in renal transplant recipients maintained on cyclosporine. Kidney Int 57(3):1100–1106
25. Strozecki P, Adamowicz A, Włodarczyk Z, Manitius J (2010) Factors associated with increased arterial stiffness in renal transplant recipients. Med Sci Monit 16(6):CR301–CR306
26. Strozecki P, Adamowicz A, Wlodarczyk Z, Manitius J (2007) The influence of calcineurin inhibitors on pulse wave velocity in renal transplant recipients. Ren Fail 29(6):679–684
27. Seckinger J, Sommerer C, Hinkel UP et al (2008) Switch of immunosuppression from cyclosporine A to everolimus: impact on pulse wave velocity in stable de-novo renal allograft recipients. J Hypertens 26(11):2213–2219
28. Joannides R, Monteil C, de Ligny BH et al (2011) Immunosuppressant regimen based on sirolimus decreases aortic stiffness in renal transplant recipients in comparison to cyclosporine. Am J Transplant 11(11):2414–2422
29. Strózecki P, Adamowicz A, Kozłowski M et al (2009) Long graft cold ischemia time is associated with increased arterial stiffness in renal transplant recipients. Transplant Proc 41(9):3580–3584
30. Mikhalski D, Wissing KM, Ghisdal L et al (2008) Cold ischemia is a major determinant of acute rejection and renal graft survival in the modern era of immunosuppression. Transplantation 85(7S):S3–S9
31. Safar ME, London GM, Plante GE (2004) Arterial stiffness and kidney function. Hypertension 43(2):163–168
32. Delahousse M, Chaignon M, Mesnard L et al (2008) Aortic stiffness of kidney transplant recipients correlates with donor age. J Am Soc Nephrol 19(4):798–805
33. Kneifel M, Scholze A, Burkert A et al (2006) Impaired renal allograft function is associated with increased arterial stiffness in renal transplant recipients. Am J Transplant 6(7):1624–1630
34. Bahous S, Stephan A, Blacher J, Safar M (2006) Aortic stiffness, living donors, and renal transplantation. Hypertension 47(2):216–221
35. Van Laecke S, Maréchal C, Verbeke F et al (2011) The relation between hypomagnesaemia and vascular stiffness in renal transplant recipients. Nephrol Dial Transplant 26(7):2363–2369
36. Barenbrock M, Hausberg M, Kosch M et al (1998) Effect of hyperparathyroidism on arterial distensibility in renal transplant recipients. Kidney Int 54(1):210–215
37. Bartels V, Hillebrand U, Kosch M et al (2012) Influence of erythropoietin on arterial stiffness and endothelial function in renal transplant recipients. Am J Nephrol 36(4):355–361
38. Metzger RA, Delmonico FL, Feng S et al (2003) Expanded criteria donors for kidney transplantation. Am J Transplant 3:114–125
39. Pascual J, Zamora J, Pirsch JD (2008) A systematic review of kidney transplantation from expanded criteria donors. Am J Kidney Dis 52(3):553–586
40. Singh SK, Kim SJ (2013) Does expanded criteria donor status modify the outcomes of kidney transplantation from donors after cardiac death? Am J Transplant 13(2):329–336
41. Bahous S, Stephan A, Blacher J, Safar M (2012) Cardiovascular and renal outcome in recipients of kidney grafts from living donors: role of aortic stiffness. Nephrol Dial Transplant 27(5):2095–2100
42. Opazo Saez A, Kos M, Witzke O et al (2008) Effect of new-onset diabetes mellitus on arterial stiffness in renal transplantation. Transpl Int 21(10):930–935
43. Verbeke F, Maréchal C, Van Laecke S et al (2011) Aortic stiffness and central wave reflections predict outcome in renal transplant recipients. Hypertension 58(5):833–838
44. Zoungas S, Kerr PG, Chadban S et al (2004) Arterial function after successful renal transplantation. Kidney Int 65(5):1882–1889
45. Hostetter TH, Olson JL, Rennke HG et al (1981) Hyperfiltration in remnant nephrons: a potentially adverse response to renal ablation. Am J Physiol 241(1):F85–F93
46. Anderson S, Meyer TW, Rennke HG, Brenner BM (1985) Control of glomerular hypertension limits glomerular injury in rats with reduced renal mass. J Clin Invest 76(2):612–619
47. Mueller TF, Luyckx VA (2012) The natural history of residual renal function in transplant donors. J Am Soc Nephrol 23(9):1462–1466

48. Ibrahim HN, Foley R, Tan L et al (2009) Long-term consequences of kidney donation. N Engl J Med 360(5):459–469
49. Mjøen G, Hallan S, Hartmann A et al (2013) Long-term risks for kidney donors. Kidney Int. doi:10.1038/ki.2013.460
50. Muzaale AD, Massie AB, Wang M et al (2014) Risk of end-stage renal disease following live kidney donation. JAMA 311(6):579–586
51. Segev DL, Muzaale AD, Caffo BS et al (2010) Perioperative mortality and long-term survival following live kidney donation. JAMA 303(10):959–966
52. Garg AX, Prasad GV, Thiessen-Philbrook HR et al (2008) Cardiovascular disease and hypertension risk in living kidney donors: an analysis of health administrative data in Ontario, Canada. Transplantation 86(3):399–406
53. Garg AX, Meirambayeva A, Huang A et al (2012) Cardiovascular disease in kidney donors: matched cohort study. BMJ 344:e1203
54. Lewington S, Clarke R, Qizilbash N et al (2002) Age-specific relevance of usual blood pressure to vascular mortality: a meta-analysis of individual data for one million adults in 61 prospective studies. Lancet 360(9349):1903–1913
55. Boudville N, Prasad GV, Knoll G et al (2006) Meta-analysis: risk for hypertension in living kidney donors. Ann Intern Med 145(3):185–196

Part V

Evaluation Procedures

Arterial Function

26

Gary F. Mitchell

26.1 A Brief Overview of Pulsatile Hemodynamics

When the heart contracts, it sets up a forward traveling flow waveform that interacts with characteristic impedance (Z_c) of the proximal aorta to produce a forward traveling pressure waveform (Fig. 26.1). This forward traveling wave propagates along the aorta and encounters impedance mismatch at the interface between the normally compliant aorta and stiff muscular arteries, which produces partial wave reflection (Fig. 26.2). Although frequently portrayed as deleterious, wave reflection plays a critical protective role that limits transmission of pulsatile energy into the microcirculation [1]. Wave reflection amplifies pressure but attenuates flow pulsatility and reduces the amount of energy transmitted into small vessels [1–3]. The abrupt interface between the normally compliant aorta and stiff muscular arteries represents the first stage barrier against penetration of excessive pulsatility into the microcirculation (Fig. 26.2). A second major barrier to penetration of pulsatile energy into the microcirculation is provided by the high impedance of the resistance vessels, which may increase further in the setting of increased aortic stiffness and excessive pressure pulsatility (Fig. 26.2).

With advancing age, the aorta stiffens to a highly variable degree for reasons that are only partially elucidated but may be related to mechanical fatigue of elastic fibers [4], inflammation [5], fibrosis, cross-linking of structural proteins within the aortic wall [6], and smooth muscle cell hypertrophy [7] or stiffening [8]. As a result, Z_c and forward wave amplitude (P_f) increase after midlife [9], resulting in an increase in the pulsatile energy content of the advancing waveform. In addition, stiffening of the aorta with age greatly exceeds stiffening of the muscular arteries, which reduces impedance mismatch and wave reflection at this critical interface

G.F. Mitchell, MD
Cardiovascular Engineering, Inc., 1 Edgewater Drive, Suite 201, Norwood, MA 02062, USA
e-mail: GaryFMitchell@mindspring.com

© Springer International Publishing Switzerland 2015
A. Berbari, G. Mancia (eds.), *Arterial Disorders:*
Definition, Clinical Manifestations, Mechanisms and Therapeutic Approaches,
DOI 10.1007/978-3-319-14556-3_26

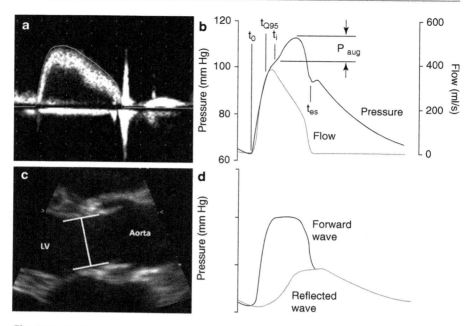

Fig. 26.1 Central aortic pressure-flow relations. Volumetric flow into the aorta is assessed by multiplying left ventricular outflow tract flow velocity (**a**) and area computed from diameter (**b**). The resulting volumetric flow waveform is paired with carotid artery tonometry and used to compute input impedance (**c**). Characteristic impedance (Z_c) is estimated by taking the ratio of change in pressure and change in flow prior to flow reaching 95 % of the peak value (t_{Q95}), which is prior to the inflection point (t_i) indicating arrival of the global reflected wave. Once Z_c is known, it is possible to separate forward and reflected pressure and flow waves (**d**)

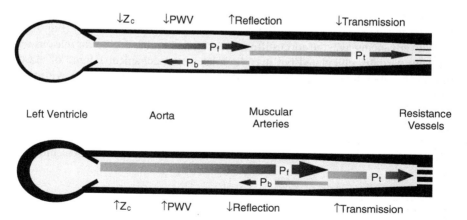

Fig. 26.2 Protective effect of wave reflection. Normal aortic stiffness is much lower than muscular artery stiffness (portrayed as differences in wall thickness). The resulting impedance mismatch produces proximal wave reflection, resulting in reflection of a component of waveform power (P_b), which limits the proportion of forward pulsatile power (P_f) that is transmitted (P_t) into the periphery, where it may cause damage (**a**). When aortic stiffness exceeds muscular artery stiffness, impedance mismatch is reduced, and a greater proportion of the pulsatile power is transmitted into the periphery (**b**)

[10]. Loss of wave reflection means that a greater percentage of pulsatile energy is transmitted into the periphery (Fig. 26.2), which is particularly deleterious for obligate high-flow organs such as the brain and kidney [1]. High-flow organs are necessarily of low impedance, meaning that a greater proportion of the pulsatility that passes through the critical first stage barrier at the aorta-muscular artery interface will be transmitted across the second stage barrier provided by the resistance vessels and may damage the microcirculation [2].

A number of measures of arterial function have been proposed to characterize the hemodynamic abnormalities summarized above. Aortic wall stiffness is readily assessed by measuring carotid-femoral pulse wave velocity, which is strongly related to incident hypertension [11] and cardiovascular disease (CVD) events [12]. The balance between aortic diameter, stiffness, and flow can be assessed by measuring forward pressure wave amplitude and Z_c. The amount of flow pulsatility penetrating into peripheral organs can be assessed by analysis of flow using Doppler ultrasound or magnetic resonance imaging [2, 3]. Wave reflection can be assessed by examining the central pressure waveform to determine augmented pressure and augmentation index (AI) or more precisely by measuring central pressure and flow waveforms [13]. Measured central aortic pressure and flow allows for separation of forward (P_f) and backward (P_b) pressure waves in order to determine relative wave reflection, for example, by calculating the global reflection coefficient, $\mathrm{RC} = P_b/P_f$ [14]. In addition, one can measure carotid intima-media thickness (CIMT) and ankle-brachial index (ABI) as measures of large artery wall hypertrophy and atherosclerotic disease. Finally, one can use multidetector computerized tomography (MDCT) to evaluate calcification in the aorta and coronary arteries as measures of structural damage and atherosclerosis.

26.2 Measures of Aortic Stiffness and Pressure Pulsatility

26.2.1 Carotid-Femoral Pulse Wave Velocity

CFPWV has been associated with CVD risk and risk reclassification in various studies and in a recent individual participant meta-analysis and has emerged as the reference standard measure of aortic stiffness [12]. In part, the ability of CFPWV to reclassify risk stems from the observation that CFPWV is only modestly associated with standard risk factors [15], although there are modest associations of higher CFPWV with greater age, mean arterial pressure, heart rate, inflammation, and components of the metabolic syndrome. In addition, CFPWV is moderately heritable and various genetic loci may contribute to increased aortic stiffness [16]. In the Framingham Offspring Study, having CFPWV in the highest (>12 m/s) as compared to the lowest (<8 m/s) quartile was associated with markedly increased risk for a first major CVD event (HR=3.4; 95 % CI, 1.4–8.3; $P < 0.008$) in a model that adjusted for standard risk factors [17]. Prevalence of CFPWV >12 m/s is low prior to 50 years of age but increases to >60 % after 70 years of age [18], suggesting that a substantial and growing burden of disease may be attributable to excessive aortic stiffness in our aging society.

CFPWV is readily measured in a clinical setting in just a few minutes with relatively modest requirements for specialized equipment and expertise. Transit time is measured by performing tonometry of the carotid and femoral arteries. The distance between recording sites is measured and CFPWV is computed as transit distance divided by transit time. Transit distance must account for parallel transmission of the advancing wavefront around the aortic arch and up the brachiocephalic and carotid arteries. The linear distance from carotid to femoral artery overestimates true transit distance. Compensation for parallel transmission is commonly achieved by using the suprasternal notch as a fiducial point for the waveform separation site and measuring upward to the carotid site and downward to the femoral site. The difference between these distances represents the corrected transit distance. An alternative approach measures the linear distance from carotid to femoral site and then rescales the distance by an empirically derived factor of 0.8 [19]. The latter approach has the potential limitation of not accounting for variability in individual anthropomorphic factors and operator positioning of the tonometer on the neck.

26.2.2 Pressure and Flow Pulsatility

European guidelines recommend consideration of pulse pressure (PP, the difference between systolic and diastolic blood pressure) when evaluating risk for CVD and when managing CVD and hypertension; $PP \geq 60$ mmHg is considered evidence of target organ damage in older patients [20]. PP and CFPWV are related but distinct measures of aortic function that contribute separately to risk. CFPWV is closely related to aortic wall stiffness but is relatively insensitive to the lumen area. In contrast, determinants of PP, such as Z_c and P_f, are strongly dependent on the aortic lumen area and matching between the aortic lumen area and ambient flow. Individuals with higher PP have higher aortic flow and ventricular dimensions and yet a smaller aortic lumen area, resulting in mismatch between the resting peak systolic flow and lumen area of the aorta, increased P_f amplitude, and increased PP [21].

Central as compared to peripheral PP has been recommended as a potentially superior tool for risk stratification. However, although absolute values for central and peripheral PP may differ because of the effects of variable timing of wave reflection, differences are modest from midlife onward, and the two values are highly correlated [22]. As a result, it is difficult to demonstrate that one or the other provides superior risk prediction. Placing the focus on increased awareness of the clinical implications of wide PP and other independent measures of aortic stiffness, such as CFPWV, rather than minor potential differences between central and peripheral PP, seems warranted.

26.2.3 Global Wave Reflection, AI, and Augmented Pressure

Measures of wave reflection are among the most frequently misunderstood and misinterpreted indicators of arterial system function. Relative wave reflection is often assessed from pressure alone by evaluating AI from a central aortic pressure wave-form (Fig. 26.1c). Higher AI was originally attributed to premature arrival of the reflected pressure wave because of increased aortic PWV. However, subsequent studies in large community-based samples have demonstrated modest relations between AI and CFPWV. In particular, after 50 years of age, when CFPWV increases dramatically, AI plateaus or falls [10, 13]. These seemingly counterintuitive rela-tions between AI and aortic stiffness are attributable in part to a reduction in imped-ance mismatch and amount of wave reflection after midlife, when aortic stiffness increases to the point that CFPWV reaches and then exceeds muscular artery PWV, resulting in reversal of the arterial stiffness gradient that normally gives rise to prox-imal wave reflection (Fig. 26.2).

In contrast to AI, augmented pressure continues to rise after midlife [13]. However, augmented pressure (or the separated P_b) amplitude depends strongly on P_f amplitude. If one rearranges the expression for global RC, one finds that $P_b = P_f$ * RC. Given that P_f increases dramatically after midlife, whereas RC falls modestly, it is clear that the increase in P_b after midlife is primarily attributable to larger P_f rather than increased wave reflection per se, as assessed by the RC. Thus, a late life increase in augmented pressure represents ratiometric rescaling of the central pres-sure waveform, with a constant percentage of PP attributable to augmentation. In addition, recent studies have shown that AI and augmented pressure amplitude are related to left ventricular function [23, 24]. P_b augments pressure and decelerates flow. The net effect on augmented pressure depends on left ventricular function and the left ventricular ejection pattern [13, 23]. Factors that limit ventricular ejection in late systole can therefore have a major effect on augmented pressure and AI even in the absence of alterations in P_b. Relations between ventricular function and aug-mentation may offer a mechanism for reducing central pressure that is not depen-dent on transferring the excess pulsatile energy into the microcirculation, as occurs with peripheral vasodilator drugs.

Measures of wave reflection have similarly complex relations with CVD risk. Early studies demonstrated relations between AI and clinical events in select sam-ples comprised of patients on dialysis [25] or with known coronary artery disease [26]. In addition, some recent community-based samples have found relations between measures of wave reflection and CVD outcomes [27–29], whereas others have not [17]. However, studies that found relations focused on P_b rather than a measure of relative wave reflection such as AI or the RC. As a result, the relation between P_b and events may be heavily dependent on P_f. Others used an imputed or estimated flow waveform rather than measured flow [27, 29], which may contribute to misclassification of wave reflection because of the dependence of the flow wave-form shape on left ventricular function [30].

In contrast to the question of risk stratification, when evaluating the effects of various interventions on blood pressure and clinical events, consideration of the dif-ferential effects of therapy on central as compared to peripheral blood pressure may be important. Drugs that reduce the amount of wave reflection or the ventricular response to a given reflected wave may have a greater effect on central as compared to peripheral systolic and PP. However, no study performed to date has demonstrated that differential lowering of central as compared to peripheral blood pressure is associated with a differential response to therapy that can be attributed to a more favorable effect of therapy on central as compared to peripheral blood pressure.

26.3   Measures of Atherosclerosis and Arterial Remodeling

26.3.1 Carotid Intima-Media Thickness (CIMT)

Carotid artery imaging provides a direct assessment of arterial wall remodeling and hypertrophy and the presence and severity of atherosclerosis. CIMT is measured in regions of the artery that are free of identifiable focal plaque, most often in the common carotid artery. CIMT represents a variable combination of medial hypertrophy and intimal thickening. Focal plaque provides clear evidence of atherosclerosis [31]. Plaque volume and characteristics may contribute separate information regarding risk. Echolucent plaques are lipid-rich and confer higher risk, whereas echogenic, fibrous plaques tend to be more stable [32, 33]. A recent individual participant data meta-analysis evaluated CVD risk reclassification offered by IMT of the common carotid based on data from 14 cohorts and 45,828 individuals with 4,007 events [34]. CIMT was associated with modestly higher risk for myocardial infarction and stroke. However, reclassification analysis demonstrated minimal net reclassification improvement in 10-year risk classification. Even in the subgroup at intermediate risk, net reclassification was small (3.6 %, 95 % CI, 2.7–4.6 %) and not likely to be clinically relevant [34].

26.3.2 Coronary Artery and Aortic Calcification

Calcification in the coronary arteries is located mostly within complex atherosclerotic plaques and associated with increased risk for adverse atherosclerotic events. Importantly, lack of calcification does not rule out the presence of disease because some plaques are not calcified; thus, coronary calcification should be used for risk stratification in the appropriate patient group (asymptomatic, intermediate risk) [35, 36]. Recent guidelines have included evaluation of coronary calcification as an option that may upstage CVD risk in those at intermediate risk [37]. However, evaluation of calcification requires exposure to radiation and therefore carries a risk that must be considered in the context of potential benefits of screening. To date, no prospective, randomized study has shown that a strategy of therapy guided by the presence of coronary calcium improves clinical outcomes.

Calcification in the aorta can occur in the intimal plaque or the media. Medial calcification is a complex, regulated process that is dysfunctional in various disease states and conditions, such as diabetes and chronic kidney disease [38]. Medial calcification may represent a cause and a consequence of arterial stiffness, leading to a potential vicious cycle that could contribute to the accelerated rate of aortic stiffening and calcification after midlife. Aortic stiffening and calcification may contribute to difficulty treating systolic hypertension in older people [39].

26.3.3 Ankle-Brachial Index (ABI)

The presence of flow-limiting lower extremity peripheral artery disease (PAD) can be confirmed noninvasively by an ABI <0.9. ABI is calculated by taking the maximum of systolic pressures in the posterior tibialis and dorsalis pedis arteries of each leg and dividing by the maximum systolic pressure in the arms, which is used as a common denominator in order to minimize confounding of ABI by upper extremity stenoses. Since PAD is often asymptomatic or associated with atypical symptoms, using ABI to screen for disease seems logical. However, studies performed to date have failed to demonstrate that ABI screening substantively reclassifies CVD risk [40–42]. Failure of ABI to fulfill criteria for a new risk biomarker is likely a consequence of strong relations between standard risk factors and abnormal ABI, i.e., rather than identifying a novel causal mechanism that contributes to CVD pathogenesis, abnormal ABI signifies rather advanced downstream consequence of risk factor exposure. For example, in the PARTNERS (PAD Awareness, Risk, and Treatment: New Resources for Survival) Study, screening of 6,979 adults >70 years of age or 50–69 years of age with diabetes identified 1,865 (29 %) with an ABI <0.9 [43]. However, the majority of participants with ABI <0.9 had clinically evident CVD or diabetes, indicating that they were already known to be high risk. The Aspirin for Asymptomatic Atherosclerosis trial used ABI to screen nearly 30,000 community-dwelling adults aged 50–75 years with no history of CVD and identified 3,350 participants with ABI <0.9 who were randomly assigned to receive aspirin or placebo [44]. There was no difference in CVD outcomes, indicating that screening was not an effective means for identifying risk and directing preventive therapy.

26.4   Dynamic Testing of Arterial Function

26.4.1 Brachial Artery Flow-Mediated Dilation

In contrast to the structural information provided by CIMT, brachial FMD provides a dynamic assessment of endothelial function in the brachial artery. The test is performed by measuring baseline brachial artery diameter and assessing change in diameter during reactive hyperemia induced by inflating a cuff on the proximal forearm to suprasystolic pressures for 5 min [45]. In healthy individuals, vigorous brachial artery dilation of 10 % or more may be seen, whereas in older individuals with CVD risk factors, little or no dilation may be seen.

FMD results must be interpreted in the context of the associated hyperemic stimulus, which provokes the FMD response and is highly variable. In the Framingham Heart Study Offspring cohort, various CVD risk factors were related to FMD in models that did not consider hyperemic flow. However, when variability in the flow response was considered, FMD-risk factor relations were attenuated or eliminated, whereas overall model R^2 improved [46]. Thus, variability in the flow response, rather than variability in the degree of local brachial FMD for a given flow stimulus, accounted for much of the observed relation between FMD and CVD risk factors. Postischemic microvascular reactivity is related to a number of CVD risk factors, including arterial stiffness [47]. Subsequent studies have shown that the level of hyperemia, rather than FMD, is associated with CVD risk [48].

26.5   Summary

The past two decades have witnessed the introduction of numerous noninvasive measures of vascular function. Hemodynamic tests offer measures of pressure pulsatility, arterial stiffness, and wave reflection. Noninvasive measures of subclinical disease include CIMT, coronary and aortic calcification, and ABI. Noninvasive measures of dynamic function include FMD and reactive hyperemia. These various tests and derived measures are related but provide complementary information. For example, data from the Framingham Offspring Study demonstrated that measures of aortic stiffness (CFPWV, P_f), wave reflection (AI), and dynamic function (FMD, resting forearm flow) were jointly associated in a single model with risk for developing hypertension in an initially normotensive subset of this community-based, middle-aged, and older cohort [11]. Complex diseases, such as hypertension and common downstream sequelae, including coronary artery disease, heart failure, stroke, dementia, and chronic kidney disease, have diverse etiologies that include specific pathologies at the parenchymal level in each affected organ and indirect effects of abnormalities in local and global vascular function. Thus, it seems unlikely that any single test will provide a comprehensive summary of arterial function and related risk. However, in light of the number of tests available, it is important to develop a strategy for integrating tests of vascular function into clinical practice. Brachial PP is a widely available measure of stiffness that should be examined further as a means for stratifying risk and as a potential target of therapy. CFPWV, a direct measure of aortic stiffness, assessed by carotid and femoral tonometry, is noninvasive and easily acquired using relatively inexpensive equipment and is supported by strong evidence from multiple studies and two large meta-analyses. Thus, CFPWV merits further consideration for routine use as a tool for risk stratification. Clinical trials are needed to determine whether use of CFPWV as a measure of risk or target of treatment results in improved survival. In addition to providing prognostic information, direct measures of aortic function, such as PP and CFPWV, may inform the development of novel therapies that are more effective at preventing or treating hypertension and related diseases.

References

1. Mitchell GF (2008) Effects of central arterial aging on the structure and function of the peripheral vasculature: implications for end-organ damage. J Appl Physiol 105:1652–1660
2. Mitchell GF, van Buchem MA, Sigurdsson S et al (2011) Arterial stiffness, pressure and flow pulsatility and brain structure and function: the age, gene/environment susceptibility–Reykjavik study. Brain 134:3398–3407
3. Woodard T, Sigurdsson S, Gotal J et al. (2014) Mediation analysis of aortic stiffness and renal microvascular function. J Am Soc Nephrol (in press). doi: 10.1681/ASN.2014050450
4. O'Rourke MF, Nichols WW (2005) Aortic diameter, aortic stiffness, and wave reflection increase with age and isolated systolic hypertension. Hypertension 45:652–658
5. Schnabel R, Larson MG, Dupuis J et al (2008) Relations of inflammatory biomarkers and common genetic variants with arterial stiffness and wave reflection. Hypertension 51:1651–1657
6. Santhanam L, Tuday EC, Webb AK et al (2010) Decreased S-nitrosylation of tissue transglutaminase contributes to age-related increases in vascular stiffness. Circ Res 107:117–125
7. Owens GK (1987) Influence of blood pressure on development of aortic medial smooth muscle hypertrophy in spontaneously hypertensive rats. Hypertension 9:178–187
8. Sehgel NL, Zhu Y, Sun Z et al (2013) Increased vascular smooth muscle cell stiffness: a novel mechanism for aortic stiffness in hypertension. Am J Physiol Heart Circ Physiol 305:H1281–H1287
9. Mitchell GF, Wang N, Palmisano JN et al (2010) Hemodynamic correlates of blood pressure across the adult age spectrum: noninvasive evaluation in the Framingham heart study. Circulation 122:1379–1386
10. Mitchell GF, Parise H, Benjamin EJ et al (2004) Changes in arterial stiffness and wave reflection with advancing age in healthy men and women: the Framingham heart study. Hypertension 43:1239–1245
11. Kaess BM, Rong J, Larson MG et al (2012) Aortic stiffness, blood pressure progression, and incident hypertension. JAMA 308:875–881
12. Ben-Shlomo Y, Spears M, Boustred C et al (2014) Aortic pulse wave velocity improves cardiovascular event prediction: an individual participant meta-analysis of prospective observational data from 17,635 subjects. J Am Coll Cardiol 63:636–646
13. Torjesen AA, Wang N, Larson MG et al (2014) Forward and backward wave morphology and central pressure augmentation in men and women in the Framingham heart study. Hypertension 64:259–265
14. Westerhof N, Sipkema P, Van Den Bos GC, Elzinga G (1972) Forward and backward waves in the arterial system. Cardiovasc Res 6:648–656
15. Cecelja M, Chowienczyk P (2009) Dissociation of aortic pulse wave velocity with risk factors for cardiovascular disease other than hypertension: a systematic review. Hypertension 54:1328–1336
16. Mitchell GF, Verwoert GC, Tarasov KV et al (2012) Common genetic variation in the 3'-BCL11B gene desert is associated with carotid-femoral pulse wave velocity and excess cardiovascular disease risk: the AortaGen consortium. Circ Cardiovasc Genet 5:81–90
17. Mitchell GF, Hwang SJ, Vasan RS et al (2010) Arterial stiffness and cardiovascular events: the Framingham heart study. Circulation 121:505–511
18. Mitchell GF, Guo CY, Benjamin EJ et al (2007) Cross-sectional correlates of increased aortic stiffness in the community: the Framingham heart study. Circulation 115:2628–2636
19. The Reference Values for Arterial Stiffness Collaboration (2010) Determinants of pulse wave velocity in healthy people and in the presence of cardiovascular risk factors: 'establishing normal and reference values'. Eur Heart J 31:2338–2350
20. Mancia G, Fagard R, Narkiewicz K et al (2013) 2013 ESH/ESC guidelines for the management of arterial hypertension: the task force for the management of arterial hypertension of the European Society of Hypertension (ESH) and of the European Society of Cardiology (ESC). J Hypertens 31:1281–1357

21. Torjesen AA, Sigurethsson S, Westenberg JJ et al (2014) Pulse pressure relation to aortic and left ventricular structure in the Age, Gene/Environment Susceptibility (AGES)-Reykjavik study. Hypertension 64:756–761

22. Narayan O, Casan J, Szarski M et al (2014) Estimation of central aortic blood pressure: a systematic meta-analysis of available techniques. J Hypertens 32:1727–1740

23. Fok H, Guilcher A, Li Y et al (2014) Augmentation pressure is influenced by ventricular contractility/relaxation dynamics: novel mechanism of reduction of pulse pressure by nitrates. Hypertension 63:1050–1055

24. Schultz MG, Davies JE, Roberts-Thomson P et al (2013) Exercise central (aortic) blood pressure is predominantly driven by forward traveling waves, not wave reflection. Hypertension 62:175–182

25. London GM, Blacher J, Pannier B et al (2001) Arterial wave reflections and survival in end-stage renal failure. Hypertension 38:434–438

26. Chirinos JA, Zambrano JP, Chakko S et al (2005) Aortic pressure augmentation predicts adverse cardiovascular events in patients with established coronary artery disease. Hypertension 45:980–985

27. Chirinos JA, Kips JG, Jacobs DR et al (2012) Arterial wave reflections and incident cardiovascular events and heart failure: MESA (Multiethnic Study of Atherosclerosis). J Am Coll Cardiol 60:2170–2177

28. Wang KL, Cheng HM, Sung SH et al (2010) Wave reflection and arterial stiffness in the prediction of 15-year all-cause and cardiovascular mortalities: a community-based study. Hypertension 55:799–805

29. Weber T, Wassertheurer S, Rammer M et al (2012) Wave reflections, assessed with a novel method for pulse wave separation, are associated with end-organ damage and clinical outcomes. Hypertension 60:534–541

30. Mitchell GF (2014) Arterial stiffness and hypertension. Hypertension 64:13–18

31. Polak JF, Pencina MJ, Pencina KM et al (2011) Carotid-wall intima-media thickness and cardiovascular events. N Engl J Med 365:213–221

32. Gronholdt ML, Nordestgaard BG, Schroeder TV et al (2001) Ultrasonic echolucent carotid plaques predict future strokes. Circulation 104:68–73

33. Polak JF, Shemanski L, O'Leary DH et al (1998) Hypoechoic plaque at US of the carotid artery: an independent risk factor for incident stroke in adults aged 65 years or older. Cardiovascular health study. Radiology 208:649–654

34. Den Ruijter HM, Peters SA, Anderson TJ et al (2012) Common carotid intima-media thickness measurements in cardiovascular risk prediction: a meta-analysis. JAMA 308:796–803

35. Blaha MJ, Blumenthal RS, Budoff MJ, Nasir K (2011) Understanding the utility of zero coronary calcium as a prognostic test: a Bayesian approach. Circ Cardiovasc Qual Outcomes 4:253–256

36. Kalra DK, Heo R, Valenti V et al (2014) Role of computed tomography for diagnosis and risk stratification of patients with suspected or known coronary artery disease. Arterioscler Thromb Vasc Biol 34:1144–1154

37. Goff DC Jr, Lloyd-Jones DM, Bennett G et al (2014) 2013 ACC/AHA guideline on the assessment of cardiovascular risk: a report of the American College of Cardiology/American Heart Association Task Force on practice guidelines. Circulation 129:S49–S73

38. Towler DA, Demer LL (2011) Thematic series on the pathobiology of vascular calcification: an introduction. Circ Res 108:1378–1380

39. McEniery CM, McDonnell BJ, So A et al (2009) Aortic calcification is associated with aortic stiffness and isolated systolic hypertension in healthy individuals. Hypertension 53:524–531

40. Lin JS, Olson CM, Johnson ES, Whitlock EP (2013) The ankle-brachial index for peripheral artery disease screening and cardiovascular disease prediction among asymptomatic adults: a systematic evidence review for the U.S. Preventive Services Task Force. Ann Intern Med 159:333–341

41. Moyer VA (2013) Screening for peripheral artery disease and cardiovascular disease risk assessment with the ankle-brachial index in adults: U.S. Preventive Services Task Force recommendation statement. Ann Intern Med 159:342–348

42. McDermott MM (2013) Ankle-brachial index screening to improve health outcomes: where is the evidence? Ann Intern Med 159:362–363

43. Hirsch AT, Criqui MH, Treat-Jacobson D et al (2001) Peripheral arterial disease detection, awareness, and treatment in primary care. JAMA 286:1317–1324
44. Fowkes FG, Price JF, Stewart MC et al (2010) Aspirin for prevention of cardiovascular events in a general population screened for a low ankle brachial index: a randomized controlled trial. JAMA 303:841–848
45. Corretti MC, Anderson TJ, Benjamin EJ et al (2002) Guidelines for the ultrasound assessment of endothelial-dependent flow-mediated vasodilation of the brachial artery: a report of the International Brachial Artery Reactivity Task Force. J Am Coll Cardiol 39:257–265
46. Mitchell GF, Parise H, Vita JA et al (2004) Local shear stress and brachial artery flow-mediated dilation: the Framingham heart study. Hypertension 44:134–139
47. Mitchell GF, Vita JA, Larson MG et al (2005) Cross-sectional relations of peripheral microvascular function, cardiovascular disease risk factors, and aortic stiffness: the Framingham heart study. Circulation 112:3722–3728
48. Anderson TJ, Charbonneau F, Title LM et al (2011) Microvascular function predicts cardiovascular events in primary prevention: long-term results from the Firefighters and Their Endothelium (FATE) study. Circulation 123:163–169

Doppler-Based Renal Resistive Index: Clinical and Prognostic Significance

27

David Schnell and Michael Darmon

Abbreviations

AKI   Acute kidney injury
RI   Doppler-based renal resistive index
US   Ultrasonography

27.1   Introduction

Ultrasonography (US) is performed routinely to assess renal and collecting system morphology [1]. B-mode US provides valuable information on anatomic features including kidney size (longitudinal diameter and parenchyma thickness) and appearance (kidney margins and echogenicity of the parenchyma, cortex, medulla, and papillae) and also on the presence and degree of hydronephrosis and the presence of stones, calcifications, cysts or solid masses. However, B-mode US does not evaluate kidney function. In contrast, renal Doppler US helps to assess vasculature of both native and transplanted kidneys [2]. Renal Doppler is valuable for

D. Schnell, MD
Medical Intensive Care Unit, Nouvel Hôpital Civil – Hôpitaux Universitaires de Strasbourg, 1 place de l'hôpital - BP 426, 67091 Strasbourg, France
e-mail: david.schnell@chru-strasbourg.fr

M. Darmon, MD, PhD (✉)
Medical-Surgical Intensive Care Unit, Saint-Etienne University Hospital, Avenue Albert Raimond, 42270 Saint-Priest-en-Jarez, Saint-Etienne, France

Jacques Lisfranc Medical School, Jean Monnet University, Saint-Etienne, France
e-mail: michael.darmon@chu-st-etienne.fr

© Springer International Publishing Switzerland 2015
A. Berbari, G. Mancia (eds.), *Arterial Disorders:*
Definition, Clinical Manifestations, Mechanisms and Therapeutic Approaches,
DOI 10.1007/978-3-319-14556-3_27

assessing large arterial or venous abnormalities and has been suggested for evaluating changes in intrarenal perfusion due to hypertension, diabetes or other diseases of the renal parenchyma [3–8]. Doppler-based renal resistive index (RI) has also been suggested as a performant tool in assessing renal allograft status [9, 10], changes in renal perfusion in critically ill patients [11–13] and for predicting the reversibility of an acute kidney injury (AKI) [14, 15]. However, many factors influence the RI and should be taken into account when interpreting RI values at the patient's bedside [16]. Indeed, ex vivo and clinical data suggest vascular compliance rather than renal perfusion to be the main factor influencing Doppler-based RI [10, 17]. The recently developed contrast-enhanced US might hold promises in assessing renal perfusion although only few data are currently available to evaluate its interest at bedside [18, 19].

The present chapter will discuss the technical requirements for Doppler assessment of the small intrarenal vessels, factors influencing Doppler-based renal resistive index and the potential interest of RI in hypertensive patients or selected renal diseases.

27.2 Technique

Although not technically difficult, Doppler assessment of the small intrarenal vessels must be carefully performed in order to obtain high-quality data [2, 20]. In most studies of renal Doppler, 2- to 5-MHz transducers were used [2, 20]. In our experience, convex transducer used for abdominal exploration usually allows to perform renal US. A small-phased array transducer can however be used. B-mode US in the posterolateral approach allows location of the kidneys and detection of signs of chronic renal damage. Although assessment of both kidneys is preferable, the right kidney is generally more accessible, and some authors have proposed to limit the investigation to this side especially if repeated measures are needed [1]. The renal artery divides in segmental and lobar arteries, which further divide in interlobar arteries, running adjacent to the medullary pyramids, which then branch into arcuate arteries encompassing the corticomedullary junction. Colour-Doppler or power-Doppler US allows vessels' localization (Fig. 27.1a) [2]. A semi-quantitative evaluation of renal perfusion using colour-Doppler has been proposed (Table 27.1) [1], and preliminary report suggests a good correlation of this index with RI [21]. Either the arcuate arteries or the interlobar arteries are then insonated with pulsed-wave Doppler using a Doppler gate as low as possible between 2 and 5 mm [2, 20]. The waveforms should be optimized for the measurements using the lowest pulse repetition frequency (usually 1.2–1.4 kHz) without aliasing (to maximize waveform size), the highest gain without obscuring background noise, and the lowest wall filter [2, 20]. A spectrum is considered optimal when three to five consecutive similar-appearing waveforms are noted [2, 20]. When measured from the main renal arteries to the arcuate arteries, renal blood flow velocities progressively decrease with a relative increase of the diastolic part of the flow. This leads to a progressive decrease in RI, which is minimal at the level of interlobar and arcuate arteries [22].

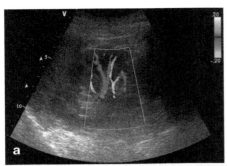

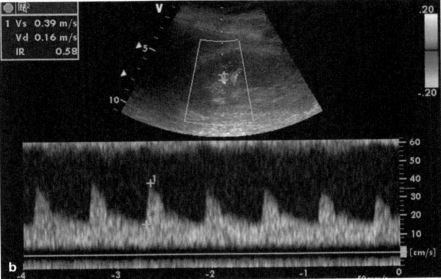

Fig. 27.1 Results of a renal colour-Doppler ultrasonography showing renal vascularization (**a**). RI measurement using pulsed-wave Doppler (**b**)

Table 27.1 Colour-Doppler for a semi-quantitative evaluation of intrarenal vascularisation [1]

Stage	Quality of renal perfusion by colour-Doppler
0	Unidentifiable vessels
1	Few vessels in the vicinity of the hilum
2	Hilar and interlobar vessels in most of the renal parenchyma
3	Renal vessels identifiable until the arcuate arteries in the entire field of view

To characterize the intrarenal Doppler waveform, most investigators have used the resistive index (RI) so-called Pourcelot index (Fig. 27.1b). Three to five reproducible waveforms are obtained, and RIs from these waveforms are averaged to compute the mean RI for each kidney. This easily calculated parameter is defined as follows:

$$RI = [peak\,systolic\,shift - minimum\,diastolic\,shift] / peak\,systolic\,shift$$

RI can theoretically range from 0 to 1. It is normally lower than 0.70. In several studies, mean RI (±SD) in healthy subjects ranged from 0.58 (±0.05) to 0.64 (±0.04) [23, 24]. The normal RI range is however age dependent. Thus, RI values greater than 0.70 have been described in healthy children younger than 4 years [25] and in individuals older than 60 years and considered healthy [26]. When the RI is measured for both kidneys, the side-to-side difference is usually less than 5 % [27].

Since RI depends in part on the minimum diastolic shift, it may be influenced by the heart rate [28]. According to observations performed by Mostbeck and colleagues regarding RI changes as consequences of heart rate variations, a formula has been developed to correct the RI value for heart rate: [corrected RI = observed RI $-0.0026 \times (80$-heart rate)] [28]. However, the influence of heart rate per se on RI remains unclear, and this formula is not used in most of the studies evaluating interest of RI [29, 30]. Arrhythmias and especially atrial fibrillation may impact renal RI measurement and interpretation.

Renal RI is a simple and non-invasive tool easy to use at the patient's bedside. Feasibility of the measure has been shown to be good, even in the settings of critically ill patients, and a recent study suggested a short (half-day) training session might allow inexperienced operators to perform renal Doppler [21]. Interobserver reproducibility of RI measurement by senior radiologist or senior intensivist is considered excellent [14, 31]. In critically ill patients, the interobserver reproducibility between senior and inexperienced operator is good, and measures seem accurate although associated with a lack of precision [21].

Renal pulsatility index is another parameter derived from renal blood flow velocities and is calculated as follows:

$$PI = [peak\,systolic\,velocity - minimum\,diastolic\,velocity] / mean\,velocity$$

Both RI and pulsatility index are however closely correlated ($r=0.92$; $P<0.001$) [13], and RI might be more adapted to the study of high-resistance vascular territories explaining why most authors report RI. Additionally, pulsatility index has been shown to be subject to wider variations than RI (reproducibility 9–22 % vs. 4–7 %) [32].

Contrast-enhanced US is believed to allow an accurate quantification of regional and global renal blood flow [19]. This technique relies on the intravascular injection of specific contrast agents that create a signal of high echogenicity, thus allowing macro- and microvascular structure visualization when using specific imaging techniques. These specific contrast agents consist in gas-filled microbubbles that oscillate in response to US waves, therefore creating a non-linear signal of high echogenicity [33]. It has been validated in humans to evaluate coronary blood flow [34], and its safety has been largely documented in this context [35]. When adding this technique to recently developed softwares, this technique is believed to allow an accurate quantification of regional blood flow, such as renal blood flow [19]. A recent study has confirmed feasibility of this technique in cardiac surgery patients, and additional studies are ongoing and should help in more clearly assessing input of this technique [36].

27.3   Physiological Significance of the Renal Resistive Index

Although renal Doppler has been the focus of many studies, the physiological significance of the RI remains debated. As suggested by its name, the RI was initially considered an indicator of renal vascular resistance and blood flow [7]. However, experimental and clinical studies have suggested correlation of RI with vascular resistance and blood flow to be weak [16, 17]. In fact, several hemodynamic and physiological factors influence the intrarenal arterial Doppler waveform patterns and, therefore, the RI value (Table 27.2).

Several studies established that vascular compliance is crucial to the interpretation of RI values [16, 17, 29]. In an in vitro study, the relationship between vascular resistance and RI was linear only when vascular compliance was normal and progressively disappeared when vascular compliance decreased [17]. This was confirmed in studies in ex vivo rabbit kidney models [16, 29]. In addition, the observed RI changes in response to pharmacologically induced changes in renal vascular resistance were modest [29]. In this model, large, non-physiological, pharmacologically induced changes in renal vascular resistances translated into slight changes in RI (RI changes of 0.047 IU (+/−0.008) per logarithmic increase in renal resistances) [29]. In the same model, changes in pulse pressure index [(systolic pressure − diastolic pressure/systolic pressure)] had direct and dramatic effects on RI values [29]. Clinical data supporting influence of impaired vascular compliance in determination of RI are scarce. However, a recent longitudinal cohort study performed in renal

Table 27.2 Physiological and pathological factors influencing the Doppler-based renal resistive index [14, 24, 34–38, 40]	Physiological factors	Vascular compliance (arterial stiffness)
		Vascular resistances
		Pulse pressure
		Renal blood flow
		Heart rate
		Oxygen and carbon dioxide levels
		Age
	Pathological factors	Interstitial pressure
		Ureteral pressure
		Intra-abdominal pressure
		Mechanical ventilation with positive pressure

allograft recipients gave interesting information as regards to this relationship [10]. Hence, the main factor associated with elevated RI in renal transplant recipient was found to be characteristics of both donor and receiver rather than renal transplant function or outcome [10]. In addition to these factors, both oxygen and carbon dioxide levels can affect RI. Several studies have demonstrated RI, or pulsatility index or RI, to vary according to PaO_2 and $PaCO_2$ levels [37–39]. These studies performed in healthy subject, patients with chronic obstructive respiratory disease, renal transplant recipients or patients with acute respiratory distress syndrome suggest that hypoxemia and hypercapnia may increase RI [37–40].

As stated above, RI has been shown to increase with age [26]. Age-related arterial stiffening may explain this phenomenon mainly by increasing central pulse pressure (i.e. increased central arterial stiffness) and maybe by decreasing intrarenal arterial compliance (i.e. increased intrarenal arterial stiffness) [41]. Similarly, elevated RI observed in several pathological states such as diabetes mellitus and hypertension may also be related to influence these diseases on arterial stiffness [42, 43]. It must be pointed out that renovascular disease is common in older subjects and might greatly influence RI. Some authors suggested an increased peak systolic velocity (more than 1 m per second) to be highly sensitive and specific to detect renal artery stenosis [42].

Besides vascular and hemodynamic factors, kidney interstitial pressure has been shown to be associated with RI in ex vivo studies [16]. An increase in interstitial pressure reduces the transmural pressure of renal arterioles, thereby diminishing arterial distensibility and, consequently, decreasing overall flow and vascular compliance. Similarly, intra-abdominal pressure may affect RI via the same mechanisms. Thus, incremental changes in intra-abdominal pressure correlated linearly with RI in a porcine model [44], and reduction in intra-abdominal pressure with paracentesis was followed by a decrease in RI in cirrhotic patients with tense ascites [45]. Finally, ureteral pressure, likely acting via interstitial pressure, also affects RI [6].

27.4 Doppler-Based Renal Resistive Index and Hypertension

As stated in the previous paragraph, the Doppler-based renal RI is an integrated index of arterial compliance, resistance, pulsatility and perfusion [17, 29]. In addition, RI has been demonstrated to be correlated with renal arteriosclerosis in numerous studies [10, 46]. Potential interest of Doppler-based renal RI has therefore been evaluated in assessing renal function or risk of end-organ damage in patients with hypertension or diabetes mellitus.

In patients with never-treated essential hypertension, a weak but significant correlation was observed between RI and both intima-media thickness ($r=0.25$; $P<0.0001$) and ambulatory arterial stiffness index ($r=0.27$; $P<0.0001$) suggesting a correlation between RI and early organ damage in hypertensive patients [47]. Other studies found similar results [48, 49]. Additionally, elevated RI was found to be associated with other targeted organ damage, namely, left ventricular hypertrophy, aortic stiffness or albuminuria [48, 50–53]. Furthermore, elevated RI was also found to be associated with mild reduction in glomerular filtration rate [42, 52]. These findings suggest Doppler-based resistive index to be a potent predictor of

Fig. 27.2 Probability of survival free of cardiovascular and renal event (all-cause death, stroke, myocardial infarction, congestive heart failure requiring hospitalization, aortic dissection or end-stage renal failure) in patients with hypertension and normal (RI <0.65 or <0.68 in patients of male gender and female gender, respectively) or elevated RI (Reproduced with permission from Doi et al. [54])

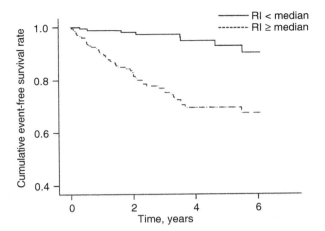

preclinical organ damage and of preclinical arteriosclerosis and therefore a predictor of cardiovascular risk profile [49].

Subsequently, several studies evaluated relationship between Doppler-based RI and outcome. Hence, Doi and colleagues demonstrated RI higher than 0.7 to be associated with cardiovascular events, end-stage renal disease or death in patients with hypertension (Fig. 27.2) [54]. Similarly, Pearce and colleagues found Doppler-based end-diastolic velocities to be associated with cardiovascular event or death in elderly patients [55]. In this study, however, only end-diastolic velocities (and not RI) were found to be associated with these events [55]. Although these studies give interesting insight as regards the potential interest of Doppler-based RI, no study to date gave an adequate cut-off or an estimation of RI performance in predicting adverse events. Additional studies in this field are therefore needed before implementing Doppler-based RI in assessing prognosis of hypertensive patients.

Interestingly, a preliminary report suggested Doppler-based RI to decrease accordingly to urine albumin excretion in patients receiving ACE inhibitors [56]. Similarly, RI was found to be decreased in parallel to blood pressure and urine albumin excretion following renal denervation [57]. Last, some authors found Doppler-based RI to be a predictor of renal outcome following renal revascularization in patients with unilateral renal artery stenosis [58]. In this study, however, blood pressure outcome was not associated with RI [58]. Although some confirmation studies are needed in this field, these findings might suggest Doppler-based RI to be of help in choosing, adapting and optimizing treatment in hypertensive patients.

27.5 Doppler-Based Renal Resistive Index in Selected Renal Diseases

Studies started in 1990 have evaluated the performance of RI measurement as a tool for assessing renal perfusion [59]. A preliminary study evaluated correlations between RI values and renal biopsy findings in patients with renal diseases requiring renal biopsy [60]. In this preliminary work, patients with interstitial, tubular, or vascular nephritis had markedly increased RI values (mean, 0.73–0.87), whereas patients with isolated glomerular disease had normal RI values (mean, 0.58) [60]. However, subsequent studies did not confirm these findings. Thus, in non-transplanted patients, RI failed to distinguish among five groups of predefined renal parenchymal diseases [61]. Similarly, several studies found that RI contributed to predict recovery from haemolytic and uremic syndrome [5], to detect renal involvement in systemic sclerosis [62], to predict renal outcomes in lupus nephritis [63] or to evaluate the progression of chronic renal diseases [64]. However, most of these studies were preliminary studies, and validation studies are still lacking in these different settings.

Several studies have evaluated the usefulness of RI measurement for assessing the risk of renal dysfunction after renal transplantation [4, 9, 10, 65]. Preliminary reports suggested that RI elevation might be highly specific of acute rejection [4, 8]. However, these findings were invalidated by subsequent studies [9, 10]. Nevertheless, several studies found that RI elevation predicted poor long-term outcomes [9, 10, 66] and accurately predicted early vascular and non-vascular renal complications (e.g., acute kidney injury, rejection and obstructive kidney disease) [67]. In a recent large prospective study, the main contributor to elevated RI was found to be characteristics of the donor or the recipient rather than renal histological features and that RI might be an integrative parameter of risk factors rather than the reflect of an acute renal events [10].

Lastly, renal Doppler has been evaluated for the early detection of AKI and for monitoring renal perfusion in critically ill patients [12]. Hence, in a preliminary study conducted in septic critically ill patients, RI measured at admission was significantly higher in patients who developed subsequently AKI [14]. This finding was recently confirmed in the post-operative setting of cardiopulmonary bypass [68]. Moreover, several studies have suggested that renal resistive index (RI) may help to discriminate between patients with transient AKI and those with persistent AKI [15, 69–71]. However, most of these studies are once again preliminary reports performed in limited population of patients, and confirmation studies are still lacking. In addition, a recent study reported discrepant results and a poor performance of RI in assessing renal dysfunction reversibility [72]. Lastly, significance of elevated RI in this population of patients remains questionable. Indeed, elevated RI might reflect renal interstitial oedema, decrease in renal perfusion, or reflect pre-existing preclinical renal arteriosclerosis and therefore a risk factor of persistent AKI.

Conclusion

Renal Doppler is a rapid, non-invasive and repeatable technique that may help in assessing renal preclinical dysfunction or vascular damages, in evaluating risk of subsequent renal dysfunction and evaluating severity of an acute kidney injury. This integrative parameter neither constitutes a substitute for renal biopsy nor provides reliable information on renal blood flow. Nevertheless, renal Doppler is a promising tool that might help in monitoring patients with hypertension, risk of cardiovascular diseases or acutely ill patients. Despite the promising preliminary results, validation studies are still awaited, and clinical relevancy of this technique is still uncertain. In addition, numerous factors have been shown to influence renal Doppler, each of them being also a potential confounder. Additional studies with larger population of unselected patients and pragmatic evaluation of the input of Doppler-based resistive index are therefore mandatory before implementing this test in clinical practice.

References

1. Barozzi L, Valentino M, Santoro A et al (2007) Renal ultrasonography in critically ill patients. Crit Care Med 35:S198–S205. doi:10.1097/01.CCM.0000260631.62219.B9
2. Platt JF (1997) Doppler ultrasound of the kidney. Semin Ultrasound CT MR 18:22–32
3. Krumme B, Blum U, Schwertfeger E et al (1996) Diagnosis of renovascular disease by intra- and extrarenal Doppler scanning. Kidney Int 50:1288–1292
4. Buckley AR, Cooperberg PL, Reeve CE, Magil AB (1987) The distinction between acute renal transplant rejection and cyclosporine nephrotoxicity: value of duplex sonography. AJR Am J Roentgenol 149:521–525. doi:10.2214/ajr.149.3.521
5. Patriquin HB, O'Regan S, Robitaille P, Paltiel H (1989) Hemolytic-uremic syndrome: intrarenal arterial Doppler patterns as a useful guide to therapy. Radiology 172:625–628. doi:10.1148/radiology.172.3.2672090
6. Platt JF (1992) Duplex Doppler evaluation of native kidney dysfunction: obstructive and non-obstructive disease. AJR Am J Roentgenol 158:1035–1042
7. Platt JF, Rubin JM, Ellis JH, DiPietro MA (1989) Duplex Doppler US of the kidney: differentiation of obstructive from nonobstructive dilatation. Radiology 171:515–517
8. Allen KS, Jorkasky DK, Arger PH et al (1988) Renal allografts: prospective analysis of Doppler sonography. Radiology 169:371–376. doi:10.1148/radiology.169.2.3051114
9. Radermacher J, Mengel M, Ellis S et al (2003) The renal arterial resistance index and renal allograft survival. N Engl J Med 349:115–124. doi:10.1056/NEJMoa022602
10. Naesens M, Heylen L, Lerut E et al (2013) Intrarenal resistive index after renal transplantation. N Engl J Med 369:1797–1806. doi:10.1056/NEJMoa1301064
11. Deruddre S, Cheisson G, Mazoit J-X et al (2007) Renal arterial resistance in septic shock: effects of increasing mean arterial pressure with norepinephrine on the renal resistive index assessed with Doppler ultrasonography. Intensive Care Med 33:1557–1562. doi:10.1007/s00134-007-0665-4
12. Duranteau J, Deruddre S, Vigue B, Chemla D (2008) Doppler monitoring of renal hemodynamics: why the best is yet to come. Intensive Care Med 34:1360–1361. doi:10.1007/s00134-008-1107-7
13. Lauschke A, Teichgräber UKM, Frei U, Eckardt K-U (2006) "Low-dose" dopamine worsens renal perfusion in patients with acute renal failure. Kidney Int 69:1669–1674. doi:10.1038/sj.ki.5000310
14. Lerolle N, Guérot E, Faisy C et al (2006) Renal failure in septic shock: predictive value of Doppler-based renal arterial resistive index. Intensive Care Med 32:1553–1559. doi:10.1007/s00134-006-0360-x
15. Darmon M, Schortgen F, Vargas F et al (2011) Diagnostic accuracy of Doppler renal resistive index for reversibility of acute kidney injury in critically ill patients. Intensive Care Med 37:68–76. doi:10.1007/s00134-010-2050-y
16. Murphy ME, Tublin ME (2000) Understanding the Doppler RI: impact of renal arterial distensibility on the RI in a hydronephrotic ex vivo rabbit kidney model. J Ultrasound Med Off J Am Inst Ultrasound Med 19:303–314
17. Bude RO, Rubin JM (1999) Relationship between the resistive index and vascular compliance and resistance. Radiology 211:411–417

18. Le Dorze M, Bouglé A, Deruddre S, Duranteau J (2012) Renal Doppler ultrasound: a new tool to assess renal perfusion in critical illness. Shock 37:360–365. doi:10.1097/SHK.0b013e3182467156
19. Schneider A, Johnson L, Goodwin M et al (2011) Bench-to-bedside review: contrast enhanced ultrasonography–a promising technique to assess renal perfusion in the ICU. Crit Care Lond Engl 15:157. doi:10.1186/cc10058
20. Schnell D, Darmon M (2012) Renal Doppler to assess renal perfusion in the critically ill: a reappraisal. Intensive Care Med 38:1751–1760. doi:10.1007/s00134-012-2692-z
21. Schnell D, Reynaud M, Venot M et al (2014) Resistive index or color-Doppler semi-quantitative evaluation of renal perfusion by inexperienced physicians: results of a pilot study. Minerva Anestesiol 80:1273–1281
22. Knapp R, Plötzeneder A, Frauscher F et al (1995) Variability of Doppler parameters in the healthy kidney: an anatomic-physiologic correlation. J Ultrasound Med Off J Am Inst Ultrasound Med 14:427–429
23. Keogan MT, Kliewer MA, Hertzberg BS et al (1996) Renal resistive indexes: variability in Doppler US measurement in a healthy population. Radiology 199:165–169
24. Norris CS, Pfeiffer JS, Rittgers SE, Barnes RW (1984) Noninvasive evaluation of renal artery stenosis and renovascular resistance. Experimental and clinical studies. J Vasc Surg 1: 192–201
25. Bude RO, DiPietro MA, Platt JF et al (1992) Age dependency of the renal resistive index in healthy children. Radiology 184:469–473
26. Terry JD, Rysavy JA, Frick MP (1992) Intrarenal Doppler: characteristics of aging kidneys. J Ultrasound Med Off J Am Inst Ultrasound Med 11:647–651
27. El Helou N, Hélénon O, Augusti M et al (1993) Renal Doppler ultrasonography in the diagnosis of acute obstructions of the upper urinary tract. J Radiol 74:499–507
28. Mostbeck GH, Gössinger HD, Mallek R et al (1990) Effect of heart rate on Doppler measurements of resistive index in renal arteries. Radiology 175:511–513
29. Tublin ME, Tessler FN, Murphy ME (1999) Correlation between renal vascular resistance, pulse pressure, and the resistive index in isolated perfused rabbit kidneys. Radiology 213: 258–264
30. Vade A, Dudiak C, McCarthy P et al (1999) Resistive indices in the evaluation of infants with obstructive and nonobstructive pyelocaliectasis. J Ultrasound Med Off J Am Inst Ultrasound Med 18:357–361
31. London NJ, Aldoori MI, Lodge VG et al (1993) Reproducibility of Doppler ultrasound measurement of resistance index in renal allografts. Br J Radiol 66:510–513
32. Mastorakou I, Lindsell DR, Piepoli M et al (1994) Pulsatility and resistance indices in intrarenal arteries of normal adults. Abdom Imaging 19:369–373
33. Raisinghani A, Rafter P, Phillips P et al (2004) Microbubble contrast agents for echocardiography: rationale, composition, ultrasound interactions, and safety. Cardiol Clin 22:171–180. doi:10.1016/j.ccl.2004.02.001
34. Vogel R, Indermühle A, Reinhardt J et al (2005) The quantification of absolute myocardial perfusion in humans by contrast echocardiography: algorithm and validation. J Am Coll Cardiol 45:754–762. doi:10.1016/j.jacc.2004.11.044
35. Dolan MS, Gala SS, Dodla S et al (2009) Safety and efficacy of commercially available ultrasound contrast agents for rest and stress echocardiography a multicenter experience. J Am Coll Cardiol 53:32–38. doi:10.1016/j.jacc.2008.08.066
36. Schneider AG, Goodwin MD, Schelleman A et al (2013) Contrast-enhanced ultrasound to evaluate changes in renal cortical perfusion around cardiac surgery: a pilot study. Crit Care Lond Engl 17:R138. doi:10.1186/cc12817
37. Sharkey RA, Mulloy EM, O'Neill SJ (1999) The acute effects of oxygen and carbon dioxide on renal vascular resistance in patients with an acute exacerbation of COPD. Chest 115: 1588–1592
38. Sharkey RA, Mulloy EM, O'Neill SJ (1998) Acute effects of hypoxaemia, hyperoxaemia and hypercapnia on renal blood flow in normal and renal transplant subjects. Eur Respir J Off J Eur Soc Clin Respir Physiol 12:653–657

39. Darmon M, Schortgen F, Leon R et al (2009) Impact of mild hypoxemia on renal function and renal resistive index during mechanical ventilation. Intensive Care Med 35:1031–1038. doi:10.1007/s00134-008-1372-5
40. Sharkey M, Long ON (1999) The effect of continuous positive airway pressure (CPAP) on renal vascular resistance: the influence of renal denervation. Crit Care Lond Engl 3:33–37
41. Mitchell GF (2008) Effects of central arterial aging on the structure and function of the peripheral vasculature: implications for end-organ damage. J Appl Physiol Bethesda Md 1985 105:1652–1660. doi:10.1152/japplphysiol.90549.2008
42. Derchi LE, Leoncini G, Parodi D et al (2005) Mild renal dysfunction and renal vascular resistance in primary hypertension. Am J Hypertens 18:966–971. doi:10.1016/j.amjhyper.2005.01.018
43. Ohta Y, Fujii K, Arima H et al (2005) Increased renal resistive index in atherosclerosis and diabetic nephropathy assessed by Doppler sonography. J Hypertens 23:1905–1911
44. Kirkpatrick AW, Colistro R, Laupland KB et al (2007) Renal arterial resistive index response to intraabdominal hypertension in a porcine model. Crit Care Med 35:207–213. doi:10.1097/01.CCM.0000249824.48222.B7
45. Umgelter A, Reindl W, Franzen M et al (2009) Renal resistive index and renal function before and after paracentesis in patients with hepatorenal syndrome and tense ascites. Intensive Care Med 35:152–156. doi:10.1007/s00134-008-1253-y
46. Ikee R, Kobayashi S, Hemmi N et al (2005) Correlation between the resistive index by Doppler ultrasound and kidney function and histology. Am J Kidney Dis Off J Natl Kidney Found 46:603–609. doi:10.1053/j.ajkd.2005.06.006
47. Florczak E, Januszewicz M, Januszewicz A et al (2009) Relationship between renal resistive index and early target organ damage in patients with never-treated essential hypertension. Blood Press 18:55–61. doi:10.1080/08037050902864078
48. Pontremoli R, Viazzi F, Martinoli C et al (1999) Increased renal resistive index in patients with essential hypertension: a marker of target organ damage. Nephrol Dial Transpl Off Publ Eur Dial Transpl Assoc – Eur Ren Assoc 14:360–365
49. Ratto E, Leoncini G, Viazzi F et al (2006) Ambulatory arterial stiffness index and renal abnormalities in primary hypertension. J Hypertens 24:2033–2038. doi:10.1097/01.hjh.0000244953.62362.41
50. Doi Y, Iwashima Y, Yoshihara F et al (2012) Association of renal resistive index with target organ damage in essential hypertension. Am J Hypertens 25:1292–1298. doi:10.1038/ajh.2012.113
51. Hashimoto J, Ito S (2011) Central pulse pressure and aortic stiffness determine renal hemodynamics: pathophysiological implication for microalbuminuria in hypertension. Hypertension 58:839–846. doi:10.1161/HYPERTENSIONAHA.111.177469
52. Kawai T, Kamide K, Onishi M et al (2011) Usefulness of the resistive index in renal Doppler ultrasonography as an indicator of vascular damage in patients with risks of atherosclerosis. Nephrol Dial Transpl Off Publ Eur Dial Transpl Assoc – Eur Ren Assoc 26:3256–3262. doi:10.1093/ndt/gfr054
53. Raff U, Schmidt BMW, Schwab J et al (2010) Renal resistive index in addition to low-grade albuminuria complements screening for target organ damage in therapy-resistant hypertension. J Hypertens 28:608–614. doi:10.1097/HJH.0b013e32833487b8
54. Doi Y, Iwashima Y, Yoshihara F et al (2012) Renal resistive index and cardiovascular and renal outcomes in essential hypertension. Hypertension 60:770–777. doi:10.1161/HYPERTENSIONAHA.112.196717
55. Pearce JD, Craven TE, Edwards MS et al (2010) Associations between renal duplex parameters and adverse cardiovascular events in the elderly: a prospective cohort study. Am J Kidney Dis Off J Natl Kidney Found 55:281–290. doi:10.1053/j.ajkd.2009.10.044
56. Leoncini G, Martinoli C, Viazzi F et al (2002) Changes in renal resistive index and urinary albumin excretion in hypertensive patients under long-term treatment with lisinopril or nifedipine GITS. Nephron 90:169–173
57. Mahfoud F, Cremers B, Janker J et al (2012) Renal hemodynamics and renal function after catheter-based renal sympathetic denervation in patients with resistant hypertension. Hypertension 60:419–424. doi:10.1161/HYPERTENSIONAHA.112.193870

58. Bruno RM, Daghini E, Versari D et al (2014) Predictive role of renal resistive index for clinical outcome after revascularization in hypertensive patients with atherosclerotic renal artery stenosis: a monocentric observational study. Cardiovasc Ultrasound 12:9. doi:10.1186/1476-7120-12-9

59. Platt JF, Rubin JM, Ellis JH (1989) Distinction between obstructive and nonobstructive pyelocaliectasis with duplex Doppler sonography. AJR Am J Roentgenol 153:997–1000

60. Platt JF, Ellis JH, Rubin JM et al (1990) Intrarenal arterial Doppler sonography in patients with nonobstructive renal disease: correlation of resistive index with biopsy findings. AJR Am J Roentgenol 154:1223–1227

61. Mostbeck GH, Kain R, Mallek R et al (1991) Duplex Doppler sonography in renal parenchymal disease. Histopathologic correlation. J Ultrasound Med Off J Am Inst Ultrasound Med 10:189–194

62. Aikimbaev KS, Canataroğlu A, Ozbek S, Usal A (2001) Renal vascular resistance in progressive systemic sclerosis: evaluation with duplex Doppler ultrasound. Angiology 52:697–701

63. Platt JF, Rubin JM, Ellis JH (1997) Lupus nephritis: predictive value of conventional and Doppler US and comparison with serologic and biopsy parameters. Radiology 203:82–86

64. Sari A, Dinc H, Zibandeh A et al (1999) Value of resistive index in patients with clinical diabetic nephropathy. Invest Radiol 34:718–721

65. Aghel A, Shrestha K, Mullens W et al (2010) Serum neutrophil gelatinase-associated lipocalin (NGAL) in predicting worsening renal function in acute decompensated heart failure. J Card Fail 16:49–54. doi:10.1016/j.cardfail.2009.07.003

66. Łebkowska U, Malyszko J, Łebkowski W et al (2007) The predictive value of arterial renal blood flow parameters in renal graft survival. Transplant Proc 39:2727–2729. doi:10.1016/j.transproceed.2007.08.043

67. Zahedi K, Wang Z, Barone S et al (2004) Identification of stathmin as a novel marker of cell proliferation in the recovery phase of acute ischemic renal failure. Am J Physiol Cell Physiol 286:C1203–C1211. doi:10.1152/ajpcell.00432.2003

68. Bossard G, Bourgoin P, Corbeau JJ et al (2011) Early detection of postoperative acute kidney injury by Doppler renal resistive index in cardiac surgery with cardiopulmonary bypass. Br J Anaesth 107:891–898. doi:10.1093/bja/aer289

69. Platt JF, Rubin JM, Ellis JH (1991) Acute renal failure: possible role of duplex Doppler US in distinction between acute prerenal failure and acute tubular necrosis. Radiology 179:419–423

70. Izumi M, Sugiura T, Nakamura H et al (2000) Differential diagnosis of prerenal azotemia from acute tubular necrosis and prediction of recovery by Doppler ultrasound. Am J Kidney Dis Off J Natl Kidney Found 35:713–719

71. Schnell D, Deruddre S, Harrois A et al (2012) Renal resistive index better predicts the occurrence of acute kidney injury than cystatin C. Shock (Augusta, Ga) 38:592–597. doi:10.1097/SHK.0b013e318271a39c

72. Dewitte A, Coquin J, Meyssignac B et al (2012) Doppler resistive index to reflect regulation of renal vascular tone during sepsis and acute kidney injury. Crit Care Lond Engl 16:R165. doi:10.1186/cc11517

Retinal Circulation in Arterial Disease

Christian Ott and Roland E. Schmieder

Hypertension has profound effect on the structure and function of the eye. In this chapter, we will focus on hypertensive retinopathy. Only for the sake of completeness, it should be mentioned that hypertension-related changes also include hypertensive optic neuropathy and hypertensive choroidopathy. Moreover, there are ocular diseases where hypertension is a potential risk factor, e.g., age-related macular degeneration and glaucoma. Most importantly, hypertension causes structural and functional vascular changes. We elaborate on the current knowledge of these processes, including innovative findings related to new applied technologies.

28.1 Vascular Remodeling

Since the pathophysiological concept of vascular remodeling was in detail described in Chap. 5, only few words will be mentioned. Remodeling can be of two types – eutrophic and hypertrophic, but both types result in an increase in the media-to-lumen ratio of small arterioles. In eutrophic remodeling, both the outer and the lumen diameter are reduced, but the media cross-sectional area is not increased because the increase in the wall thickness-to-lumen diameter ratio is caused by a rearrangement of the smooth muscle cells around a narrowed lumen [1]. In contrast, in hypertrophic remodeling, an enhanced growth response resulting in an increased media cross-sectional area was documented. Eutrophic remodeling predominates in patients with essential hypertension, and hypertrophic remodeling was found in patients with severe and long-standing hypertension.

C. Ott • R.E. Schmieder (✉)
Department of Nephrology and Hypertension, Friedrich-Alexander University
Erlangen-Nürnberg (FAU), Ulmenweg 18, Erlangen 91054, Germany
e-mail: christian.ott@uk-erlangen.de; roland.schmieder@uk-erlangen.de

© Springer International Publishing Switzerland 2015
A. Berbari, G. Mancia (eds.), *Arterial Disorders:*
Definition, Clinical Manifestations, Mechanisms and Therapeutic Approaches,
DOI 10.1007/978-3-319-14556-3_28

Table 28.1 Traditional Keith-Wagener-Barker classification and simplified (Wong-Mitchell) classification

Keith-Wagener-Barker classification		Simplified (Wong-Mitchell) classification	
Grade	Features	Grade	Features
1	Mild generalized retinal arteriolar narrowing	None	No detectable signs
2	Definite focal narrowing and arteriovenous nipping	Mild	Generalized arteriolar narrowing, focal arteriolar narrowing, arteriovenous nicking, opacity ("copper wiring") of arteriolar wall or a combination of these signs
3	Signs of grade 2 retinopathy plus retinal hemorrhages, exudates, and cotton wool spots	Moderate	Retinal hemorrhages (blot, dot, or flame-shaped), microaneurysm, cotton wool spot, hard exudates, or a combination of these signs
4	Severe grade 3 retinopathy plus papilledema	Malignant	Signs of moderate retinopathy plus swelling of the optic disk

The importance of vascular remodeling is based on a finding that it is one of the early (or even the earliest) processes that occurs in response to increased blood pressure (BP) and leads to hypertensive end-organ damage [2], but also that effective antihypertensive treatment is capable to reverse these vascular adaptive processes [3].

The exceptional position of retinal vasculature is known for a long time. Already in 1939, Keith et al. has stated "because the arterioles are small and are difficult to visualize in the peripheral organs, for example, in the skin, mucous membranes, and voluntary muscle, the retina, as seen through the ophthalmoscope, offers a unique opportunity for observing these small vessels from time to time. Therefore, we think that certain visible changes of the retinal arterioles have been of exceptional value in affording a clearer clinical conception of altered arteriolar function throughout the body." [4]. Based on the pioneering work of Keith, Wagener and Barker, their four-group grading system with increasing severity (Table 28.1) was widely applied in the last decades for the stratification of risk in hypertensive patients [4]. However, the clinical usefulness, and hence relevance to current clinical practice, has been questioned, because of poor reproducibility (e.g., 20–40 % interobserver variability) and weak association with other target organ damage (TOD) in grade I and II retinopathy, respectively [5].

Subsequently, a simplified three-grade classification system according to the severity of the retinal signs was proposed by Wong and Mitchell [6] (Table 28.1, Fig. 28.1), based on the evidence that certain hypertensive retinopathy signs (e.g., arteriolar narrowing or arteriovenous nicking) are independently associated with cardiovascular (CV) risk. In a small study comprising 50 normal and 50 hypertensive fundi, respectively, inter- and intraobserver reliabilities of the simplified three-grade classification system and the traditional four-grade classification system introduced by Keith, Wagener and Barker were reported to be comparable [7].

In the ESH/ESC guidelines, it is no longer recommended in general [8]. However, the retinal circulation offers the unique opportunity to visualize repeatedly the

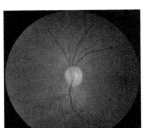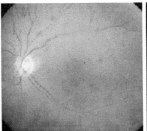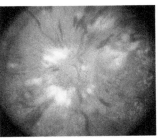

Fig. 28.1 Funduscopy (grade none, moderate, and malignant)

body's microcirculation directly, noninvasively, and safely in vivo. Hence, in the last decade, new and more specific approaches were introduced to overcome these shortcomings and to detect reliable early changes of the retinal circulation.

28.2 Retinal Photographs/Funduscopy (Static)

In the last two decades, several large-scale, population-based studies assessing retinal photographs were conducted, including patients with and without hypertension. In (most of) these studies, standardized protocols of retinal photographs (45° non-stereoscopic color retinal photograph centered between the optic disk and the macula) were used to define specific signs of retinopathy, but not regarding a prespecified grading system. In part, retinal abnormalities were described based solely on qualitative parameters, such as tortuosity, arteriovenous crossing, caliber, and optic disk, but due to limited clinical usefulness, these data will not be reviewed. As further improvement, the imaging software "Interactive Vessels Analysis" (IVAN) (University of Wisconsin, Madison, WI, USA) has been established. This system conducts semiautomated measurement of retinal arterioles and venules, and hence its ratio (A/V ratio); however, it is not able to evaluate the retinal vascular wall directly.

Based on this approach, these studies have analyzed the relationship between retinal vascular alterations and their association with BP, TOD, and CV events which are (in part) summarized in Table 28.2.

It has been repeatedly shown that retinal alterations are strongly correlated with past, current, and incident hypertension. In most of these large-scale studies, associations with directly assessed (generalized) arteriolar narrowing or a decreased A/V ratio, indirectly indicative of proposed arteriolar narrowing, and hypertension were reported (for details, see Table 28.2). In contrast, conflicting results according to retinal venules and hypertension were found. For example, in the Blue Mountains Eye Study, venular narrowing was associated with current hypertension [19]. In accordance, in the Rotterdam Study, venular narrowing was found to be predictive of current and incident blood pressure [28], but in the Multi-Ethnic Study of

Table 28.2 Large scale, population-based studies (in alphabetical order) assessing associations between retinal vascular caliber (based on retinal photography) and blood pressure, target organ damage, and cardiovascular risk (in chronological order)

Study	Country	Ethnicity	Year	Sample size	Retinal vascular	Finding
Atherosclerosis Risk In Communities Study (ARIC)	USA	White, black	1999	9,300	A/V ratio	Past and current blood pressure [9]
			2001	10,358	A/V ratio	Incident stroke [10]
			2002	9,648	A/V ratio	Incident CHD, acute MI (only in women) [11]
			2004	5,628	A/V ratio	Incident hypertension [12]
		(Only) black	2008	1,439	Generalized arteriolar narrowing	Left ventricular hypertrophy [13]
					A/V ratio	Left ventricular hypertrophy [13]
		White, black	2010	10,496	Generalized arteriolar narrowing	Incident lacunar stroke [14]
					Generalized venular widening	Incident lacunar stroke [14]
Beaver Dam Eye Study (BDES)	USA	White	2003	1,611	A/V ratio	CV mortality (43–74 years) [15]
			2003	4,926	Retinal arteriolar diameter	Current blood pressure [16]
					A/V ratio	Current blood pressure [16]
			2004	2,451	A/V ratio	Incident hypertension [17]
			2007	4,926	Smaller arterioles	CHD death [18]
					Larger venules	CHD death [18]

Study	Country	Ethnicity	Year	Sample size	Retinal vascular	Finding
Blue Mountains Eye Study (BMES)	Australia	White	2003	3,654	Arteriolar narrowing	Current blood pressure [19]
					Venular narrowing	Current blood pressure [19]
					A/V ratio	Current blood pressure [19]
			2004	2,335	Arteriolar narrowing	Past and current systolic/diastolic blood pressure [20]
					AV ratio	Past diastolic and current systolic/diastolic blood pressure [20]
			2004	1,319	Arteriolar narrowing	Incident severe hypertension [21]
					A/V ratio	Incident severe hypertension [21]
			2006	3,654	Venular caliber increase	CHD death (men and women, 49–75 years) [22]
					Arteriolar caliber decrease	CHD death (women, 49–75 years) [22]
					A/V ratio	CHD death (women, 49–75 years) [22]
Cardiovascular Health Study (CHS)	USA	White, black	2002	2,405	Arteriolar narrowing	Past and current blood pressure [23]
					A/V ratio	Current blood pressure [23]
			2006	1,992	Smaller arteriolar caliber	Incident CHD [24]
					Larger venular caliber	Incident CHD and stroke [24]
					A/V ratio	Incident CHD [24]
Multi-Ethnic Study of Atherosclerosis (MESA)	USA	White, Hispanics, Black, Chinese	2006	5,979	Smaller arteriolar caliber	Current blood pressure [25]
			2009	2,583	Narrower arteriolar diameter	Incident hypertension [26]
					Wider venular diameter	Incident hypertension [26]
			2011	4,594	Arteriolar narrowing	Incident CKD stage 3 (only whites) [27]

(continued)

Table 28.2 (continued)

Study	Country	Ethnicity	Year	Sample size	Retinal vascular	Finding
Rotterdam Study	Netherlands	White	2004	5,674	Arteriolar diameter decrease	Current blood pressure [28]
					Venular diameter decrease	Current blood pressure [28]
					A/V ratio	Current blood pressure [28]
			2006	1,900	Arteriolar narrowing	Incident hypertension [29]
					Venular narrowing	Incident hypertension [29]
					A/V ratio	Incident hypertension [29]
			2006	5,540	Larger venular diameter	Incident stroke, cerebral infarction [30]
			2010	5,518	Larger venular caliber	Incident stroke, cerebral infarction, intracerebral hemorrhage [31]
Singapore Malay Eye Study (SiMES)	Singapore	Malay	2008	3,019	Smaller arteriolar caliber	Current blood pressure [32]
			2009	2,581	Arteriolar narrowing	Prevalent CKD, micro-/macroalbuminuria [33]
Singapore Prospective Study Program (SP2)	Singapore	Chinese, Malay, Indian	2009	3,749	Arteriolar caliber decrease	Current blood pressure [34]
					Venular caliber increase	Current blood pressure [34]
					A/V ratio	Current blood pressure [34]
			2009	3,602	Arteriolar caliber decrease	Prevalent CKD [35]
Sydney Childhood Eye Study	Australia	White, Chinese, and others	2007	1,572	Arteriolar narrowing	Current blood pressure [36]

Atherosclerosis, venular widening was associated with incident hypertension [26]. While arteriolar narrowing can easily be harmonized with hypertension, it may be more difficult to explain why wider retinal venular caliber is associated with development of hypertension. A recent meta-analysis, comprising 10,229 patients without prevalent hypertension, diabetes, or CV disease, proposed that 2,599 patients developed new-onset hypertension during follow-up of 2.9–10 years. Both arteriolar narrowing (OR per 20 µm difference 1.29, 95 % CI 1.20–1.39) and venular widening (OR per 20 µm difference 1.14, 95 % CI 1.06–1.23) were independently associated with incident hypertension [37].

Importantly, in a population-based cohort comprising 1,572 children aged 6–8 years, each 10 mmHg increase of systolic BP was associated with arteriolar narrowing by 2.08 µm (95 % CI: 1.38–2.79, $p < 0.0001$), indicative that effects of elevated BP manifest early in life [36].

Regarding TOD data are even more limited. In 1,439 middle-aged African-Americans participants of the Atherosclerosis Risk in Communities Study A/V ratio was associated with measures of left ventricular hypertrophy, which was partly explained by additional CV risk factors and hypertension [13]. In contrast, in an Italian study comprising 386 untreated and treated hypertensive patients, no intergroup differences in A/V ratio was found between presence and absence of acknowledged TOD like left ventricular hypertrophy, carotid intima-media thickness, or microalbuminuria, hence indicating limited value of A/V ratio for identifying patients with high CV risk based on cardiac and extracardiac TOD [38].

There is also an ambiguous picture of arteriolar and venular diameter and different components of CV events. Regarding incident stroke, associations of both arteriolar narrowing and venular widening were reported in some studies, whereas in the Rotterdam Study, only an association of venular widening was found, but not for arteriolar narrowing [30]. Moreover, in the latter Rotterdam Study, venular widening was also associated with intracerebral hemorrhage [31]. These conflicting results are supported based on meta-analyses performed mainly by the META-EYE study group and published in the last years [18, 39].

These conflicting results of the individual components (with respect to arteriolar and venular diameter) have also to be taken into account, when interpreting reported findings about A/V ratio. An altered A/V ratio can be due to single and concurrent changes and their individual amount, and vice versa nonfindings can be seen, for example, by diverging changes.

28.3 Global Geometrical and Branching Parameters (Retinal Vascular Network)

The vasculature is a branching system, and alterations from optimal architecture are proposed to impair function and hence increased vascular damage. Thus, interest has gained on further developments in computer-assisted programs enabling the assessment of several quantitative parameters of retinal vascular network. Using these newly developed retinal vascular parameters, analysis of the Singapore Malay

Eye Study has shown that a combination of smaller retinal vascular fractal dimensions (D_f), proposed to be a global measure of the geometric complexity, and evidence of straighter retinal arterioles indicate poor BP control in treated hypertensive patients [40]. Therefore, retinal alterations can be assumed as pathophysiological markers not only for the severity of hypertension, but also on the effectiveness of drug therapy in hypertension.

Utilizing data from the multiethnic Singapore Prospective Study Program (SP2), the same group has shown that retinal D_f was inversely correlated with BP level in all three ethnic groups. Notably, this was the case in patients with uncontrolled as well as untreated hypertension, but not in patients with controlled hypertension [41].

However, by applying again and again several new parameters, and analyzing these new parameters in the same studies, it is still missing the differentiation which is the most promising and reliable parameter to detect early retinal involvement in the clinical course of hypertension.

28.4   Scanning Laser Doppler Flowmetry (Dynamic)

Funduscopic photographs have the limitation that arteriolar and venular alterations cannot be quantified separately and the vascular wall precisely visualized. Moreover, the term remodeling if assessed in vivo takes two aspects into account, which were interrelated and indistinguishable, namely, morphological changes (i.e., rearrangement of vascular smooth muscle cells) as well as changes of the vascular tone (i.e., endothelial function). To overcome these limitations, one promising approach introduced by our study group about 10 years ago allows the dynamic assessment of both functional and structural parameters by using scanning laser Doppler flowmetry (SLDF) [42]. In brief, SLDF is performed in the juxtapapillary area of the right eye, 2–3 mm temporal superior of the optic nerve at 670 nm (Heidelberg Retina Flowmeter, Heidelberg Engineering, Germany). An arteriole (80–140 μm) of the superficial retinal layer in a retinal sample of $2.56 \times 0.64 \times 0.30$ nm is scanned within 2 s (one systolic and one diastolic phase) and measured every 10 μm of this specific length of the arteriole. The confocal technique of the device ensures that only capillary flow of the superficial layer of 300 μm is measured. The outer arteriole diameter (AD) is measured by reflection images, and the lumen diameter (LD) is measured by perfusion images. Wall-to-lumen ratio (WLR) is calculated using the formula (AD – LD)/LD (Fig. 28.2). Analyses are performed offline with automatic full-field perfusion imaging analysis (AFFPIA) (SLDF Version 4.0 by Welzenbach with improved resolution) [43].

It is noteworthy to mention that assessing both retinal function and structure by SLDF does not require applying any mydriatic drug, which is not only important from the scientific point of view – local application of tropicamide profoundly affects the retinal perfusion [44], but also for patient management perspective (i.e., no constriction of daily routine).

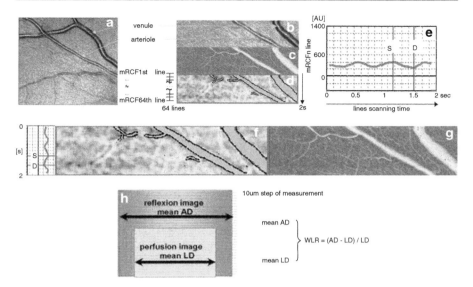

Fig. 28.2 Scanning laser Doppler flowmetry (SLDF). (**a**) Differentiation between retinal arteriole and venule (SLDF live image before measurement). (**b**) Scanned area – reflection image. (**c**) Scanned area – perfusion image. (**d**) Scanned area – corrected and analyzed flow image. (**e**) Pulse curve run as mean retinal capillary flow (*RCF*) and time plot.(**f**) Localization of systolic and diastolic RCF on the image **d**. (**g**) Localization of systolic and diastolic RCF on the image **c**. (**h**) Calculation of wall-to-lumen ratio (*WLR*)

28.5   Retinal Capillary Flow

Due to its common origin from the internal carotid artery, the retinal microcirculation is morphologically and functionally related to the cerebral circulation [45].

Further dynamic information (e.g., basal nitric oxide [NO] activity) of the retinal capillaries can be assessed by measuring changes of retinal capillary flow (RCF) due to nonpharmacological and pharmacological tools. Flicker light increases at least in part via a NO-dependent mechanism and represents a nonpharmacological tool to investigate vasodilatory capacity of retinal capillaries. Notably, flicker light exposure has no effects on systemic BP, thereby minimizing potential systemic hemodynamic influences on RCF. Moreover, basal NO activity is assessed by administration of the NO synthase inhibitor N^G-monomethyl-L-arginine (L-NMMA). Findings in normo- and hypertensive patients are summarized in Table 28.3.

In young hypertensive patients, baseline RCF was similar to normotensive controls. However, assessment of basal NO activity (L-NMMA) revealed an impaired endothelial function in young hypertensive patients, which was improved after treatment with an ARB [42], whereas in elderly hypertensive men treatment with an ARB did not improve RCF at least after short-term treatment of 8 days [46]. Notably, even in

Table 28.3 Studies of our research group, analyzing hypertensive patients and/or patients with cardiovascular event, using scanning laser Doppler flowmetry to assess early vascular changes (in chronological order)

Reference	Patients	Retinal endothelial function	Retinal arteriolar structure
Delles et al. [42]	19 hypertensive men 19 normotensive men	Endothelial function[a] is impaired in essential hypertension and is improved after ARB treatment	
Oehmer et al. [46]	20 (elderly) hypertensive men	Short-term treatment (8 days) with an ARB did not improve retinal endothelial function[a] in elderly hypertensive men	
Harazny et al. [47] (Study 1)	182 normotensive men 117 hypertensive men		WLR is correlated with age in normo- and hypertensive men
Harazny et al. [47] (Study 2)	74 normotensive men 47 hypertensive men 18 men with cerebrovascular event		WLR is higher in subjects with cerebrovascular event than in normo- and hypertensive men Treated patients with poor BP control have higher WLR than patients with good BP control (<140/90 mmHg)
Ritt et al. [48]	21 hypertensive men 19 normotensive men		Systolic and diastolic BP were positively related with WLR, independent from other various cardiovascular risk factors WLR is higher in hypertensive men, but WCSA did not differ between the groups (suggesting eutrophic remodeling)
Baleanu [49]	16 normotensives 83 hypertensives 23 patients with cerebrovascular event		*Arteriovenous ratio were similar between the three groups* Both WLR and WCSA are higher in patients with cerebrovascular event than in normo- and hypertensives *Arteriovenous ratio was not correlated with WLR*

Reference	Patients	Retinal endothelial function	Retinal arteriolar structure
Ritt et al. [50]	89 normotensive men 52 hypertensive men	In normotensive men, vasodilatory capacity[b] was greater in patients above compared to below median RCF In hypertensive men, this was not evident	In hypertensive men, vasodilatory capacity[b] was negatively related to WLR In normotensive men, this was not evident
Raff et al. [51]	40 patients with TRH		WLR, WT, and WCSA were strongly associated with 24-h urinary sodium excretion
Ritt et al. [52]	96 normotensive men 50 hypertensive men	Vasodilatory capacity[b] was higher in normotensive compared to hypertensive patients	
Ott et al. [53]	135 patients with wide BP range		Central PP was an independent determinant of WLR
Harazny et al. [54]	20 hypertensives 19 patients with TRH	Pulsed RCF, but not mean RCF, was higher in patients with TRH compared to hypertensive patients	WT remained unchanged between systole and diastole in patients with TRH, whereas WT changed dynamically in hypertensive patients
Ott et al. [55]	51 patients with TRH	Pulsed RCF, but not mean RCF was reduced by RDN Vasodilatory capacity[b] was increased after RDN	

[a]Change of RCF to L-NMMA infusion

[b]Change in RCF to flicker-light exposure

hypercholesterolemic patients, treatment with an ARB led to a marked BP reduction, which was associated with an improved vasodilatory capacity (flicker light) [56]. In accordance, it was previously shown that vasodilatory capacity (flicker light) was lower in untreated hypertensive patients compared to normotensive controls. Systolic BP was inversely related to the percent increase of RCF due to flicker light exposure, independent of other CV risk factors [52].

Recently, we have shown that also individual pulsatile pattern of RCF (and structural parameters, see below) of retinal arterioles in systole and diastole can be reliably assessed. By doing so, we could show that with advanced stage of hypertensive disease, namely, patients with treatment-resistant hypertension (TRH), pulsed RCF (difference in RCF between systole and diastole) is exaggerated compared to patients with hypertension stages 1–2 [54].

Moreover, further data of our group reveal that BP and hence pulse pressure (PP) changes have an impact on pulsed RCF. In patients with TRH, we observed a decrease of systolic and pulsed RCF 6 and 12 months after renal denervation (RDN), in parallel to decreases of BP and heart rate. The reduction of pulsed RCF after RDN transfers into less shear stress on the vascular wall and, thereby, suggests an improvement of retinal (and potentially cerebral) microcirculation [55].

The importance of these findings is supported by prospective studies showing that, among others, carotid PP and pulsatility index were each associated with an increased risk for silent subcortical infarcts and with lower memory scores [57]. These data suggest that excessive flow pulsatility damages the microcirculation, clinically detectable by impaired cognitive function. Moreover, in a longitudinal study, PP significantly predicted the incidence of stroke (HR 1.33, 95 % CI 1.16–1.51 for each 10 mmHg of PP), which still remained borderline significant ($p = 0.1$) after adjustment for classical CV risk factors [58].

28.6   Structural Parameters of Retinal Arterioles

By using SLDF, also structural parameters of retinal arterioles can be assessed with high reliability [43].

We could show that WLR of retinal arterioles is positively related with systolic and diastolic BP, independent of various other CV risk factors. WLR was higher in never-treated hypertensive patients compared to normotensive controls [48]. Regarding blood pressure control, we found that in patients with poor BP control, WLR is higher than in controlled hypertensive patients [47]. These data are similar to published findings in large-scale population-based studies using retinal funduscopy (see above).

However, in a small cross-sectional study, A/V ratio was not able to discriminate between patients with cerebral event (transient ischemic attack or lacunar cerebral infarct) and normotensive as well as hypertensive patients. In contrast, WLR was significantly higher and could therefore discriminate between patients with cerebrovascular event compared to both normotensive controls and hypertensive patients without cerebrovascular event [49].

In a study comprising patients with wide range of BP values, it was shown that central PP is a strong and independent predictor of WLR (vascular remodeling) beyond "classical" CV risk factors and additional factors that are proposed to have an impact on vascular structure [53]. Such a relationship indicates coupling and intensive cross talk between the micro- and macrovascular changes due to hypertension.

Similar to our RCF analysis, also structural parameters can be assessed according to different heart phases (systole and diastole). In patients with TRH, a stiffer wall of retinal arterioles can be assumed, since wall thickness (WT) remained unchanged between systole and diastole, whereas in patients with hypertension grade 1–2, WT changed dynamically between systole and diastole [54].

Although no data from prospective studies regarding SLDF-assessed WLR and CV events are yet available, indirect, but strong, evidence of the validity for measuring WLR was demonstrated by Rizzoni et al. WLR assessed by SLDF (retinal arterioles in vivo) and media-to-lumen ratio measured with the myograph ex vivo (subcutaneous small arteries taken from a biopsy) showed a close correlation in hypertensive patients, suggesting that SLDF may provide similar information about microcirculation alterations compared to acknowledged prognostic measurement of subcutaneous small arteries, which represent the "gold standard" and prognostically relevant approach to the evaluation of small artery morphology in humans [59]. The absolute values differ due to the different methodologies, e.g., the analysis with myograph takes place ex vivo whereas the SLDF measures the parameters in vivo. The SLDF may underestimate the true internal diameter, since flow diameter does not include any endothelial plasma layer [49].

Nowadays, several other approaches (e.g., adaptive optics and optical coherence tomography) as well as SLDF with another software (e.g., data from Rizzoni et al.) focused on the assessment of WLR of retinal arterioles. It is notable to respect that the methodology of vascular measurements differs between the individual techniques. Therefore, a simple transfer of research findings into clinical practice may not be possible without further validation (see below). An overview of the recent available data is given in Table 28.4.

28.7   Adaptive Optics

Nowadays, available adaptive optics-based fundus cameras are able to assess semi-automatically focal vascular changes (e.g., focal arteriolar narrowing). Moreover, arteriolar morphometry can be applied with a resolution up to near two micrometers, thereby visualizing (among others) vascular wall of retinal arterioles. The feasibility and reproducibility of retinal arterioles imaging was demonstrated in untreated hypertensive patients [62]. Following these pilot investigations, the same authors could show that adaptive optics-based assessment of WLR was positively correlated with mean BP and age which accounted for 43 % of variability of WLR [60]. Although the results on WLR measurements by adaptive optics are close to those reported by SLDF (Table 28.4), it has to be taken into account that no

Table 28.4 Comparison of retinal structural parameters assessed with scanning laser Doppler flowmetry (SLDF), adaptive optics, and optical coherence tomography (OCT)

	SLDF (Ritt et al. [48])		SLDF (Rizzoni et al. [59])		Adaptive optics (Koch et al. [60])		OCT (Muraoka et al. [61])	
	Normotensive (n=29)	Hypertensive (n=21)	Normotensive (n=16)	Hypertensive (n=24)	Normotensive (n=30)	Hypertensive (n=19)	Normotensive (n=83)	Hypertensive (n=103)
Age (years)	36.7±5.9	39.1±5.4	59.3±14	57.7±15	42.3±15	48±11	68.5±7.8	69.1±8.1
BMI (kg/m²)	31.5±2.3	33.1±4.4	25.6±4.4	27.4±5.1	23.8±4.5	26.4±4		
Systolic BP (mmHg)	129±6.9	145±6.8	125±17	139±17	118±13	154±14		
Diastolic BP (mmHg)	78±7.6	88±8.3	71±12	89±10	74±9.5	96±10		
WLR (-)	0.28±0.1	0.36±0.1	0.26±0.1	0.37±0.1	0.29±0.1	0.36±0.1	0.41[b] (mean)	0.41[b] (mean)
Outer (vessel) diameter (μm)	109±15	111±9.6	93.6±19	81.7±20	107[a] (mean)	100[a] (mean)	123±9.3	125±11
Inner (lumen) diameter (μm)	85.3±11	81.8±7.8	74.4±16	59.6±13	83.5±11	74±13	87.3±8.3	88.5±11

[a]Calculated on the published mean values (lumen diameter + parietal thickness)

[b]Calculated on the published mean values ([outer diameter – inner diameter]/inner diameter)

validation of the method in respect to other available techniques is yet provided. Adaptive optics needs to be directly compared with SLDF measurement or even better, with the media-to-lumen ratio of subcutaneous small resistance arteries assessed by the myographic approach. Adaptive optics examinations may be possible without mydriasis in most but not all cases. Only limited data ($n = 9$) are so far published investigating vascular morphometry before and after locally applied tropicamide. Mean vascular diameter increased only slightly (about 1 %), but data on individual diameters or wall properties are missing [60]. Hence, the effect of locally administered tropicamide cannot be fully excluded.

The major limitation of adaptive optics is that in contrast to SLDF, it cannot measure RCF.

28.8 Optical Coherence Tomography

The optical coherence tomography (OCT) allows the assessment of retinal circulation in an enhanced resolution within an acceptable time period. However, data about the retinal circulation in arterial hypertension are limited. In an analysis of patients (aged over 50 years), it was shown that mean arteriolar outer and inner diameter did not differ between patients with hypertension ($n = 103$, defined by use of antihypertensive medication or physician's diagnosis) and without hypertension ($n = 83$), but mean arterial wall thickness was significantly larger [61]. This is in line with previous findings (unchanged outer and lumen diameter, but higher wall thickness of retinal arterioles) using SLDF in never-treated hypertensive patients compared to controls [48]. However, OCT-measured WLR was higher than previosuly measured with SLDF, perhaps likely attributable to age differences [48], but no direct comparison has so far been made.

Additional features, which can be assessed using OCT, like retinal nerve fiber layer and its importance in hypertension is not determined yet.

28.9 Perspective

Exciting new technologies emerged and offered the opportunities to directly visualize vascular remodeling of small retinal arterioles. The clinical perspective is that the physician may be enabled to diagnose early vascular remodeling to hypertension and tailor the antihypertensive strategy for individual patients. The findings may go beyond the retinal arterioles since the changes in the retinal circulation mirror these in cerebrovascular circulation, one of the major targets of hypertensive disease.

References

1. Schiffrin EL (2004) Remodeling of resistance arteries in essential hypertension and effects of antihypertensive treatment. Am J Hypertens 17:1192–1200

2. Mulvany MJ (2008) Small artery remodelling in hypertension: causes, consequences and therapeutic implications. Med Biol Eng Comput 46:461–467
3. Feihl F, Liaudet L, Levy BI, Waeber B (2008) Hypertension and microvascular remodelling. Cardiovasc Res 78:274–285
4. Keith NM, Wagener HP, Barker NW (1939) Some different types of essential hypertension: their course and prognosis. Am J Med Sci 197:332–343
5. Dimmitt SB, West JN, Eames SM et al (1989) Usefulness of ophthalmoscopy in mild to moderate hypertension. Lancet 1:1103–1106
6. Wong TY, Mitchell P (2004) Hypertensive retinopathy. N Engl J Med 351:2310–2317
7. Downie LE, Hodgson LA, Dsylva C et al (2013) Hypertensive retinopathy: comparing the Keith-Wagener-Barker to a simplified classification. J Hypertens 31:960–965
8. Mancia G, Fagard R, Narkiewicz K et al.; Task Force Members (2013) 2013 ESH/ESC guidelines for the management of arterial hypertension: the task force for the management of arterial hypertension of the European Society of Hypertension (ESH) and of the European Society of Cardiology (ESC). J Hypertens 31:1281–1357
9. Sharrett AR, Hubbard LD, Cooper LS et al (1999) Retinal arteriolar diameters and elevated blood pressure: the Atherosclerosis Risk in Communities Study. Am J Epidemiol 150:263–270
10. Wong TY, Klein R, Couper DJ et al (2001) Retinal microvascular abnormalities and incident stroke: the Atherosclerosis Risk in Communities Study. Lancet 358:1134–1140
11. Wong TY, Klein R, Sharrett AR et al (2002) Retinal arteriolar narrowing and risk of coronary heart disease in men and women. The Atherosclerosis Risk in Communities Study. JAMA 287:1153–1159
12. Wong TY, Klein R, Sharrett AR et al.; Atherosclerosis Risk in Communities Study (2004) Retinal arteriolar diameter and risk for hypertension. Ann of Intern Med 140:248–255
13. Tikellis G, Arnett DK, Skelton TN et al (2008) Retinal arteriolar narrowing and left ventricular hypertrophy in African Americans. The Atherosclerosis Risk In Communities (ARIC) Study. Am J Hypertens 21:352–359
14. Yatsuya H, Folsom AR, Wong TY, Investigators AS et al (2010) Retinal microvascular abnormalities and risk of lacunar stroke: Atherosclerosis Risk in Communities Study. Stroke 41:1349–1355
15. Wong TY, Klein R, Nieto FJ et al (2003) Retinal microvascular abnormalities and 10-year cardiovascular mortality: a population-based case-control study. Ophthalmology 110:933–940
16. Wong TY, Klein R, Klein BE et al (2003) Retinal vessel diameters and their associations with age and blood pressure. Invest Ophthalmol Vis Sci 44:4644–4650
17. Wong TY, Shankar A, Klein R et al (2004) Prospective cohort study of retinal vessel diameters and risk of hypertension. BMJ 329:79
18. Wang JJ, Liew G, Klein R et al (2007) Retinal vessel diameter and cardiovascular mortality: pooled data analysis from two older populations. Eur Heart J 28:1984–1992
19. Leung H, Wang JJ, Rochtchina E et al (2003) Relationships between age, blood pressure, and retinal vessel diameters in an older population. Invest Ophthalmol Vis Sci 44:2900–2904
20. Leung H, Wang JJ, Rochtchina E et al (2004) Impact of current and past blood pressure on retinal arteriolar diameter in an older population. J Hypertens 22:1543–1549
21. Smith W, Wang JJ, Wong TY et al (2004) Retinal arteriolar narrowing is associated with 5-year incident severe hypertension: the Blue Mountains Eye Study. Hypertension 44:442–447
22. Wang JJ, Liew G, Wong TY et al (2006) Retinal vascular calibre and the risk of coronary heart disease-related death. Heart 92:1583–1587
23. Wong TY, Hubbard LD, Klein R et al (2002) Retinal microvascular abnormalities and blood pressure in older people: the cardiovascular health study. Br J Ophthalmol 86:1007–1013
24. Wong TY, Kamineni A, Klein R et al (2006) Quantitative retinal venular caliber and risk of cardiovascular disease in older persons: the cardiovascular health study. Arch Intern Med 166:2388–2394
25. Wong TY, Islam FM, Klein R et al (2006) Retinal vascular caliber, cardiovascular risk factors, and inflammation: the multi-ethnic study of atherosclerosis (mesa). Invest Ophthalmol Vis Sci 47:2341–2350

26. Kawasaki R, Cheung N, Wang JJ et al (2009) Retinal vessel diameters and risk of hypertension: the multiethnic study of atherosclerosis. J Hypertens 27:2386–2393
27. Yau JW, Xie J, Kawasaki R et al (2011) Retinal arteriolar narrowing and subsequent development of CKD stage 3: the multi-ethnic study of atherosclerosis (MESA). Am J Kidney Dis 58:39–46
28. Ikram MK, de Jong FJ, Vingerling JR et al (2004) Are retinal arteriolar or venular diameters associated with markers for cardiovascular disorders? The Rotterdam Study. Invest Ophthalmol Vis Sci 45:2129–2134
29. Ikram MK, Witteman JC, Vingerling JR et al (2006) Retinal vessel diameters and risk of hypertension: the Rotterdam Study. Hypertension 47:189–194
30. Ikram MK, de Jong FJ, Bos MJ et al (2006) Retinal vessel diameters and risk of stroke: the Rotterdam Study. Neurology 66:1339–1343
31. Wieberdink RG, Ikram MK, Koudstaal PJ et al (2010) Retinal vascular calibers and the risk of intracerebral hemorrhage and cerebral infarction: the Rotterdam Study. Stroke 41:2757–2761
32. Sun C, Liew G, Wang JJ et al (2008) Retinal vascular caliber, blood pressure, and cardiovascular risk factors in an Asian population: the Singapore Malay Eye Study. Invest Ophthalmol Vis Sci 49:1784–1790
33. Sabanayagam C, Shankar A, Koh D et al (2009) Retinal microvascular caliber and chronic kidney disease in an Asian population. Am J Epidemiol 169:625–632
34. Jeganathan VS, Sabanayagam C, Tai ES et al (2009) Effect of blood pressure on the retinal vasculature in a multi-ethnic Asian population. Hypertens Res 32:975–982
35. Sabanayagam C, Tai ES, Shankar A et al (2009) Retinal arteriolar narrowing increases the likelihood of chronic kidney disease in hypertension. J Hypertens 27:2209–2217
36. Mitchell P, Cheung N, de Haseth K et al (2007) Blood pressure and retinal arteriolar narrowing in children. Hypertension 49:1156–1162
37. Ding J, Wai KL, McGeechan K et al (2014) Retinal vascular caliber and the development of hypertension: a meta-analysis of individual participant data. J Hypertens 32:207–215
38. Masaidi M, Cuspidi C, Giudici V et al (2009) Is retinal arteriolar-venular ratio associated with cardiac and extracardiac organ damage in essential hypertension? J Hypertens 27:1277–1283
39. McGeechan K, Liew G, Macaskill P et al (2009) Meta-analysis: retinal vessel caliber and risk for coronary heart disease. Ann Int Med 151:404–413
40. Cheung CY, Tay WT, Mitchell P et al (2011) Quantitative and qualitative retinal microvascular characteristics and blood pressure. J Hypertens 29:1380–1391
41. Sng CC, Wong WL, Cheung CY et al (2013) Retinal vascular fractal and blood pressure in a multiethnic population. J Hypertens 31:2036–2042
42. Delles C, Michelson G, Harazny J et al (2004) Impaired endothelial function of the retinal vasculature in hypertensive patients. Stroke 35:1289–1293
43. Harazny JM, Raff U, Welzenbach J et al (2011) New software analyses increase the reliability of measurements of retinal arterioles morphology by scanning laser Doppler flowmetry in humans. J Hypertens 29:777–782
44. Harazny JM, Schmieder RE, Welzenbach J, Michelson G (2013) Local application of tropicamide 0.5% reduces retinal capillary blood flow. Blood Press 22:371–376
45. Patton N, Aslam T, Macgillivray T et al (2005) Retinal vascular image analysis as a potential screening tool for cerebrovascular disease: a rationale based on homology between cerebral and retinal microvasculatures. J Anat 206:319–348
46. Oehmer S, Harazny J, Delles C et al (2006) Valsartan and retinal endothelial function in elderly hypertensive patients. Blood Press 15:185–191
47. Harazny JM, Ritt M, Baleanu D et al (2007) Increased wall: lumen ratio of retinal arterioles in male patients with a history of a cerebrovascular event. Hypertension 50:623–629
48. Ritt M, Harazny JM, Ott C et al (2008) Analysis of retinal arteriolar structure in never-treated patients with essential hypertension. J Hypertens 26:1427–1434
49. Baleanu D, Ritt M, Harazny J et al (2009) Wall-to-lumen ratio of retinal arterioles and arteriole-to-venule ratio of retinal vessels in patients with cerebrovascular damage. Invest Ophthalmol Vis Sci 50:4351–4359

50. Ritt M, Harazny JM, Ott C et al (2012) Influence of blood flow on arteriolar wall-to-lumen ratio in the human retinal circulation in vivo. Microvasc Res 83:111–117
51. Raff U, Harazny JM, Titze SI et al (2012) Salt intake determines retinal arteriolar structure in treatment resistant hypertension independent of blood pressure. Atherosclerosis 222:235–240
52. Ritt M, Harazny JM, Ott C et al (2012) Impaired increase of retinal capillary blood flow to flicker light exposure in arterial hypertension. Hypertension 60:871–876
53. Ott C, Raff U, Harazny JM et al (2013) Central pulse pressure is an independent determinant of vascular remodeling in the retinal circulation. Hypertension 61:1340–1345
54. Harazny JM, Ott C, Raff U et al (2014) First experience in analysing pulsatile retinal capillary flow and arteriolar structural parameters measured noninvasively in hypertensive patients. J Hypertens 32:2246–2252
55. Schmieder RE, Ott C, Uder M et al (2014) Retinal microperfusion one year after renal artery denervation in treatment resistant hypertensive patients. J Hypertens 32 (Suppl 1): e69
56. Ott C, Schlaich MP, Harazny J et al (2008) Effects of angiotensin ii type 1-receptor blockade on retinal endothelial function. J Hypertens 26:516–522
57. Wohlfahrt P, Krajcoviechova A, Jozifova M et al (2014) Large artery stiffness and carotid flow pulsatility in stroke survivors. J Hypertens 32:1097–1103; discussion 1103
58. Laurent S, Katsahian S, Fassot C et al (2003) Aortic stiffness is an independent predictor of fatal stroke in essential hypertension. Stroke 34:1203–1206
59. Rizzoni D, Porteri E, Duse S et al (2012) Relationship between media-to-lumen ratio of subcutaneous small arteries and wall-to-lumen ratio of retinal arterioles evaluated noninvasively by scanning laser Doppler flowmetry. J Hypertens 30:1169–1175
60. Koch E, Rosenbaum D, Brolly A et al (2014) Morphometric analysis of small arteries in the human retina using adaptive optics imaging: relationship with blood pressure and focal vascular changes. J Hypertens 32:890–898
61. Muraoka Y, Tsujikawa A, Kumagai K et al (2013) Age- and hypertension-dependent changes in retinal vessel diameter and wall thickness: an optical coherence tomography study. Am J Ophthalmol 156:706–714
62. Rosenbaum D, Koch E, Girerd X et al (2013) Imaging of retinal arteries with adaptative optics, feasibility and reproducibility. Ann Cardiol Angeiol 62:184–188

Part VI
Therapeutic Options

Therapeutic Options: Lifestyle Measures and Pharmacological Approaches

29

Ian B. Wilkinson and Bronwen G. King

29.1 Introduction

Preventing cardiovascular disease by lifestyle and therapeutic intervention is a broad topic, which encompasses an enormous amount of published research. This chapter shall focus largely on the primary prevention of atherosclerosis and arteriosclerosis. Although frequently confused, these are in reality distinct disorders, differing in their underlying pathophysiology. As such preventative therapeutic strategies are likely to differ.

29.2 Atherosclerosis

The main risks factors for atherosclerotic disease have been firmly established by a wealth of research over the last 60 years. These include smoking, hypertension, hyperlipidaemia and diabetes mellitus, each of which can be addressed by both lifestyle and pharmacological interventions.

29.2.1 Lifestyle

Modification of the major lifestyle risk factors is potentially a very powerful form of intervention, which can benefit a substantial proportion of the population. However, there are significant challenges in implementation at an individual level,

I.B. Wilkinson, DM, FRCP (✉) • B.G. King
Division of Experimental Medicine and Immunotherapeutics, University of Cambridge,
Addenbrooke's Hospital, Cambridge CB2 2QQ, UK
e-mail: ibw20@cam.ac.uk

© Springer International Publishing Switzerland 2015
A. Berbari, G. Mancia (eds.), *Arterial Disorders:*
Definition, Clinical Manifestations, Mechanisms and Therapeutic Approaches,
DOI 10.1007/978-3-319-14556-3_29

and some interventions may be better addressed through government-led public health initiatives, e.g. forcing companies to reduce the amount of salt and trans fats added to food, increasing taxes and banning cigarette advertising. Recent research suggests that such measures can have a significant benefit to the population [1].

29.2.2 Smoking

Smoking is a well-established risk factor for atherosclerosis; it causes a number of vascular changes including endothelial dysfunction, which contribute to both the formation and acceleration of atheroma. There are many epidemiology cohort studies that link cigarette smoking to atherosclerosis and to cardiovascular diseases per se. Current cigarette smoking gives a ~50 % risk of atherosclerosis compared to a non-smoker; an even greater increase in risk of atherosclerosis is found in smokers who also suffered from diabetes and/or hypertension [2]. This is supported by a 50-year observational cohort study of British doctors finding greater mortality among smokers compared to non-smokers [3].

Intervention studies show that quitting reduces the chances of cardiovascular disease [4]. It can be said that a patient who has smoked for a long time may never fully decrease their risk to that of a non-smoker, and there is mixed evidence on how advantageous the benefits of quitting are [5]. Smokers commonly gain weight initially after smoking cessation; an increased BMI is a risk factor for cardiovascular disease itself. Despite this, ex-smokers perform better on an exercise stress test than current smokers, indicating that the positive health and fitness benefits of quitting smoking outweigh the negative health effects of an increased BMI [6].

In ex-smokers who have smoked for a long period of time, there is still a significant increased risk of mortality even after quitting compared to never smokers. For example, individuals who have smoked more than 20 years have a significant excess of cardiovascular deaths 10–29 years after quitting compared to individuals who smoked for less than 19 years [4]. Nevertheless, there is a fall in mortality risk from coronary heart disease in the first 19 years after quitting, but after this the risk is almost unchanged. On average, former cigarette smokers have a greater risk of cardiovascular disease than never smokers but a smaller risk than current smokers. Smoking, therefore, has a dose-dependent effect.

The progressive popularity of e-cigarettes raises the question of how safe smokeless tobacco actually is [7]. Unfortunately, there are relatively few studies on the matter, but a meta-analysis of the available data, including case control and cohort studies, concluded that there was an increased risk of cardiovascular disease, 40 % excess risk, in smokeless tobacco (e-cigarettes and chewing tobacco) users compared to non-smokers. In smokeless tobacco users there was less evidence of atherosclerotic plaques than in smokers but more than in non-smokers. There is also a lot of evidence to suggest that passive smoking can be almost as damaging as active smoking [8], but like smoking, this is dose dependent.

There are many measures that can help increase rates of quitting, including social and pharmacological measures. In a meta-analysis of randomised clinical trials, all three licensed quitting therapies, bupropion (an antidepressant), varenicline (a nicotine receptor partial agonist) and nicotine replacement, were effective [9]. Bupropion and varenicline do not increase cardiovascular disease, but nicotine replacement studies showed an elevated risk compared to the other two; relative risk is 2.29 for non-serious cardiovascular events, but for serious cardiovascular events, none of the methods increase the risk [10].

29.2.3 Alcohol

There is a paradox revolving around alcohol consumption. Alcohol has a linear relationship with blood pressure; the more alcohol consumed, the greater the person's blood pressure. However, alcohol consumption has a U-shaped relationship with cardiac deaths. So although alcohol raises blood pressure, mild to moderate drinking is seemingly protective against cardiovascular events.

The French paradox is a well-known phenomenon, in which the French, although not consuming perhaps the healthiest diet (high in saturated fats) and drinking a lot of red wine, have a much lower risk of cardiovascular disease. A lower cardiovascular risk is seen with moderate alcohol intake of all forms, but alcohols rich in polyphenols appear to have a particularly protective effect. In a meta-analysis of prospective cohort studies, it was found that the relative risk of drinkers of alcohol to non-drinkers for cardiovascular disease mortality was 0.75. The authors concluded that mild–moderate alcohol intake was associated with reduced cardiac death and stroke deaths [11].

Those who consumed between 2.5 and 14.9 g alcohol a day were protected against all cardiovascular events, but those who consumed more than 60 g/day were at a greater risk of stroke than non-drinkers. Alcohol consumption lowers the risk of ischemic stroke but slightly raises the risk of haemorrhagic strokes, giving an overall reduction in risk of stroke in those who drink moderately [11].

In some in vitro studies, the effects of gin and wine on LDL levels and oxidation were observed, and while both reduced oxidation, wine had the greater effect [12]. Red wine also reduces inflammation, gin does so too but to a lesser extent.

29.2.4 Salt

One of the well-known dietary risk factors towards atherosclerosis is salt (NaCl) intake. High sodium intake is associated with hypertension, a leading risk factor for atherosclerosis. In 2010 it was estimated that 1.65 million people died as a consequence of excess NaCl intake [13], and daily intake of salt is above recommended guidelines in almost all countries [14].

The INTERSALT study showed that the amount of sodium excretion was positively correlated with systolic pressure. Sodium intake was also positively correlated with raised diastolic pressure, but this was also related to confounding factors such as body mass index and alcohol intake [15]. In England from 2003 to 2011, there was a population fall in blood pressure of 2.7/1.1 mmHg and corresponding drop in rates of stroke and ischemic heart disease of about 40 %, which may have been related to an concomitant fall in salt consumption [16]. In a meta-analysis the authors concluded that high salt intake was associated with an increased risk of stroke [17].

There are many interventional studies of the short-term effect of reduced salt on blood pressure; a meta-analysis of randomised clinical trials shows that a modest reduction of salt intake, 4.4 g/day, for 4 weeks can cause a significant decrease in blood pressure, a mean fall of 4.18/2.06 mmHg. This was associated with no adverse effects on lipid and hormone level [18]. Other studies have reported similar results [19]. A fall in blood pressure was seen with salt reduction across all ethnicities [20]. Theoretically a fall in blood pressure should result in a reduction in atherosclerosis and cardiovascular events. This has been reported in some small studies [21], but a recent meta-analysis suggested that the data were still inconclusive and that more randomised trials were still required [22].

There is evidence that nationwide intervention could be beneficial. From 2001 to 2011 the amount of salt in UK bread has been reduced [23]. This corresponds with the reduction in daily salt intake seen over this time period. Thus, public health initiatives, e.g. reduction of salt in readymade foods, could lead to a significant decrease in population blood pressure and resultant cardiovascular disorders.

29.2.5 Potassium

From the INTERSALT study there appears to be an inverse relationship between potassium concentration and sodium concentration in the urine [24]. A high sodium to potassium ratio was associated with an increased systolic and, although less strong an association, increased diastolic pressure [15]. Potassium supplementation is linked to a reduction in postprandial brachial artery flow-mediated dilatation (FMD) [25]. An increased potassium intake is associated with a drop in blood pressure in both epidemiological studies and clinical trials; the mechanism behind this decrease in blood pressure is unclear [26]. However, it may be related to swelling and softening of the endothelium leading to an increase in nitric oxide a vasodilator, whereas sodium causes the stiffening of endothelium cells resulting in less nitric oxide production and thus an increased blood pressure [27].

29.2.6 Diet

Much has been written about the potential cardiovascular and anti-atherosclerotic benefits of many different diets. Men who follow a Mediterranean diet, rich in unsaturated fats, tomatoes and fresh fruit/vegetables, appear to be less at risk from coronary artery disease and death from cardiovascular disease [28]. The dietary approaches to stop hypertension, or DASH diet, is rich in fruit, vegetables and low-fat dairy product and is low in saturated fat and total fat. The DASH diet was found to lead to a reduction in blood pressure [29].

Those who eat large amounts of fruit and vegetables have a reduced risk of myocardial infarction and other cardiovascular diseases, with adjustment for history of diabetes, hypertension or high cholesterol; there was a relative risk for CVD of 0.45 between the extremes of vegetable intakes [30]. The effect of low-carbohydrate, high-protein diets on a wide range of surrogate phenotypes and biomarkers has been widely investigated, but a recent meta-analysis suggested that they may have no effect of mortality [31]. However, they appear effective in aiding weight loss in the long term [32].

29.2.7 Exercise

Exercise is associated with a reduced risk of atherosclerosis and cardiovascular disease. However, some studies have reported that high levels of exercise can actually be associated with cardiovascular disease.

Perhaps the most famous epidemiology study on the relationship between (self-reported) exercise and mortality and cardiovascular disease is the Harvard alumni study. This showed that those who undertake more exercise have an extra 1.5 years of life compared to those who did not. However, participation in light exercise did not correlate with mortality, whereas participating in moderate activity and vigorous activity was associated with reduced mortality [33] and reduced carotid arterial thickness. Interestingly, however, the Harvard alumni study also found an association between high levels of vigorous activity and slightly higher risk of cardiac death (a U-shaped curve) [34].

Vigorous exercise is known to be a protector against carotid artery calcification (an indicator for atherosclerosis) as well as decreasing the relative risk of cardiovascular diseases as a whole [35]. At least 120 min a week of moderate activity is all that is necessary for a clinically relevant benefit [36]. Exercise as a primary prevention method should be started in the young for the best results [37].

However, in interventional studies exercise has been shown to reduce blood pressure over 6 weeks by about 5.5/3.5 mmHg in the elderly (over 65) [38]. In the young exercise undertaken for 180 min a week leads to a decreased blood pressure, improves fitness and delays arterial remodelling [39].

29.3   Pharmacological

29.3.1 Hypertension Treatment

Hypertension is a major risk factor for atherosclerosis. There is a linear relationship between blood pressure and cardiovascular risk and as such there are no hard and fast limits as to what is a 'safe' blood pressure to have [40]. The main classes of antihypertensive drugs in current common use are diuretics, beta blockers, ACE inhibitors, calcium channel blockers and alpha blockers. There has been considerable debate as to whether decreasing blood pressure is of most importance or whether there are differences between drug classes.

The largest study to compare classes and drugs was the ALLHAT study. This compared ACE inhibitors (lisinopril), calcium channel blockers (amlodipine), diuretics (chlorthalidone) and alpha blockers. The alpha blocker (doxazosin) arm of the ALLHAT terminated early due to a twofold higher risk of congestive heart failure for patients on doxazosin compared to chlorthalidone [41]. This was largely based on a clinical diagnosis of heart failure not lab defined results and debate continues as to the clinical benefits/harm of alpha blockers, but mostly they are not now used first line. All other agents reduced the risk of the trial's primary outcomes of fatal CHD or nonfatal myocardial infarction and secondary outcomes of all-cause mortality, fatal and nonfatal stroke, combined CHD and combined CVD. However, thiazide diuretics were slightly more effective both at lowering blood pressure and reducing clinical events as well as being the most accepted as well as being low cost [42].

Beta blockers were not included in the ALLHAT study, and a meta-analysis by Lindhlom et al. showed that atenolol was inferior to other agents in preventing CVD and that there was a lack of evidence to support their first-line use [43]. This, and the results of the ASCOT study, which showed that atenolol plus thiazide was inferior to a calcium channel antagonist and ACE inhibitor in reducing total and cardiovascular mortality, led to the demotion of beta blockers to fourth line [44]. However, it is unclear as to whether some newer beta blockers, e.g. nebivolol, which have vasodilating properties may be as effective as other agents in reducing events. Certainly nebivolol lowers central blood pressure and left ventricular mass more effectively than traditional agents [45, 46].

In patients who are black, thiazide diuretics have a more noticeable effect compared to other drugs tested in the ALLHAT study at preventing cardiovascular events, such as myocardial infarction and stroke, or renal events [47].

Combination therapy may be preferable to single therapy. This is due in part to synergism between the two therapies but also because one drug's side effects offset that of the other, as well as lower doses of both being needed [26]. Studies comparing combination versus initial monotherapy are ongoing.

29.3.1.1 Hyperlipidaemia

There is a well-established positive relationship between LDL cholesterol, and inverse relationship between HDL cholesterol, and atherosclerosis. The most effective drug class for lowering LDL cholesterol are statins, and they are one of the most commonly prescribed pills.

There is overwhelming evidence that statins decrease the risk of cardiovascular events. In a meta-analysis of studies, statins reduced the risk of myocardial infarction by 39.4 % and stroke by 23.8 % in elderly patient who have had no pre-existing cardiovascular diseases; therefore, statins may be a very good primary prevention method [48]. In a meta-analysis of adults with both no past history of cardiovascular disease (CVD) and those with a past history of CVD, statins gave an odds ratio of all-cause mortality of 0.86 compared to controls, as well as relative risks of CVD 0.75, CHD 0.73 and stroke 0.78 (all both fatal and nonfatal) [49]. Statins are also known to have few adverse effects, although they may slightly increase the risk of diabetes mellitus [50]. Benefits of statins are rapid as assessed by improvements in FMD [51].

Niacin or vitamin B has been examined for its use in raising HDL levels. In some clinical trials niacin appears to give a reduction in the risk of cardiovascular disorders and major coronary heart disease (but does not cause a reduction in stroke risk) [52, 53]. When niacin and statins are combined, there is an even greater increase in the number of HDLs present in the blood [54]. However, this evidence remains controversial and some studies are to the contrary [55]. Therefore, the effectiveness of niacin requires further study. Niacin may even increase risk in some high-CVD-risk individuals [56].

A variety of other cholesterol modifying have been, or are, in current development. CEPT inhibitors such as torcetrapib were developed to raise HDL cholesterol, but development has now largely ceased as torcetrapib was linked with an excess cardiovascular mortality [57] and other related agents appeared not to improve surrogate end points [58]. PCSK9 antagonists offer more promise and initial data suggest impressive reductions in LDL cholesterol [59]. However, these are given by infusion, which may limit their widespread applicability for primary prevention of atherosclerosis.

Diabetes Mellitus

Suffering from diabetes greatly increases the risks of cardiovascular disease. Diabetic patients without previous myocardial infarction have as high a risk of myocardial infarction as non-diabetic patients with a history of previous myocardial infarction [60].

Diabetics benefit as much if not more so than non-diabetics by targeting other cardiovascular risk factors. Diabetics may gain a greater benefit from blood pressure and cholesterol treatment than nondiabetics [61]. Therefore, it is of benefit to treat other risk factors in diabetics rather than focusing exclusively on tight glycaemia control. Indeed, multifactorial, long-term, aggressive treatment reduces risk of cardiovascular and microvascular events by 50 % compared to conventional treatment [62]. However, interventions in obese and overweight diabetics focusing on weight loss do not reduce the risk of cardiovascular disease [63].

The UK PDS study showed that reducing glucose reduced the risk of 'any diabetes-related end point' by 12 % but did not significantly reduce macrovascular complications [64, 65]. Likewise, subsequent randomised trials failed to show cardiovascular benefit of intensive glycaemic control, as did a recent meta-analysis of published trial data [66]. Nevertheless, intensive control does appear to reduce microvascular events [66]. There is still a debate about whether cardiovascular outcome varies between classes of hypoglycaemic agent. A recent meta-analysis suggested that sulphonylureas have a relative risk of 1.27 for cardiovascular death and 1.18 for cardiovascular events [67]. Metformin appears safe, but does not reduce events when added to insulin, compared to insulin alone [68]. The combination with incretins also appears not to increase events.

29.4   Arteriosclerosis

Arteriosclerosis is a general thickening and stiffening of the arteries with the loss of elasticity, caused by mainly fatigue fracture of the elastic fibres within the arterial wall. It is an independent risk factor for cardiovascular disease and mortality [69]. The literature surrounding arteriosclerosis is difficult to assess because stiffness of a vessel is dependent on the pressure at which stiffness is measured; i.e. blood pressure is a confounding factor, as may also be the case for heart rate. Therefore, any intervention that changes heart rate or blood pressure may indirect effect stiffness without altering isobaric stiffness. Stiffness is often accessed in a variety of different ways, which are not always comparable. The gold standard is the aortic pulse wave velocity (aPWV), as it has the most evidence of independent predictive value, and so studies employing aPWV should be given more weighting. An addition issue is that many of the published studies are very small and no doubt underpowered. All of these factors make interpreting the published data challenging.

29.5   Lifestyle

29.5.1 Smoking

Smoking is associated with atherosclerosis, but there is also some evidence to suggest that smoking is also associated with arteriosclerosis and arterial stiffness. Epidemiological data suggest that smoking in youth may be associated with increased aPWV [70, 71] and other studies have reported a positive association between aPWV and smoking in adults [72, 73]. However, the data are inconsistent [74, 75] and longitudinal data do not support a strong role for smoking [76–80].

There is little evidence concerning smoking cessation. One study did report a lowering of brachial-ankle pulse wave velocity after 12 months cessation, but brachial-ankle index increased [81]. There is also some evidence to suggest that flavonoids such as those found in chocolate and grape juice may have a protective effect against arterial stiffness in smokers [82].

29.5.2 Alcohol

Moderate, chronic alcohol consumption is associated with a lowered risk of cardiovascular disease, compared to no alcohol consumption and heavy alcohol consumption. In women there is evidence that moderate alcohol consumption is linked to decreased arterial stiffness in a J-shaped correlation; drinking between 4 and 20 glasses a week reduces arterial stiffness but greater than 21 results in an increase in arterial stiffness [83]. A similar association was seen in men; when adjusted for other factors effecting PWV, this association was unchanged [84].

29.5.3 Diet

There is epidemiological evidence that salt intake is related to arterial stiffness. Avolio et al. completed a study comparing arterial distensibility between rural Chinese and urban Chinese populations. This study found that those individuals in rural communities have less age-related arterial stiffening, likely due to differences in salt consumption between the two groups, with the rural group consuming less sodium than the urban group, resulting in a lower blood pressure [85]. Similar results were seen in studies comparing urban and rural pygmies, showing the impact of environment vs. genetics on arterial stiffness [86].

Consuming a low-salt diet results in a lower AASI (ambulatory arterial stiffness index), whereas high-salt intervention results in a raised AASI [87]. The effect of salt consumption is not purely a long-term progressive effect; salt can also have an acute effect on arterial stiffness. A high-sodium meal can increase arterial stiffness for a short time period as assessed by augmentation index (AIx) [88]. Interestingly, however, this study did not find an association between blood pressure and acute salt consumption. This is backed by a study of salt consumption in the Portuguese which used the gold standard aPWV to conclude that the association with salt consumption was, independently of blood pressure [89], linked to arterial stiffness. In clinical trials salt reduction may have a greater impact on black people's pulse wave velocity than whites or Asians [20].

29.5.4 Exercise

There is mixed evidence as to whether exercise is of benefit against arterial stiffness. The evidence remains largely inconclusive over how much and what sort of exercise should be undertaken. High-intensity exercise may be harmful rather than beneficial.

In heart failure patients with reduced ejection fraction, 8 weeks of exercise increases arterial compliance [90]. Resistance training may be linked to arterial stiffness, but this is more likely to be restricted to high-intensity resistance training [90]. Long-distance endurance training may be associated with pathological structural remodelling of arteries [91]. However, again this is generally only with high-intensity training.

However, both endurance and resistance training have in some studies led to a significant decrease in arterial stiffness as well as blood pressure in pre-hypertensive students [92]. Exercise is associated with increased total systemic arterial compliance [93]. Exercise can be combined with weight loss to increase the endothelial-dependent flow-mediated dilatation (FMD) in patient with coronary heart disease greater than that of weight loss alone [94]. Therefore, exercise appears to be beneficial provided it is not undertaken to excess. However, in the majority, it is unclear as to whether isobaric stiffness is affected. Larger randomised studies, with adequate controls/blinding and correction for changes in blood pressure, are clearly required.

29.6   Pharmacology

A number of small studies have assessed the effect of antihypertensive drugs on measures of arterial stiffness including aPWV. Many of these suggest that aPWV is lowered, but it is difficult to know the effect on isobaric stiffness. One meta-analysis suggested that ACE inhibitors in particular may reduce aPWV independently of blood pressure. However, this was based on data from only 294 subjects [95]. Several head-to-head comparisons suggest that beta blockers may reduce stiffness more than other drugs and that vasodilating agents may be even better [96], but again sample sizes are very small [97, 98]. There is also a lack of data concerning the long-term effects of BP lowering per se. If fatigue fracture of the elastic elements is largely driven by pulsatile load and heart rate, then lowering average pressure, pulsatility and heart rate may retard age-related arterial stiffening, but this hypothesis remains to be formally tested.

Matrix proteins are another target for therapies designed to alter stiffness. ALT711 is an advanced glycation end point (ACE) breaker meaning that it has the potential to reverse the stiffening of arteries due to cross-linking of elastic elements. This hypothesis was supported by an animal data [99], and early human studies reported a lowering of reduced left ventricular stiffness and systolic pressure compared to placebo [100]. However, development was discontinued and no other similar agents are currently available for trials.

Statins may have pleomorphic effects beyond simply cholesterol lowering, including improving endothelial function and acting as a modest but clinically apparent anti-inflammatory. There have also been many studies demonstrating that statins decrease arterial stiffness [101]. However, these invariably included only tiny numbers of subjects, and the much larger CAFE sub-study of ASCOT did not find any difference in estimated aPWV between those randomised to a statin compared to placebo, all be it in a hypertensive population.

Acute inflammation can increase stiffness. In one study, using *Salmonella typhi* vaccine to induce an inflammatory response in healthy individuals, there was a modest increase in aortic pulse wave velocity (aPWV), a marker of arterial stiffness. This aPWV increase was not seen in the aspirin-pretreated patients.

Chronic inflammation is another potential target for de-stiffening therapies. Mounting data suggests a link between inflammation and stiffness, particularly in individuals with chronic systemic inflammatory conditions such as rheumatoid arthritis [102]. Anti-inflammatory therapy with anti-TNF-alpha drugs leads to a reduction in aPWV [103], and this appears to be related to a reduction in aortic inflammation per se [104]. Similar results have been reported in inflammatory bowel disease [105]. However, whether less potent anti-inflammatories can modify stiffness in patients with cardiovascular disease or in a primary prevention setting is unclear.

Additional potential targets are the factors regulating vascular calcification, which has previously been linked with stiffening, and other components with the matrix. Gene expression studies and proteomics may help identify targets in this respect, but it is important to remember that the animal aorta is contractile and that the human is not, so specifies differences may be important.

References

1. Freeman B, Gartner C, Hall W, Chapman S (2010) Forecasting future tobacco control policy: where to next? Aust N Z J Public Health 34(5):447–450
2. Howard G, Wagenknecht LE, Burke GL et al (1998) Cigarette smoking and progression of atherosclerosis: the Atherosclerosis Risk in Communities (ARIC) study. JAMA 279(2):119–124
3. Doll R, Peto R, Boreham J, Sutherland I (2004) Mortality in relation to smoking: 50 years' observations on male British doctors. BMJ 328(7455):1519
4. Alvarez LR, Balibrea JM, Surinach JM et al (2013) Smoking cessation and outcome in stable outpatients with coronary, cerebrovascular, or peripheral artery disease. Eur J Prev Cardiol 20(3):486–495
5. Munafo MR, Tilling K, Ben-Shlomo Y (2009) Smoking status and body mass index: a longitudinal study. Nicotine Tob Res 11(6):765–771
6. Asthana A, Piper ME, McBride PE et al (2012) Long-term effects of smoking and smoking cessation on exercise stress testing: three-year outcomes from a randomized clinical trial. Am Heart J 163(1):81–87.e1
7. Critchley JA, Unal B (2004) Is smokeless tobacco a risk factor for coronary heart disease? A systematic review of epidemiological studies. Eur J Cardiovasc Prev Rehabil 11(2):101–112
8. Diez-Roux AV, Nieto FG, Comstock GW et al (1995) The relationship of active and passive smoking to carotid atherosclerosis 12–14 years later. Prev Med 24(1):48–55
9. Cahill K, Srevens S, Perera R, Lancaster T (2013) Pharmacological interventions for smoking cessation: an overview and network meta-analysis. Cochrane Database Syst Rev (5): CD009329
10. Mills EJ, Thorlund K, Eapen S et al (2014) Cardiovascular events associated with smoking cessation pharmacotherapies: a network meta-analysis. Circulation 129(1):28–41
11. Ronksley PE, Brien SE, Turner BJ et al (2011) Association of alcohol consumption with selected cardiovascular disease outcomes: a systematic review and meta-analysis. BMJ 342:d671
12. Estruch R, Sacanella E, Mota F et al (2011) Moderate consumption of red wine, but not gin, decreases erythrocyte superoxide dismutase activity: a randomised cross-over trial. Nutr Metab Cardiovasc Dis 21(1):46–53
13. Mozaffarian D, Fahimi S, Singh GM et al (2014) Global sodium consumption and death from cardiovascular causes. N Engl J Med 371(7):624–634
14. Powles J, Fahimi S, Micha R et al (2013) Global, regional and national sodium intakes in 1990 and 2010: a systematic analysis of 24 h urinary sodium excretion and dietary surveys worldwide. BMJ Open 3(12):e003733
15. Zimmers T, Golomb RI (1991) Cases in electrocardiography. Am J Emerg Med 9(6):588–591
16. He FJ, Pombo-Rodrigues S, Macgregor GA (2014) Salt reduction in England from 2003 to 2011: its relationship to blood pressure, stroke and ischaemic heart disease mortality. BMJ Open 4(4):e004549
17. Li XY, Cai XL, Bian PD, Hu LR (2012) High salt intake and stroke: meta-analysis of the epidemiologic evidence. CNS Neurosci Ther 18(8):691–701
18. He FJ, Li J, Macgregor GA (2013) Effect of longer-term modest salt reduction on blood pressure. Cochrane Database Syst Rev (4):CD004937
19. He FJ, MacGregor GA (2004) Effect of longer-term modest salt reduction on blood pressure. Cochrane Database Syst Rev (3):CD004937
20. He FJ, Marciniak M, Visagie E et al (2009) Effect of modest salt reduction on blood pressure, urinary albumin, and pulse wave velocity in white, black, and Asian mild hypertensives. Hypertension 54(3):482–488
21. Cook NR, Cutler JA, Obarzanek E et al (2007) Long term effects of dietary sodium reduction on cardiovascular disease outcomes: observational follow-up of the trials of hypertension prevention (TOHP). BMJ 334(7599):885–888
22. Taylor RS, Ashton KE, Moxham T et al (2011) Reduced dietary salt for the prevention of cardiovascular disease. Cochrane Database Syst Rev (7):CD009217
23. Brinsden HC, He FJ, Jenner KH, Macgregor GA (2013) Surveys of the salt content in UK bread: progress made and further reductions possible. BMJ Open 3:e002936

24. Brown IJ, Dyer AR, Chan Q et al (2013) Estimating 24-hour urinary sodium excretion from casual urinary sodium concentrations in Western populations: the INTERSALT study. Am J Epidemiol 177(11):1180–1192
25. Blanch N, Clifton PM, Keogh JB (2014) Postprandial effects of potassium supplementation on vascular function and blood pressure: a randomised cross-over study. Nutr Metab Cardiovasc Dis 24(2):148–154
26. Cheriyan J, McEniery CM, Wilkinson IB (2010) Hypertension, Oxford specialist handbooks. Oxford University Press, Oxford, p 322
27. Oberleithner H, Callies C, Kusche-Vihrog (2009) Potassium softens vascular endothelium and increases nitric oxide release. Proc Natl Acad Sci U S A 106(8):2829–2834
28. Atkins JL, Whincup PH, Morris RW et al (2014) High diet quality is associated with a lower risk of cardiovascular disease and all-cause mortality in older men. J Nutr 144(5): 673–680
29. Sacks FM, Svetkey LP, Vollmer WM et al (2001) Effects on blood pressure of reduced dietary sodium and the Dietary Approaches to Stop Hypertension (DASH) diet. DASH-Sodium Collaborative Research Group. N Engl J Med 344(1):3–10
30. Liu S, Manson JE, Lee IM et al (2000) Fruit and vegetable intake and risk of cardiovascular disease: the women's health study. Am J Clin Nutr 72(4):922–928
31. Noto H, Goto A, Tsujimoto T et al (2013) Low-carbohydrate diets and all-cause mortality: a systematic review and meta-analysis of observational studies. PLoS One 8(1):e55030
32. Bueno NB, de Melo IS, de Oliveira SL, da Rocha Ataide T (2013) Very-low-carbohydrate ketogenic diet v. low-fat diet for long-term weight loss: a meta-analysis of randomised controlled trials. Br J Nutr 110(7):1178–1187
33. Lee IM, Paffenbarger RS Jr (2000) Associations of light, moderate, and vigorous intensity physical activity with longevity. The Harvard alumni health study. Am J Epidemiol 151(3): 293–299
34. Sesso HD, Paffenbarger RS Jr, Lee IM (2000) Physical activity and coronary heart disease in men: the Harvard alumni health study. Circulation 102(9):975–980
35. Delaney JA, Jensky NE, Criqui MH et al (2013) The association between physical activity and both incident coronary artery calcification and ankle brachial index progression: the multi-ethnic study of atherosclerosis. Atherosclerosis 230(2):278–283
36. Newby DE, Cockcroft JR, Wilkinson IB (2005) Coronary heart disease: your questions answered. Elsevier/Churchill, Livingstone
37. Walther C, Gaede L, Adams V et al (2009) Effect of increased exercise in school children on physical fitness and endothelial progenitor cells: a prospective randomized trial. Circulation 120(22):2251–2259
38. Chomiuk T, Folga A, Mamcarz A (2013) The influence of systematic pulse-limited physical exercise on the parameters of the cardiovascular system in patients over 65 years of age. Arch Med Sci 9(2):201–209
39. Farpour-Lambert NJ, Aggoun Y, Marchand LM et al (2009) Physical activity reduces systemic blood pressure and improves early markers of atherosclerosis in pre-pubertal obese children. J Am Coll Cardiol 54(25):2396–2406
40. Lewington S, Clarke R, Qizilbash N et al (2002) Age-specific relevance of usual blood pressure to vascular mortality: a meta-analysis of individual data for one million adults in 61 prospective studies. Lancet 360(9349):1903–1913
41. Vidt DG (2000) Alpha-blockers and congestive heart failure: early termination of an arm of the ALLHAT trial. Cleve Clin J Med 67(6):429–433
42. The ALLHAT Officers and Coordinators for the ALLHAT Collaborative Research Group. The Lipid-Lowering Treatment to Prevent Heart Attack Trial (2002) Major outcomes in high-risk hypertensive patients randomized to angiotensin-converting enzyme inhibitor or calcium channel blocker vs diuretic: The Antihypertensive and Lipid-Lowering Treatment to Prevent Heart Attack Trial (ALLHAT). JAMA 288(23):2981–2997
43. Lindholm LH, Carlberg B, Samuelsson O (2005) Should beta blockers remain first choice in the treatment of primary hypertension? A meta-analysis. Lancet 366(9496):1545–1553

44. van den Meiracker AH, van Montfrans GA (2006) The most recent study into blood pressure lowering by amlodipine: the beginning of the end for the beta-blockers. Ned Tijdschr Geneeskd 150(16):886–888

45. Kampus P, Serg M, Kals J et al (2011) Differential effects of nebivolol and metoprolol on central aortic pressure and left ventricular wall thickness. Hypertension 57(6):1122–1128

46. Dhakam Z, Yasmin, McEniery CM et al (2008) A comparison of atenolol and nebivolol in isolated systolic hypertension. J Hypertens 26(2):351–356

47. Einhorn PT, Davis BR, Wright JT et al (2010) ALLHAT: still providing correct answers after 7 years. Curr Opin Cardiol 25(4):355–365

48. Savarese G, Gotto AM Jr, Paolillo S et al (2013) Benefits of statins in elderly subjects without established cardiovascular disease: a meta-analysis. J Am Coll Cardiol 62(22):2090–2099

49. Taylor F, Huffman MD, Macedo AF et al (2013) Statins for the primary prevention of cardiovascular disease. Cochrane Database Syst Rev (1):CD004816

50. Naci H, Brugts J, Ades T (2013) Comparative tolerability and harms of individual statins: a study-level network meta-analysis of 246 955 participants from 135 randomized, controlled trials. Circ Cardiovasc Qual Outcomes 6(4):390–399

51. Dupuis J, Tardif JC, Cernacek P, Theroux P (1999) Cholesterol reduction rapidly improves endothelial function after acute coronary syndromes. The RECIFE (reduction of cholesterol in ischemia and function of the endothelium) trial. Circulation 99(25):3227–3233

52. Lavigne PM, Karas RH (2013) The current state of niacin in cardiovascular disease prevention: a systematic review and meta-regression. J Am Coll Cardiol 61(4):440–446

53. Duggal JK, Singh M, Attri N et al (2010) Effect of niacin therapy on cardiovascular outcomes in patients with coronary artery disease. J Cardiovasc Pharmacol Ther 15(2):158–166

54. Sibley CT, Vavere AL, Gottlieb I et al (2013) MRI-measured regression of carotid atherosclerosis induced by statins with and without niacin in a randomised controlled trial: the NIA plaque study. Heart 99(22):1675–1680

55. Zambon A, Zhao XQ, Brown BG et al (2014) Effects of niacin combination therapy with statin or bile acid resin on lipoproteins and cardiovascular disease. Am J Cardiol 113(9):1494–1498

56. HPS2-THRIVE Collaborative Group, Landrey MJ, Haynes R et al (2014) Effects of extended-release niacin with laropiprant in high-risk patients. N Engl J Med 371(3):203–212

57. Barter PJ, Caulfield M, Eriksson M et al (2007) Effects of torcetrapib in patients at high risk for coronary events. N Engl J Med 357(21):2109–2122

58. Luscher TF, Taddei S, Kaski JC et al (2012) Vascular effects and safety of dalcetrapib in patients with or at risk of coronary heart disease: the dal-VESSEL randomized clinical trial. Eur Heart J 33(7):857–865

59. Stein EA, Mellis S, Yancopoulos GD et al (2012) Effect of a monoclonal antibody to PCSK9 on LDL cholesterol. N Engl J Med 366(12):1108–1118

60. Haffner SM, Lehto S, Ronnemaa T et al (1998) Mortality from coronary heart disease in subjects with type 2 diabetes and in nondiabetic subjects with and without prior myocardial infarction. N Engl J Med 339(4):229–234

61. Collins R, Armitage J, Parish S et al (2003) MRC/BHF Heart Protection Study of cholesterol-lowering with simvastatin in 5963 people with diabetes: a randomised placebo-controlled trial. Lancet 361(9374):2005–2016

62. Gaede P, Vedel P, Larsen N et al (2003) Multifactorial intervention and cardiovascular disease in patients with type 2 diabetes. N Engl J Med 348(5):383–393

63. Look ARG, Wing RR, Bolin P et al (2013) Cardiovascular effects of intensive lifestyle intervention in type 2 diabetes. N Engl J Med 369(2):145–154

64. UK Prospective Diabetes Study (UKPDS) Group (1998) Intensive blood-glucose control with sulphonylureas or insulin compared with conventional treatment and risk of complications in patients with type 2 diabetes (UKPDS 33). UK Prospective Diabetes Study (UKPDS) Group. Lancet 352(9131):837–853

65. UKPDS Office, DTU (2014) UK prospective diabetes study (completed). https://www.dtu.ox.ac.uk/UKPDS/trialresults.php

66. Hemmingsen B, Lund SS, Gluud C et al (2013) Targeting intensive glycaemic control versus targeting conventional glycaemic control for type 2 diabetes mellitus. Cochrane Database Syst Rev (11):CD008143
67. Phung OJ, Schwartzman E, Allen RW et al (2013) Sulphonylureas and risk of cardiovascular disease: systematic review and meta-analysis. Diabet Med 30(10):1160–1171
68. Hemmingsen B, Christensen LL, Wetterslev J et al (2012) Comparison of metformin and insulin versus insulin alone for type 2 diabetes: systematic review of randomised clinical trials with meta-analyses and trial sequential analyses. BMJ 344:e1771
69. Ben-Shlomo Y, Spears M, Boustred C et al (2014) Aortic pulse wave velocity improves cardiovascular event prediction: an individual participant meta-analysis of prospective observational data from 17,635 subjects. J Am Coll Cardiol 63(7):636–646
70. van de Laar RJ, Stehouwer CD, Boreham CA et al (2011) Continuing smoking between adolescence and young adulthood is associated with higher arterial stiffness in young adults: the Northern Ireland Young Hearts Project. J Hypertens 29(11):2201–2209
71. Lerant B, Christina S, Olah L et al (2012) The comparative analysis of arterial wall thickness and arterial wall stiffness in smoking and non-smoking university students. Ideggyogy Sz 65(3–4):121–126
72. Jain S, Mathur S, Mathur A et al (2012) Effect of tobacco use on arterial stiffness in community dwelling females. J Assoc Physicians India 60:20–23
73. Hata K, Nakagawa T, Mizuno M et al (2012) Relationship between smoking and a new index of arterial stiffness, the cardio-ankle vascular index, in male workers: a cross-sectional study. Tob Induc Dis 10(1):11
74. Cecelja M, Chowienczyk P (2009) Dissociation of aortic pulse wave velocity with risk factors for cardiovascular disease other than hypertension: a systematic review. Hypertension 54(6):1328–1336
75. McEniery CM, Yasmin, Maki-Petaja KM et al (2010) The impact of cardiovascular risk factors on aortic stiffness and wave reflections depends on age: the Anglo-Cardiff Collaborative Trial (ACCT III). Hypertension 56(4):591–597
76. Johansen NB, Vistisen D, Brunner EJ et al (2012) Determinants of aortic stiffness: 16-year follow-up of the Whitehall II study. PLoS One 7(5):e37165
77. Wildman RP, Farhat GN, Patel AS et al (2005) Weight change is associated with change in arterial stiffness among healthy young adults. Hypertension 45(2):187–192
78. El Khoudary SR, Barinas-Mitchell E, White J et al (2012) Adiponectin, systolic blood pressure, and alcohol consumption are associated with more aortic stiffness progression among apparently healthy men. Atherosclerosis 225(2):475–480
79. Kaess BM, Rong J, Larson MG et al (2012) Aortic stiffness, blood pressure progression, and incident hypertension. JAMA 308(9):875–881
80. AlGhatrif M, Strait JB, Morrell CH et al (2013) Longitudinal trajectories of arterial stiffness and the role of blood pressure: the Baltimore longitudinal study of aging. Hypertension 62(5):934–941
81. Yu-Jie W, Hui-Liang L, Bing L et al (2013) Impact of smoking and smoking cessation on arterial stiffness in healthy participants. Angiology 64(4):273–280
82. Siasos G, Tousoulis D, Kokkou E et al (2014) Favorable effects of concord grape juice on endothelial function and arterial stiffness in healthy smokers. Am J Hypertens 27(1):38–45
83. Mattace-Raso FU, van der Cammen TJ, van den Elzen AP et al (2005) Moderate alcohol consumption is associated with reduced arterial stiffness in older adults: the Rotterdam study. J Gerontol A Biol Sci Med Sci 60(11):1479–1483
84. Sierksma A, Muller M, van der Schouw YT et al (2004) Alcohol consumption and arterial stiffness in men. J Hypertens 22(2):357–362
85. Avolio AP, Deng FQ, Li WQ et al (1985) Effects of aging on arterial distensibility in populations with high and low prevalence of hypertension: comparison between urban and rural communities in China. Circulation 71(2):202–210
86. Lemogoum D, Ngatchou W, Janssen C et al (2012) Effects of hunter-gatherer subsistence mode on arterial distensibility in Cameroonian pygmies. Hypertension 60(1):123–128

87. Liu Z, Peng J, Lu F et al (2013) Salt loading and potassium supplementation: effects on ambulatory arterial stiffness index and endothelin-1 levels in normotensive and mild hypertensive patients. J Clin Hypertens (Greenwich) 15(7):485–496
88. Dickinson KM, Clifton PM, Burrell LM et al (2014) Postprandial effects of a high salt meal on serum sodium, arterial stiffness, markers of nitric oxide production and markers of endothelial function. Atherosclerosis 232(1):211–216
89. Polonia J, Maldonado J, Ramos R et al (2006) Estimation of salt intake by urinary sodium excretion in a Portuguese adult population and its relationship to arterial stiffness. Rev Port Cardiol 25(9):801–817
90. Sacre JW, Jennings GL, Kingwell BA (2014) Exercise and dietary influences on arterial stiffness in cardiometabolic disease. Hypertension 63(5):888–893
91. O'Keefe JH, Patil HR, Lavie CJ et al (2012) Potential adverse cardiovascular effects from excessive endurance exercise. Mayo Clin Proc 87(6):587–595
92. Beck DT, Martin JS, Casey DP, Braith RW (2013) Exercise training reduces peripheral arterial stiffness and myocardial oxygen demand in young prehypertensive subjects. Am J Hypertens 26(9):1093–1102
93. Cameron JD, Dart AM (1994) Exercise training increases total systemic arterial compliance in humans. Am J Physiol 266(2 Pt 2):H693–H701
94. Ades PA, Savage PD, Lischke S et al (2011) The effect of weight loss and exercise training on flow-mediated dilatation in coronary heart disease: a randomized trial. Chest 140(6):1420–1427
95. Ong KT, Delerme S, Pannier B et al (2011) Aortic stiffness is reduced beyond blood pressure lowering by short-term and long-term antihypertensive treatment: a meta-analysis of individual data in 294 patients. J Hypertens 29(6):1034–1042
96. McEniery CM, Schmitt M, Qasem A et al (2004) Nebivolol increases arterial distensibility in vivo. Hypertension 44(3):305–310
97. Dhakam Z, McEniery CM, Yasmin (2006) Atenolol and eprosartan: differential effects on central blood pressure and aortic pulse wave velocity. Am J Hypertens 19(2):214–219
98. Pannier BM, Guerin AP, Marchais SJ, London GM (2001) Different aortic reflection wave responses following long-term angiotensin-converting enzyme inhibition and beta-blocker in essential hypertension. Clin Exp Pharmacol Physiol 28(12):1074–1077
99. Vaitkevicius PV, Lane M, Spurgeon H et al (2001) A cross-link breaker has sustained effects on arterial and ventricular properties in older rhesus monkeys. Proc Natl Acad Sci U S A 98(3):1171–1175
100. Fujimoto N, Hastings JL, Carrick-Ranson G et al (2013) Cardiovascular effects of 1 year of alagebrium and endurance exercise training in healthy older individuals. Circ Heart Fail 6(6):1155–1164
101. Wilkinson I, Cockroft J (2007) Cholesterol, lipids and arterial stiffness. In: Safar ME, Frohlich ED (eds) Atherosclerosis, large arteries and cardiovascular risk, vol 44, Advances in cardiology. Karger, Basel, pp 261–277
102. Maki-Petaja KM, McEniery CM, Franklin SS, Wilkinson IB (2014) Arterial stiffness in chronic inflammation. In: Safar ME, O'Rourke MF, Frohlich ED (eds) Blood pressure and arterial wall mechanics in cardiovascular diseases. Springer, London, pp 435–444
103. Maki-Petaja KM, Hall FC, Booth AD et al (2006) Rheumatoid arthritis is associated with increased aortic pulse-wave velocity, which is reduced by anti-tumor necrosis factor-alpha therapy. Circulation 114(11):1185–1192
104. Maki-Petaja KM, Elkhawad M, Cheriyan J et al (2012) Anti-tumor necrosis factor-alpha therapy reduces aortic inflammation and stiffness in patients with rheumatoid arthritis. Circulation 126(21):2473–2480
105. Zanoli L, Rastelli S, Inserra G et al (2014) Increased arterial stiffness in inflammatory bowel diseases is dependent upon inflammation and reduced by immunomodulatory drugs. Atherosclerosis 234(2):346–351

CPSIA information can be obtained
at www.ICGtesting.com
Printed in the USA
LVOW02*2139300316

481456LV00001B/2/P